Pancreatic Surgery: Clinical Principles and Practice

Pancreatic Surgery: Clinical Principles and Practice

Edited by Clark Porter

hayle
medical

New York

Hayle Medical,
750 Third Avenue, 9th Floor,
New York, NY 10017, USA

Visit us on the World Wide Web at:
www.haylemedical.com

ISBN: 978-1-63241-601-8

Cataloging-in-Publication Data

Pancreatic surgery : clinical principles and practice / edited by Clark Porter.
    p. cm.
Includes bibliographical references and index.
ISBN 978-1-63241-601-8
1. Pancreas--Surgery. 2. Pancreas--Diseases. 3. Pancreatectomy.
4. Endocrine glands--Diseases. I. Porter, Clark.
RD546 .P36 2019
617.556--dc23

Table of Contents

Permissions

List of Contributors

Index

Preface

Over the recent decade, advancements and applications have progressed exponentially. This has led to the increased interest in this field and projects are being conducted to enhance knowledge. The main objective of this book is to present some of the critical challenges and provide insights into possible solutions. This book will answer the varied questions that arise in the field and also provide an increased scope for furthering studies.

The pancreas is an important organ of the body, critical for digestion and endocrine function. Pancreatic surgery is performed either to address conditions causing inflammation such as pancreatitis or to treat tumors. Pancreatitis may either be acute or chronic, and may require surgery when pancreatic tissue atrophies or becomes infected. Pancreatic tumors can be benign or malignant. The surgical management of these typically involves removing the diseased section of the pancreas. The most common form of pancreatic surgery is Whipple surgery, which is done to remove cancerous tumors from the head of the pancreas. Pancreas transplantation may be performed in an insulin-dependent diabetic patient. After the successful completion of pancreatic surgery, post-surgical difficulties may arise which require careful monitoring by a health care team. This book provides comprehensive insights into the clinical principles and practices of pancreatic surgery. It will also provide interesting topics for research, which interested readers can take up. Scientists and students actively engaged in this field will find this book full of crucial and unexplored concepts.

I hope that this book, with its visionary approach, will be a valuable addition and will promote interest among readers. Each of the authors has provided their extraordinary competence in their specific fields by providing different perspectives as they come from diverse nations and regions. I thank them for their contributions.

Editor

Evaluation of survival in patients after pancreatic head resection for ductal adenocarcinoma

Marius Distler[1*†], Felix Rückert[2†], Maximilian Hunger[1], Stephan Kersting[1], Christian Pilarsky[1], Hans-Detlev Saeger[1] and Robert Grützmann[1]

Abstract

Background: Surgery remains the only curative option for the treatment of pancreatic adenocarcinoma (PDAC). The goal of this study was to investigate the clinical outcome and prognostic factors in patients after resection for ductal adenocarcinoma of the pancreatic head.

Methods: The data from 195 patients who underwent pancreatic head resection for PDAC between 1993 and 2011 in our center were retrospectively analyzed. The prognostic factors for survival after operation were evaluated using multivariate analysis.

Results: The head resection surgeries included 69.7% pylorus-preserving pancreatoduodenectomies (PPPD) and 30.3% standard Kausch-Whipple pancreatoduodenectomies (Whipple). The overall mortality after pancreatoduodenectomy (PD) was 4.1%, and the overall morbidity was 42%. The actuarial 3- and 5-year survival rates were 31.5% (95% CI, 25.04%-39.6%) and 11.86% (95% CI, 7.38%-19.0%), respectively. Univariate analyses demonstrated that elevated CEA (p = 0.002) and elevated CA 19–9 (p = 0.026) levels, tumor grade (p = 0.001) and hard texture of the pancreatic gland (p = 0.017) were significant predictors of a poor survival. However, only CEA >3 ng/ml (p < 0.005) and tumor grade 3 (p = 0.027) were validated as significant predictors of survival in multivariate analysis.

Conclusions: Our results suggest that tumor marker levels and tumor grade are significant predictors of poor survival for patients with pancreatic head cancer. Furthermore, hard texture of the pancreatic gland appears to be associated with poor survival.

Keywords: Pancreatic cancer, Tumor marker, Surgery, Whipple procedure, Pylorus-preserving pancreatoduodenectomy (PPPD)

Background

The prognosis for patients with cancer of the pancreatic head remains poor. Currently, tumor resection is the only therapeutic option to achieve long-term survival.

However, only a small number of patients (30-40%) present a resectable tumor at the time of diagnosis. The overall 5-year survival after pancreatic head resection for cancer ranges between 10 and 25% [1-3]. Adjuvant chemotherapy, which improves patient survival, is routinely used [4,5]. The following characteristics have been reported to be significant prognostic factors for patient survival after tumor resection: age, tumor size, nodal and margin status and tumor grade [2,6-8]. Pancreatic surgery, specifically pancreatoduodenectomy (PD), has been identified to be a 'formidable' operation in earlier years [9]. The operation can be performed safely, and postoperative mortality in some specialized pancreatic centers is currently less than 5% [10,11].

Reduced mortality was achieved by concentrating pancreatic surgeries in specialized centers because pancreatic surgery is technically demanding and places high demands on the perioperative management [12,13]. Another important factor for reducing mortality and morbidity is better patient selection. Clinical decision-

* Correspondence: marius.distler@uniklinikum-dresden.de
†Equal contributors
[1]Department of General, Thoracic and Vascular Surgery, University Hospital Carl Gustav Carus, Technical University Dresden, Fetscherstrasse 74, Dresden 01307, Germany
Full list of author information is available at the end of the article

making will be increasingly influenced by evidence-based medicine [14].

The 5-year survival rate can be significantly improved for patients with pancreatic cancer when surgery is possible. However, some patients relapse shortly after the resection and exhibit a limited life span even after R0 resection.

To better assess the risks and benefits of surgical treatment, it is necessary to analyze the factors that might influence or determine which patients have limited survival.

The present study reports the short- and long-term outcome of 195 consecutive pancreatic head resections due to pancreatic cancer from a single German pancreatic center. Univariate and multivariate analyses were performed to examine the factors affecting survival.

Methods
Patients
Eight fellowship-trained pancreatobiliary surgeons performed 672 consecutive PDs between October 1993 and November 2008 in our department; the period of observation was 1993 to 2011. We excluded patients who underwent palliative bypass or pancreatic resections for pancreatic cancer in the body and tail of the pancreas, distal cholangiocarcinoma, duodenal carcinoma, neuroendocrine tumors, cyst-adenocarcinoma, solid and papillary tumors, and metastatic tumors. The final pathological diagnosis confirmed ductal pancreatic adenocarcinoma (PDAC) in 195 (29%) of the remaining patients. The demographic characteristics are summarized in Table 1.

Table 1 Patient cohort demographic and clinical data (n = 195)

	n=
Sex (m/f)	103 (53%)/92 (47%)
Age y (±SD)	67.0 (± 9.7) 95% CI 63.3-66.1
Hypertension (yes/no)	100 (51.3%)/95 (48.7%)
Preoperative diabetes mellitus	
(yes/no)	69 (35.4%)/126 (64.6%)
Obstructive jaundice (yes/no)	159 (81.5%)/36 (18.5%)
Preoperative biliary stent (yes/no)	139 (71.3%)/56 (28.7%)
Alcohol abuse (yes/no)	64 (32.8%)/131 (67.2%)
Nicotine abuse (yes/no)	35 (17.9%)/160 (82.1%)
Pack-years (±SD)	20 (± 6.5 y)
BMI (m/kg^2)	24.8 (± 3.6) 95% CI 24.5-25.5
General condition	
Good	150 (76.9%)
Mediocre	43 (22.1%)
Poor	2 (1.0%)

Operations
The head resection surgeries analyzed in the study included 69.7% pylorus-preserving pancreatoduodenectomies (PPPD) and 30.3% standard Kausch-Whipple pancreatoduodenectomies (Whipple). The decision for one of the approaches (either Whipple or PPPD) was made during the operation. The primary goal of every operation was en bloc R0 tumor resection. In all the patients, a lymphadenectomy was performed along the hepatoduodenal ligament, common hepatic artery, vena cava, interaortocaval and right side of the superior mesenteric artery. In cases with portal vein involvement, a venous resection was performed to achieve R0-resection. Patients with arterial infiltration by the tumor were stated to be locally irresectable. Thrombosis of the portal vein was always a contraindication for pancreatic head resection. The two-layer invagination technique was used for pancreatic anastomosis in all the cases as previously described [14]. We routinely placed drains intraoperatively. All the patients were staged preoperatively with CT and/or MRI and transabdominal ultrasound, and the PD patients were routinely observed at the Intensive Care Unit (ICU). The drains were removed after exclusion of a postoperative pancreatic fistula (POPF). Postoperative complications were treated symptomatically.

Data collection
The medical records from a prospective database of patients who underwent PDs for PDAC were analyzed retrospectively for each case. In accordance with the guidelines for human subject research, approval was obtained from the Ethics Committee at the Carl Gustav Carus University Hospital. All the operated patients singed inform consent agreements before surgery. The survey data were complemented with the clinical notes of the patients' physicians and surgeons. Details regarding the deceased patients were obtained from family members or from the general practitioner. The postoperative follow-up time was three years or until the death of the patient.

Patient characteristics and parameters used for statistical analysis are listed in the supplementary information (Additional file 1: Table S1). The postoperative events and clinical outcomes were recorded prospectively and analyzed retrospectively. The tumor-stage designation was categorized according to the TNM system of the Union Internationale Contre le Cancer (UICC 2007).

Definitions
Perioperative mortality was defined as in-hospital mortality. Postoperative pancreatic hemorrhage (PPH) was categorized according to the ISGPS consensus definition. [15]. Delayed gastric emptying (DGE) was classified according to the definition suggested by the ISGPS [16].

Postoperative pancreatic fistula (POPF) was defined according to the ISGPF criteria [17].

Statistical analysis
The statistical analyses were performed using SPSS for Windows, version 15.0 (SPSS, Inc., Chicago, IL). All clinical and pathological characteristics were stratified to build categorical or nominal variables. CEA and CA19-9 were grouped according to the cutoff values used in our center (cut-off levels CEA and CA 19–9: ≤3 ng/ml and ≤75 U/ml). Other variables such as age and BMI were grouped according to previous publications [8]. The thresholds used for categorization were based on previously described thresholds in the literature and/or recursive partitioning as previously described [18]. Continuous data are presented as 95% confidence intervals (95% CI) and standard deviation (SD). The univariate examination of the relationship between the assessed criteria and survival was performed with a χ^2-test. To assess the impact of the different parameters on survival, we utilized a 3-year survival rate. The estimates of patient survival were generated using the Kaplan-Meier method. The comparisons of survival were performed using the log-rank test. Student's t-tests (ratio scale) and Fisher's exact tests (ordinal scale) were utilized for comparisons between groups. Ordinal-scaled variables were compared using the chi-square test. Significant factors (at P < 0.10) at the univariate level were entered into the multivariate model. A Cox regression analysis with stepwise backwards elimination based on the likelihood ratios was employed to test for independent predictors of survival. A p-value <0.05 was considered significant.

Results
Patient demographics and preoperative parameters
From 1993 to 2008, 195 patients underwent pancreatic head resections (PD) due to ductal adenocarcinoma of the pancreas at our institution. The patients were observed from 1993 to 2011. The patient characteristics are described in Table 1. An obstructive jaundice appeared on average 4 weeks before the operation (± 2.3 weeks) in 159 patients (81.5%), and 139 of the patients were preoperatively treated with a biliary stent (71.3%). The maximal bilirubin concentration was 17.26 mg/dl (± 15.9 mg/dl). Weight loss was observed in 119 (61.0%) patients, and the average preoperative weight loss was 8.55 kg (± 4.57 kg). The average onset of weight loss was 8.0 weeks before the operation (± 9.8 weeks).

Intraoperative parameters
In most of the cases, the indication for operation was suspicion of malignancy (98.5%). The median postoperative hospital stay was 19.02 days (range 7–100) and included a median postoperative ICU stay of 5.2 days (range 0–69). In 29.7% of the cases, a partial resection of the portal vein (or superior mesenteric vein) was necessary. The mean duration of the pancreatic resection was 420.88 ± 99.0 minutes (range: 234–874 min) (Table 2).

Morbidity and mortality
The occurrence of perioperative mortality was 4.1% (8 patients) in the 195 patients who underwent resection for pancreatic cancer. During the postoperative course, 81 patients (42%) developed one or more complications. Most of the complications were minor (30%).

Grade B delayed gastric emptying was observed in 13 patients (6.7%), and grade C delayed gastric emptying was observed in 5 patients (2.6%). Ten patients developed grade B (5.1%) POPF, and 3 patients developed grade C POPF (1.5%). Grade B PPH was observed in 5 patients (2.6%), and grade C PPH was observed in three patients (1.5%). Table 3 presents the morbidity and mortality after PD.

Forty-eight of the patients developed one complication, 18 patients developed two complications, seven patients developed three complications, and eight patients developed more than three complications.

Histological analysis of the specimen
The tumor stage was pT1 in 7 (3.6%) patients, pT2 in 12 (6.1%) patients, pT3 in 173 (88.8%) patients and pT4 in 3 (1.5%) patients; the most frequent postoperative UICC 2002 stages were IIa and IIb. In 138 cases (70.8%), an R0 resection was certified by pathohistological examination of the specimen (R1: n = 42 (21.5%); R2: n = 10 (5.1%); Rx: n = 5 (2.6%)). Nodal disease was diagnosed in 129 (66.2%) of the 195 patients, 66 (33.8%) patients were

Table 2 Indications for operations and performed procedures (n = 195)

Indication for operation*	
Pain (%)	1.5
Suspicion of malignancy (%)	98.5
Obstructive jaundice (%)	20.0
Gastric outlet obstruction (%)	1.0
Performed procedures	
Whipple (%)	30.3
PPPD (%)	69.7
Resection of the SMV/portal vein (%)	29.7
Mean operative time (minutes) SD	420.88 ± 99.0
Postoperative hospital stay (days)	19.02 (range 7–100)
Postoperative ICU stay (days)	5.24 (range 0–69)

*Multiple answers were possible.
(SMV, Superior mesenteric vein; PPPD, Pylorus-preserving pancreaticoduodenectomy; ICU, Intensive care unit).

Table 3 Morbidity/outcome after PD due to PDAC of the pancreatic head

Complication/morbidity	Patients with complication*
	n = 81 (42%)
POPF	
Grade B	n = 10 (5.1%)
Grade C	n = 3 (1.5%)
PPH	
Grade B	n = 5 (2.6%)
Grade C	n = 3 (1.5%)
DGE	
Grade B	n = 13 (6.7%)
Grade C	n = 5 (3.6%)
Other complications	
Wound infections	n = 30 (15.4%)
Postoperative pneumonia	n = 10 (5.1%)
Pancreatitis	n = 8 (4.1%)
Cholangitis	n = 3 (1.5%)
Urinary tract infection	n = 7 (3.6%)
Anastomotic leakage	
Hepaticojejunostomy	n = 8 (4.1%)
Pancreatojejunostomy	n = 16 (8.2%)
In-hospital mortality	n = 8 (4.1%)

*Multiple answers were possible.

Table 4 Pathological features and tumor classification (n = 195)

TNM (2007)	
Tumor stage	
pT1	7 (3.6%)
pT2	12 (6.1%)
pT3	173 (88.8%)
pT4	3 (1.5%)
Nodal status	
pN0	66 (33.8%)
pN1	124 (63.6%)
pN1b	5 (2.6%)
Interaortocaval metastasis	
M1	15 (7.7%)
Resectional status	
R0	138 (70.8%)
R1	42 (21.5%)
R2	10 (5.1%)
Rx	5 (2.6%)
Perineural invasion	
PN0	76 (39.0%)
PN1	116 (59.5%)
PNx	3 (1.5%)
Tumor differentiation	
G1	6 (3.1%)
G2	102 (52.3%)
G3	82 (42.0%)
G4	5 (2.6%)

node negative, 124 (63.6%) patients had a pN1 status, and 5 (2.6%) patients had a pN1b status. In 15 patients, an M1 situation was confirmed in the final pathological evaluation. In all the cases, the M1 status was due to interaortocaval lymph nodes (Table 4).

The PDAC was well differentiated (G1) in 6 (3.1%) patients, intermediately differentiated (G2) in 102 (52.3%) patients, poorly differentiated (G3) in 82 (42.0%) patients and undifferentiated (G4) in 5 (2.6%) patients (Table 4).

Survival

To date, 163 of the 195 patients have died; 16 of the patients have died due to other causes and were censored for the survival analysis. The actuarial 3- and 5-year survival rates were 31.5% (95% CI, 25.04%-39.6%) and 11.86% (95% CI, 7.38%-19.0%), respectively. The median overall survival was 17.08 months (95% CI, 14.0%-20.1%) (Figure 1).

Adjuvant therapy was not routinely used in our center until 2003. Seventy-nine (40.5%) of the patients received postoperative adjuvant therapy. The median survival for patients without adjuvant CTx was 16.4 months (95% CI, 11.6- 21.2), and the median survival was 21.0 months (95% CI, 14.2-27.9) for patients with adjuvant CTx, which was not significant ($p = 0.931$).

Univariate survival analysis

In the univariate analysis, we correlated different parameters with the 3-year survival rate. CEA >3 ng/ml (p = 0.002), CA 19–9 >75 U/ml (p = 0.026) levels, tumor grade 3 (p = 0.001) and hard texture of the pancreatic gland (p = 0.017) were identified as significant predictive factors of poor patient survival. The lymph node ratio, T-stage or R-status (R1/R2 resection) were not found to be significant factors in univariate analysis. Table 5 summarizes the findings of the univariate analysis.

Multivariate survival analysis

All the factors that were significant in the univariate analyses at the p < 0.10 level (CEA, CA 19–9, age, texture of the pancreas and tumor grade) were tested using multivariate analysis. However, only the CEA level >3 ng/ml (p < 0.001) and tumor grade 3 (p = 0,013) could be identified as independent risk factors for patient survival (HR 2.350 and 1.346, respectively) (Table 6).

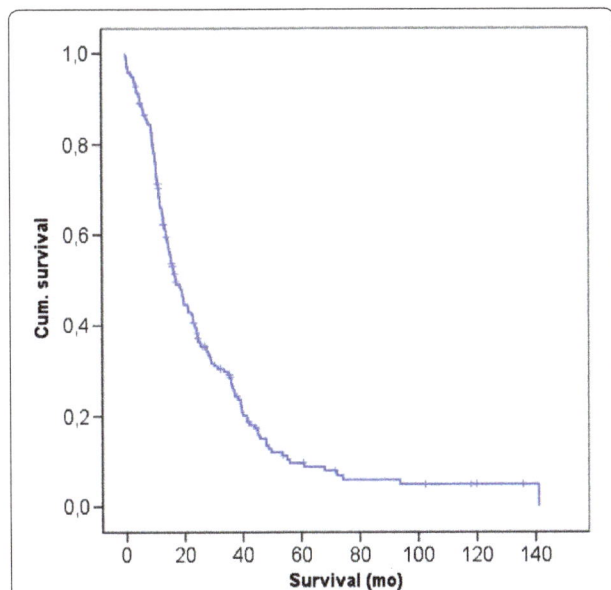

Figure 1 Kaplan-Meier analysis of overall survival of patients with PDAC of the pancreatic head after PD; the 3- and 5-year survival rates were 31.5% (95% CI, 25.04%-39.6%) and 11.86% (95% CI, 7.38%-19.0%), respectively.

Table 5 Univariate analysis of factors that influenced 3-year survival after PD due to PDAC of the pancreatic head

	3-year survival	p Value
Age (years)		0.073
<60 (n = 74)	n = 22 (30%)	
61-65 (n = 100)	n = 18 (18%)	
>65 (n = 21)	n = 2 (9%)	
CEA (ng/ml)		*0.002*
<4 (n = 151)	*n = 39 (26%)*	
>4 (n = 36)	*n = 1 (3%)*	
CA 19–9 (U/ml)		*0.026*
<24 (n = 39)	*n = 13 (33%)*	
>24 (n = 151)	*n = 26 (17%)*	
T- stage		0.894
pT1 n = 7	n = 2 (28%)	
pT2 n = 12	n = 2 (17%)	
pT3 n = 173	n = 37 (21%)	
pT4 n = 3	n = 1 (33%)	
R-status		0.155
R0 n = 138	n = 30 (22%)	
R1 n = 42	n = 8 (19%)	
R2 n = 10	n = 1 (10%)	
Lymph node-ratio		0.709
<0.2 (n = 134)	n = 30 (22%)	
≥0.2 (n = 60)	n = 12 (20%)	
Tumor grade		*0.001*
G1 (n = 6)	*n = 4 (67%)*	
G2 (n = 102)	*n = 21 (20%)*	
G3 (n = 82)	*n = 12 (15%)*	
G4 (n = 5)	*n = 2 (40%)*	
Pancreas texture		*0.017*
Hard n = 33	*n = 2 (6%)*	
Soft n = 161	*n = 40 (25%)*	
Preoperative diabetes (n = 69)	n = 12 (17%)	0.365
Nicotine abuse (n = 35)	n = 6 (17%)	0.651
Hypertension (n = 100)	n = 18 (18%)	0.163
BMI >35 (n = 3)	0	0.631
POPF grade B (n = 10)	n = 4 (40%)	0.228
POPF grade C (n = 3)	n = 1 (33%)	0.387

Discussion

In the present study, we retrospectively analyzed the long-term survival of patients undergoing PD for carcinoma of the pancreatic head in a single, high-volume center. The aim of this study was to identify predictive factors for long-term survival. The characteristics of the patient cohort were similar to previous reports [12,19]. The head resections included PPPD and Whipple procedures. The most common indication for operation was suspected malignancy, and most of the patients presented obstructive jaundice due to a tumor in the pancreatic head. All the patients exhibited histologically confirmed PDAC in the final examination of the specimen.

We observed a perioperative mortality of 4.1% in our study group, which was within the range of previous reports and indicates that the procedure is safe when performed in a hospital setting [12,19,20]. Surgical complications were observed in 42% of the patients undergoing PD. The high morbidity might have resulted from our comprehensive data acquisition. Our prospective pancreatic database includes surgical and unspecific complications. Most of the analyzed complications exhibited only minor effects on patient health such as wound infection, which was the most common surgical complication, or delayed gastric emptying (DGE). Severe complications (as defined by the ISGPS), such as grade C POPF, PPH or anastomotic leakage, were observed in 10% (n = 19) of the patients (Table 3). The complication rate is similar to previous studies [12,19]. Considering the complication rate, the indication for pancreatic resection should be performed carefully.

During univariate analyses, the elevated tumor marker levels of CEA and CA 19–9, the texture of the pancreas (hard) and the tumor grade (grade 3) were identified as significant factors with negative prognostic effects on patient survival. Multivariate analysis demonstrated that a

Table 6 Multivariate analysis of factors that influenced 3-year survival in patients after PD for PDAC of the pancreatic head

		HR	95% Confidence Interval HR		P value
			Lower	Upper	
Step 1	Age	1.205	0,916	1,549	0.162
	CEA >3 ng/ml	2.293	1,488	3,628	<0.001
	CA 19–9 >75 U/ml	1.130	0,721	1,671	0.560
	Tumor-grade 3	1.312	1,032	1,685	0.027
	Pan. Texture (hard)	1.046	0,590	1,713	0.866
Step 2	Age	1.203	1,489	3,626	0.164
	CEA >3 ng/ml	2.297	0,916	1,547	<0.001
	CA 19–9 >75 U/ml	1.136	0,724	1,667	0.539
	Tumor-grade 3	1.313	1,032	1,685	0.027
Step 3	Age	1.215	0,917	1,547	0.142
	CEA >3 ng/ml	2.258	1,490	3,627	<0.001
	Tumor-grade 3	1.330	1,035	1,683	0.565
Step 4					
	CEA >3 ng/ml	2.350	1,518	3,639	<0.001
	Tumor-grade 3	1.346	1,064	1,702	0.013

CEA level > 3 ng/ml (p < 0,005) and tumor grade 3 (p = 0,027) were independent predictive factors for patient survival. CEA and CA19-9 are the most studied serum tumor markers for the diagnosis and prognosis of pancreatic adenocarcinoma [21]. CEA is known to exhibit low sensitivity in screening PDAC [22]. However, other authors hypothesized that high levels might be associated with the existence of occult metastasis or locally advanced diseases in patients with PDAC. Therefore, previously high levels of CEA could be associated with incurability in patients with pancreatic cancer [23,24]. Although CEA might not be appropriate for screening, its serum level should be determined in patients prior to operation. High serum levels of CEA should be considered by the surgeon in cases where respectability or operability is questionable.

Levels of carbohydrate antigen (CA) 19–9, a tumor-associated glycoprotein, are elevated in approximately 85% of patients with PDAC [25], and serum CA19-9 measurements can be used for diagnostic purposes (i.e., as a predictor of resectability or as a marker of recurrent disease after resection) [26]. Both CA19-9 and CEA can be used to predict survival after pancreatic resection [27,28]. In an analysis by Hartwig et al., CA-19-9 levels greater than 400 U/ml were identified as one of the strongest negative survival predictors [29]. However, cholestasis is known to influence serum tumor marker concentrations. Both CA19-9 and CEA undergo biliary excretion, and serum levels may artificially increase due to biliary obstruction caused by cancer masses [30]. Because many patients experienced obstructive jaundice in

our study cohort, our results, particularly the CA19-9 results, may be biased. However, in multivariate analysis, CA19-9 could not be identified as a significant predictor of survival in patients with PDAC.

According to our data, tumor differentiation plays a prominent role for survival in pancreatic cancer, as already shown in other tumor entities. Tumor differentiation was an independent prognostic factor in multivariate analysis [1,8,31]. Contrary to these results, we did not observe an influence of the TNM classification or the resectional status, similarly to previous publications [1,8]. It is unclear why these parameters were not correlated with survival. Data published by Esposito et al. suggest that most resections in pancreatic cancer are R1 resections [32]. As a result, other researchers in this field refer to pancreatic cancer as a "systemic disease". While the classification as a systemic disease may be immoderate for a solid tumor, it shows that aggressive infiltration and metastasizing are important hallmarks of pancreatic cancer. These hallmarks might be more pronounced in tumors with poor differentiation, which might also explain why our results did not identify the lymph node ratio as a significant factor as previously published by Riediger et al. The lymph node ratio may be diagnostically relevant similar to other tumor entities. However, tumor grading appears be a more relevant indicator of the patient's prognosis as shown in our analysis.

Furthermore, the texture of the pancreas was identified to be a predictor of survival in our analysis. Soft texture of the gland was related to a good prognosis (p < 0.017). This sudden finding is especially difficult to interpret because pancreatojejunal anastomosis is safer in a fibrotic pancreas compared with a soft and friable normal pancreas with a narrow main pancreatic duct [14,33]. In patients with a soft pancreas, chronic pancreatitis is usually not present, and the patients may exhibit better organ function, which results in a better prognosis. Tumors derived from a chronic pancreatitis (associated with hard texture) were more aggressive or exhibited more aggressive pathophysiology than carcinomas arising from a normal pancreas. Because no significance for the texture was shown in the multivariate analysis, the parameter might be a surrogate for another variable influencing outcome. Furthermore, the evaluation of pancreatic texture must be considered, especially in retrospective analyses, because it is very subjective and easy to overestimate.

The actuarial overall 3- and 5-year survival rates were 31.5% (95% CI, 25.04%-39.6%) and 11.86% (95% CI, 7.38%-19.0%), respectively. These findings are similar to those reported in the literature [1,12,29]. There was no statistical significance between the subgroups of patients with or without adjuvant chemotherapy [median survival: without adjuvant CTx 16.4 months (95% CI, 11.6-21.2 months) vs. with adjuvant CTx 21.0 months (95% CI, 14.2-27.9 months) (p = 0.931)], which may be due to the heterogeneity of the chemotherapeutic regimes. Approximately 50% of our patients received adjuvant chemotherapy (i.e., mainly with gemcitabine). Although long-term survival may be achieved in only a minority of patients, the complete surgical resection of pancreatic adenocarcinoma represents the only potential curative option.

Conclusion

In our single-center analysis, CEA tumor marker levels and tumor grade were identified as significant predictors for poor survival in patients with pancreatic head cancer. However, hard texture of the pancreatic gland appears to exhibit an indirect positive effect on patient survival after pancreatic head resection, but the reason for the effect remains unclear.

Abbreviations
ICU: Intensive care unit; PDAC: Pancreatic ductal adenocarcinoma; ISGPS: International study group of pancreatic surgery; POPF: Postoperative pancreatic fistula; PPH: Post pancreatic hemorrhage; DGE: Delayed gastric emptying; PD: Pancreatoduodenectomy; MRI: Magnetic resonance imaging; CTx: Chemotherapy; PPPD: Pylorus-preserving pancreatoduodenectomy.

Competing interests
The authors declare no competing interests. This research received no specific grant from any funding agency in public, commercial, or not-for-profit sectors.

Authors' contributions
DM wrote the manuscript, collected the data, interpreted the results and statistically analyzed the data, RF and KS analyzed the data statistically, interpreted the results and critically revised the manuscript, HM collected the data and wrote parts of the manuscript, RF analyzed the data statistically and corrected the manuscript, EF statistically analyzed the data, interpreted the results and critically revised the manuscript, PC gave important manuscript corrections, SHD designed the concept of the manuscript operations and critically revised the manuscript, and GR designed the study, collected data, and drafted the manuscript. All authors read and approved the final manuscript.

Acknowledgments
We thank Heike Berthold for her support in data preparation and for servicing our prospective pancreatic database.

Author details
[1]Department of General, Thoracic and Vascular Surgery, University Hospital Carl Gustav Carus, Technical University Dresden, Fetscherstrasse 74, Dresden 01307, Germany. [2]Surgical Department, University Hospital Mannheim, Heidelberg University, Mannheim, Germany.

References
1. Sommerville CA, Limongelli P, Pai M, et al: Establishment of a preclinical ovine model for tibial segmental bone defect repair by applying bone tissue engineering strategies. J Surg Oncol 2009, 100(8):651–656.
2. Richter A, Niedergethmann M, Sturm JW, et al: Long-term results of partial pancreaticoduodenectomy for ductal adenocarcinoma of the pancreatic head: 25-year experience. World J Surg 2003, 27(3):324–329. Epub 2003 Feb 27.
3. Winter JM, Cameron JL, Campbell KA, et al: 1423 Pancreaticoduodenectomies for pancreatic cancer: a single-institution experience. J Gastrointest Surg 2006, 10(9):1199–1210. discussion 1210–1.
4. Neoptolemos JP, Stocken DD, Tudur Smith C, et al: Adjuvant 5-fluorouracil and folinic acid vs observation for pancreatic cancer: composite data from the ESPAC-1 and −3(v1) trials. Br J Cancer 2009, 100(2):246–250.
5. Oettle H, Post S, Neuhaus P, Gellert K, et al: Adjuvant chemotherapy with gemcitabine vs observation in patients undergoing curative-intent resection of pancreatic cancer: a randomized controlled trial. JAMA 2007, 297(3):267–277.
6. Lim JE, Chien MW, Earle CC: Prognostic factors following curative resection for pancreatic adenocarcinoma: a population-based, linked database analysis of 396 patients. Ann Surg 2003, 237(1):74–85.
7. Sohn TA, Yeo CJ, Cameron JL, et al: Resected adenocarcinoma of the pancreas-616 patients: results, outcomes, and prognostic indicators. J Gastrointest Surg 2000, 4(6):567–579.
8. Riediger H, Keck T, Wellner U, et al: The lymph node ratio is the strongest prognostic factor after resection of pancreatic cancer. J Gastrointest Surg 2009, 13(7):1337–1344.
9. Yeo CJ, Cameron JL, Sohn TA, et al: Six hundred fifty consecutive pancreaticoduodenectomies in the 1990s: pathology, complications, and outcomes. Ann Surg 1997, 226(3):248–257.
10. Cameron JL, Riall TS, Coleman J, Belcher KA: One thousand consecutive pancreaticoduodenectomies. Ann Surg 2006, 244(1):10–15.
11. Andrén-Sandberg A, Neoptolemos JP: Resection for pancreatic cancer in the new millennium. Pancreatology 2002, 2(5):431–439.
12. Yeo CJ, Cameron JL, Lillemoe KD, et al: Pancreaticoduodenectomy with or without distal gastrectomy and extended retroperitoneal lymphadenectomy for periampullary adenocarcinoma, part 2: randomized controlled trial evaluating survival, morbidity, and mortality. Ann Surg 2002, 236(3):355–366.
13. Ho CK, Kleeff J, Friess H, Büchler MW: Complications of pancreatic surgery. HPB (Oxford) 2005, 7(2):99–108.

14. Rückert F, Kersting S, Fiedler D, *et al*: Chronic pancreatitis: early results of pancreatoduodenectomy and analysis of risk factors. *Pancreas* 2011, **40**(6):925–930.

15. Wente MN, Veit JA, Bassi C, *et al*: Postpancreatectomy hemorrhage (PPH): an international study group of pancreatic surgery (ISGPS) definition. *Surgery* 2007, **142**(1):20–25.

16. Wente MN, Bassi C, Dervenis C, *et al*: Delayed gastric emptying (DGE) after pancreatic surgery: a suggested definition by the international study group of pancreatic surgery (ISGPS). *Surgery* 2007, **142**(5):761–768.

17. Bassi C, Dervenis C, Butturini G, *et al*: Postoperative pancreatic fistula: an international study group (ISGPF) definition. *Surgery* 2005, **138**(1):8–13.

18. Rückert F, Distler M, Hoffmann S, *et al*: Quality of life in patients after pancreaticoduodenectomy for chronic pancreatitis. *J Gastrointest Surg* 2011, **15**(7):1143–1150.

19. Farnell MB, Pearson RK, Sarr MG, *et al*: A prospective randomized trial comparing standard pancreatoduodenectomy with pancreatoduodenectomy with extended lymphadenectomy in resectable pancreatic head adenocarcinoma. *Surgery* 2005, **138**(4):618–628.

20. Trede M, Schwall G, Saeger HD: Survival after pancreatoduodenectomy. 118 consecutive resections without an operative mortality. *Ann Surg* 1990, **211**(4):447–458.

21. Rückert F, Pilarsky C, Grützmann R: Serum tumor markers in pancreatic cancer-recent discoveries. *Cancers* 2010, **2**(2):1107–1124.

22. Lundin J, Roberts PJ, Kuusela P, *et al*: The prognostic value of preoperative serum levels of CA 19–9 and CEA in patients with pancreatic cancer. *Br J Cancer* 1994, **69**(3):515–519.

23. Fujioka S, Misawa T, Okamoto T, *et al*: Preoperative serum carcinoembryonic antigen and carbohydrate antigen 19–9 levels for the evaluation of curability and resectability in patients with pancreatic adenocarcinoma. *J Hepatobiliary Pancreat Surg* 2007, **14**(6):539–544. Epub 2007 Nov 30.

24. Schlieman MG, Fahy BN, Ramsamooj R, *et al*: Incidence, mechanism and prognostic value of activated AKT in pancreas cancer. *Br J Cancer* 2003, **89**(11):2110–2115.

25. Safi F, Schlosser W, Falkenreck S, *et al*: Prognostic value of CA 19–9 serum course in pancreatic cancer. *Hepatogastroenterology* 1998, **45**(19):253–259.

26. Katz MH, Varadhachary GR, Fleming JB, *et al*: Serum CA 19–9 as a marker of resectability and survival in patients with potentially resectable pancreatic cancer treated with neoadjuvant chemoradiation. *Ann Surg Oncol* 2010, **17**(7):1794–1801.

27. Ferrone CR, Finkelstein DM, Thayer SP, *et al*: Perioperative CA19-9 levels can predict stage and survival in patients with resectable pancreatic adenocarcinoma. *J Clin Oncol* 2006, **24**(18):2897–2902.

28. Smith RA, Bosonnet L, Ghaneh P, *et al*: Preoperative CA19-9 levels and lymph node ratio are independent predictors of survival in patients with resected pancreatic ductal adenocarcinoma. *Dig Surg* 2008, **25**(3):226–232.

29. Hartwig W, Hackert T, Hinz U, *et al*: Pancreatic cancer surgery in the new millennium: better prediction of outcome. *Ann Surg* 2011, **254**(2):311–319.

30. Basso D, Fabris C, Plebani M, *et al*: Alterations in bilirubin metabolism during extra- and intrahepatic cholestasis. *Clin Investig* 1992, **70**(1):49–54.

31. Vincent A, Herman J, Schulick R, *et al*: Pancreatic cancer. *Lancet* 2011, **378**(9791):607–620.

32. Esposito I, Kleeff J, Bergmann F, *et al*: Most pancreatic cancer resections are R1 resections. *Ann Surg Oncol* 2008, **15**(6):1651–1660.

33. Hamanaka Y, Nishihara K, Hamasaki T, *et al*: Pancreatic juice output after pancreatoduodenectomy in relation to pancreatic consistency, duct size, and leakage. *Surgery* 1996, **119**(3):281–287.

2

Adult pancreatic hemangioma in pregnancy – concerns and considerations of a rare case

Jon Arne Søreide[1,4*], Ole Jakob Greve[2] and Einar Gudlaugsson[3]

Abstract

Background: Pancreatic tumors in pregnancy are rare but clinically challenging. Careful diagnostic workup, including appropriate imaging examinations, should be performed to evaluate surgery indications and timing . In the present case a diagnosis of an adult pancreatic hemangioma was made. We were not able to identify a similar case in the very sparse literature on this rare disease.

Case presentation: A 30-year-old woman at 12 weeks of gestation was diagnosed with a large pancreatic tumor having a cystic pattern based on imaging. Although the preoperative diagnosis was uncertain, patient preference and clinical symptoms and signs suggested surgery. Open distal pancreatic resection including splenectomy was performed, and complete resection of the large cystic tumor was successfully achieved, with no postoperative complications. Although a solid pseudopapillary epithelial neoplasm (SPEN) was suspected, specimen morphology, including immunohistochemistry, supported the diagnosis of an adult benign pancreatic hemangioma.

Conclusion: Although mucinous cystic neoplasm (MCN) and adenocarcinoma are the most common pancreatic tumors during pregnancy, various other malignant and benign lesions can be encountered. This report adds to the very small number of pancreatic hemangiomas reported in the literature and involves the first patient diagnosed with this rare condition during pregnancy. Careful clinical considerations regarding diagnostic workup and treatments are required to ensure that mother and child receive the best possible care.

Keywords: Cystic lesion, Hemangioma, Pancreas, Pregnancy

Background

In pregnant women, the acute abdomen is often a challenge. Careful clinical evaluation, close cooperation between the surgeon and the gynecologist as needed, and the application of appropriate diagnostic tools and educated judgment remain the cornerstones of standard care [1–6]. Although the diagnostic workup can be demanding in these cases, a responsible surgeon might regard appropriate surgical treatment as stressful for the relatively common diseases encountered during pregnancy such as appendicitis [7, 8] and acute cholecystitis [9, 10]. A surgeon is confronted by even greater responsibility for a mother and her child in clinical settings involving rare acute abdominal conditions of pregnancy, which include acute severe pancreatitis [11], gastrointestinal bleeding [12, 13], and suspected tumors in various locations [14–19]. In cases involving a cystic lesion, the nature of the lesion, including its malignant potential and the risk of a spontaneous rupture, must be considered when discussing indications for and the timing of surgery [15, 20]. In this situation, the surgical approach, which varies depending on the pregnancy trimester is a particularly concerning issue.

In this report, we discuss clinical considerations related to the unexpected finding of a large cystic lesion that appears to be related to the pancreas in a pregnant woman with acute abdomen.

Ethics

Written informed consent was obtained from the patient for publication of this Case report and any accompanying images. A copy of the written consent is available for review by the Editor of this journal.

* Correspondence: jonarne.soreide@uib.no
[1]Department of Gastrointestinal Surgery, Stavanger University Hospital, N-4068 Stavanger, Norway
[4]Department of Clinical Medicine, University of Bergen, Bergen, Norway
Full list of author information is available at the end of the article

Case presentation

An otherwise healthy, non-obese 30-year-old woman, para 0, at 12 weeks gestation was admitted to our hospital's Department of Gastrointestinal Surgery with a history of 3 weeks of varying but increasing pain in the left upper quadrant of her abdomen and nausea without vomiting. A palpable left subcostal mass was detected by clinical examination, which revealed no other notable findings except for her pregnant status. Ultrasound (US) examination (Fig. 1) revealed a large cystic lesion (size, 17 × 10 cm) with septa related to the tail of the pancreas and spleen. Magnetic resonance imaging (MRI) depicted a multicystic lesion related to the pancreatic tail, between the spleen and left kidney, with moderate dislocation of both the kidney and spleen (Fig. 2). Routine biochemistry was normal, and tumor markers carcinoembryomic antigen (CEA = 4 μg/l), cancer antigen 125 (CA125 = 42kU/l), carbohydrate antigen 19–9 (CA19–9 < 5 kU/l), and chromogranin A(CgA = 2.8 nmol/l) were all within normal ranges. The preoperative diagnosis was uncertain; however, based on imaging findings and the patient's young age, a solid pseudopapillary epithelial neoplasm (SPEN) was considered. A gynecologist evaluated the patient's pregnancy as normal. Relevant factors when considering indications for surgery included the presence of increasing clinical symptoms in a pregnant woman, the uncertain nature of the rather large cystic pancreatic tumor, and the possible risk and undesirable consequences of a rupture of this tumor during the second or third trimester. In accordance with the patient's preferences, surgical treatment was recommended. Open resection of the most distal portion of the pancreas, including the large cystic tumor and spleen, was performed. Frozen sections of the pancreas resection border confirmed that the resected tissue was benign. The patient's postoperative course was uneventful, and she was able to leave the hospital on the 6th postoperative day without complications.

The multicystic tumor (Fig. 3) measured 19.5 × 10 × 7 cm and exhibited close adherence to the distal pancreas but without infiltration in the pancreas parenchyma or any communication with the pancreatic ducts. Microscopically, benign pancreatic tissue was confirmed, and the tumor was multicystic with extremely thin septa, fibrosis and a pattern of chronic inflammation, but no epithelial tissue indicating that SPEN was unlikely. Additional immunohistochemistry (IHC) with CD34 and CD 31 (Fig. 4) provided information to support a large-vessel hemangioma lined with single endothelial layer without cytologic atypia, and with focal degenerative changes in septa and the cystic wall. This endothelial lining was negative for cytokeratins and calretinin, excluding epitehelial and mestothelial nature of the lesion Taken together, the tumor morphological findings were characteristic of a truly benign lesion most consistent with adult pancreatic hemangioma, which was resected completely without any ruptures.

After surgery, the patient's pregnancy proceeded uneventfully, and she spontaneously delivered a healthy child

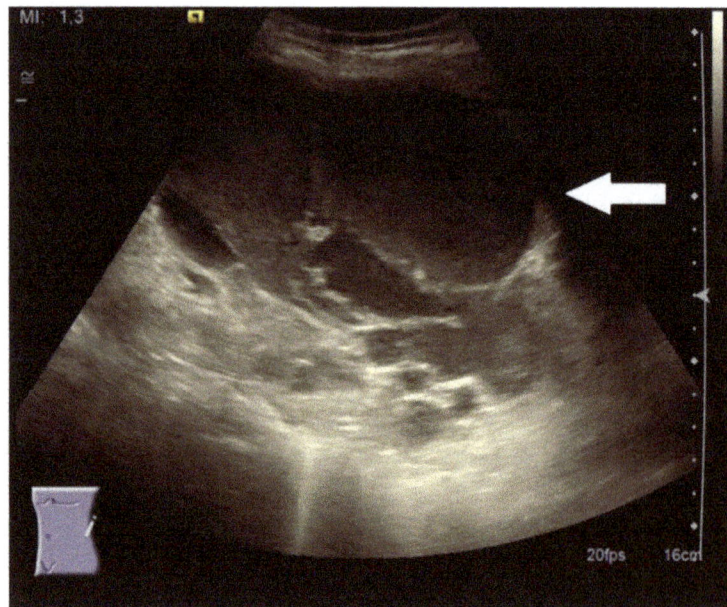

Fig. 1 Ultrasound showed a large cystic lesion with septa and some sedimentation. Minimal Doppler signal of the large tumor (18 × 10 cm). Spleen, pancreas and left kidney without focal lesions

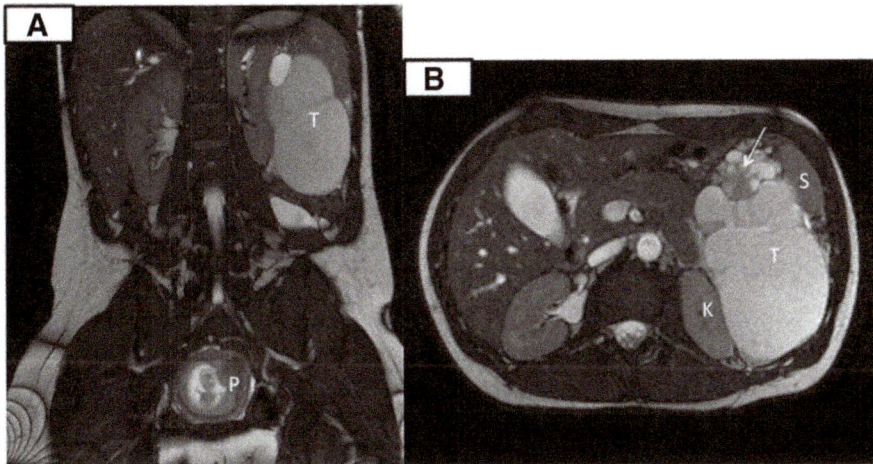

Fig. 2 Coronal (**a**) and transversal (**b**) MRI T2 (FIESTA) view. Large tumor (T) medial to the spleen (S) and adjacent to the pancreatic tail dislocating the left kidney (K) medial and cranial. Mostly high signal intensity at T2 and intermediate to high at T1, indicating cystic components with protein or blood. A smaller part of the lesion had lower signal and diffusion restriction indicating more solid parts. (P) is the pregnant uterus. A solid pseudopapillary epithel neoplasia (SPEN) of the pancreas was suspected in this young woman with an encapsulated lesion with cystic, solid and hemorrhagic components

at the calculated gestational time. During follow-up of at least 12 postoperative months, the patient has expressed no complaints or concerns related to her treatment.

Discussion

While hemangiomas are rarely found in the pancreas, they are very common in the liver. Mundinger et al. reviewed the literature and found only 9 cases with confirmed adult pancreatic hemangiomas reported between 1939 and 2009 [21]. The lesions were most commonly located in the head, or head/body of the gland, with a size varying from 3 cm to 20 cm in diameter. Recently, Bursics and coworkers [22] reported on another patient (a 72-year-old man) surgically treated for a confirmed adult hemangioma of the pancreas, and presented relevant data on the 12 reported cases, including their own, published until 2013. Male:female ratio was found to be 2:1, and the median age was 61 (range, 30–79) years. As demonstrated by these 12 reported cases in the world literature [21, 22], pain was the most common clinical symptom which was also the case in our patient. The pattern of a suggested cystic lesion by imaging was

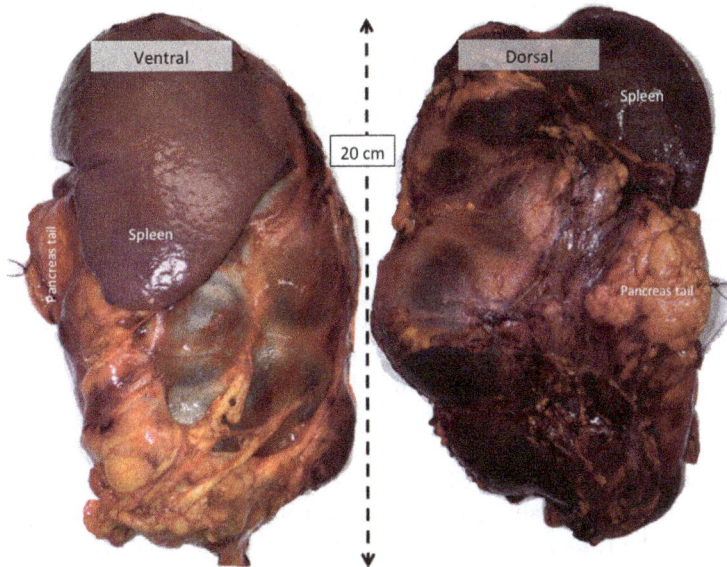

Fig. 3 Operative specimen with the cystic tumor and the spleen seen from the ventral (*left*) and the dorsal (*right*) side. The cystic tumor measured 19.5 × 10 × 7 cm

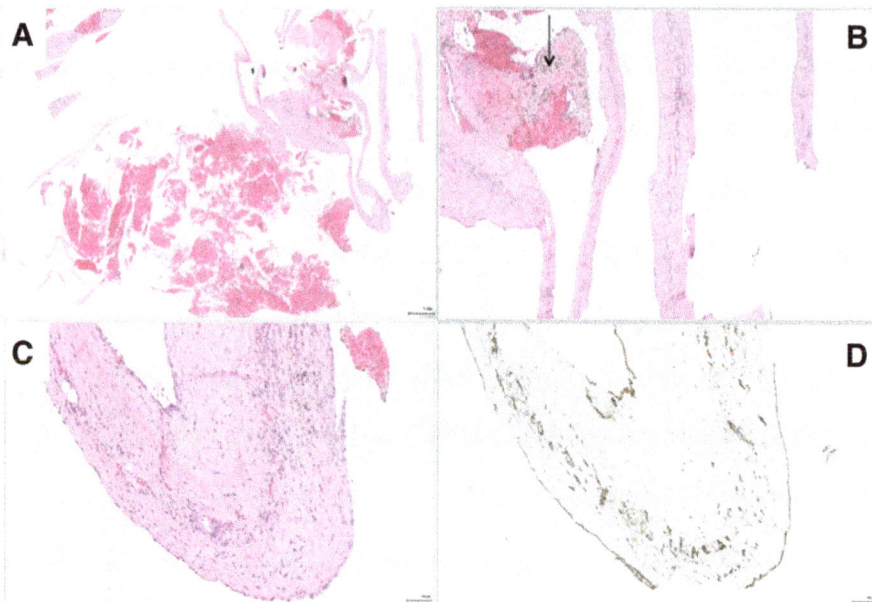

Fig. 4 a Large dilated vascular structures lined by endothelial cells filled with red blood cells. The thickened vessel walls are composed of fibrous or spindle cell stroma with mild chronic inflammation. (H and E; original magnification: ×10). **b** Large dilated vascular structures lined by endothelial cells filled with red blood cells. The thickened vessel walls are composed of fibrous or spindle cell stroma with mild chronic inflammation and hemosiderin loaded macrophages (arrow) (H and E; original magnification: ×20). **c** Microscopy showing large dilated vascular structure lined by endothelial cells. The wall is infiltrated with mild chronic inflammation. (H and E; original magnification: ×100). **d**. Immunohistochemical expression of CD31 (brown) depicting the endothelial lining of larger vascular spaces and small vessels in the stroma (original magnification, ×20)

found in most patients with available information in this regard. Notably, the CT patterns of a pancreatic hemangioma are different from the CT signs of a liver hemangioma, as a typical early peripheral contrast-enhancement during the arterial phase is missing in the former [23]. Therefore, this imaging modality is ineffective for ruling out pancreatic hemangioma.

Our patient was definitely in the younger range of age, and importantly, we report on the first pregnant patient diagnosed with an adult pancreas hemangioma. Although the final morphologic diagnosis of this rare condition can be challenging, CD 31 and CD 34 immunohistochemical labeling adds valuable support to the diagnosis of a neoplasm of vascular origin [21].

Both benign and malignant pancreatic neoplasms are rarely diagnosed during pregnancy; in particular, pancreatic cancer during pregnancy is extremely rare, with fewer than 10 described cases to date [15, 16]. However, a number of dilemmas can be encountered when attempting to determine an accurate diagnosis to enable appropriate treatment. Within this context, both US and MRI are reliable and useful imaging modalities [5, 20] without known health risks for the fetus [24]. When indicated, CT can also contribute to imaging findings. Of note, the risk that the fetus will develop congenital abnormalities due to the side effects of radiation exposure

(via repeat and/or multiphase CT scans) is considered to be extremely low [25], nonetheless, due to concerns regarding the potential for deleterious side effects, radiation and various contrast agents should be limited and used with care [24, 25].

Del Chiaro et al. [26] recently demonstrated that the overall accuracy of preoperative diagnoses of cystic pancreatic lesions is only approximately 60 %, with similar accuracies for asymptomatic and symptomatic lesions. Thus, inaccurate preoperative assessments of pancreatic cystic lesions are common; however, diagnostic errors are clinically relevant in less than 10 % of these cases. Data regarding lesion size, patient gender, and the patient's prior history (with respect to pancreatitis or other relevant diseases) could be valuable information for reaching appropriate decisions and thereby preventing the overutilization of operative resection in patients with these lesions [27]. For non-pregnant patients, additional imaging (e.g., contrast CT scans) and endoscopic ultrasound (EUS)-guided aspiration of the cystic lesion for analyses of DNA mutations and proteins within pancreatic cyst fluid can contribute to the diagnostic workup [20, 28]. However, due to potential risks for a biopsy related bleeding, rupture of the lesion or peritoneal seeding of biopsy material, we did not regard our symptomatic pregnant patient with a large pancreatic lesion as a candidate for this diagnostic approach. Her subjective and increasing complaints, the uncertain nature of the lesion, and the risk of tumor rupture with undesired side effects or complications later during her pregnancy, were all important considerations for the timing of treatment. The preoperative diagnosis of a possible SPEN was not definitively determined. As recently suggested [29] SPENs are rare cystic lesions that frequently occur in young women and patients with these lesions exhibit good prognoses if radical surgical resection can be achieved. Despite the challenging nature of a definite diagnosis, the only feature of the described case that could be associated with malignancy was a large tumor size at diagnosis [20, 29]. Thus fare, malignancy has not been reported for pancreatic hemangiomas. Based on the rarity of this condition, the lack of reliable follow-up data, and the sparse literature on this topic, an understanding of the pathophysiology and natural history of these lesions remains at an early stage [21].

Conclusion

Although reports have described a number of anecdotes involving worrisome histories of pregnant women with malignant tumors, including carcinomas of the pancreas [16, 30, 31], pancreatic neuroendocrine tumors [14], and bleeding neoplasms [32], or spontaneous SPEN rupture [33], these cases are generally exceptions rather than the rule. Nevertheless, given the objective of providing optimal care to both mother and child, the determination of an appropriate treatment schedule for any young pregnant woman requires the consideration of a wide range of diagnoses and a number of important factors. Although the second trimester is considered to be the most favorable time for surgical intervention for pancreatic tumors [15], multidisciplinary consultation should occur with respect to a pregnant patient's diagnosis, indications and timing to ensure that the best possible outcomes for both the mother and the child are achieved [15, 18, 19, 22, 26].

Abbreviations
CT: Computer tomography; EUS: Endoscopic ultrasound; IHC: Immunohistochemistry; MCN: Mucinous cystic neoplasm; MRI: Magnetic resonance imaging; SPEN: Solid pseudopapillary epithelial neoplasm.

Competing interests
The authors declare they have no competing interests.

Authors' contributions
Study conception and design: JAS. Data acquision: JAS, OJG, EG. Data interpretation: JAS, OJG, EG. Drafting of the manuscript: JAS. Manuscript editing and final approval: JAS, OJG, EG.

Acknowledgements
The authors appreciate the patient's consent to present this case.

Author details
[1]Department of Gastrointestinal Surgery, Stavanger University Hospital, N-4068 Stavanger, Norway. [2]Department of Radiology, Stavanger University Hospital, Stavanger, Norway. [3]Department of Pathology, Stavanger University Hospital, Stavanger, Norway. [4]Department of Clinical Medicine, University of Bergen, Bergen, Norway.

References

1. Ackerman SJ, Irshad A, Anis M. Ultrasound for pelvic pain II: nongynecologic causes. Obstet Gynecol Clin North Am. 2011;38:69–83. viii.
2. Boregowda G, Shehata HA. Gastrointestinal and liver disease in pregnancy. Best Pract Res Clin Obstet Gynaecol. 2013;27:835–53.
3. Dewhurst C, Beddy P, Pedrosa I. MRI evaluation of acute appendicitis in pregnancy. J Magn Reson Imaging. 2013;37:566–75.
4. Katz DS, Khalid M, Coronel EE, Mazzie JP. Computed tomography imaging of the acute pelvis in females. Can Assoc Radiol J. 2013;64:108–18.
5. Khandelwal A, Fasih N, Kielar A. Imaging of acute abdomen in pregnancy. Radiol Clin North Am. 2013;51:1005–22.
6. Kilpatrick CC, Orejuela FJ. Management of the acute abdomen in pregnancy: a review. Curr Opin Obstet Gynecol. 2008;20:534–9.
7. Flexer SM, Tabib N, Peter MB. Suspected appendicitis in pregnancy. Surgeon. 2014;12:82–6.
8. Teixeira PG, Demetriades D. Appendicitis: changing perspectives. Adv Surg. 2013;47:119–40.
9. Knab LM, Boller AM, Mahvi DM. Cholecystitis. Surg Clin North Am. 2014;94:455–70.
10. Sucandy I, Tellagorry J, Kolff JW. Minimally invasive surgical management of acute cholecystitis during pregnancy: what are the recommendations? Am Surg. 2013;79:E251–2.
11. Abdullah B, Kathiresan Pillai T, Cheen LH, Ryan RJ. Severe acute pancreatitis in pregnancy. Case Rep Obstet Gynecol. 2015;2015:239068.
12. Friedel D, Stavropoulos S, Iqbal S, Cappell MS. Gastrointestinal endoscopy in the pregnant woman. World J Gastrointest Endosc. 2014;6:156–67.
13. Knez J, Day A, Jurkovic D. Ultrasound imaging in the management of bleeding and pain in early pregnancy. Best Pract Res Clin Obstet Gynaecol. 2014;28:621–36.
14. Besemer B, Mussig K. Insulinoma in pregnancy. Exp Clin Endocrinol Diabetes. 2010;118:9–18.
15. Boyd CA, Benarroch-Gampel J, Kilic G, Kruse EJ, Weber SM, Riall TS. Pancreatic neoplasms in pregnancy: diagnosis, complications, and management. J Gastrointest Surg. 2012;16:1064–71.
16. Kakoza RM, Vollmer Jr CM, Stuart KE, Takoudes T, Hanto DW. Pancreatic adenocarcinoma in the pregnant patient: a case report and literature review. J Gastrointest Surg. 2009;13:535–41.
17. Onuma T, Yoshida Y, Yamamoto T, Kotsuji F. Diagnosis and management of pancreatic carcinoma during pregnancy. Obstet Gynecol. 2010;116 Suppl 2:518–20.
18. Wiseman JE, Yamamoto M, Nguyen TD, Bonadio J, Imagawa DK. Cystic pancreatic neoplasm in pregnancy: a case report and review of the literature. Arch Surg. 2008;143:84–6.
19. Dunkelberg JC, Barakat J, Deutsch J. Gastrointestinal, pancreatic, and hepatic cancer during pregnancy. Obstet Gynecol Clin North Am. 2005;32:641–60.
20. Choi JY, Kim MJ, Kim JH, Kim SH, Lim JS, Oh YT et al. Solid pseudopapillary tumor of the pancreas: typical and atypical manifestations. AJR Am J Roentgenol. 2006;187:W178–86.
21. Mundinger GS, Gust S, Micchelli ST, Fishman EK, Hruban RH, Wolfgang CL. Adult pancreatic hemangioma: case report and literature review. Gastroenterol Res Pract. 2009;2009:839730.
22. Bursics A, Gyokeres T, Bely M, Porneczi B. Adult hemangioma of the pancreas: difficult diagnosis of a rare disease. Clin J Gastroenterol. 2013;6:338–43.
23. Kobayashi H, Itoh T, Murata R, Tanabe M. Pancreatic cavernous hemangioma: CT, MRI, US, and angiography characteristics. Gastrointest Radiol. 1991;16:307–10.
24. Baysinger CL. Imaging during pregnancy. Anesth Analg. 2010;110:863–7.
25. Patel SJ, Reede DL, Katz DS, Subramaniam R, Antskatlis A. Imaging the pregnant patient for nonobstetric conditions: algorithms and radiation dose considerations. Radiographics. 2007;27:1705–22.
26. Del Chiaro M, Segersvard R, Pozzi Mucelli R, Rangelova E, Kartalis N, Ansorge C, et al. Comparison of preoperative conference-based diagnosis with histology of cystic tumors of the pancreas. Ann Surg Oncol. 2014;21:1539–44.

27. Allen PJ. Operative resection is currently overutilized for cystic lesions of the pancreas. J Gastrointest Surg. 2014;18:182–3.

28. Kwon RS. Advances in the diagnosis of cystic neoplasms of the pancreas. Curr Opin Gastroenterol. 2012;28:494–500.

29. Butte JM, Brennan MF, Gonen M, et al. Solid pseudopapillary tumors of the pancreas. Clinical features, surgical outcomes, and long-term survival in 45 consecutive patients from a single center. J Gastrointest Surg. 2011;15:350–7.

30. Gundling F, Nerlich A, Heitland W, Schepp W. Neuroendocrine pancreatic carcinoma after initial diagnosis of acute postpartal coeliac disease in a 37-year old woman - fatal coincidence or result of a neglected disease? Anticancer Res. 2014;34:2449–54.

31. Hakamada K, Miura T, Kimura A, Nara M, Toyoki Y, Narumi S, et al. Anaplastic carcinoma associated with a mucinous cystic neoplasm of the pancreas during pregnancy: report of a case and a review of the literature. World J Gastroenterol. 2008;14:132–5.

32. Brown TH, Menon VS, Richards DG, Griffiths AP. Gastrointestinal bleeding in a pregnant woman: mucinous cystic neoplasm of pancreas mimicking gastrointestinal stromal tumor of stomach. J Hepatobiliary Pancreat Surg. 2009;16:681–3.

33. Huang SC, Wu TH, Chen CC, Chen TC. Spontaneous rupture of solid pseudopapillary neoplasm of the pancreas during pregnancy. Obstet Gynecol. 2013;121:486–8.

3

The evidence based dilemma of intraperitoneal drainage for pancreatic resection – a systematic review and meta-analysis

Ulrich Nitsche[1], Tara C Müller[1], Christoph Späth[1], Lynne Cresswell[2], Dirk Wilhelm[1], Helmut Friess[1], Christoph W Michalski[3†] and Jörg Kleeff[1*†]

Abstract

Background: Routine placement of intraperitoneal drains has been shown to be ineffective or potentially harmful in various abdominal surgical procedures. Studies assessing risks and benefits of abdominal drains for pancreatic resections have demonstrated inconsistent results. We thus performed a systematic review of the literature and meta-analyzed outcomes of pancreatic resections with and without intraoperative placement of drains.

Methods: A database search according to the PRISMA guidelines was performed for studies on pancreatic resection with and without intraperitoneal drainage. The subgroup 'pancreaticoduodenectomy' was analyzed separately. The quality of studies was assessed using the MINORS and STROBE criteria. Pooled estimates of morbidity, mortality and length of hospital stay were calculated using random effects models.

Results: Only two randomized trials were identified. Their results were contradictory. We thus included six further, retrospective studies in the meta-analysis. However, with $I^2 = 68\%$ for any kind of complication, the estimate of inter-study heterogeneity was high. While overall morbidity after any kind of pancreatic resection was lower without drains ($p = 0.04$), there was no significant difference in mortality rates. In contrast, pooled estimates of outcomes after pancreaticoduodenectomy demonstrated no differences in morbidity ($p = 0.40$) but increased rates of intraabdominal abscesses ($p = 0.04$) and mortality ($p = 0.04$) without intraperitoneal drainage.

Conclusion: Although drains are associated with slightly increased morbidity for pancreatic resections, routine omission of drains cannot be advocated, especially after pancreaticoduodenectomy. While selective drainage seems reasonable, further efforts to generate more reliable data are questionable because of the current studies and the presumed small differences in outcomes.

Keywords: Pancreas, Pancreatic, Resection, Drainage, Drain, Intraperitoneal

Background

Intraperitoneal drains are frequently placed at the end of complex abdominal operations [1]. These drains were initially thought to enable the early identification of hemorrhage or anastomotic dehiscence, allowing timely re-operations. It has also been hypothesized that prophylactic intraperitoneal drainage can prevent additional

interventions for intraabdominal fluid collections [2]. However, many studies, including randomized controlled trials, systematic reviews and meta-analyses have shown that routine drainage after various general surgical procedures such as appendectomy, cholecystectomy, hepatectomy, colectomy and gastrectomy does not reduce the number of complications [1]. Some of these studies even found an increased risk of complications with drains [2,3]. This is thought to be a result of an artificial access to the peritoneal cavity, of an inflammatory response to the drain as a foreign body, and of increased pain

* Correspondence: kleeff@tum.de
†Equal contributors
[1]Department of Surgery, Klinikum rechts der Isar, Technische Universität München, Ismaninger Strasse 22, 81675 Munich, Germany
Full list of author information is available at the end of the article

due to the drain itself. Despite a high level of evidence favoring the omission of drains, clinical practice has only slowly changed [1].

The evidence for or against intraperitoneal drainage after pancreatic resection is much less clear. Here, drains are placed to detect hemorrhage in the immediate postoperative period, but are also frequently left in place for an extended period of time to allow for detection of leakage of the pancreatic anastomosis/pancreatic stump [2]. Though this concept has not been substantiated by reliable evidence, it is the standard of care all over the world. Interestingly, it had already been challenged in 1992, when Jeekel and co-authors published a series of 22 patients without intraperitoneal drainage [4]. Here, omission of drains was not associated with an increased rate of complications. In 1998, the first retrospective study from the Memorial Sloan Kettering Cancer Center (MSKCC) was published, comparing patients with intraperitoneal drainage to those without. There was "no statistical difference in the rate of fistula, abscess, CT drainage, or length of hospital stay" [5]. Because of these findings, the MSKCC group at that time designed and conducted a randomized controlled trial to generate better evidence. The results were published in the Annals of Surgery in 2001 [6]. 179 patients with pancreaticoduodenectomy or distal pancreatectomy had been randomized to the drain or no drain group. There was no significant difference in the number or type of complications between the groups. Thus, for the first time, level 1b evidence had shown that intraperitoneal drains may not be necessary after pancreatic resection. Several years later, the authors of this randomized study validated their promising initial results by another retrospective report on 1,122 patients of their institution. They again advocated the benefits of omitting drains [7]. However, the latter retrospective non-randomized analysis also revealed that the participating surgeons still decided to place a drain in roughly half of all pancreatic resections.

Subsequently, with only very few exceptions, several retrospective reports did not identify significant differences between drain and no drain groups regarding morbidity, pancreatic fistula, abscess, interventional radiology procedures, re-operation, length of hospital stay, or mortality [5,7-11]. These studies demonstrated that drains could probably be safely omitted after pancreatic resections. However, the available level of evidence was still not convincingly enough to change clinical practice. A main reason for this was that the prospective, randomized trial from the Memorial Sloan Kettering Cancer Center [6] had not reported complications (and particularly, leak rates) according to current standards – owing to the lack of such reporting standards at that time. This reasoning prompted the initiation of a multi-center, randomized trial whose results have recently been reported [12]. In this study,

137 patients with pancreaticoduodenectomy for benign or malignant pancreatic pathologies were randomized to placement or no placement of an intraperitoneal drain. The study was conducted at nine academic high-volume pancreas surgery centers in the United States. Randomization by demographics and clinical characteristics was performed thoroughly, minimizing the risk for any systematic bias. Unexpectedly, the group of patients without a drain had a higher complication rate, a higher complication severity, and most importantly, a higher mortality rate (12% versus 3%). The trial was thus prematurely terminated by the Institutional Review Board. These results were surprising [12,13], given that the trial has been multi-centric and all institutions had a vast experience in pancreatic surgery. In addition, a recent retrospective study published by one of the authors of the trial had demonstrated less complications and comparable mortality with omission of drains after pancreaticoduodenectomy and distal pancreatectomy [8].

Because of these recent publications, we sought to provide pooled estimates of the available literature to allow for a better interpretation of the current evidence.

Methods
Literature search
This meta-analysis was performed according to the PRISMA (Preferred Reporting Items for Systematic Reviews and Meta-Analyses) statement [14]. The literature screening was conducted by two independent researchers (U.N. and T.C.M.) in January 2014, without time or language restriction for all articles mentioning the phrases "pancreas" together with "resection" and "drain". No other limits were applied. Reviewed databases were Pubmed/Medline, Science direct, The Cochrane Central register of controlled trials/Cochrane Library, and EMBASE. Congress abstracts and personal communications were not considered in order to warrant a reproducible meta-analysis of sufficient quality. Articles were included when they reported clinical studies on human subjects with any kind of benign or malignant elective pancreatic resections. The studies needed to compare a group of patients with any kind of pancreatic resection and postoperative intraperitoneal drainage (control group) versus a group of patients with comparable pancreatic resections but no postoperative intraperitoneal drainage (intervention group). Studies reporting on enucleation or drainage for pancreatitis without resection were excluded. We included studies regardless of their design (prospective/retrospective, randomized controlled/non randomized controlled, cohort/case–control) and length of follow up. Identified studies were evaluated by title, abstract, or full reading until inclusion or exclusion criteria were met, respectively. In addition, references of included studies were screened.

Outcome variables

Eligible studies were evaluated regarding study design, patient population, underlying pancreatic diseases, surgical procedures, and time of recruitment, as reported in Table 1. The primary outcome was overall morbidity after pancreatic resection with or without an intraperitoneal drain. A subgroup analysis was performed for pancreaticoduodenectomy. Secondary outcomes that were not reported in all studies were rates of minor and major complications (according to the Clavien/Dindo classification system [15] grade I-II and III-V, respectively), pancreatic fistulas (according to the ISGPF classification system [16] grade B-C), intraabdominal abscesses, the need for interventional radiology procedures (insertion of drainage catheters), the need for re-operations, the length of hospital stay, and mortality (Table 2). To assess study quality and reporting bias, the MINORS [17] and STROBE [18] criteria were applied. Each study was evaluated for the 12 MINORS items with 0, 1, or 2 points, and for all 34 STROBE items with 0 or 1 point, respectively. The results of the MINORS as well as STROBE questions were added and reported in percentages to allow for a review of the individual study quality (Table 1). Zero percent depicts the worst possible study design and 100% depicts a perfectly conducted study. This meta-analysis was registered at the PROSPERO international prospective register of systematic reviews with the number CRD42014007497, as reported on www.crd.york.ac.uk/PROSPERO. Because all original data of this study has already been published in individual reports and no kind of research has been performed on living individuals, no ethics approval was requested at the institutional review board.

Statistical analysis

The dichotomous data on morbidity and mortality were analyzed in random effects meta-analyses by the Mantel-Haenszel method, using odds ratios (OR) and 95% confidence intervals (CI) as the effect measures. To estimate a pooled mean difference regarding the length of hospital stay using a random effects meta-analysis required the mean and standard deviation of length of stay for each group in each study. If the studies reported on median and interquartile range (Fisher et al. [8], Van Buren et al. [12]) or median and range (Paulus et al. [10], Adham et al. [9]), but not mean and standard deviation, it was estimated as suggested by the Cochrane Handbook for Systematic Reviews of Interventions [19]. Due to the applied approximations, the results regarding length of hospital stay should be interpreted with caution. Inter-study heterogeneity for the respective analyses is shown in the figures as I^2. Data are displayed in total numbers and are illustrated by Forest plots with p-values and 95% confidence intervals. Publication bias was assessed by a funnel plot. All statistical tests were performed two-sided, and p-values less than 0.05 were considered to be statistically significant. No correction of p-values was applied to adjust for multiple comparisons. However, results of all statistical tests conducted were thoroughly reported, so that an informal adjustment of p-values can be performed while reviewing the data [20]. No additional analyses other than the reported ones were performed. All analyses were performed using the software Revman 5.2.7 for Windows, available online for free at http://ims.cochrane.org/revman/download (downloaded January 04, 2014).

Results

Identified studies

Based on the search criteria, 4,682 articles were screened and assessed for eligibility. Of those, duplicates were omitted and 82 abstracts were reviewed in more detail. All abstracts were available either in English or were translated into English. Twenty one studies (all in English) required

Table 1 Characteristics, patient numbers, and quality of the eight studies that were included in this meta-analysis

Year	Author	Study design	Patients	Inclusion year (from - until)	Age (years)	Gender (men, women)	Disease (malignant, benign)	Type of resection (PD, distal, others)	Study quality	
									MINORS	STROBE
1998	Heslin [5]	Retrospective	89	1994 - 1996	65 (mean)	50, 39	78, 11	89, 0, 0	83%	58%
2001	Conlon [6]	Prospective randomized	179	n.s. - n.s.	65 (mean)	89, 90	176, 3	139, 40, 0	79%	77%
2011	Fisher [8]	Time cohort	226	2004 - 2010	62 (median)	97, 129	113, 113	153, 73, 0	60%	69%
2012	Paulus [10]	Retrospective	69	1997 - 2011	55 (median)	n.s., n.s.	52, 17	0, 69, 0	65%	55%
2013	Adham [9]	Retrospective	242	2005 - 2012	62 (median)	127, 115	180, 62	148, 66, 28	58%	66%
2013	Mehta [11]	Retrospective	709	2005 - 2012	62 (mean)	352, 357	451, 258	709, 0, 0	70%	69%
2013	Correa-Gallego [7]	Retrospective	1122	2006 - 2011	65 (mean)	548, 574	786, 336	739, 350, 33	50%	60%
2014	Van Buren [12]	Prospective randomized	137	2011 - 2012	63 (mean)	75, 62	95, 42	137, 0, 0	88%	90%

If not indicated otherwise, numbers of patients are stated. For the explanation of study quality according to MINORS and STROBE criteria, see in the text. n.s., not specified, PD, pancreaticoduodenectomy.

Table 2 Numbers of included patients, complication rates, intervention rates, length of hospital stay, and mortality for the drain and no drain group

Year	Author	All patients		Any complication		Minor complication		Major complication		Fistula (grade B/C)		Abscess		Rad. Intervention		Re-operation		Length of hospital stay (d, estimated mean ± SD)		Mortality	
		Drain	No drain	Drain	No drain	Drain	No drain	Drain	No drain	Drain	No drain	Drain	No drain	Drain	No drain	Drain	No drain	Drain	No drain	Drain	No drain
1998	Heslin [5]	51	38	23	15	13	9	14	8	3	1	3	0	2	1	1	3	12±7	12±6	n.s.	n.s.
2001	Conlon [6]	88	91	66	57	93*	83*	43**	39**	11	0	6	6	11	7	8	4	n.s.	n.s.	2	2
2011	Fisher [8]	179	47	117	22	171***	23***	38	7	21	5	10	2	4	5	8	0	7±2	7±1	1	1
2012	Paulus [10]	39	30	15	20	n.s.	n.s.	n.s.	n.s.	6	0	8	7	5	7	11	8	9±2.5	6.5±1	1	0
2013	Adham [9]	130	112	83	45	46	27	32	48	12	13	16	15	8	14	16	17	16.2±24	17.8±31	7	5
2013	Mehta [11]	251	458	171	248	n.s.	n.s.	62	75	41	35	n.s.	n.s.	21	29	14	26	n.s.	n.s.	5	11
2013	Correa-Gallego [7]	553	569	301	272	n.s.	n.s.	185	150	149	102	n.s.	n.s.	103****	83*****	3****	2*****	n.s.	n.s.	6****	12*****
2014	Van Buren [12]	68	69	50	55	n.s.	n.s.	21	28	8	14	8	18	6	16	2	6	7±2	8±5	2	8

These values were used for the meta-analysis. Consider the difficulty of comparing the length of hospital stay due to its varying specifications, as mentioned in the text. d, days, SD, standard deviation, n.s., not specified.

*Out of 176 (multiple mentions).
**Out of 82 (multiple mentions).
***Out of 194 (multiple mentions).
****Out of 540 (subgroup).
*****Out of 549 (subgroup).

full reading to decide on inclusion. The remaining 61 studies were excluded because the abstracts revealed that the inclusion criteria were not met. Subsequently, the reference lists of all reviewed articles were checked manually, which did not lead to the identification of additional studies. Figure 1 displays the flow diagram of the screening and inclusion process according to the PRISMA statement [14]. Eight studies met the full inclusion criteria and were included in the meta-analysis. Table 1 gives an overview of the included studies, patient numbers, time spans of recruitment, clinical data, and estimation of the methodological study quality according to MINORS [17] and STROBE [18] criteria. The methodological quality of all studies was at least 50% (of a maximal possible 100%), and

assessment regarding MINORS versus STROBE criteria did not show any relevant discrepancies for the individual studies (mean value MINORS: 69%, mean value STROBE: 68%; p = 0.80, paired t test). The smallest study [10] reported on 69 patients, while the largest study [7] reported on 1,122 patients. The two prospective randomized studies were from the years 2001 [6] (n = 179 patients) and 2014 [12] (n = 137 patients). The latter was the only multi-center study [12]; all other studies were single center reports. In total, 1,414 patients without drain were compared to 1,359 patients with drain. Three of all eight studies reported only on pancreaticoduodenectomy and were thus eligible for subgroup analysis [5,11,12]. Additionally, Correa-Gallego et al. [7] reported separately on

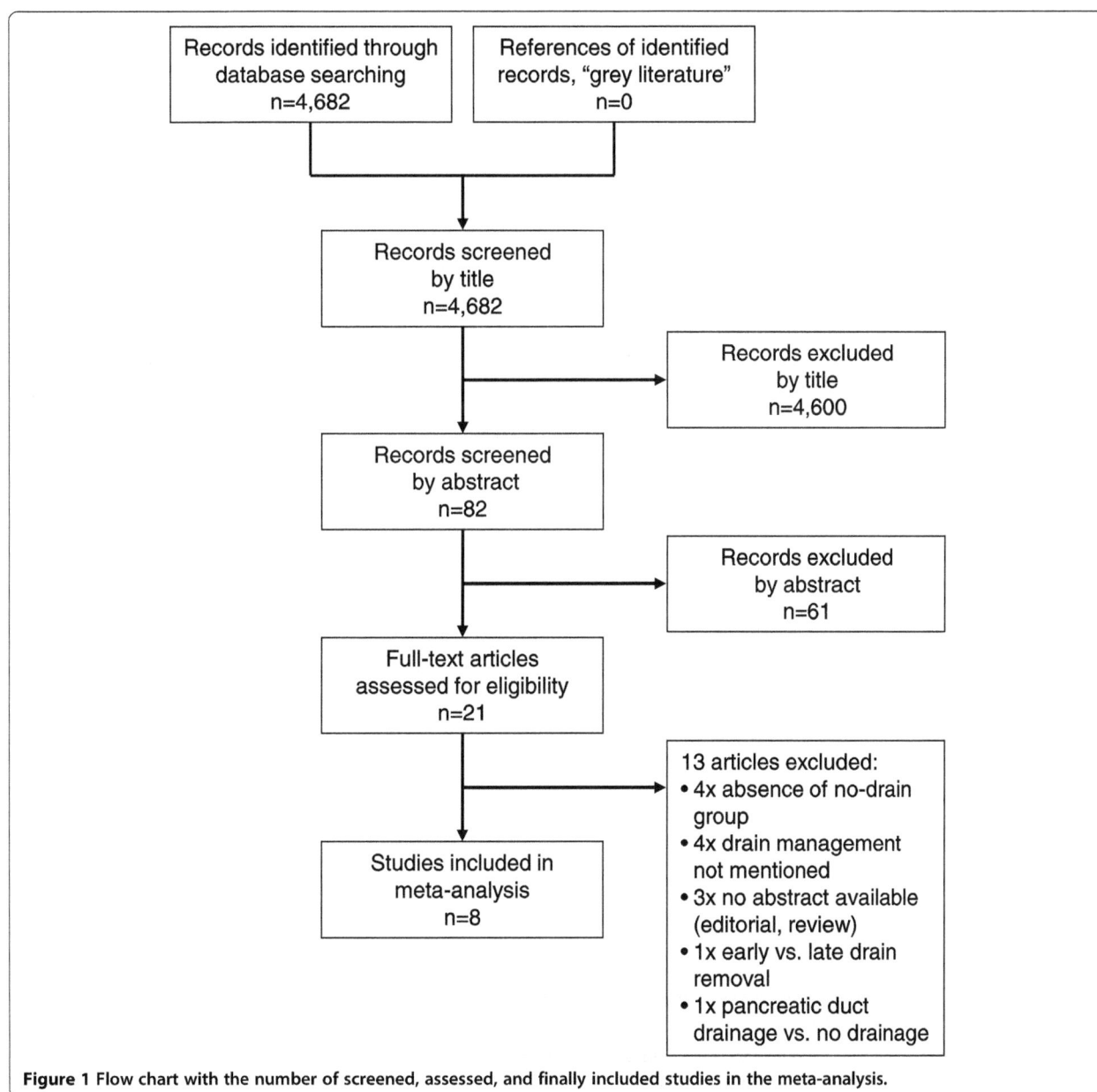

Figure 1 Flow chart with the number of screened, assessed, and finally included studies in the meta-analysis.

pancreaticoduodenectomy. Thus, finally four studies were included in the subgroup analysis, comparing 565 patients without drain to 370 patients with drain.

Drain versus no drain: any complication

Table 2 shows the numbers of patients for the parameters that were analyzed. All eight studies and all 2,773 patients were included for the comparison of any complication. A funnel plot for potential publication bias regarding the development of any complication after pancreatic resection with and without drain is shown in Figure 2 and does not provide evidence of publication bias. All studies except for two (including one randomized controlled trial) [10,12] revealed a lower morbidity in the no drain group. Overall heterogeneity was high with $I^2 = 68\%$. Patients without drain had significantly less complications (p = 0.04, OR 0.70, 95% CI 0.51 – 0.98, Figure 3). If only the two prospective randomized studies [6,12] were taken into account, this effect was not significant (p = 0.75, OR 0.86, 95% CI 0.35 – 2.14, graph not shown).

Drain versus no drain: specific complications

Not all studies reported on the number of patients with minor complications (grade I and II [15]), major complications (grade III – V [15]), pancreatic fistulas (grade B and C [16]), intraabdominal abscesses, the need for interventional radiology procedures, and the need for re-operations.

Pooled estimates showed no differences in rates of minor and major complications (p = 0.19 and p = 0.67, respectively), pancreatic fistula, intraabdominal abscess, the numbers of interventional radiology procedures, and re-operations (Figures 3, 4 and 5).

Drain versus no drain: length of hospital stay and mortality

The length of hospital stay was reported in all eight studies. However, the days of the hospital stay were reported as mean, median, or without any specification, making a robust comparison difficult. Using the estimations as described in the Methods section, there was no significant difference in the length of hospital stay. Postoperative mortality was reported in seven studies, with an observation period of up to three months. Pooled estimates of mortality rates did not show a significant difference (Figure 5).

Subgroup analysis: pancreaticoduodenectomy

Outcomes after pancreaticoduodenectomy were analyzed separately. Here, no differences were found for any complication (p = 0.40; Figure 6), minor complications (p = 0.85), major complications (p = 0.61), pancreatic fistula (p = 0.63), the need for interventional radiology procedures (p = 0.99), re-operation rates (p = 0.39), or the length of hospital stay (p = 0.16; data not shown). However, without drains the number of intraabdominal

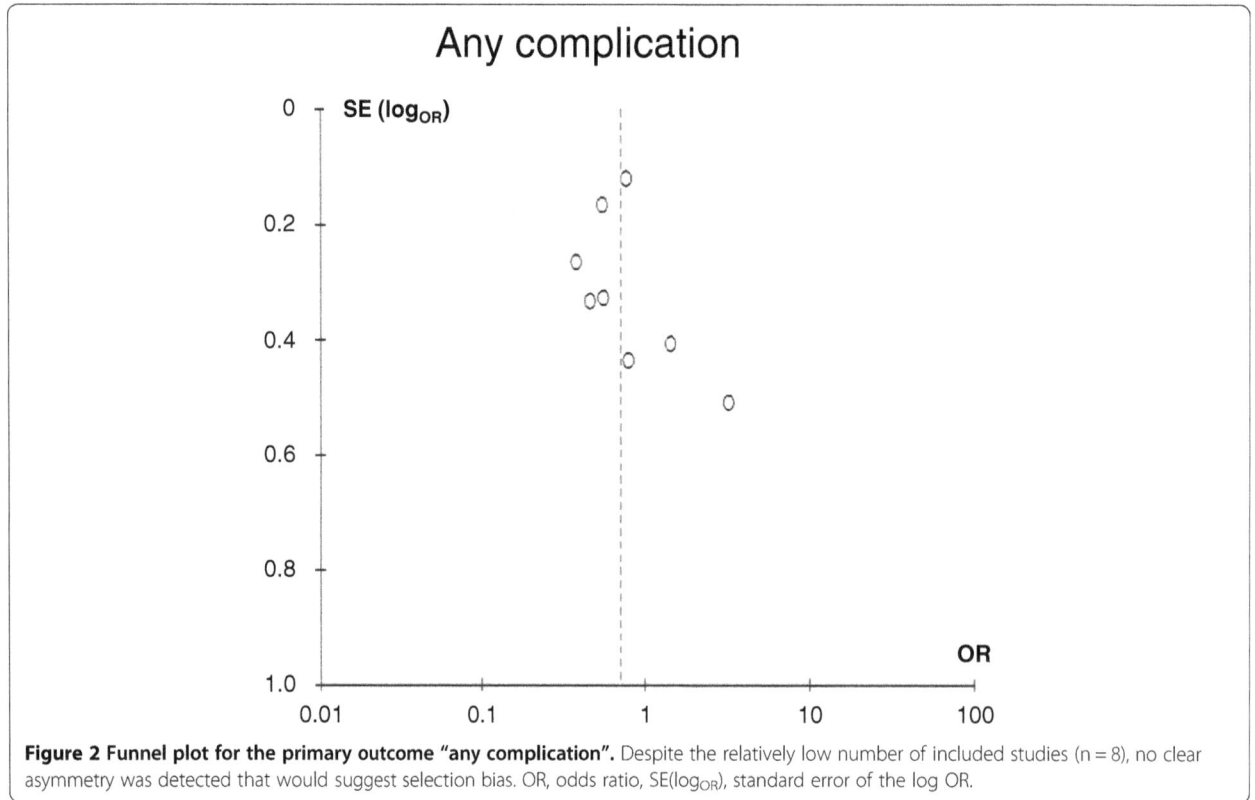

Figure 2 Funnel plot for the primary outcome "any complication". Despite the relatively low number of included studies (n = 8), no clear asymmetry was detected that would suggest selection bias. OR, odds ratio, SE(log$_{OR}$), standard error of the log OR.

Any complication

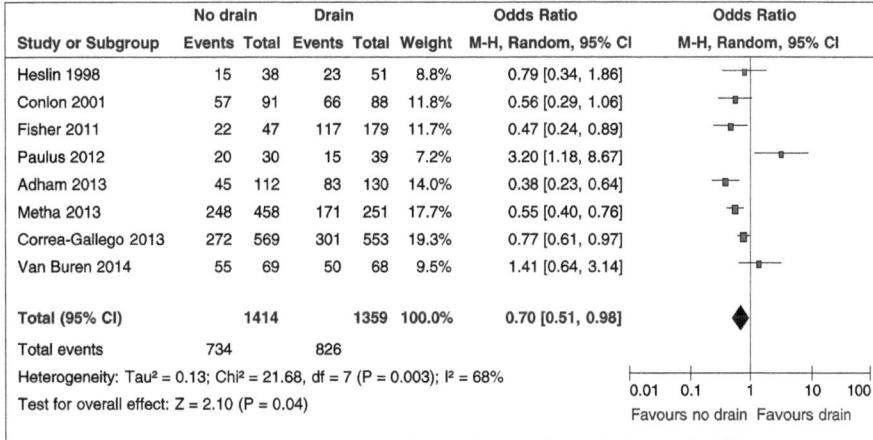

Study or Subgroup	No drain Events	No drain Total	Drain Events	Drain Total	Weight	Odds Ratio M-H, Random, 95% CI
Heslin 1998	15	38	23	51	8.8%	0.79 [0.34, 1.86]
Conlon 2001	57	91	66	88	11.8%	0.56 [0.29, 1.06]
Fisher 2011	22	47	117	179	11.7%	0.47 [0.24, 0.89]
Paulus 2012	20	30	15	39	7.2%	3.20 [1.18, 8.67]
Adham 2013	45	112	83	130	14.0%	0.38 [0.23, 0.64]
Metha 2013	248	458	171	251	17.7%	0.55 [0.40, 0.76]
Correa-Gallego 2013	272	569	301	553	19.3%	0.77 [0.61, 0.97]
Van Buren 2014	55	69	50	68	9.5%	1.41 [0.64, 3.14]
Total (95% CI)		1414		1359	100.0%	0.70 [0.51, 0.98]
Total events	734		826			

Heterogeneity: Tau² = 0.13; Chi² = 21.68, df = 7 (P = 0.003); I² = 68%
Test for overall effect: Z = 2.10 (P = 0.04)

Odds Ratio M-H, Random, 95% CI
0.01 0.1 1 10 100
Favours no drain Favours drain

Minor complication

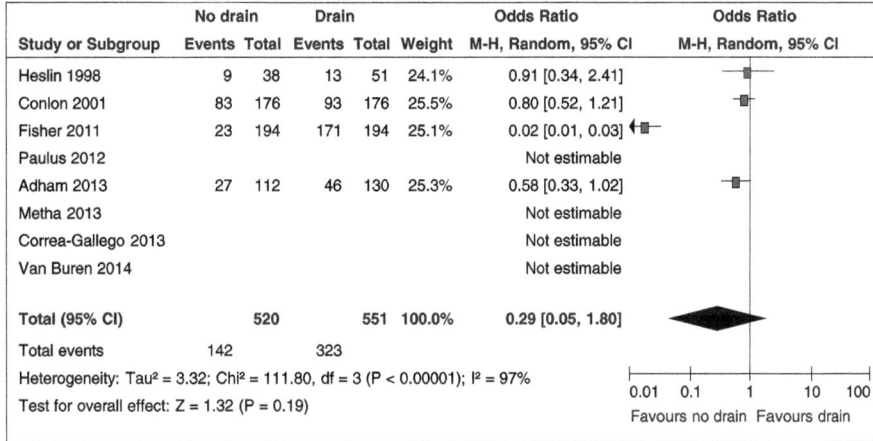

Study or Subgroup	No drain Events	No drain Total	Drain Events	Drain Total	Weight	Odds Ratio M-H, Random, 95% CI
Heslin 1998	9	38	13	51	24.1%	0.91 [0.34, 2.41]
Conlon 2001	83	176	93	176	25.5%	0.80 [0.52, 1.21]
Fisher 2011	23	194	171	194	25.1%	0.02 [0.01, 0.03]
Paulus 2012						Not estimable
Adham 2013	27	112	46	130	25.3%	0.58 [0.33, 1.02]
Metha 2013						Not estimable
Correa-Gallego 2013						Not estimable
Van Buren 2014						Not estimable
Total (95% CI)		520		551	100.0%	0.29 [0.05, 1.80]
Total events	142		323			

Heterogeneity: Tau² = 3.32; Chi² = 111.80, df = 3 (P < 0.00001); I² = 97%
Test for overall effect: Z = 1.32 (P = 0.19)

Odds Ratio M-H, Random, 95% CI
0.01 0.1 1 10 100
Favours no drain Favours drain

Major complication

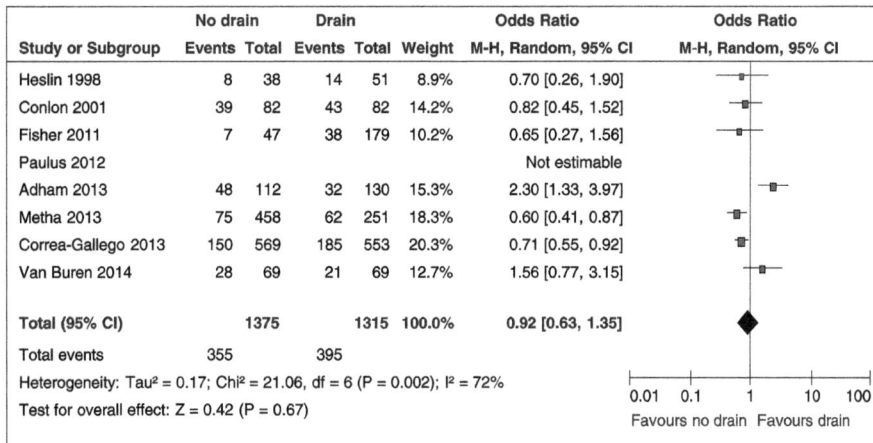

Study or Subgroup	No drain Events	No drain Total	Drain Events	Drain Total	Weight	Odds Ratio M-H, Random, 95% CI
Heslin 1998	8	38	14	51	8.9%	0.70 [0.26, 1.90]
Conlon 2001	39	82	43	82	14.2%	0.82 [0.45, 1.52]
Fisher 2011	7	47	38	179	10.2%	0.65 [0.27, 1.56]
Paulus 2012						Not estimable
Adham 2013	48	112	32	130	15.3%	2.30 [1.33, 3.97]
Metha 2013	75	458	62	251	18.3%	0.60 [0.41, 0.87]
Correa-Gallego 2013	150	569	185	553	20.3%	0.71 [0.55, 0.92]
Van Buren 2014	28	69	21	69	12.7%	1.56 [0.77, 3.15]
Total (95% CI)		1375		1315	100.0%	0.92 [0.63, 1.35]
Total events	355		395			

Heterogeneity: Tau² = 0.17; Chi² = 21.06, df = 6 (P = 0.002); I² = 72%
Test for overall effect: Z = 0.42 (P = 0.67)

Odds Ratio M-H, Random, 95% CI
0.01 0.1 1 10 100
Favours no drain Favours drain

Figure 3 Forrest plots for risk of any complication, minor and major complications for patients after all kinds of pancreatic resection, with and without intraperitoneal drain. The overall effect is shown by the diamond, with level of significance (p-value), 95% confidence intervals (CIs), and diversity between studies (Heterogeneity, I²).

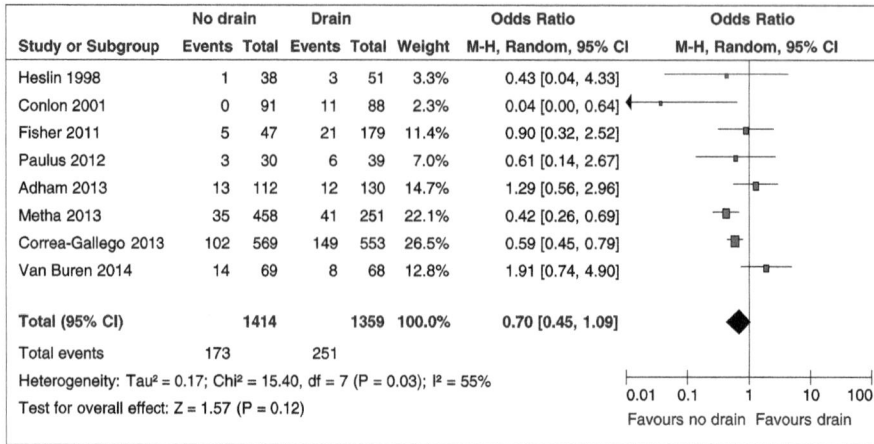

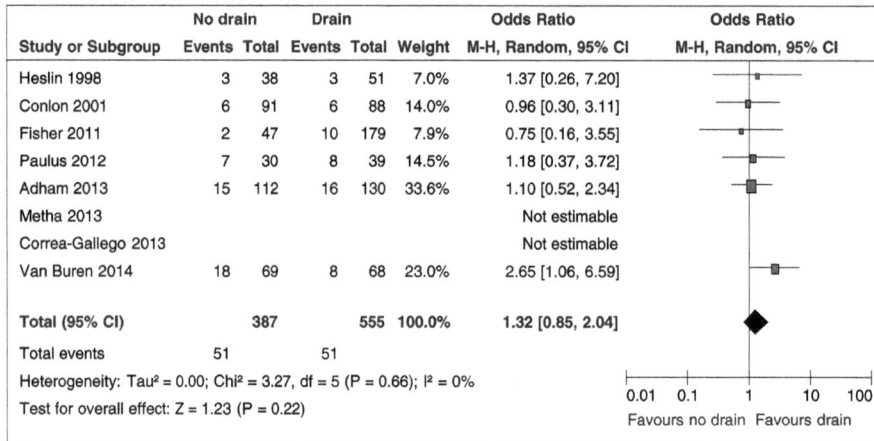

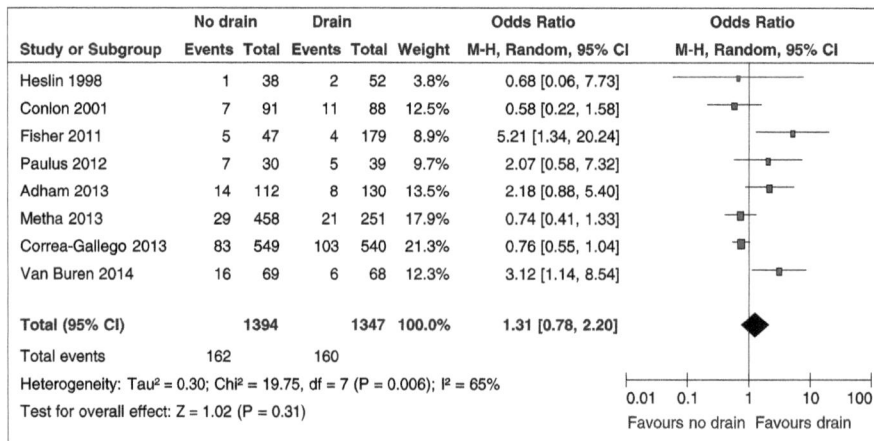

Figure 4 Forrest plots for risk of fistula, abscess, and interventional radiology procedures for patients after all kinds of pancreatic resection, with and without intraperitoneal drain. The overall effect is shown by the diamond, with level of significance (p-value), 95% confidence intervals (CIs), and diversity between studies (Heterogeneity, I²).

Re-operation

Study or Subgroup	No drain Events	No drain Total	Drain Events	Drain Total	Weight	Odds Ratio M-H, Random, 95% CI
Heslin 1998	3	38	1	51	2.8%	4.29 [0.43, 42.92]
Conlon 2001	4	91	8	88	9.9%	0.46 [0.13, 1.59]
Fisher 2011	0	47	8	179	1.8%	0.21 [0.01, 3.75]
Paulus 2012	8	30	11	39	13.3%	0.93 [0.32, 2.69]
Adham 2013	17	112	16	130	28.0%	1.27 [0.61, 2.66]
Metha 2013	26	458	14	251	33.8%	1.02 [0.52, 1.99]
Correa-Gallego 2013	2	549	3	540	4.7%	0.65 [0.11, 3.93]
Van Buren 2014	6	69	2	68	5.6%	3.14 [0.61, 16.16]
Total (95% CI)		**1394**		**1346**	**100.0%**	**1.05 [0.71, 1.54]**
Total events	66		63			

Heterogeneity: Tau² = 0.00; Chi² = 6.65, df = 7 (P = 0.47); I² = 0%
Test for overall effect: Z = 0.23 (P = 0.82)

Favours no drain Favours drain

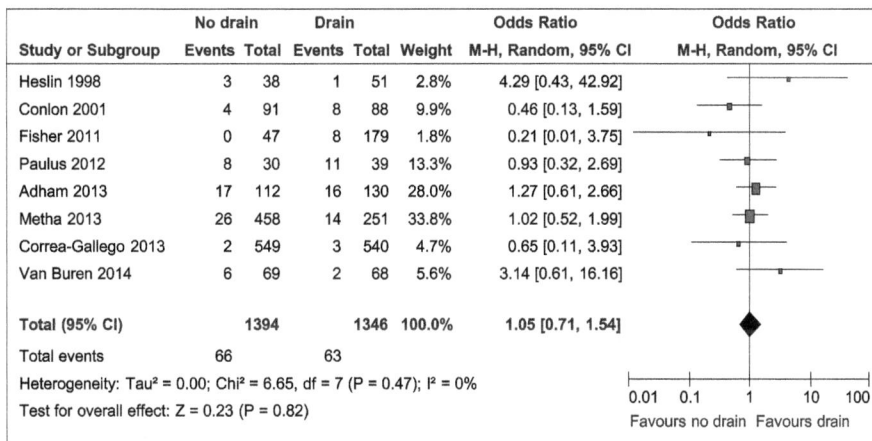

Length of hospital stay

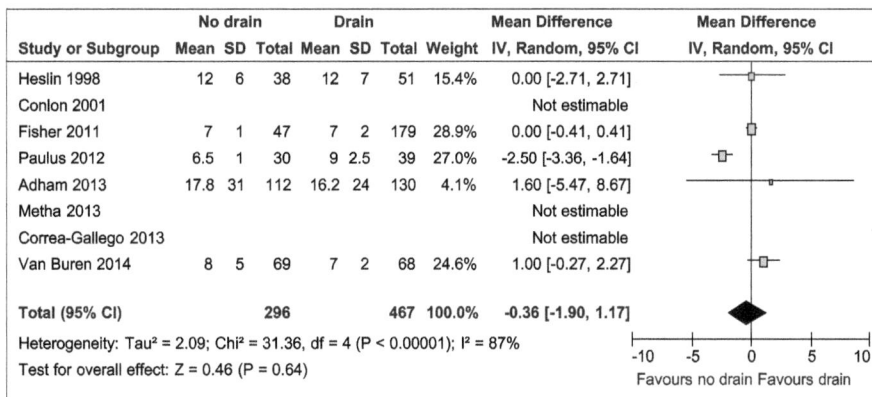

Study or Subgroup	No drain Mean	SD	Total	Drain Mean	SD	Total	Weight	Mean Difference IV, Random, 95% CI
Heslin 1998	12	6	38	12	7	51	15.4%	0.00 [-2.71, 2.71]
Conlon 2001								Not estimable
Fisher 2011	7	1	47	7	2	179	28.9%	0.00 [-0.41, 0.41]
Paulus 2012	6.5	1	30	9	2.5	39	27.0%	-2.50 [-3.36, -1.64]
Adham 2013	17.8	31	112	16.2	24	130	4.1%	1.60 [-5.47, 8.67]
Metha 2013								Not estimable
Correa-Gallego 2013								Not estimable
Van Buren 2014	8	5	69	7	2	68	24.6%	1.00 [-0.27, 2.27]
Total (95% CI)			**296**			**467**	**100.0%**	**-0.36 [-1.90, 1.17]**

Heterogeneity: Tau² = 2.09; Chi² = 31.36, df = 4 (P < 0.00001); I² = 87%
Test for overall effect: Z = 0.46 (P = 0.64)

Favours no drain Favours drain

Mortality

Study or Subgroup	No drain Events	No drain Total	Drain Events	Drain Total	Weight	Odds Ratio M-H, Random, 95% CI
Heslin 1998						Not estimable
Conlon 2001	2	91	2	88	7.3%	0.97 [0.13, 7.01]
Fisher 2011	1	47	1	179	3.7%	3.87 [0.24, 63.04]
Paulus 2012	0	30	1	39	2.7%	0.42 [0.02, 10.70]
Adham 2013	5	112	7	130	20.6%	0.82 [0.25, 2.66]
Metha 2013	11	458	5	251	25.0%	1.21 [0.42, 3.52]
Correa-Gallego 2013	12	549	6	540	29.3%	1.99 [0.74, 5.34]
Van Buren 2014	8	69	2	68	11.3%	4.33 [0.88, 21.18]
Total (95% CI)		**1356**		**1295**	**100.0%**	**1.49 [0.87, 2.54]**
Total events	39		24			

Heterogeneity: Tau² = 0.00; Chi² = 4.41, df = 6 (P = 0.62); I² = 0%
Test for overall effect: Z = 1.46 (P = 0.14)

Favours no drain Favours drain

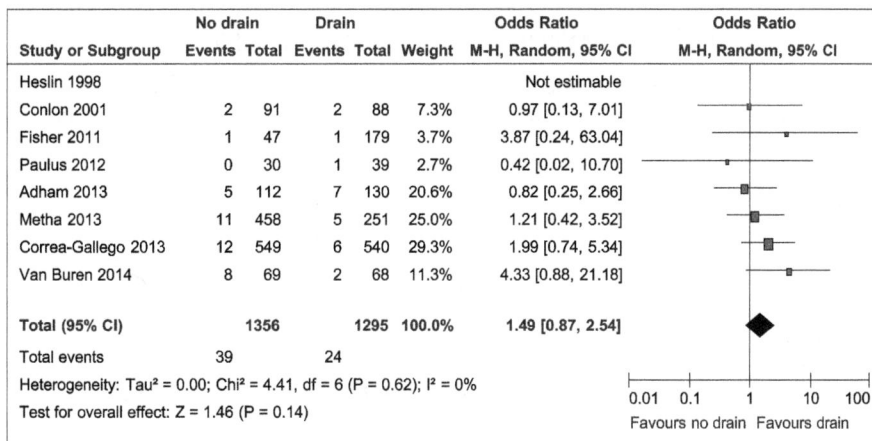

Figure 5 Forrest plots for risk of re-operation and mortality, and difference in the length of hospital stay for patients after all kinds of pancreatic resection, with and without intraperitoneal drain. The overall effect is shown by the diamond, with level of significance (p-value), 95% confidence intervals (CIs), and diversity between studies (Heterogeneity, I²).

Any complication (pancreaticoduodenectomy)

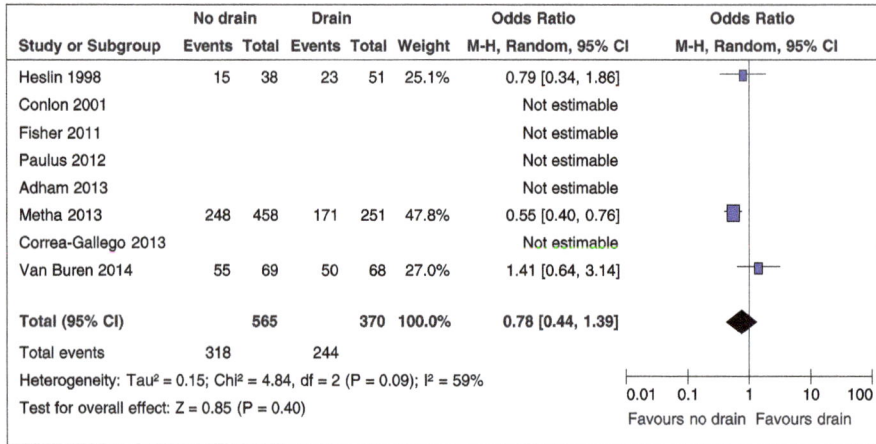

Study or Subgroup	No drain Events	Total	Drain Events	Total	Weight	Odds Ratio M-H, Random, 95% CI
Heslin 1998	15	38	23	51	25.1%	0.79 [0.34, 1.86]
Conlon 2001						Not estimable
Fisher 2011						Not estimable
Paulus 2012						Not estimable
Adham 2013						Not estimable
Metha 2013	248	458	171	251	47.8%	0.55 [0.40, 0.76]
Correa-Gallego 2013						Not estimable
Van Buren 2014	55	69	50	68	27.0%	1.41 [0.64, 3.14]
Total (95% CI)		565		370	100.0%	0.78 [0.44, 1.39]
Total events	318		244			

Heterogeneity: Tau² = 0.15; Chi² = 4.84, df = 2 (P = 0.09); I² = 59%
Test for overall effect: Z = 0.85 (P = 0.40)

0.01 0.1 1 10 100
Favours no drain Favours drain

Abscess (pancreaticoduodenectomy)

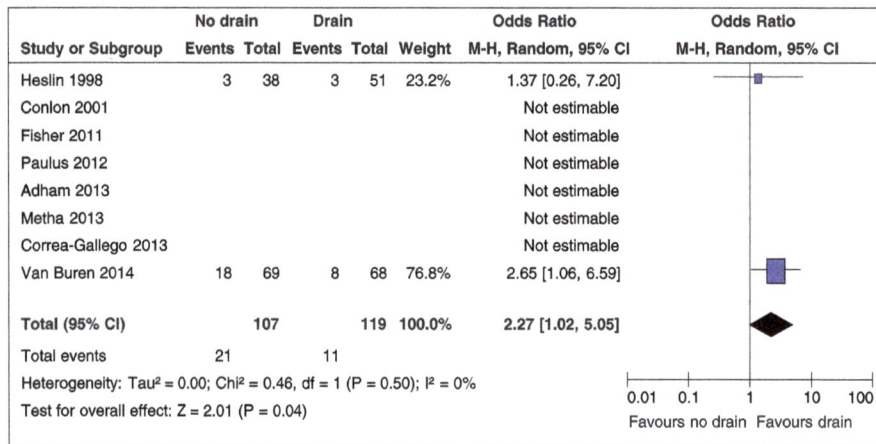

Study or Subgroup	No drain Events	Total	Drain Events	Total	Weight	Odds Ratio M-H, Random, 95% CI
Heslin 1998	3	38	3	51	23.2%	1.37 [0.26, 7.20]
Conlon 2001						Not estimable
Fisher 2011						Not estimable
Paulus 2012						Not estimable
Adham 2013						Not estimable
Metha 2013						Not estimable
Correa-Gallego 2013						Not estimable
Van Buren 2014	18	69	8	68	76.8%	2.65 [1.06, 6.59]
Total (95% CI)		107		119	100.0%	2.27 [1.02, 5.05]
Total events	21		11			

Heterogeneity: Tau² = 0.00; Chi² = 0.46, df = 1 (P = 0.50); I² = 0%
Test for overall effect: Z = 2.01 (P = 0.04)

0.01 0.1 1 10 100
Favours no drain Favours drain

Mortality (pancreaticoduodenectomy)

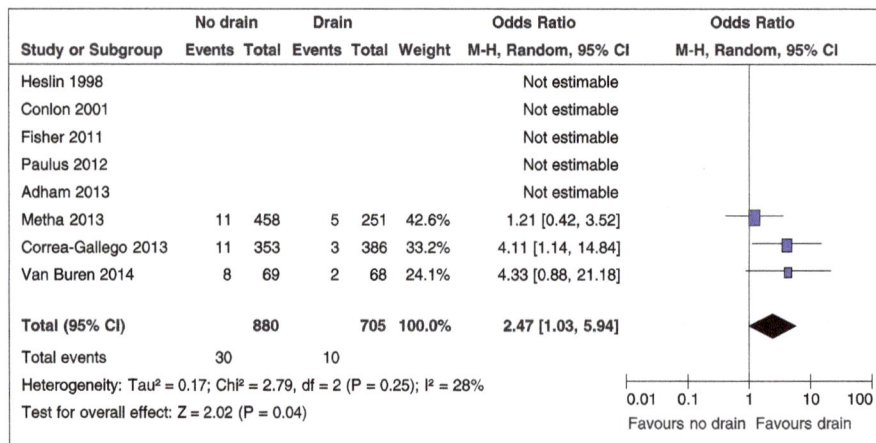

Study or Subgroup	No drain Events	Total	Drain Events	Total	Weight	Odds Ratio M-H, Random, 95% CI
Heslin 1998						Not estimable
Conlon 2001						Not estimable
Fisher 2011						Not estimable
Paulus 2012						Not estimable
Adham 2013						Not estimable
Metha 2013	11	458	5	251	42.6%	1.21 [0.42, 3.52]
Correa-Gallego 2013	11	353	3	386	33.2%	4.11 [1.14, 14.84]
Van Buren 2014	8	69	2	68	24.1%	4.33 [0.88, 21.18]
Total (95% CI)		880		705	100.0%	2.47 [1.03, 5.94]
Total events	30		10			

Heterogeneity: Tau² = 0.17; Chi² = 2.79, df = 2 (P = 0.25); I² = 28%
Test for overall effect: Z = 2.02 (P = 0.04)

0.01 0.1 1 10 100
Favours no drain Favours drain

Figure 6 Forrest plots for risk of any complication, abscess, and mortality for patients after pancreaticoduodenectomy, with and without intraperitoneal drain. The overall effect is shown by the diamond, with level of significance (p-value), 95% confidence intervals (CIs), and diversity between studies (Heterogeneity, I²).

abscesses was significantly increased (p = 0.04, OR 2.27, 95% CI 1.02 – 5.05; Figure 6) and mortality was considerably higher (p = 0.04, OR 2.47, 95% CI 1.03 – 5.94; Figure 6).

Discussion

In this meta-analysis, prophylactic intraperitoneal drainage after pancreatic resection increased the risk of complications, but not the rate of mortality. Pooled estimates of outcomes in the subgroup 'pancreaticoduodenectomy' demonstrated different results. Here, the rate of complications was comparable with or without a drain; however, mortality was increased by omission of intraperitoneal drains.

It could be argued that drains following pancreatic resection (as in other abdominal operations) are associated with an, albeit small 1.4-fold (OR 1.43, 95% CI 1.02 – 1.96), increased risk of morbidity without significantly influencing mortality. In the case of pancreaticoduodenectomy, leakage/dehiscence of the pancreatic-intestinal anastomosis is a potentially dreadful complication significantly contributing to the overall mortality following this procedure. From the clinical experience as well as from the data of the included studies, it is possible to conceive that a drain could help to detect a leak earlier and to drain this potentially hazardous fluid (leading to haemorrhage etc.) earlier and more efficiently than an interventional placed drain. Thus, omission of a routine drain following pancreaticoduodenectomy results in a 2.5-fold (OR 2.47, 95% CI 1.03 – 5.94) increased risk of mortality.

These conclusions are supported by the eight included studies, making this meta-analysis the most comprehensive so far. Despite the proper methodological quality of all includes trials, this study has limitations. Because of the different surgical approaches, we performed a subgroup analysis for pancreaticoduodenectomy. In general, there are few studies available investigating the use of drains for pancreatic resections, and only two prospective randomized trials exist. Especially in consideration of the results of the most recent prospective multicenter trial [12], future randomized studies may be ethically difficult to conduct.

The latter trial by Van Buren et al. [12] was stopped preliminary due to the unexpectedly high rate of mortality after pancreaticoduodenectomy in the no drain group. Unfortunately, the reasons for this outcome remain unclear, especially since it was highly contradictory to prior studies. A thorough analysis of the potential factors contributing to these results is beyond the scope of this review. However, it has to be acknowledged that this was the first multicenter study with a well-planned study protocol and the participation of only highly experienced centers. Certainly, the results cannot be explained by the multicentric character, flaws in the study protocol or the lack of experience in the participating centers. As such, the data of the trial by Van Buren et al. have to be taken as high quality evidence.

Recently, a meta-analysis by Rondelli et al. was published, which also meta-analyzed the results of intraperitoneal drainage after pancreatic resection [21]. In contrast to our meta-analysis, the results of the study by Paulus et al. [10] were not included. Comparable to our results, intraperitoneal drainage was identified to be associated with an increase in the total post-operative complication rate (OR 1.52, 95% CI 1.30 – 1.78), and mortality did not differ significantly between the drain/no drain group. Rondelli et al. also performed a subgroup analysis for pancreaticoduodenectomy. As for our analysis, four studies were eligible and the authors found no difference in mortality when analyzing the available randomized study, or the remaining retrospective studies separately. However, when analyzing all studies on pancreaticoduodenectomy together, there was still no significant difference identified in the mentioned meta-analysis, which is in contrast to our results.

Conclusion

Taking together the data for all pancreatic resections and the subgroup analysis, intraperitoneal drains seem not to be harmful, but may not be beneficial in general either. This would argue for a concept of selective abdominal drain application with placement of a prophylactic drain according to patient factors (e.g. comorbidity, perioperative risk, anticoagulation), pancreatic texture (e.g., small pancreatic duct, soft tissue), surgeon (level of experience, type of operation), and setting (e.g., missing 24/7 availability of interventional radiology procedures) [13]. However, mortality is increased if drains are omitted after pancreaticoduodenectomy. Though this result is driven by the inclusion of the most recent randomized trial into this meta-analysis, it should certainly be taken seriously. Thus, it is very difficult to argue for an omission of drains after a pancreaticoduodenectomy – even under circumstances where anastomotic complications are unlikely. With a reduction of morbidity after any kind of pancreatic resection however, omission of drains after distal pancreatectomy may truly be an option. The results of a currently ongoing randomized trial on distal pancreatectomy are eagerly awaited.

Competing interests
The authors declare that they have no competing interests.

Authors' contributions
UN carried out the review of the literature, participated in performing the meta-analysis and drafted the first version of the manuscript. TCM carried out the independent review of the literature. CS collected data and drafted the manuscript. LC performed and validated the statistical analyses. DW participated in the design of the study and drafted the manuscript. HF

interpreted and reviewed the data. CWM made the study concept and drafted the manuscript. JK planned the study, coordinated the drafting of the manuscript, and edited the manuscript. All authors read and approved the final manuscript.

Author details
[1]Department of Surgery, Klinikum rechts der Isar, Technische Universität München, Ismaninger Strasse 22, 81675 Munich, Germany. [2]Institute of Medical Statistics and Epidemiology, Klinikum rechts der Isar, Technische Universität München, Munich, Germany. [3]Division of Surgical Oncology, Department of Surgery, Oregon Health and Science University, Portland, OR, USA.

1. Buchler MW, Friess H: Evidence forward, drainage on retreat. still we ignore and drain!? Ann Surg 2006, 244(1):8–9.
References
2. van der Wilt AA, Coolsen MM, de Hingh IH, van der Wilt GJ, Groenewoud H, Dejong CH, van Dam RM: To drain or not to drain: a cumulative meta-analysis of the use of routine abdominal drains after pancreatic resection. HPB 2013, 15(5):337–344.
3. Kaminsky PM, Mezhir JJ: Intraperitoneal drainage after pancreatic resection: a review of the evidence. J Surg Res 2013, 184(2):925–930.
4. Jeekel J: No abdominal drainage after Whipple's procedure. Br J Surg 1992, 79(2):182.
5. Heslin MJ, Harrison LE, Brooks AD, Hochwald SN, Coit DG, Brennan MF: Is intra-abdominal drainage necessary after pancreaticoduodenectomy? J Gastrointest Surg 1998, 2(4):373–378.
6. Conlon KC, Labow D, Leung D, Smith A, Jarnagin W, Coit DG, Merchant N, Brennan MF: Prospective randomized clinical trial of the value of intraperitoneal drainage after pancreatic resection. Ann Surg 2001, 234(4):487–493. discussion 493–484.
7. Correa-Gallego C, Brennan MF, D'Angelica M, Fong Y, Dematteo RP, Kingham TP, Jarnagin WR, Allen PJ: Operative drainage following pancreatic resection: analysis of 1122 patients resected over 5 years at a single institution. Ann Surg 2013, 258(6):1051–1058.
8. Fisher WE, Hodges SE, Silberfein EJ, Artinyan A, Ahern CH, Jo E, Brunicardi FC: Pancreatic resection without routine intraperitoneal drainage. HPB 2011, 13(7):503–510.
9. Adham M, Chopin-Laly X, Lepilliez V, Gincul R, Valette PJ, Ponchon T: Pancreatic resection: drain or no drain? Surgery 2013, 154(5):1069–1077.
10. Paulus EM, Zarzaur BL, Behrman SW: Routine peritoneal drainage of the surgical bed after elective distal pancreatectomy: is it necessary? Am J Surg 2012, 204(4):422–427.
11. Mehta VV, Fisher SB, Maithel SK, Sarmiento JM, Staley CA, Kooby DA: Is it time to abandon routine operative drain use? A single institution assessment of 709 consecutive pancreaticoduodenectomies. J Am Coll Surg 2013, 216(4):635–642. discussion 642–634.
12. Van Buren G 2nd, Bloomston M, Hughes SJ, Winter J, Behrman SW, Zyromski NJ, Vollmer C, Velanovich V, Riall T, Muscarella P, Trevino J, Nakeeb A, Schmidt CM, Behrns K, Ellison EC, Barakat O, Perry KA, Drebin J, House M, Abdel-Misih S, Silberfein EJ, Goldin S, Brown K, Mohammed S, Hodges SE, McElhany A, Issazadeh M, Jo E, Mo Q, Fisher WE: A Randomized Prospective Multicenter Trial of Pancreaticoduodenectomy With and Without Routine Intraperitoneal Drainage. Ann Surg 2014, 259(4):605–612.
13. Strobel O, Buchler MW: Drainage after pancreaticoduodenectomy: controversy revitalized. Ann Surg 2014, 259(4):613–615.
14. Liberati A, Altman DG, Tetzlaff J, Mulrow C, Gotzsche PC, Ioannidis JP, Clarke M, Devereaux PJ, Kleijnen J, Moher D: The PRISMA statement for reporting systematic reviews and meta-analyses of studies that evaluate health care interventions: explanation and elaboration. PLoS Med 2009, 6(7):e1000100.
15. Dindo D, Demartines N, Clavien PA: Classification of surgical complications: a new proposal with evaluation in a cohort of 6336 patients and results of a survey. Ann Surg 2004, 240(2):205–213.
16. Bassi C, Dervenis C, Butturini G, Fingerhut A, Yeo C, Izbicki J, Neoptolemos J, Sarr M, Traverso W, Buchler M: Postoperative pancreatic fistula: an international study group (ISGPF) definition. Surgery 2005, 138(1):8–13.
17. Slim K, Nini E, Forestier D, Kwiatkowski F, Panis Y, Chipponi J: Methodological index for non-randomized studies (minors): development and validation of a new instrument. ANZ J Surg 2003, 73(9):712–716.
18. Vandenbroucke JP, von Elm E, Altman DG, Gotzsche PC, Mulrow CD, Pocock SJ, Poole C, Schlesselman JJ, Egger M: Strengthening the reporting of observational studies in epidemiology (STROBE): explanation and elaboration. PLoS Med 2007, 4(10):e297.
19. Higgins JPT, Green S: Cochrane Handbook for Systematic Reviews of Interventions Version 5.1.0 [updated March 2011]. The Cochrane Collaboration. 2011. Available from www.cochrane-handbook.org.
20. Saville DJ: Multiple comparison procedures - the practical solution. Am Stat 1990, 44(2):174–180.
21. Rondelli F, Desio M, Vedovati MC, Balzarotti Canger RC, Sanguinetti A, Avenia N, Bugiantella W: Intra-abdominal drainage after pancreatic resection: is it really necessary? A meta-analysis of short-term outcomes. Int J Surg 2014, 12(Supplement 1):S40–S47.

4

Neuroendocrine tumors of the pancreas: a retrospective single-center analysis using the ENETS TNM-classification and immunohistochemical markers for risk stratification

Stefan M Brunner[1*], Florian Weber[2], Jens M Werner[1], Ayman Agha[1], Stefan A Farkas[1], Hans J Schlitt[1] and Matthias Hornung[1]

Abstract

Background: This study was performed to assess the 2006 introduced ENETS TNM-classification with respect to patient survival and surgical approach for patients who underwent surgery for a neuroendocrine tumor of the pancreas (PNET).

Methods: Between 2001 and 2010 38 patients after resection of a PNET were investigated regarding tumor localization and size. Further, patient survival with regards to the new TNM-classification, the operation methods and immunohistochemical markers was analyzed.

Results: The estimated mean survival time of the 38 patients was 91 ± 10 months (female 116 ± 9, male 56 ± 14 months; $p = 0.008$). The 5-year survival rate was 63.9%. Patient survival differed significantly depending on tumor size (pT1 107 ± 13, pT2 94 ± 16, pT3 44 ± 7 and pT4 18 ± 14 months; $P = 0.006$). Patients without lymph node metastasis survived significantly longer compared to patients with positive lymph node status (108 ± 9 vs. 19 ± 5 months; $P < 0.001$). However, survival in patients with and without distant metastasis did not differ significantly (92 ± 11 vs. 80 ± 23 months; $P = 0.876$). Further, the tumor grading significantly influenced patient survival (G1 111 ± 12, G2 68 ± 12 and G3 21 ± 14 months; $P = 0.037$).

Conclusions: As part of the TNM-classification especially lymph node status and also tumor size and grading were identified as important factors determining patient survival. Further, gender was demonstrated to significantly influence survival time. If an R0 resection was achieved in patients with distant metastases patient survival was comparable to patients without metastasis.

Keywords: Neuroendocrine Tumors Of The Pancreas, Tnm Classification, Risk Stratification, Lymph Node Metastasis, E-Cadherin, B-Catenin, Cyclin D1, Il-17a

* Correspondence: stefan.brunner@ukr.de
[1]Department of Surgery, University Medical Center Regensburg,
Franz-Josef-Strauss-Allee 11, 93053 Regensburg, Germany
Full list of author information is available at the end of the article

Background

Neuroendocrine tumors represent a heterogenous group of neoplasms regarding biological features and clinical behavior [1-3]. These tumors are rare with an incidence between 3.24 and 6.5 per 100,000 [4]. However, over the last years there has been a remarkable increase in frequency with predominant localization of the neuroendocrine tumors in the gastrointestinal tract or the bronchopulmonary system [4]. Approximately 5% of all neuroendocrine tumors develop in the pancreas with one of the poorest outcomes (35% 5-year survival rate) [3,5-8]. The WHO classification published in 2000 and modified by Kloeppel at al. in 2004 distinguishes between well-differentiated neuroendocrine tumors, well-differentiated neuroendocrine carcinomas and poorly-differentiated neuroendocrine carcinomas [7]. Because of the wide variety in clinical behavior between these tumor entities, a tailored surgical and medical therapy based on this classification was challenging [9]. A new TNM classification with a grading system based on the mitotic count and the Ki-67 index was established by the European Neuroendocrine Tumor Society (ENETS) to address this problem in 2006. In this system PNETs with a size <2 cm are classified as T1, with a size from 2–4 cm as T2, with >4 cm or invasion of duodenum or bile duct as T3, and all tumors invading adjacent organs or the wall of large vessels as T4 [10]. The status of regional lymph nodes and distant metastasis were taken into account analogously to the TNM classification system of other tumors in combination with a grading system according to mitotic count and the Ki-67-index. Based on these criteria, a risk stratification of patients using different disease stages was proposed. Stage I includes pT1 tumors, stage IIa pT2 tumors, stage IIb pT3 tumors and stage IIIa pT4 tumors all without lymph node or distant metastasis. Tumors of any pT stage with lymph node metastasis are classified in stage IIIb and all tumors with distant metastasis are characterized as stage IV [10]. In 2010 the UICC/AJCC/WHO 2010 TNM staging system was introduced which differs significantly from the 2006 ENETS TNM staging. Due to the fact that Rindi et al. demonstrated that the 2006 ENETS TNM staging system is superior to the UICC/AJCC/WHO 2010 TNM staging system we decided to use the 2006 ENETS TNM staging for our study [11]. Since the 2006 ENETS TNM classification is based on the published experience of single centers and not on a uniform database, the purpose of this study was to analyze neuroendocrine tumors of the pancreas that were resected in our center with regards to clinicopathological characteristics that influence patient survival. Further, we wanted to assess the new 2006 ENETS TNM classification system and its prognostic value for long-term survival.

Additionally to Ki-67 that as marker for proliferation is included in the TNM classification systems it has been shown previously that pancreatic endocrine neoplasms and adenocarcinoma of the pancreas express E-cadherin and β-catenin, both being important for cell-cell contact, and that cyclin D1 and IL-17A contribute to malignant transformation in pancreatic tumors [12-17]. In our study we tested if different expression levels of these markers influence patient survival.

Methods

Study setting

The study was performed at the University Medical Center of Regensburg, Germany in the Department of Surgery in compliance with the Helsinki Declaration and was approved by the ethics committee of the University Medical Center Regensburg, Germany (Nr. 13-180-0248).

Study cohort

Patients with PNETs confirmed by histology who underwent surgery at our center between 2001 and 2010 were identified using the hospital computer data base (access available with permission of the University Medical Center Regensburg, Germany). Only patients with a surgically possible R0 resection were included (N = 38). If a distant metastasis was present these metastases were resected simultaneously which was achieved in 6 out of the 7 patients with distant metastases. General patient information like age and gender were documented. Tumor localization was categorized as pancreas head, corpus or tail based on intraoperative findings and histology. Partial pancreatoduodenectomy (Kausch-Whipple operation), pancreas tail resection with and without splenectomy and localized resection were used as operation methods, individually adapted for tumor size, localization and extent of tumor infiltration into other organs. In case of a localized resection a systematic lymphadenectomy was only performed in case of suspicious lymph nodes in the preoperative diagnostic. Survival data were obtained using the database of the regional tumor center of East Bavaria, Germany (access freely available for hospitals in the region of East Bavaria, Germany). Two patients were lost to follow-up and were excluded from the survival analysis.

Histology

The specimens were fixed in 4% paraformaldehyde and embedded in paraffin. The tumor tissue sections were reevaluated by a pathologist based on the 2006 ENETS TNM classification [10]. Additionally, tissue sections from the tumor region were also stained for endocrine markers and the proliferation marker Ki-67 and a mitotic count was conducted for each specimen. Therefore, positive nuclear staining (MIB-1 antibody) in 10 subsequent high power fields in areas with highest proliferative activity was counted. Further, immunohistochemistry of tissue microarray sections was performed. 2 μm tissue microarray sections were first deparaffinized and then automated stained for cyclin D1 (RM-9104-R7, NeoMarkers Inc., Fremont, CA, USA; Dilution 1:25), E-cadherin (M3612, Dako North America Inc., Carpinteria, CA, USA; Dilution 1:50), β-catenin (sc-7963, Santa Cruz Biotechnology Inc., Santa Cruz, CA, USA; Dilution 1:50) and IL-17A (AF-317-NA, R&D Systems Inc. Minneapolis, MN, USA; Dilution 1:50) with a Ventana BenchMark Ultra IHC/ISH Staining Module (Ventana Medical Systems, Inc., Tucson, Arizona, USA) according to the manufacturers staining procedures. Stained tissue microarrays were analyzed by an independent pathologist blinded for patient and survival data. E-cadherin and β-catenin expression was quantified in 3 levels as low, intermediate and high, cyclin D1 and IL-17A expression was described in 2 levels as low or high.

Statistics

For statistical analysis SPSS 18.0 for Windows (Copyright SPSS Inc., Chicago, Illinois, USA) was used. The distribution of age at operation, follow-up period, tumor size and operation time was described as mean ± standard deviation and compared using Mann–Whitney-U-test due to the fact that these values do not show a normal distribution. Survival after surgery was estimated using the Kaplan-Meier method. The log rank test was used to compare survival stratified according to histological classification and grading, tumor localization, operation method, age at operation, gender and different immunohistochemical groups. Distributions of tumor stages, nodal status, metastasis, grading and operation methods were analyzed with Pearsons's chi squared test. P values < 0.05 were considered statistically significant.

Results
General characteristics

In total 38 patients (18 men, 20 women) with PNETs were included in this retrospective analysis. The mean follow-up time was 45 months. Among the 38 PNETs, twelve neoplasms (31.6%) were localized in the pancreas head, eight (21.1%) in the pancreas corpus and eighteen (47.4%) in the pancreas tail. Eight patients (21.1%) had a functional (3 glucagonomas, 5 insulinomas) and thirty patients (78.9%) a non-functional PNET. Two patients were lost during follow-up and were excluded from survival analysis. Out of the 36 persons who completed follow-up, ten (27.8%) died during this period. The mean age at operation did not significantly differ between women and men (54 ± 16 vs. 50 ± 16 years). The mean tumor size was 3.5 ± 0.5 cm (range 0.3 – 15.0 cm; women 3.2 ± 3.6 vs. 3.7 ± 2.8 cm) (Table 1).

TNM classification

According to the TNM classification, 13 of the PNETs were staged as pT1 (34%), 12 as pT2 (32%), 9 as pT3 (24%)

Table 1 General characteristics of patients with PNETs

	Female	Male	p
N	20(52.6%)	18(47.4%)	
Age at operation (years)	54±16	50±16	0.400
Tumor size (cm)	3.2±3.6	3.7±2.8	0.596
Tumor localization			0.621
Pancreas head	5	7	
Pancreas corpus	5	3	
Pancreas tail	10	8	
pT Stage			0.164
pT1	8	5	
pT2	8	4	
pT3	2	7	
pT4	1	2	
Nodal Status			0.095
N0	17	11	
N1	3	7	
Metastasis			0.024
cMO	19	12	*
cM1	1	6	*
Grading			0.023
G1	13	5	*
G2	6	10	*
G3	0	3	*

Age and tumor size presented as mean±SD.Group comparisons using the Mann-White-U-test or persons's chi-squared test (*p<0.05).

and 3 as pT4 (8%) with no statistically significant difference in gender distribution. In one patient there was not enough material left for a histological reevaluation of the tumor. Therefore, this patient was excluded from the analysis regarding T stages and grading. 28 of the patients (74%) had a negative lymph node status whereas in 10 patients (26%) the lymph nodes were infiltrated by tumor cells. Though there was a trend towards increased lymph node infiltration in male patient the level of significance was not reached. Distant metastases were present in seven patients (18%) with a statistically significant higher ratio of men (P = 0.024), in the remaining 31 patients (82%) no metastasis were found. Eighteen of the 37 PNETs were graded as G1 (47%), 16 as G2 (42%) and 3 as G3 (8%) tumors with a statistically significant higher tumor grading in male patients (P = 0.023). (Additional file 1: Table S1; detailed TNM staging of individual patients in Additional file 1: Table S1).

Operation methods

Eight patients (21%) were treated with a localized resection either as enucleation of the tumor or as pancreas segment resection. Five patients (13%) received a spleen preserving pancreas tail resection, fourteen patients (37%) had a pancreas tail resection with splenectomy and in eleven patients (29%) a partial pancreatoduodenectomy (Kausch-Whipple operation) was performed. For a tumor localization in the pancreas head only in 1 out of 12 patients (8%) a localized resection was used compared to a higher rate of a limited surgical approach in the pancreas corpus (3 out of 8 localized resections; 38%) and in the pancreas tail (4 out of 18 localized resections (22%) and 5 out of 18 (28%) spleen preserving pancreas tail resections.

Gender but not tumor localization influences patient survival

Survival curves were calculated using the Kaplan-Meier method. The mean overall survival time was 91 ± 10 months and the 5-year overall survival rate was 64%. Women had an estimated mean survival time of 116 ± 9 months which was significantly longer compared to men with 56 ± 14 months (P = 0.008) (Figure 1).

The mean survival time for PNETs localized in the pancreas head was 49 ± 9 months, in the pancreas corpus 70 ± 18 months and in the pancreas tail 105 ± 12 without significant differences.

T stage, nodal status and grading but not distant metastasis influence survival of resected patients

Further, the influence of the tumor size on patient survival after resection of the PNETs was assessed. In this analysis pT1 tumors showed a mean survival of 107 ± 13 months, pT2 tumors of 94 ± 16 months, pT3 tumors of 44 ± 7 months and pT4 tumors of 18 ± 14 months. Survival of pT1, pT2 and pT3 stages was statistically significant different to survival of patients with pT4 tumors (pT1 vs. pT4 P = 0.001; pT2 vs. pT4 P = 0.026; pT3 vs. pT4 P = 0.047) (Figure 2A).

Additionally, the influence of the lymph node status on patient survival was tested using the Kaplan-Meier method. Patients with negative lymph node status had a statistically significant longer estimated mean survival time of 108 ± 9 months compared to patients with tumor infiltrated lymph nodes with an estimated mean survival time of 19 ± 5 months (P < 0.001) (Figure 2B).

Furthermore, a survival analysis with regards to distant metastasis was performed. Interestingly, mean survival time of cM1 tumors (N = 7) was not significantly different compared to cM0 tumors (N = 31) (80 ± 23 months vs. 92 ± 11 months; P = 0.876) (Figure 3A). Notably, within the patients that developed distant metastases the distribution of tumor grading (2 G1, 4 G2, 1 G3) was

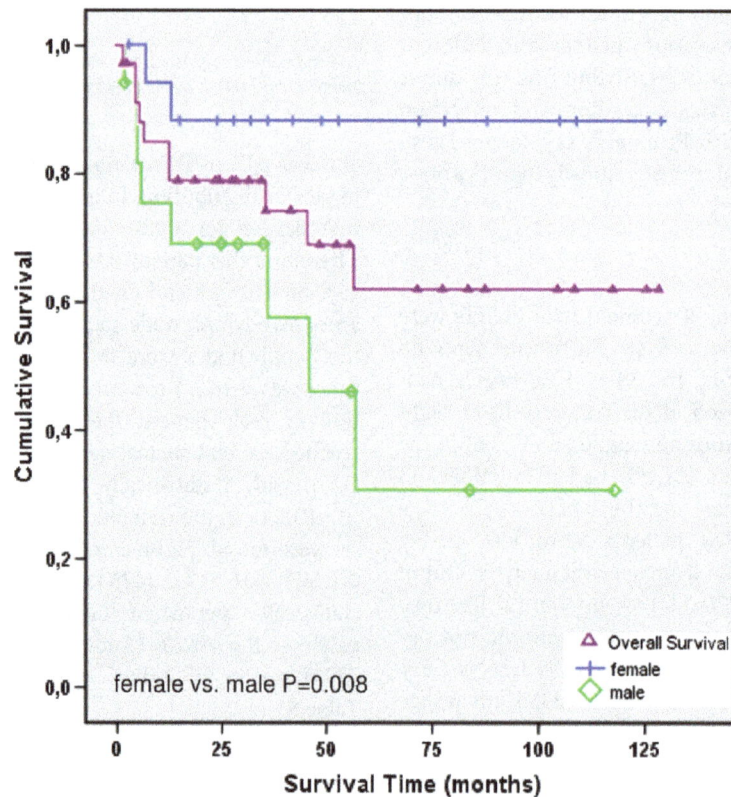

Figure 1 Overall survival and survival stratified for gender. The mean overall survival time was 92 ± 10 months and the 5-year overall survival rate was 63.9%. Women showed a significantly longer mean survival time compared to men (116 ± 9 versus 56 ± 14 months; P = 0.008).

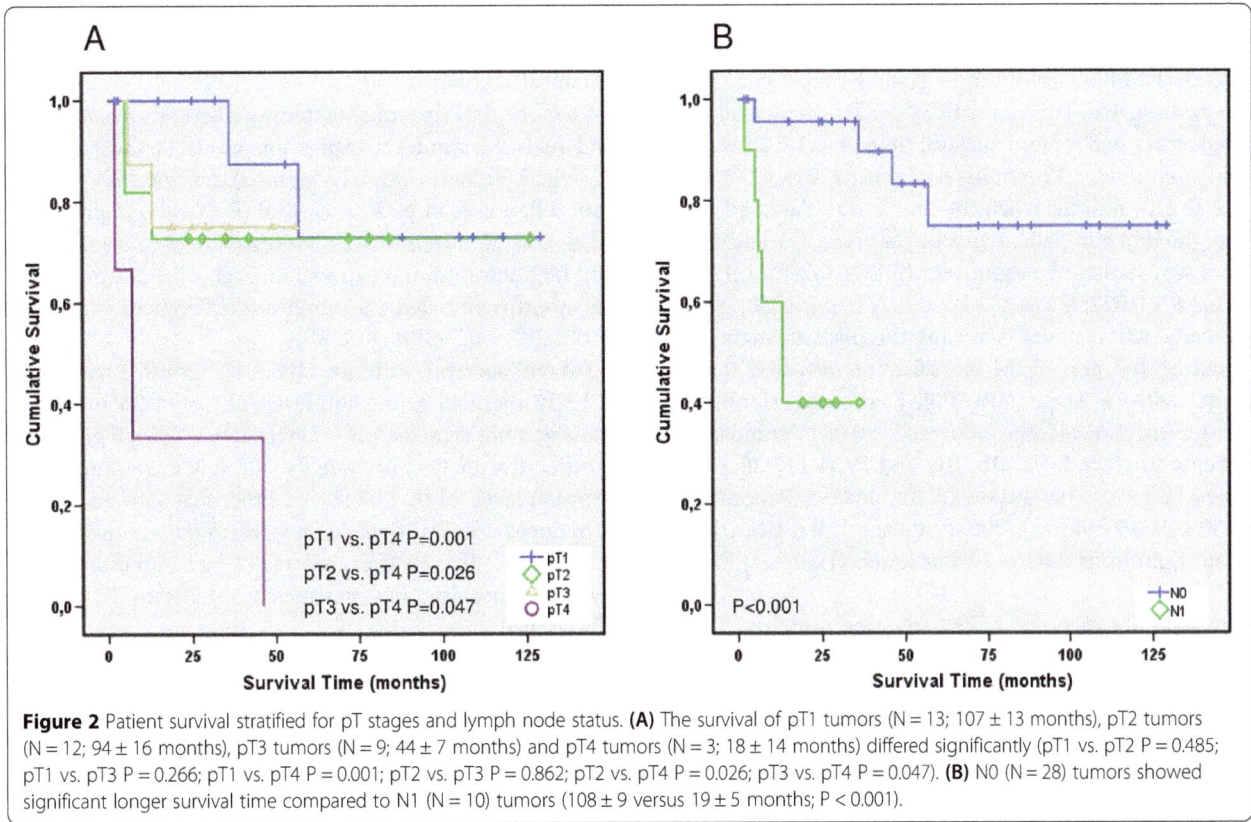

Figure 2 Patient survival stratified for pT stages and lymph node status. **(A)** The survival of pT1 tumors (N = 13; 107 ± 13 months), pT2 tumors (N = 12; 94 ± 16 months), pT3 tumors (N = 9; 44 ± 7 months) and pT4 tumors (N = 3; 18 ± 14 months) differed significantly (pT1 vs. pT2 P = 0.485; pT1 vs. pT3 P = 0.266; pT1 vs. pT4 P = 0.001; pT2 vs. pT3 P = 0.862; pT2 vs. pT4 P = 0.026; pT3 vs. pT4 P = 0.047). **(B)** N0 (N = 28) tumors showed significant longer survival time compared to N1 (N = 10) tumors (108 ± 9 versus 19 ± 5 months; P < 0.001).

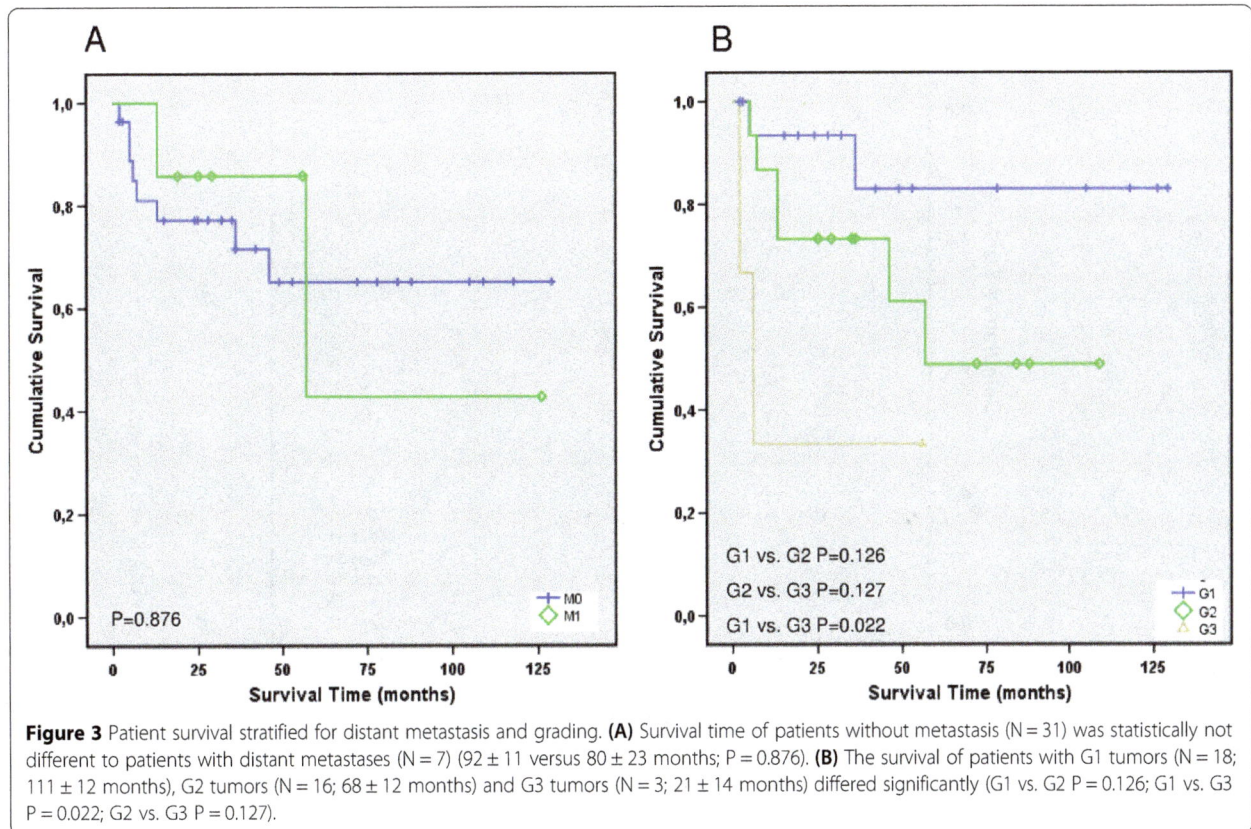

Figure 3 Patient survival stratified for distant metastasis and grading. **(A)** Survival time of patients without metastasis (N = 31) was statistically not different to patients with distant metastases (N = 7) (92 ± 11 versus 80 ± 23 months; P = 0.876). **(B)** The survival of patients with G1 tumors (N = 18; 111 ± 12 months), G2 tumors (N = 16; 68 ± 12 months) and G3 tumors (N = 3; 21 ± 14 months) differed significantly (G1 vs. G2 P = 0.126; G1 vs. G3 P = 0.022; G2 vs. G3 P = 0.127).

not different to patients without distant metastases (16 G1, 12 G2, 2 G3; P = 0.471).

Next, the influence of tumor grading on patient survival was investigated. Patients with a PNET histologically classified as G1 had a mean survival time of 111 ± 12 months, compared to 68 ± 12 months for patients with a G2 tumor and 21 ± 14 months when the tumor was classified as G3. The difference in patient survival between G1 and G3 tumors was statistically significant (G1 vs. G2 P = 0.126; G1 vs. G3 P = 0.022; G2 vs. G3 P = 0.127) (Figure 3B).

Finally, survival analysis using the disease staging proposed by the new TNM classification revealed that patients with a stage IIIb PNET showed significantly shorter survival (12 ± 5 months; P < 0.001) compared to patients in stage I, IIa, IIb, IIIa and IV (I 117.38 ± 10.87; IIa 74.12 ± 9.24; IIb 49.00 ± 0; IIIa 46.00 ± 0 months; IV 80.30 ± 23.35 months). Between stage I, IIa, IIb, IIIa and IV no significant difference was found (Figure 4).

Intratumoral expression of cell adhesion proteins E-cadherin and β-catenin and expression of cyclin D1 and IL-17A do not influence patient survival

To test if E-cadherin, β-catenin, cyclin D1 and IL-17A influence patient survival, these markers were additionally used to stain the PNET tissue samples. Kaplan-Meier analysis was performed for the respective immunohistochemical staining.

Low (67 ± 21 months), intermediate (91 ± 16 months) and high intratumoral expression levels of the adhesion protein E-cadherin (82 ± 16 months) did not show significant differences in patient survival (P = 0.855) (Figure 5A). Also, low (70 ± 18 months), intermediate (97 ± 16 months) and high intratumoral expression levels of β-catenin (77 ± 16 months) revealed no significant differences in patient survival (P = 0.795) (Figure 5B).

Patient survival with low (86 ± 11 months) and high (92 ± 15 months) expression levels of Cyclin D1 in the tumors was not significantly different (P = 0.795) (Figure 6A). Further, the analysis of patients with low intratumoral expression levels of IL-17A (87 ± 14 months) showed a trend to reduced survival times compared to patients with high intratumoral IL-17A expression (117 ± 11 months) though the difference was not statistically significant (P = 0.211) (Figure 6B).

Discussion

In this study the lymph node status was detected to be an important and statistically significant factor for patient

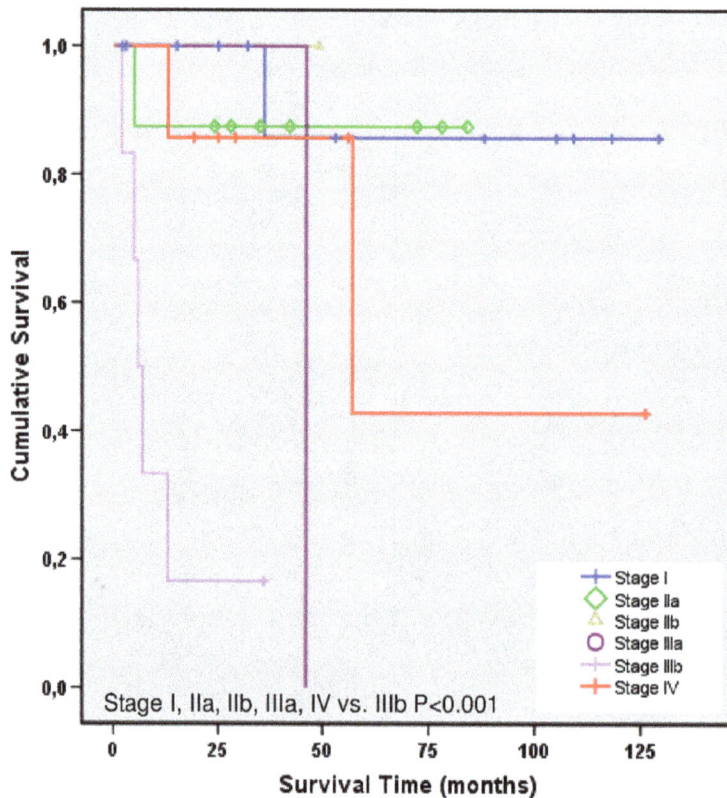

Figure 4 Patient survival stratified for disease stages. Patients with stage IIIb disease showed significant shorter survival (12 ± 5 months; P < 0.001) compared to patients in stage I (117 ± 11 months), IIa (74 ± 9 months), IIb (49 ± 0 months), IIIa (46 ± 0 months) and IV (80 ± 23 months). Between stage I, IIa, IIb, IIIa and IV no statistically significant difference could be found.

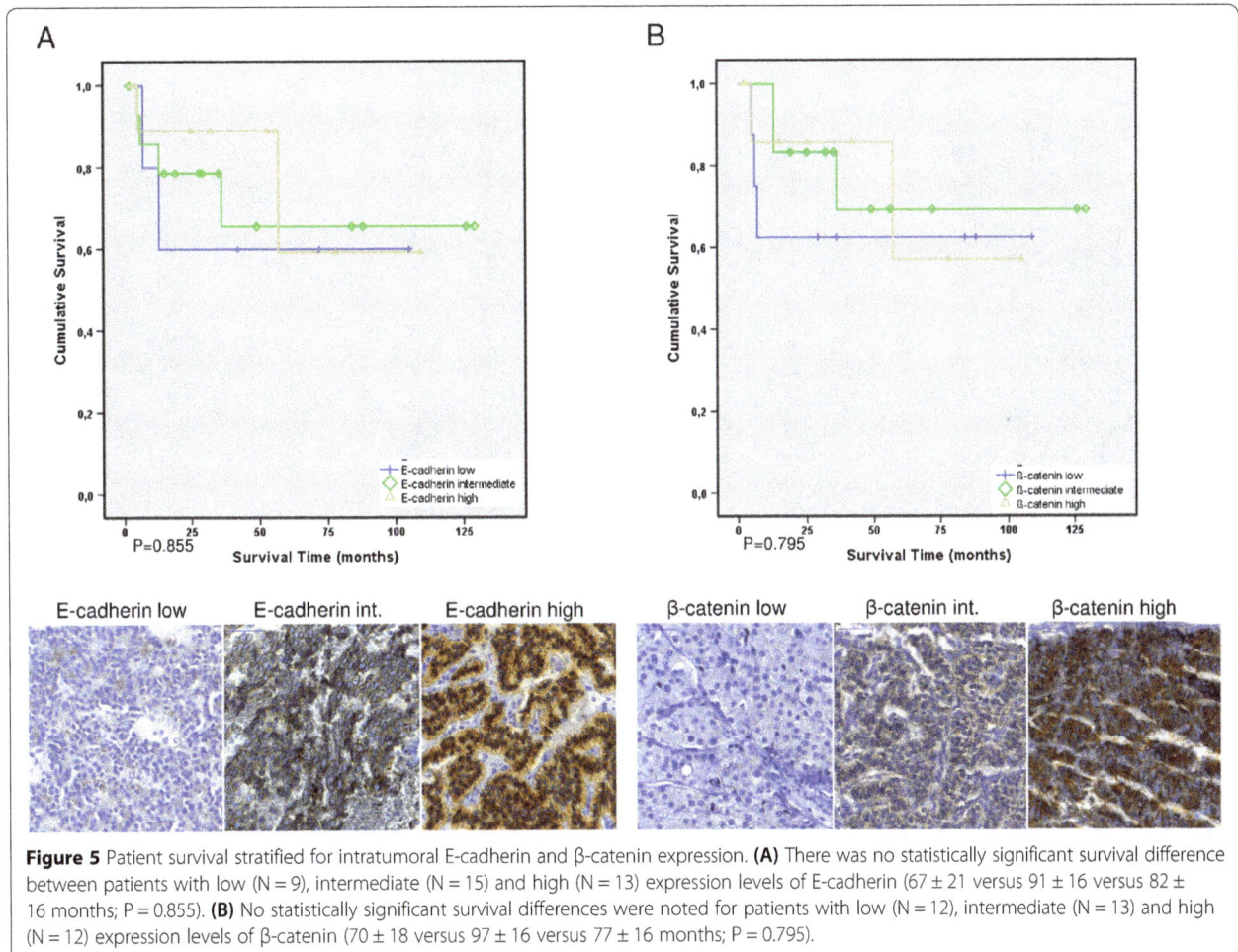

Figure 5 Patient survival stratified for intratumoral E-cadherin and β-catenin expression. **(A)** There was no statistically significant survival difference between patients with low (N = 9), intermediate (N = 15) and high (N = 13) expression levels of E-cadherin (67 ± 21 versus 91 ± 16 versus 82 ± 16 months; P = 0.855). **(B)** No statistically significant survival differences were noted for patients with low (N = 12), intermediate (N = 13) and high (N = 12) expression levels of β-catenin (70 ± 18 versus 97 ± 16 versus 77 ± 16 months; P = 0.795).

survival after resection of a PNET with a mean survival time of 108 ± 9 months for N0 in contrast to 19 ± 5 months for N1 tumors (P < 0.001). This is supported by reports from Ito and Scarpa et al. who both also identified lymph node metastasis as relevant prognostic factor [9,18]. However, a large study with 3851 patients by Bilimoria et al. using the National Cancer Data Base found the nodal status not to be associated with survival [19]. A possible explanation for these contrary findings may be the use of different surgical approaches in these studies and also the rather long time of patient recruitment between 1985 and 2004 in the epidemiologic study by Bilimoria et al. Similar to previously published results, in this study the pT staging and grading provided a statistically significant prognostic stratification of patients [9,18,20].

Different to other tumor entities, in our study distant metastasis had no impact on patient survival. This is supported by the study of Fischer et al. who also found no statistical influence of distant metastasis on survival [2]. However, Scarpa et al. observed distant metastasis to be a statistically significant factor for survival [9]. These contrary findings may be explained by very diverging

patient cohorts and low number of cases in our study, which is one limitation of this study additionally to the fact that data were analyzed retrospectively at a single-center. However, these critical result of our study can be explained since in the study by Scarpa et al. also palliative patients without resection were included whereas in ours and Fischer's study only patients with surgical resection of the tumor were analyzed [2,9]. Taken together, these results suggest that distant metastasis may have no impact on patient survival if they are properly resected.

As a consequence of the findings that positive lymph nodes but not distant metastasis influence survival of resected patients, we were not able to get a good survival stratification using the proposed 2006 ENETS TNM stages which stands in contrast to other studies [10,18]. Only patients suffering from stage IIIb tumors showed significantly worse survival in our analysis. Also the modified staging system proposed by Scarpa et al. would not result in a better risk stratification in our patient cohort [9]. However, this most probable is due to low case numbers in our study since a large study by Rindi et al. demonstrated that this ENETS TNM stages

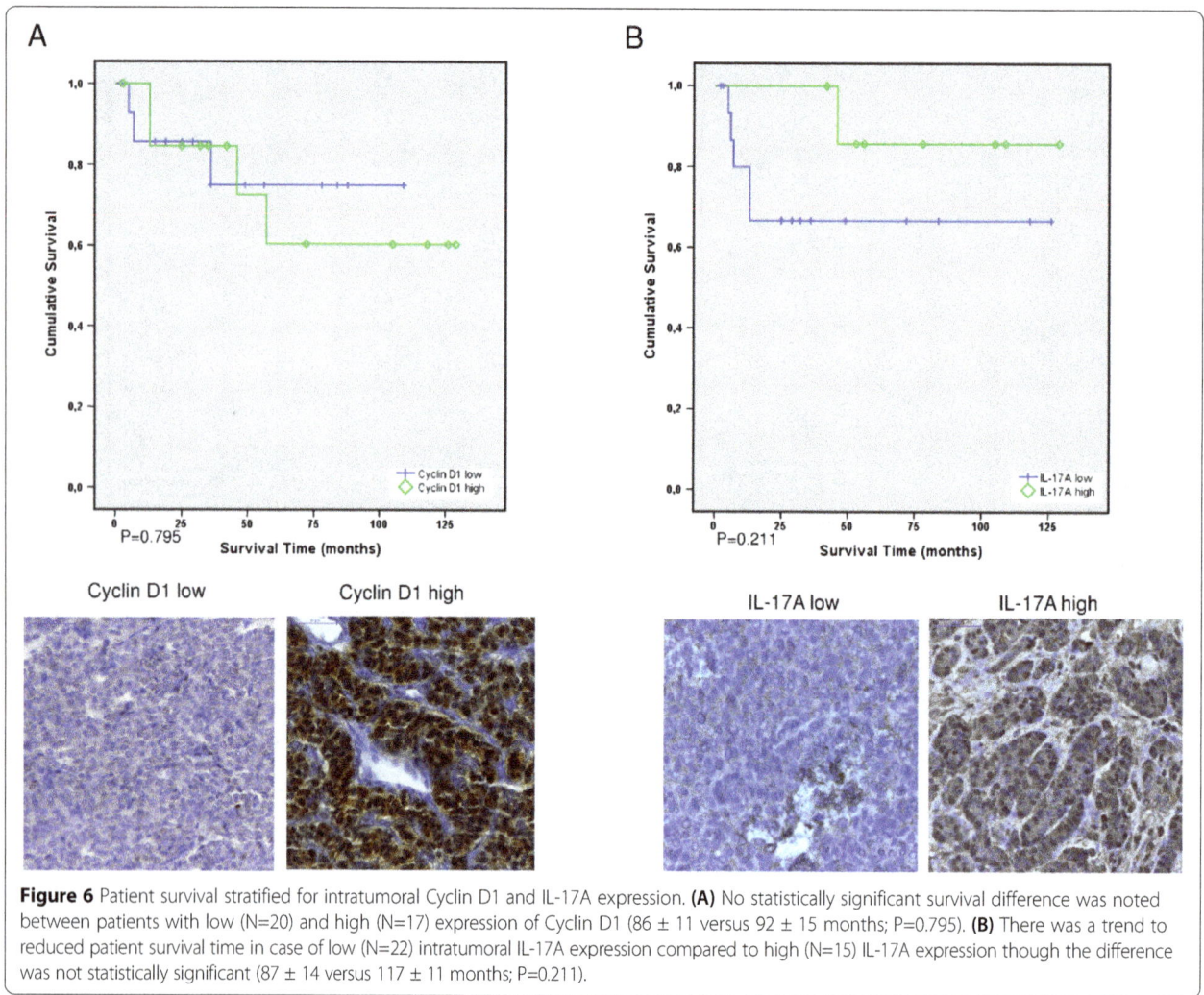

Figure 6 Patient survival stratified for intratumoral Cyclin D1 and IL-17A expression. **(A)** No statistically significant survival difference was noted between patients with low (N=20) and high (N=17) expression of Cyclin D1 (86 ± 11 versus 92 ± 15 months; P=0.795). **(B)** There was a trend to reduced patient survival time in case of low (N=22) intratumoral IL-17A expression compared to high (N=15) IL-17A expression though the difference was not statistically significant (87 ± 14 versus 117 ± 11 months; P=0.211).

work well and are even superior to the UICC/AJCC/WHO 2010 TNM staging system [11].

Very interesting was the fact, that we found statistically significant differences in survival between women and men (116 ± 9 months vs. 56 ± 14 months; P = 0.008). This is supported by a recent study from Kim et al. who found gender to be a prognostic factor for disease free survival of neuroendocrine tumors and also by Rindi et al. who also shows male patients being at higher risk [11,21]. One reason for shorter survival of male patients may be the trend to more tumor positive lymph nodes and the higher tumor grading in our patient cohort, however, these differences between men and women were not statistically significant and therefore both groups were comparable. Possible explanations for these differences in tumor biology and survival may be gender imbalances for risk factors like smoking and alcohol, a different constitution or hormonal influences as suggested by Kim et al. [21].

Since previous studies demonstrated that pancreatic endocrine neoplasms and adenocarcinoma of the pancreas express E-cadherin and β-catenin and that further cyclin D1 and IL-17A contribute to malignant transformation in pancreatic tumors, these markers were used to stain PNET tissue samples [12-17]. Cell adhesion proteins like E-cadherin and β-catenin have also been shown to promote tumor progression and are associated with poor patient survival in colorectal adenocarcinoma and in a subgroup of patients with non-small cell lung cancer if expressed at low levels [22-25]. However, no influence on patient survival was found in our PNET cohort. Further, no correlation of Cyclin D1 with patient survival was shown in the investigated PNETs in contrast to other reports with different tumor entities before [26,27]. In the analysis of intratumoral IL-17A expression a trend towards reduced patient survival in case of low IL-17A expression was noted, however, the differences were not statistically significant. So far, there have been conflicting reports about the effects of IL-17A expression in tumor microenvironment on survival [28-31]. In our cohort of PNET patients the patient number might be too small to conclude if intratumoral IL-17A expression is beneficial. Also, the other tested factors were not suitable for patient risk stratification.

The surgical approach in this study was based on the individual preoperative diagnostic results with the goal to achieve an R0 resection. Limited tumors with regards to TNM staging and grading were treated with a localized resection or a pancreas tail resection without splenectomy. If distant metastasis were present, a simultaneous resection was performed. This operation strategy is supported by reports from Hodul et al. and others [3,32,33]. According to published results, we found an overall 5-year survival rate of 63.9% [9,18,19].

Taking into account that we detected the lymph node status and the tumor grading to be the essential histopathological prognostic factors for survival of patients with surgically resected PNETs it seems to be very important to identify these patients at high risk before surgery. For this purpose, the ^{68}Ga-DOTATOC positron emission tomography/computed tomography may emerge as a useful tool not only for the evaluation of the primary tumor and the distant metastasis but also for the detection of lymph node metastasis as suggested by Kumar et al. [34]. Then an individualized surgical therapy could be performed. If an extensive lymph node dissection with the goal of achieving an R0 situation or a neoadjuvant therapy concept with [99]Y-Dotatoc as suggested by Stoelzing et al. can improve the poor outcome of these patients needs to be evaluated in future studies [34,35].

Conclusion
In conclusion, we identified the lymph node status and also tumor size and grading as important survival factors within the new ENET classification system but not distant metastasis if an R0 resection was achieved. This is important for a tailored therapy of patients with PNETs.

Competing interests
The authors declare that they have no competing interests.

Authors' contributions
SMB designed the study concept, collected and analyzed data, and wrote the manuscript. FW and JMW collected and analyzed data. SAF, AA and HJS analyzed data and reviewed the manuscript. MH designed the study concept, collected and analyzed data, and reviewed the manuscript. All authors read and approved the final manuscript.

Acknowledgments
This study was supported by the University of Regensburg, Regensburg, Germany.

Author details
[1]Department of Surgery, University Medical Center Regensburg, Franz-Josef-Strauss-Allee 11, 93053 Regensburg, Germany. [2]Institute of Pathology, University Medical Center Regensburg, Regensburg, Germany.

References
1. Bergmann F, Breinig M, Hopfner M, Rieker RJ, Fischer L, Kohler C, et al. Expression pattern and functional relevance of epidermal growth factor receptor and cyclooxygenase-2: novel chemotherapeutic targets in pancreatic endocrine tumors? Am J Gastroenterol. 2009;104(1):171–81.
2. Fischer L, Kleeff J, Esposito I, Hinz U, Zimmermann A, Friess H, et al. Clinical outcome and long-term survival in 118 consecutive patients with neuroendocrine tumours of the pancreas. Br J Surg. 2008;95(5):627–35.
3. Hodul PJ, Strosberg JR, Kvols LK. Aggressive surgical resection in the management of pancreatic neuroendocrine tumors: when is it indicated? Cancer Control. 2008;15(4):314–21.
4. Hauso O, Gustafsson BI, Kidd M, Waldum HL, Drozdov I, Chan AK, et al. Neuroendocrine tumor epidemiology: contrasting Norway and North America. Cancer. 2008;113(10):2655–64.
5. Bilimoria KY, Tomlinson JS, Merkow RP, Stewart AK, Ko CY, Talamonti MS, et al. Clinicopathologic features and treatment trends of pancreatic neuroendocrine tumors: analysis of 9,821 patients. J GastrointestSurg. 2007;11(11):1460–7.
6. Davies K, Conlon KC. Neuroendocrine tumors of the pancreas. Curr Gastroenterol Rep. 2009;11(2):119–27.
7. Kloppel G, Perren A, Heitz PU. The gastroenteropancreatic neuroendocrine cell system and its tumors: the WHO classification. Ann NY Acad Sci. 2004;1014:13–27.
8. Kloppel G, Rindi G, Anlauf M, Perren A, Komminoth P. Site-specific biology and pathology of gastroenteropancreatic neuroendocrine tumors. Virchows Arch. 2007;451 Suppl 1:S9–27.
9. Scarpa A, Mantovani W, Capelli P, Beghelli S, Boninsegna L, Bettini R, et al. Pancreatic endocrine tumors: improved TNM staging and histopathological grading permit a clinically efficient prognostic stratification of patients. Mod Pathol. 2010;23(6):824–33.
10. Rindi G, Kloppel G, Alhman H, Caplin M, Couvelard A, de Herder WW, et al. TNM staging of foregut (neuro)endocrine tumors: a consensus proposal including a grading system. Virchows Arch. 2006;449(4):395–401.
11. Rindi G, Falconi M, Klersy C, Albarello L, Boninsegna L, Buchler MW, et al. TNM staging of neoplasms of the endocrine pancreas: results from a large international cohort study. J Natl Cancer Inst. 2012;104(10):764–77.
12. Biliran Jr H, Wang Y, Banerjee S, Xu H, Heng H, Thakur A, et al. Overexpression of cyclin D1 promotes tumor cell growth and confers resistance to cisplatin-mediated apoptosis in an elastase-myc transgene-expressing pancreatic tumor cell line. Clin Cancer Res. 2005;11(16):6075–86.
13. Burford H, Baloch Z, Liu X, Jhala D, Siegal GP, Jhala N. E-cadherin/beta-catenin and CD10: a limited immunohistochemical panel to distinguish pancreatic endocrine neoplasm from solid pseudopapillary neoplasm of the pancreas on endoscopic ultrasound-guided fine-needle aspirates of the pancreas. Am J Clin Pathol. 2009;132(6):831–9.
14. El-Bahrawy MA, Rowan A, Horncastle D, Tomlinson I, Theis BA, Russell RC, et al. E-cadherin/catenin complex status in solid pseudopapillary tumor of the pancreas. Am J Surg Pathol. 2008;32(1):1–7.
15. Kim G, Khanal P, Lim SC, Yun HJ, Ahn SG, Ki SH. Interleukin-17 induces AP-1 activity and cellular transformation via upregulation of tumor progression locus 2 activity. Carcinogenesis. 2012;34(2):341–50.
16. Kim MJ, Jang SJ, Yu E. Loss of E-cadherin and cytoplasmic-nuclear expression of beta-catenin are the most useful immunoprofiles in the diagnosis of solid-pseudopapillary neoplasm of the pancreas. Hum Pathol. 2008;39(2):251–8.
17. Takahashi K, Hirano F, Matsumoto K, Aso K, Haneda M. Homeobox gene CDX2 inhibits human pancreatic cancer cell proliferation by down-regulating cyclin D1 transcriptional activity. Pancreas. 2009;38(1):49–57.
18. Ito H, Abramson M, Ito K, Swanson E, Cho N, Ruan DT, et al. Surgery and staging of pancreatic neuroendocrine tumors: a 14-year experience. J Gastrointest Surg. 2010;14(5):891–8.
19. Bilimoria KY, Talamonti MS, Tomlinson JS, Stewart AK, Winchester DP, Ko CY, et al. Prognostic score predicting survival after resection of pancreatic

neuroendocrine tumors: analysis of 3851 patients. AnnSurg. 2008;247(3):490–500.

20. Mboti FB, Loi P, Nagy N, Myriam D, Gelin M, Closset J. Neuroendocrine tumors of pancreas: how can we apply the 2006 TNM proposal? Hepatogastroenterology. 2010;57(98):344–8.

21. Kim SJ, Kim JW, Oh DY, Han SW, Lee SH, Kim DW, et al. Clinical Course of Neuroendocrine Tumors With Different Origins (the Pancreas, Gastrointestinal Tract, and Lung). Am J Clin Oncol. 2011;35(6):549–56.

22. Elzagheid A, Buhmeida A, Laato M, El-Faitori O, Syrjanen K, Collan Y, et al. Loss of E-cadherin expression predicts disease recurrence and shorter survival in colorectal carcinoma. APMIS. 2012;120(7):539–48.

23. Engelman MD, Grande RM, Naves MA, de Franco MF, de Paulo CTV. Integrin-Linked Kinase (ILK) Expression Correlates with Tumor Severity in Clear Cell Renal Carcinoma. Pathol Oncol Res. 2012;19(1):27–33.

24. Kreiseder B, Orel L, Bujnow C, Buschek S, Pflueger M, Schuett W. Hundsberger H, de MR, Wiesner C: alpha-Catulin downregulates E-cadherin and promotes melanoma progression and invasion. Int J Cancer. 2013;132(3):521–30.

25. Wu Y, Liu HB, Ding M, Liu JN, Zhan P, Fu XS, et al. The impact of E-cadherin expression on non-small cell lung cancer survival: a meta-analysis. Mol Biol Rep. 2012;39(10):9621–8.

26. Xie C, Song LB, Wu JH, Li J, Yun JP, Lai JM, et al. Upregulator of cell proliferation predicts poor prognosis in hepatocellular carcinoma and contributes to hepatocarcinogenesis by downregulating FOXO3a. PLoS One. 2012;7(7):e40607.

27. Yeh BW, Wu WJ, Li WM, Li CC, Huang CN, Kang WY, et al. Overexpression of TG-interacting factor is associated with worse prognosis in upper urinary tract urothelial carcinoma. Am J Pathol. 2012;181(3):1044–55.

28. Gnerlich JL, Mitchem JB, Weir JS, Sankpal NV, Kashiwagi H, Belt BA, et al. Induction of Th17 cells in the tumor microenvironment improves survival in a murine model of pancreatic cancer. J Immunol. 2010;185(7):4063–71.

29. Iida T, Iwahashi M, Katsuda M, Ishida K, Nakamori M, Nakamura M, et al. Tumor-infiltrating CD4+ Th17 cells produce IL-17 in tumor microenvironment and promote tumor progression in human gastric cancer. Oncol Rep. 2011;25(5):1271–7.

30. Kryczek I, Wei S, Szeliga W, Vatan L, Zou W. Endogenous IL-17 contributes to reduced tumor growth and metastasis. Blood. 2009;114(2):357–9.

31. Wilke CM, Kryczek I, Wei S, Zhao E, Wu K, Wang G, et al. Th17 cells in cancer: help or hindrance? Carcinogenesis. 2011;32(5):643–9.

32. Abu HM, McPhail MJ, Zeidan BA, Jones CE, Johnson CD, Pearce NW. Aggressive multi-visceral pancreatic resections for locally advanced neuroendocrine tumours. Is it worth it? JOP. 2009;10(3):276–9.

33. Dralle H, Krohn SL, Karges W, Boehm BO, Brauckhoff M, Gimm O. Surgery of resectable nonfunctioning neuroendocrine pancreatic tumors. World J Surg. 2004;28(12):1248–60.

34. Kumar R, Sharma P, Garg P, Karunanithi S, Naswa N, Sharma R, et al. Role of (68)Ga-DOTATOC PET-CT in the diagnosis and staging of pancreatic neuroendocrine tumours. Eur Radiol. 2011;21(11):2408–16.

35. Stoeltzing O, Loss M, Huber E, Gross V, Eilles C, Mueller-Brand J, et al. Staged surgery with neoadjuvant (90)Y-DOTATOC therapy for down-sizing synchronous bilobular hepatic metastases from a neuroendocrine pancreatic tumor. Langenbecks Arch Surg. 2010;395(2):185–92.

5

A case report of a solitary pancreatic metastasis of an adrenocortical carcinoma

Johannes Baur[1*], Ulla Schedelbeck[2], Alina Pulzer[4], Christina Bluemel[3], Vanessa Wild[5,6], Martin Fassnacht[4,5] and U. Steger[1]

Abstract

Background: Solitary metastases to the pancreas are rare. Therefore the value of resection in curative intention remains unclear. In the literature there are several promising reports about resection of solitary metastasis to the pancreas mainly of renal origin.

Case presentation: Here we report for the first time on the surgical therapy of a 1.5 cm solitary pancreatic metastasis of an adrenocortical carcinoma. The metastasis occurred almost 6 years after resection of the primary tumor. A partial pancreatoduodenectomy was performed and postoperatively adjuvant mitotane treatment was initiated. During the follow-up of 3 years after surgery no evidence of tumor recurrence occurred.

Conclusion: Resection of pancreatic tumors should be considered, even if the mass is suspicious for metastatic disease including recurrence of adrenocortical cancer.

Keywords: Adrenocortical Carcinoma, Metastases to pancreas, Surgical treatment

Background

Adrenocortical carcinoma (ACC) is a rare malignant tumor with an estimated incidence of 1 to 2 cases per million population [1]. The occurrence has a first peak in childhood and a second in the fourth and fifth decade of life. The majority of ACC are sporadic. But in some cases ACC is part of hereditary syndromes like Li-Fraumeni syndrome, Beckwith-Wiedeman syndrome, multiple endocrine neoplasia (MEN) 1, congenital adrenal hyperplasia or familial polyposis coli [2]. Therapy and prognosis strongly depend on the European Network for the Study of Adrenal Tumours (ENSAT) classification [3]. In localized disease, surgery is treatment of choice [4], whereas in advanced disease mitotane alone or in combination with cytotoxic drugs is standard of care [5]. According to the German ACC register, 5-year-survival rates are 84 %, 63 %, 51 % and 15 % for Stage I, II, III and IV respectively [6]. Management of recurrent disease is not standardized [5], but recent retrospective studies suggest that surgery is of benefit in selected cases [7].

Metastatic involvement of pancreas due to any primary malignant tumor is rare and represents about 2 % of all pancreatic tumors. Most of these patients show diffuse distant metastases of their primary tumor [8] with no opportunity of surgical treatment.

Here, we present a case of recurrent ACC with a solitary pancreatic metastasis 6 years after resection of the primary tumor.

Case presentation

A 45-year-old woman was first diagnosed in 2006 with ACC showing typical signs of Cushing's syndrome with consecutive increase of weight and body hair, acne, therapy-refractory arterial hypertension and decrease of physical working capacity. Hormonal work-up revealed elevated cortisol levels basal and after dexamethasone suppression, as well as elevated dehydroepiandrosterone sulphate (DHEA-S) and androgen levels. CT scan showed a 4.7 × 5.2 × 4.5 cm sized mass of the left adrenal gland with venous contrast enhancement suspicious for adrenocortical carcinoma (Fig. 1).

The patient underwent conventional resection of the left adrenal gland and lymphadenectomy. Pathological study of the resected tissue was performed by two independent pathologists. The tumor presented a solid growth pattern with some fibrous bands and small areas of necrosis. Tumor cells appeared monomorphic with small nuclei

* Correspondence: baur_j@ukw.de
[1]Department of General, Visceral, Vascular and Pediatric Surgery, University Hospital Wuerzburg, Wuerzburg, Germany
Full list of author information is available at the end of the article

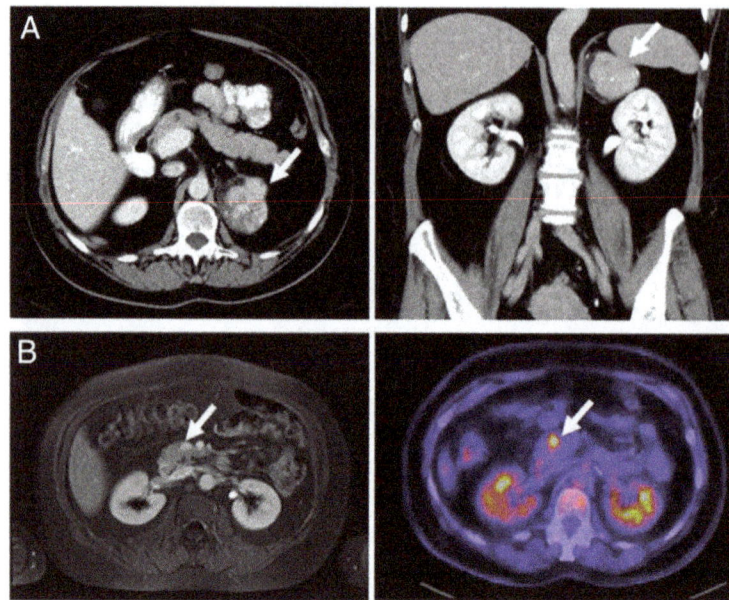

Fig. 1 Imaging of the primary adrenocortical carcinoma (**a**) and the solitary metachronous metastasis inside the pancreatic head (**b**) by MRT and FDG-PET/CT, respectively

and condensated chromatin. The rate of mitosis was under 1 in 10 high power fields. Interestingly there were large amounts of myelolipomatosis metaplastic areas. All three classic scoring systems showed results still within the value range for benign lesions. However, a high Ki-67 expression of 20 % led to the diagnosis of an adrenocortical carcinoma (ENSAT stage II). Due to a good differentiation, no adjuvant mitotane therapy has been performed. Though the patient underwent follow-up examinations periodically, including hormonal work-up and CT or MR imaging performed initially every 3 months and eventually every 6 months after a 2-year-recurrence-free survival.

Sixty-six months after surgical treatment MR imaging showed a new hyperperfused mass in the head of the pancreas with progression of size in the following studies as well as a high FDG-uptake in positron emission tomography (Fig. 1). Thus, the mass was highly suspicious of malignancy and resection was recommended by interdisciplinary consensus.

The patient underwent pylorus preserving partial pancreaticoduodenectomy. Postoperatively the patient developed a pancreatic fistula with an intraabdominal abscess formation, which had to be drained interventionally on day 10 after surgery. The drain could be removed on day 24 after surgery.

Histological and immunohistochemical examination of the resected tissue showed a 1.5 cm sized well differentiated tumor with solid growth pattern (Fig. 2a). Tumor cells presented monomorphic with eosinophilic cytoplasm and unremarkable nuclei. The metastasis

stained positive for synapthophysin, Melan A and steroidogenic factor 1 (SF-1) in consistency with the diagnosis as a metastasis of the adrenocortical carcinoma (Fig. 2b) with a Ki-67 expression in 10 % of tumor cells. There where no signs of a primary pancreatic carcinoma as the tumor cells stained negative for pan cytokeratine (pan-ck) (Fig. 2c). In addition, pathological examination by the reference pathologist of the German ACC study group was performed and confirmed the correlation between the ACC primary tumor and the unusual site of metastasis.

According to interdisciplinary consensus an adjuvant mitotane therapy was initiated after the tumor resection and is still ongoing. During follow-up, including endocrine and imaging work-up every 3 months now for more than 3 years, there is no evidence of recurrence (Time axis see Table 1).

Literature review

A literature review has been performed to identify the distribution of different tumor entities of solitary metastases inside the pancreas. A PubMed search for studies or case reports dealing with "metastases to pancreas" was performed. Articles were included in this review if 10 or more patients were investigated retrospectively or prospectively, patients suffered of metastases to pancreas (no infiltrative involvement) and only the pancreas was affected by metastases, patients received resection of pancreas metastases in curative intension and different tumor entities were included in each study. Four retrospective studies [9–12] summerized in Table 2 met the

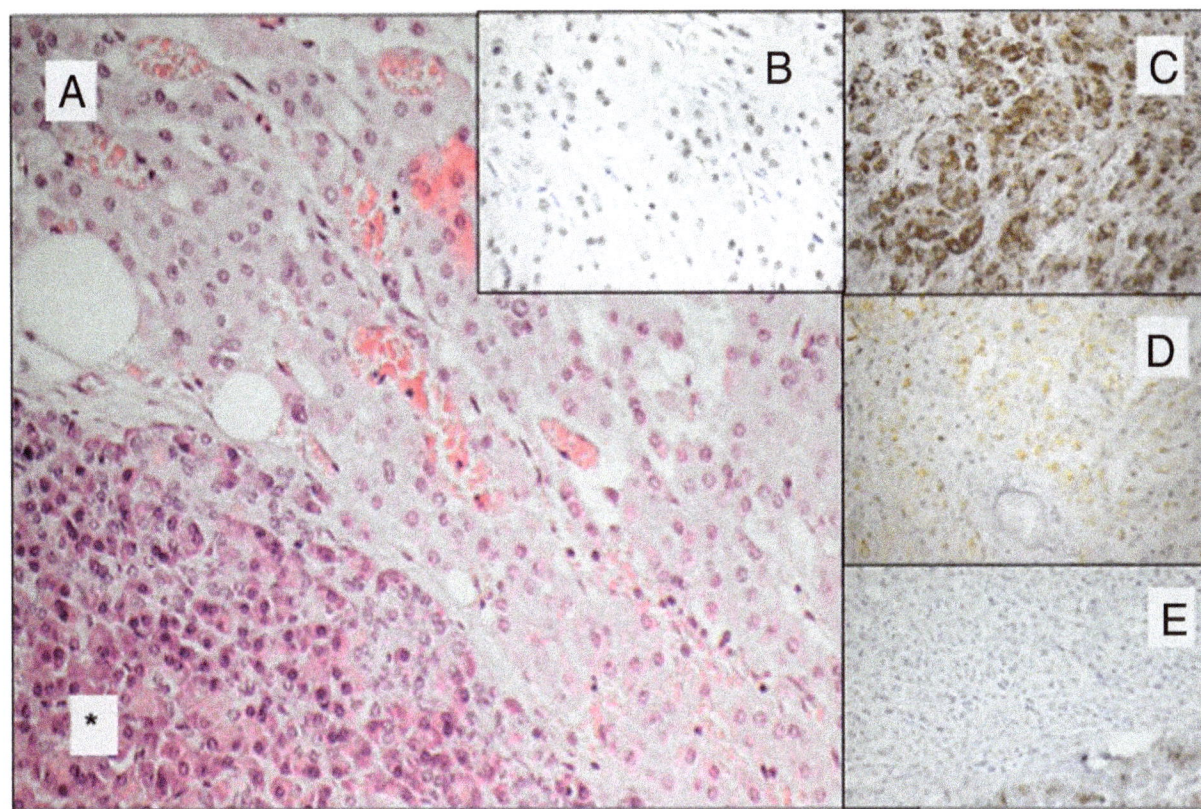

Fig. 2 Histology of pancreatic mass (**a**) metastasis with adjacent pancreatic tissue (*) (HE stain, 20x) (**b**) ACC metastasis with nuclear positive staining pattern for SF-1 (SF1, 40x) (**c**) ACC metastasis with positive cytoplasmic staining for Synaptophysin (**d**) ACC metastasis with positive cytoplasmic staining for Inhibin [E] ACC metastasis is negative for pan-ck (AE1/3, 20x), the pancreatic acini stain positive for pan-ck

inclusion criteria with a total of 92 patients. Median age of patients ranged from 59 to 64 years. Most frequent origin of pancreatic metastases was the kidney in 46 % of the cases followed by melanoma in about 10 % of the cases. Rectal and Colon carcinomas were involved in only 5 cases. One "non-pancreatic endocrine tumor" was reported but not specified in more detail [12]. Here, the distribution of metastatic origin is different to other literature reviews, where the proportion of renal cell carcinomas range between 60 and 70 % [8]. This is caused by the exclusion of studies intending to investigate a single tumor entity metastatic to the pancreas (mostly renal cell carcinomas). Median survival after curative resection of pancreatic metastases was 2.2 to 4.3 years. 5-year-survival ranged between 36 % and 61 %.

Discussion

Solitary metastases to the pancreas are rare. Only 1.3 % of patients undergoing pancreatic resection present a solitary metastasis of a primary solid tumor [12]. In our literature review singular metastasis to the pancreas was most frequent of renal origin (46 % of cases). The value of resection in curative intention remains unclear. As our literature review revealed, 5-year-survival may range between 36 % and 61 % if different tumor entities are taken together. Certain metastatic tumor entities even show better survival rates after curative resection compared to primary pancreatic carcinomas. In case of a singular pancreatic metastasis of renal cell carcinoma a 5-year-survival between 66 % and 79 % can be achieved by curative resection of pancreatic metastasis [8, 13].

Table 1 Time axis

2006	Conventional left-side Adrenalectomie of an Adrenocortical Carcinoma (stadium II, diameter 7 cm)
2006 - 2012	Unsuspicious follow-up in periodically performed cross-sectional studies
02/2012	Detection of a pancreatic mass suspicious for malignancy in PET
03/2012	Pylorus preserving partial pancreaticoduodenectomy Histological and immunhistochemic examination showed a 1.5 cm sized well differentiated metastasis of the adrenocortical carcinoma
Till present date	Mitotane Therapy, unsuspicious follow-up in periodically performed cross-sectional studies and hormonal work-up

Table 2 Literature review

Author (Year)	Years observed	No. of patients	Median age	Median survival (y)	5-year-survival (y)	RCC	Melanoma	Gall bladder	Sarcoma	Colon	Ovar	Lung	Breast	Others[a]
Reddy el al. (2008) [10]	1970–2007	49	60	3.7	36 %	21 (42.9)	3(6.1)	6 (12.2)	4 (8.2)	2 (4.1)	4(8.1)	4 (8.2)	1 (2.0)	4(8.1)
Bahra ct al. (2008) [7]	1989–2007	20	62	not reached	61 %	9 (45.0)	1 (5.0)	1 (5.0)	2 (10.0)	1 (5.0)	-	-	-	6(12.2)
Eidt ct al. (2007) [9]	1993–2005	12	64	4.3	not reported	7(58.3)	4(33.1)	-	-	1 (8.3)	-	-	-	-
Crippa ct al. (2006) [8]	1994–2005	11	59	2.2	48 %	5 (45.5)	1(9.1)	-	-	1 (9.1)	1(9.1)	-	3 (27.3)	-
		92				42(45.7)	9,(9.8)	7(7.6)	6(6.5)	5(5.4)	4(4.3)	4(4.3)	4(4.3)	10(10.9)

RCC Renal cell careinoma
[a]Schwannoma (reported twice); Seminoma, Teratocarcinoma, Hepatocellular Carcinoma, Langerhans cell histiocytosis, esophagus, mesechymal gastric tumor, non-pancreatic endocrine tumor (not specified), GIST (each one case reported)

Here we report for the first time a case of a solitary pancreatic metastasis of an adrenocortical carcinoma. ACC is one of the most aggressive endocrine tumors known so far. Resection of recurrent tumor is recommended in selected case (e.g. when the disease-free interval exceeds 12 months and complete resection seems to be feasible) [7]. In our case, the metastasis occurred almost 6 years after resection of a very well differentiated primary tumor and a R0 resection could be performed. Although known to improve recurrence-free survival after resection of primary tumor [14], it remains unclear if adjuvant mitotane therapy would have prevented recurrence of ACC. However, the patient would have suffered from mitotane side effects like adrenocortical insufficiency. As the patient is now again free of disease for more than 3 years, surgical approach to treat solitary pancreatic ACC metastasis was most likely of great benefit to her.

Conclusion

In conclusion, resection of pancreatic tumors should be considered, even if the mass is suspicious for metastatic disease including recurrence of adrenocortical cancer.

Abbreviations

ACC: Adrenocortical carcinoma; ENSAT: European Network of the Study of Adrenal Tumours; DHEA-S: Dehydroepiandrosterone sulphate; SF-1: Steroidogenic factor 1; pan-ck: Pancreatic cytoceratine.

Competing interests

The authors declare that they have no competing interests.

Authors' contributions

JB was involved in postoperative care of the patient after pancreatic resection, wrote the case report, made literature review and drafted the manuscript. US and CB were the main persons involved in preoperative detection of pancreatic mass and revised the manuscript. MF and AP were involved in diagnosis, adjuvant treatment and follow-up before and after resection of primary tumor and metastasis to the pancreas. Both revised the paper. VW performed conventional and immunohistochemical staining of pancreatic ACC metastasis and revised the manuscript. US performed pancreatic resection, was involved in postoperative care of the patient and revised the manuscript. All authors read and approved the final manuscript.

Acknowledgements

This publication was funded by the German Research Foundation (DFG) and the University of Wuerzburg in the funding program Open Access Publishing.

Author details

[1]Department of General, Visceral, Vascular and Pediatric Surgery, University Hospital Wuerzburg, Wuerzburg, Germany. [2]Institute of Radiology, University Hospital Wuerzburg, Wuerzburg, Germany. [3]Department of Nuclear Medicine, University Hospital Wuerzburg, Wuerzburg, Germany. [4]Department of Internal Medicine I, Endocrinology, University Hospital Wuerzburg, Wuerzburg, Germany. [5]Comprehensive Cancer Center Mainfranken, University of Wuerzburg, Wuerzburg, Germany. [6]Institute of Pathology, University Wuerzburg, Wuerzburg, Germany.

References

1. Fassnacht M, Kroiss M, Allolio B. Update in adrenocortical carcinoma. J Clin Endocrinol Metab. 2013;98:4551–64.
2. Fassnacht M, Libe R, Kroiss M, Allolio B. Adrenocortical carcinoma: a clinician's update. Nat Rev Endocrinol. 2011;7:323–35.
3. Fassnacht M, Johanssen S, Quinkler M, Bucsky P, Willenberg HS, Beuschlein F, et al. Limited prognostic value of the 2004 International Union Against Cancer staging classification for adrenocortical carcinoma: proposal for a Revised TNM Classification. Cancer. 2009;115:5847.
4. Berruti A, Baudin E, Gelderblom H, Haak HR, Porpiglia F, Fassnacht M, et al. Adrenal cancer: ESMO Clinical Practice Guidelines for diagnosis, treatment and follow-up. Ann Oncol. 2012;23 Suppl 7.
5. Else T, Kim AC, Sabolch A, Raymond VM, Kandathil A, Caoili EM, et al. Adrenocortical carcinoma. Endocr Rev. 2014;35:282–326.
6. Fassnacht M, Allolio B. Clinical management of adrenocortical carcinoma. Best Pract Res Clin Endocrinol Metab. 2009;23:273–89.
7. Erdogan I, Deutschbein T, Jurowich C, Kroiss M, Ronchi C, Quinkler M, et al. The role of surgery in the management of recurrent adrenocortical carcinoma. J Clin Endocrinol Metab. 2013;98:181–91.
8. Reddy S, Wolfgang CL. The role of surgery in the management of isolated metastases to the pancreas. Lancet Oncol. 2009;10:287–93.
9. Bahra M, Jacob D, Langrehr JM, Glanemann M, Schumacher G, Lopez-Hanninen E, et al. Metastatic lesions to the pancreas. When is resection reasonable? Chirurg. 2008;79:241–8.
10. Crippa S, Angelini C, Mussi C, Bonardi C, Romano F, Sartori P, et al. Surgical treatment of metastatic tumors to the pancreas: a single center experience and review of the literature. World J Surg. 2006;30:1536–42.
11. Eidt S, Jergas M, Schmidt R, Siedek M. Metastasis to the pancreas–an indication for pancreatic resection? Langenbecks Arch Surg. 2007;392:539–42.
12. Reddy S, Edil BH, Cameron JL, Pawlik TM, Herman JM, Gilson MM, et al. Pancreatic resection of isolated metastases from nonpancreatic primary cancers. Ann Surg Oncol. 2008;15:3199–206.
13. Yuasa T, Inoshita N, Saiura A, Yamamoto S, Urakami S, Masuda H, et al. Clinical outcome of patients with pancreatic metastases from renal cell cancer. BMC Cancer. 2015;15:46.
14. Terzolo M, Angeli A, Fassnacht M, Daffara F, Tauchmanova L, Conton PA, et al. Adjuvant mitotane treatment for adrenocortical carcinoma. N Engl J Med. 2007;356:2372–80.

6

Localized and systemic bacterial infections in necrotizing pancreatitis submitted to surgical necrosectomy or percutaneous drainage of necrotic secretions

Bruno Cacopardo[1]*, Marilia Rita Pinzone[1], Salvatore Berretta[2], Rossella Fisichella[2], Maria Di Vita[2], Guido Zanghì[2], Alessandro Cappellani[2], Giuseppe Nunnari[1], Antonio Zanghì[2]

Abstract

Background: Infectious complications are observed in 40-70% of all patients with severe acute pancreatitis. Infections are associated with a significant increase in mortality rates.

Methods: We evaluated the prevalence and characteristics of pancreatic and systemic infections in 46 patients with necrotizing pancreatitis submitted to surgical procedures during their hospital stay as well as the impact of such infectious complications on patient clinical outcome. Samples for microbiological cultures were taken at hospital admission from blood and bile and 2 days after invasive procedure from blood, drainage fluid, bile and necrotic tissues.

Results: 74% patients with necrotizing pancreatitis had a localized or systemic infection. At admission, 15% of subjects had positive blood cultures whereas 13% had evidence of bacterial growth from bile cultures. Two days after the invasive procedures for removal of necrotic materials and fluids, blood cultures became positive in 30% of patients in spite of antibiotic prophylaxis and bile cultures resulted positive in 22% of cases. Furthermore, bacterial growth from drainage fluids was found in 30% and from homogenized necrotic material in 44% of cases. As refers to bacterial isolates, all patients had a monomicrobial infection. Carbapenems were the drugs with the best sensitivity profile.
Mortality rate was significantly ($p < 0.05$) higher among patients with infection (17%) than subjects without infection (8%). Within the infected group, those subjects with evidence of systemic infection (positive blood cultures) developed more complications and demonstrated a higher ($p < 0.05$) mortality rate (28%) than those who had only a localized infection (10%).

Conclusions: Infectious complications significantly increase mortality in patients with necrotizing pancreatitis. In addition, subjects with systemic infections developed more complications and demonstrated a higher mortality rate in comparison with those having a localized infection. In our study, the sensitivity pattern of the isolated microorganisms suggests to consider carbapenems as the best option for empirical treatment in patients with necrotizing pancreatitis who develop a clear-cut evidence of systemic or localized bacterial infection.

* Correspondence: cacopardobruno@inwind.it
[1]Department of Clinical and Molecular Biomedicine, Division of Infectious Diseases, University of Catania, 95125 Catania, Italy
Full list of author information is available at the end of the article

Background

Infectious complications are observed in 40-70% of all patients with severe acute pancreatitis [1-3]. Mortality usually peaks within the first 7-10 days as a result of infectious complications, either limited to pancreatic necrotic areas or spread in the bloodstream [4,5].

Sterile pancreatic necrosis has a mortality rate of 20%, whereas it increases to more than 50% in the case of infected necrosis [6]. There is evidence that the involved bacteria originate from the gastrointestinal tract by transepithelial traslocation [7].

These patients are often given prophylactic antibiotics, although the use of this strategy may result in the development of an infection with resistant bacteria.

We conducted a study aimed at evaluating the prevalence and characteristics of pancreatic and systemic infections in patients with necrotizing pancreatitis submitted to surgical procedures during their hospital stay. We also evaluated the impact of such infectious complications on patient clinical outcome.

Patients and methods

46 patients affected with acute necrotizing pancreatitis were consecutively enrolled among those admitted over a five-year period (2006-2011) at the Department of Surgery, University Hospital of Catania. The diagnosis of acute pancreatitis was based on clinical features, elevated serum amylase and/or lipase levels (more than 4-fold the upper reference limit) and evidence of pancreatic abnormalities on contrast-enhanced computed tomography (CECT) of the abdomen. The most common etiologies were gallstones (21 cases), alcohol (14 cases) and pancreotoxic drugs (8 cases), whereas 3 cases originated from abdominal traumas. The CT Severity Index [8] was 10 in 22 cases, 9 in 14 patients and 8 in the remainder 10 patients. All patients were closely monitored with adequate amounts of intravenous fluids and pain management. Supportive measures such as enteral nutrition and antibiotic prophylaxis were adopted in all cases. All 46 cases were managed invasively: 16 cases were treated by open surgical removal of necrotic areas, 15 cases underwent percutaneous catheter drainage of necrotic secretions, 15 cases received minimally invasive retroperitoneal necrosectomy. Seven of 46 patients (15%) died within 3 weeks from the onset of the disease.

Samples for microbiological cultures were taken at hospital admission from blood and bile and 2 days after invasive procedure from blood, drainage fluid, bile and necrotic tissues. Necrotic tissue samples from patients undergoing necrosectomy were homogenized immediately before culture.

The protocol for the study was approved by the Ethical Committee of our institution and written informed consent was obtained from all patients. The study protocol conformed to the ethical guidelines of the Declaration of Helsinki.

Statistical analysis was carried out using the statistical software package SPSS version 17.0 (SPSS, Chicago, Illinois, USA). A two-tailed P value of less than 0.05 was considered significant. All quantitative variables were expressed as mean ± standard deviation (SD). The chi-square test and the Fisher's exact test were adopted for statistical comparisons.

Results

In our study population, mean age was 63 ± 17 years, 24 (52%) were males. Comprehensively, in 34 of 46 (74%) patients with necrotizing pancreatitis cultures demonstrated the presence of a localized or systemic infection.

In more detail, at hospital admission 7 of 46 patients (15%) already showed positive blood cultures whereas 6 (13%) had evidence of bacterial growth from bile cultures. Two days after the invasive procedures for removal of necrotic materials and fluids, blood cultures became positive in 14 of 46 patients (30%) in spite of antibiotic prophylaxis and bile cultures resulted positive in 10 patients (22%). Furthermore, bacterial growth from drainage fluids was found in 14 patients (30%) and from homogenized necrotic material in 20 (44%) cases. All those patients with positive bile or blood cultures also had infection of necrotic material.

As refers to bacterial isolates, all patients had a monomicrobial infection. Table 1 shows the cultured microorganisms with reference to the source sites. Table 2 shows the antibiotic resistance rates of the isolated strains.

As refers to the clinical outcome, mortality rate was significantly (p < 0.05) higher among patients with infection (N = 34) than subjects without infection (N = 12): 6 (17%)

Table 1 Number of isolated strains and site of isolation among 46 patients with necrotizing pancreatitis

	N. isolated strains			
	Blood	Bile	Drainage	Necrotic material
Gram-negative bacteria				
Escherichia coli	4	4	7	10
Pseudomonas aeruginosa	2	2	1	3
Klebsiella pneumoniae	2	2	1	-
Proteus mirabilis	1	2	1	1
Acinetobacter baumannii	-	-	-	1
Gram-positive bacteria				
Coagulase negative Staphylococci (CNS)	6	2	1	1
Methicillin-resistant Staphylococcus aureus (MRSA)	1	-	1	2
Enterococcus faecium	3	2	1	1
Enterococcus faecalis	2	2	1	1

Table 2 Antibiotic resistance rates (%) of all the isolated bacteria among 46 patients with necrotizing pancreatitis

	E. coli	P. aeruginosa	K. pneumoniae	P. mirabilis	A. baumannii	E. faecium/faecalis	CNS	MRSA
Amoxi/Clavulanate	22	48	60	32	100	100	50	100
Amikacin	10	20	12	18	88	44	58	100
Ampi/Sulbactam	22	48	60	36	100	40	68	100
Cefotaxime	54	68	72	44	100	42	36	92
Ceftazidime	32	38	38	20	88	100	78	100
Ceftriaxone	40	60	44	42	100	100	56	92
Ciprofloxacin	24	82	62	26	92	42	22	78
Imipenem	**2**	**12**	**8**	**0**	**24**	-	-	-
Levofloxacin	24	82	52	16	100	40	20	56
Meropenem	**0**	**6**	**2**	**0**	**16**	-	-	-
Piperacillin/Tazobactam	22	48	26	16	58	90	40	100
Linezolid	-	-	-	-	-	2	0	2
Vancomycin	-	-	-	-	-	2	0	2
Rifampicin	80	100	68	88	2	2	0	68
Cotrimoxazole	32	100	40	38	100	100	0	50

MRSA: Methicillin-resistant Staphylococcus aureus; CNS: Coagulase negative Staphylococci

vs. 1 (8%), respectively. Within the infected group, those 14 subjects with evidence of systemic infection (positive blood cultures) developed more complications (Table 3) and demonstrated a higher ($p < 0.05$) mortality rate in comparison with those who had only a localized infection (limited to necrotic material, bile or drainage fluids): 4 (28%) vs. 2 (10%), respectively.

Discussion

In the present study, we examined pancreatic and systemic infections in patients with necrotizing pancreatitis. In keeping with previous studies, the prevalence of infections in this setting usually correlates with the extent of pancreatic necrosis [9,10].

In our experience, comprehensive rate of infection was 74%, with an overall prevalence of bloodstream infections of 30% and a rate of localized infections within pancreatic necrotic areas exceeding 40%. Noor et al. [11] observed pancreatic infections in 37.3% of patients

Table 3 Complications developed among patients with evidence of systemic or localized infection

	Bloodstream infection N = 14	Infection of necrotic tissue/bile/drainage fluids N = 20
Pleural effusion	4 (28%)	2 (10%)
Pericardial effusion	3 (21%)	1 (5%)
Pneumonia	3 (21%)	0
Cerebral abscess	1 (7%)	0
Septic shock	3 (21%)	1 (5%)
DIC	1 (7%)	0

DIC: Disseminated Intravascular Coagulation

and extrapancreatic infections in 62.7% of patients with severe acute pancreatitis.

In a study by Garg et al. [12], extrapancreatic bacterial infections were found in 31.7% of 63 patients. Bourgaux et al. [13] reported extrapancreatic infections in 25% of their patients. The most common sites of infection were the peritoneal fluid (26.8%) and blood (24.4%). Finally, in a recent study by Besselink et al. [14], bacteremia was reported only in 13.4% of the enrolled cases.

Similarly to our data, in patients with pancreatic infections monomicrobial infections were reported to be more common than polymicrobial ones [11].

The most common mechanism for early infection in acute necrotizing pancreatitis involves bacterial translocation from the gut. This could explain the high frequency of pancreatic and systemic infections by Escherichia *coli* we found in our study. Recently, Su et al. [15] described Escherichia *coli* to be the most common microbe responsible for infection in patients with severe acute pancreatitis.

Infections with Gram-positive organisms could occur later due to nosocomial bloodstream spread [11]. Actually, a progressive shift from Gram-negative to Gram-positive organisms might occur either associated to the increasing length of hospital stay or related to the administration of prophylactic antibiotics mainly targeting Gram-negative bacteria [14].

Previous studies emphasized the role of pancreatic infections as unfavorable predictors of patient clinical outcome. Noor et al. [11] reported mortality to be significantly higher in patients with pancreatic infections. Also, in the study by Besselink et al. [14] patients with infected pancreatic necrotic areas had a higher mortality rate. Differently from them, our study showed that bacteremic infections throughout the course of necrotizing pancreatitis worsened the outcome of the disease much more than localized infections either in terms of development of complications or in terms of crude mortality rate. Actually, in the study by Besselink et al. [14] the highest mortality rates were found in those cases with concomitant pancreatic and bacteremic infection.

The results of the sensitivity pattern of the isolated microorganisms suggest that carbapenems should be evaluated for empirical treatment in those patients with necrotizing pancreatitis who develop a clear-cut evidence of systemic or localized bacterial infection.

Competing interests
The authors declare that they have no competing interests.

Authors' contributions
BC: conception and design, interpretation of data, statistical analysis, critical revision, given final approval of the version to be published. MRP: acquisition of data, drafting the manuscript, statistical analysis, given final approval of the version to be published. SB: acquisition of data, given final approval of the version to be published. RF: acquisition of data, given final approval of the version to be published. MDV: acquisition of data, given final approval of the version to be published. GZ: acquisition of data, given final approval of the version to be published. AC: acquisition of data, given final approval of the version to be published. GN: acquisition of data, drafting the manuscript, given final approval of the version to be published. AZ: interpretation of data, critical revision, given final approval of the version to be published.

Authors' information
BC: Associate Professor of Infectious Diseases at University of Catania
MRP: Resident in Infectious Diseases at University of Catania
SB: Full Professor of Surgery at University of Catania
RF: Resident in Surgery at University of Catania
MDV: Assistant Professor of Surgery at University of Catania
GZ: Associate Professor of Surgery at University of Catania
AC: Associate Professor of Surgery at University of Catania
GN: Assistant Professor of Infectious Diseases at University of Catania
AZ: Associate Professor of Surgery at University of Catania

Declarations
Publication of this article was funded by the Department of Clinical and Molecular Biomedicine, University of Catania.
This article has been published as part of *BMC Surgery* Volume 13 Supplement 2, 2013: Proceedings from the 26th National Congress of the Italian Society of Geriatric Surgery. The full contents of the supplement are available online at http://www.biomedcentral.com/bmcsurg/supplements/13/S2

Authors' details
[1]Department of Clinical and Molecular Biomedicine, Division of Infectious Diseases, University of Catania, 95125 Catania, Italy. [2]Department of Surgery, General Surgery Unit, University of Catania, 95100 Catania, Italy.

References
1. Gloor B, Muller CA, Worni M, Stahel PF, Redaelli C, Uhl W, Buchler MW: Pancreatic infection in severe pancreatitis: the role of fungus and multiresistant organisms. *Arch Surg* 2001, 136(5):592-596.
2. Beger HG, Bittner R, Block S, Buchler M: Bacterial contamination of pancreatic necrosis: a prospective clinical study. *Gastroenterology* 1986, 91(2):433-438.
3. Schmid SW, Uhl W, Friess H, Malfertheiner P, Buchler MW: The role of infection in acute pancreatitis. *Gut* 1999, 45(2):311-316.
4. Isenmann R, Rau B, Beger HG: Bacterial infection and extent of necrosis are determinants of organ failure in patients with acute necrotizing pancreatitis. *Br J Surg* 1999, 86(8):1020-1024.
5. Gerzof SG, Banks PA, Robbins AH, Johnson WC, Spechler SJ, Wetzner SM, Snider JM, Langevin RE, Jay ME: Early diagnosis of pancreatic infection by computed tomography guided aspiration. *Gastroenterology* 1987, 93(6):1315-1320.
6. De Beaux AC, Palmer KR, Carter DC: Factors influencing morbidity and mortality in acute pancreatitis: an analysis of 279 cases. *Gut* 1995, 37(1):121-126.
7. Capurso G, Zerboni G, Signoretti M, Valente R, Stigliano S, Piciucchi M, Delle Fave G: Role of the gut barrier in acute pancreatitis. *J Clin Gastroenterol* 2012, 46(suppl):S46-51.
8. Mir MA, Bali BS, Mir RA, Wani H: Assessment of the severity of acute pancreatitis by contrast-enhanced computerized tomography in 350 patients. *Ulus Travma Acil Cerrahi Derg* 2013, 19(2):103-108.
9. Babu RY, Gupta R, Kang M, Bhasin DK, Rana SS, Singh R: Predictors of surgery in patients with severe acute pancreatitis managed by the step-up approach. *Ann Surg* 2013, 257(4):737-750.
10. Khan GM, Li JJ, Tenner S: Association of extent and infection of pancreatic necrosis with organ failure and death in acute necrotizing pancreatitis. *Clin Gastroenterol Hepatol* 2005, 3(8):829.
11. Noor MT, Radhakrishna Y, Kochhar R, Ray P, Wig JD, Sinha SK, Singh K: Bacteriology of infection in severe acute pancreatitis. *J Pancreas* 2011, 12(1):19-25.
12. Garg PK, Khanna S, Bohidar NP, Kapil A, Tandon RK: Incidence, spectrum and antibiotic sensitivity pattern of bacterial infections among patients with acute pancreatitis. *J Gastroenterol Hepatol* 2001, 16(9):1055-1059.
13. Bourgaux JF, Defez C, Muller L, Vivancos J, Prudhomme M, Navarro F, Pouderoux P, Sotto A: Infectious complications, prognostic factors and assessment of antiinfectious management of 212 consecutive patients with acute pancreatitis. *Gastroenterol Clin Biol* 2007, 31(4):431-435.
14. Besselink MG, van Santvoort HC, Boermeester MA, Nieuwenhuijs VB, van Goor H, Dejong CH, Schaapherder AF, Gooszen HG, Dutch Acute Pancreatitis Study Group: Timing and impact of infections in acute pancreatitis. *Br J Surg* 2009, 96(3):267-273.
15. Su MS, Lin M, Zhao Q, Liu Z, He L, Jia N: Clinical study of distribution and drug resistance of pathogens in patients with severe acute pancreatitis. *Chin Med J* 2012, 125(10):1772-1776.

The short- and long-term outcomes of radical antegrade modular pancreatosplenectomy for adenocarcinoma of the body and tail of the pancreas

Masaaki Murakawa[1†], Toru Aoyama[1*†], Masahiro Asari[1], Yusuke Katayama[1], Koichiro Yamaoku[1], Amane Kanazawa[1], Akio Higuchi[1], Manabu Shiozawa[1], Satoshi Kobayashi[2], Makoto Ueno[2], Manabu Morimoto[2], Naoto Yamamoto[3], Takaki Yoshikawa[1], Yasushi Rino[3], Munetaka Masuda[3] and Soichiro Morinaga[1]

Abstract

Background: Radical antegrade modular pancreatosplenectomy (RAMPS) is a relatively new modification of the standard distal pancreatosplenectomy. In this method, dissection proceeds from right-to-left to achieve negative posterior resection margins. However, short-term and long-term outcomes of RAMPS for pancreatic cancer have not yet been clarified. The aim of this study is to evaluate short-term and long-term outcomes in the patients who have undergone RAMPS.

Methods: Consecutive 49 patients were selected from the retrospective database of the Kanagawa Cancer Center from 2000 to 2014. Data from the operative notes, pathology reports, postoperative data, and outpatient data (recurrence and survival) were entered into the database.

Results: All patients were undergone anterior RAMPS. The median operation time was 278 min (range from 140 to 625 mins). The median blood loss in operation was 850 ml (range from 60 to 2790 ml). The overall incidence of morbidity was 51.4 % and the incidence of mortality was 0 %. Forty-one patients (83.7 %) had negative resection margins. The mean number of lymph nodes harvested was 15 and 27 patients had lymph node metastasis. After the median follow-up period was 41.1 months, 1-year and 3-year overall survival rates were 84.1 and 38.6 %, respectively. Median overall survival was 22.6 months.

Conclusions: The present study results suggested that RAMPS procedure might be safe and feasible without an increase in morbidity and morbidity and have survival benefit compared with standard DP.

Keywords: RAMPS, Body and tail pancreatic adenocarcinoma, Pancreatosplenectomy

Background

Pancreatic cancer, with a five-year survival rate of 5–10 %, is the fourth leading cause of cancer-related death in developed countries [1]. Complete resection is essential for cure. Distal pancreatectomy (DP) has been the standard procedure for the resection of tumors of the body and tail of the pancreas for over 100 years [2].

Adenocarcinoma of the pancreatic body and tail are as aggressive as pancreatic head tumors in terms of local invasion and their propensity for lymph node metastasis. To achieve a cure, it is therefore essential to perform a complete resection of the tumor with a margin of normal tissue and to resect the regional lymph nodes. However, the traditional approach of left-to-right pancreatosplenectomy is associated with a high rate of tangential margin positivity [3, 4], and is not based on the lymphatic drainage of the organ.

Strasberg et al. [2, 3] described an operative technique that allows for a more complete dissection of posterior

* Correspondence: t-aoyama@lilac.plala.or.jp
†Equal contributors
[1]Department of Gastrointestinal Surgery, Kanagawa Cancer Center, 2-3-2 Nakao, Asahi-Ku, Yokohama 241-8515, Japan
Full list of author information is available at the end of the article

margin and which incorporates lymph node mapping for the resection of all of the regional nodes. Radical antegrade modular pancreatosplenectomy (RAMPS) is a relatively new modification of the standard distal pancreatosplenectomy procedure. In this method, dissection proceeds from right-to-left in 1 of 2 posterior dissection planes to achieve negative posterior resection margins. The accompanying N1 lymph node dissection is based on the established anatomy of lymph node drainage of this part of the pancreas. Recently, some literatures had been published about surgical outcomes of the RAMPS [5, 6], however, outcomes of RAMPS in the treatment of pancreatic cancer remain to be clarified.

The aim of the present study is to evaluate the short-term and long-term outcomes of 49 patients who underwent RAMPS and to compare the results with the results of previously published surgical case series in which open and laparoscopic procedures were performed in patients with adenocarcinoma of the pancreatic body and tail.

Methods
Patients
The patients were selected from the retrospective database of the Kanagawa Cancer Center from 2000 to 2014. The patients were selected according to the following criteria: (1) a histologically proven pancreatic adenocarcinoma located in the body and tail of pancreas according to the seventh edition of the International Union Against Cancer (UICC) TNM [7]; (2) the patients underwent distal pancreatosplenectomy as the primary treatment for pancreatic adenocarcinoma; (3) the patients underwent surgery that consisted of dissection of more than the N1 lymph nodes and which achieved a curative or R1 resection; (4) the patients did not have synchronous or metachronous malignancies. Patients with pancreatic cancer derived from intraductal papillary mucinous neoplasms, mucinous cystic neoplasms, and neuroendocrine tumors were excluded from the present study.

Procedure
We performed the RAMPS procedure in patients with adenocarcinoma of the pancreatic body and tail. The initial dissection in the RAMPS procedure begins medially. The splenic artery and vein are ligated and the neck of the pancreas is transected. The dissection continues posteriorly to the aorta at the celiac and superior mesenteric trunks. The resection plane is decided based on the progression of cancer. In patients in whom the tumor appears to penetrate the adrenal gland (or more deeply), the plane of dissection is deepened to the posterior plane behind the adrenal gland.

Perioperative care
In principle, all of the patients received the same perioperative care. In brief, the patients were allowed to eat until midnight on the day before the surgery and were required to drink the contents of two 500-ml plastic bottles containing oral rehydration solution until 3 h before surgery. The nasogastric tube was removed on postoperative day 1 after surgery. Oral intake was initiated on POD 2, beginning with water and an oral nutritional supplement. The patients began to eat solid food on POD 5 (starting with rice gruel and soft food on POD 3 and advancing in three steps to regular food intake on POD 7). The patients were discharged when they had achieved adequate pain relief and soft food intake, had returned to their preoperative level of mobility and exhibited normal laboratory data.

Adjuvant chemotherapy
Based on the results of CONKO-001 [8], the patients received gemcitabine adjuvant treatment from 2007 to 2011. Treatment with gemcitabine was initiated within eight weeks after surgery. The patients received a weekly dose of 1,000 mg/m^2 for three weeks, followed by one week of rest. S-1 chemotherapy was started within 10 weeks after surgery. Based on the results of JASPAC-01, the patients received S-1 adjuvant treatment from 2011 to 2014 [9]. The patients received S-1 (40 mg/m^2 of body-surface area) twice a day for four weeks, followed by two weeks of rest as one course (six-week schedule) or two weeks followed by one week of rest as one course (three-week schedule). In principle, all patients continued gemcitabine or S-1 treatment for six months.

Follow up
The patients were followed up at outpatient clinics. The levels of the CEA and CA19-9 tumor markers were measured at least every three months for five years. All patients underwent CT examinations every three months during the first three years after surgery; CT examinations were then performed every six months until five years after surgery.

Evaluations and statistical analysis
Overall survival was calculated from the date of first surgery to the date of death by any cause or the last day of follow-up. The two groups were compared by unpaired Student's t-test or the X^2 test. P values of <0.05 were considered to be statistically significant. The data are presented as medians ± ranges. Survival curves were calculated using the Kaplan-Meier method and compared using the log-rank test. This study was approved by the Institutional Review Board of Kanagawa Cancer Center

(2015.epidemiologic study 32-1). This study was in compliance with the Declaration of Helsinki.

Results

The background of the patients

Forty-nine patients were eligible for inclusion in the present study. The median patient age was 68 years (range: 46-86 years). Thirty-one patients were male, and 16 were female. The median follow-up period was 41.1 months (range: 5.6-98.3 months). Forty-six patients received adjuvant chemotherapy after surgery (gemcitabine adjuvant chemotherapy [$n = 23$], gemcitabine plus S-1 adjuvant chemotherapy [$n = 1$], and S-1 adjuvant chemotherapy [$n = 22$]. Three patients refused to undergo adjuvant chemotherapy.

Surgical findings and complications

All of the patients underwent anterior RAMPS. The median operation time was 278 min (range: 140–625 min). The median operative blood loss was 850 ml (range: 60–2790 ml). Blood transfusion was required in 11 of 49 patients (22.4 %). Postoperative complications occurred in 20 patients (40.8 %). Table 1 showed the operative findings and surgical complications. The surgical complications were graded according to the Clavien-Dindo classification system [10, 11]: grade 2 complications occurred in 18 patients (36.7 %), a grade 3a complication occurred in one patient (2.1 %), and a grade 3b occurred in one patient (2.1 %). The mean hospital stay was 21 days (range: 8–57 days).

Table 1 Operative findings and surgical complications

Operative findings		
Operation time (min)		257 (140–625)
Estimated blood loss		610 (60–2790)
Transfusion (%)		6 (15.3 %)
Length of hospital stay (day)		21 (8–57)
Surgical complications		
Clavien-Dindo Grade II	Pancreatic fistula	14 (28.6 %)
	Delayed gastric empty	3 (6.1 %)
	Surgical site infection	1 (2.1 %)
Clavien-Dindo Grade IIIa	Intraabdominal abscess	1 (2.1 %)
Clavien-Dindo Grade IIIb	Intraabdominal abscess	1 (2.1 %)
Total		20 (40.8 %)
Resection of tumor		
R0		39
R1		10
DPM positive		7/39 (17.9 %)

Pathological findings

Three patients had T1 tumors, 1 patient had a T2 tumor, 37 patients had T3 tumors and 4 patients had T4 tumors. Twenty-seven of the 49 patients had positive lymph nodes (55 %). According to American Joint Committee on Cancer Staging of Tumors, 3 patients had Stage IA disease, 15 patients had Stage IIA, 23 patients had Stage IIB, and 8 patients had Stage III. The tumors ranged from 5–83 mm in diameter (mean diameter; 38 mm). Thirteen patients had well-differentiated tumors, 22 patients had moderately differentiated tumors, 8 patients had poorly differentiated tumors, 2 patients had anaplastic carcinoma, 2 patients had papillary adenocarcinoma, and 1 patient had mucinous and adenosquamous carcinoma. The mean number of lymph nodes harvested was 15, 27 patients had lymph node metastasis. Forty-one patients (83.7 %) had negative resection margins.

Overall survival and recurrence free survival

At the time of writing, 25 of the 49 patients (51 %) are alive and 24 patients (49 %) have died. Nineteen of the 25 surviving patients (38.8 %) showed no evidence of recurrence, while 6 (12.2 %) patients are alive with recurrence. The median overall survival was 22.6 months. The 1-year and 3-year overall survival rates were 84.1 and 38.6 %, respectively (Fig. 1). Thirty of 49 patients experienced recurrence. The sites of recurrence included the liver ($n = 6$), the lymph nodes ($n = 11$), the pancreatic bed ($n = 6$), the peritoneum ($n = 5$), and the lungs ($n = 1$). Among 11 lymph nodes recurrences patients, 8 patients recurred in para-aortic lymph node, 3 patients recurred in para-superior mesenteric artery lymph node.

Discussion

We evaluated the short-term and long-term results of the RAMPS procedure for pancreatic cancer. The overall incidence of morbidity was 51.4 %, while the incidence of mortality was 0 %. Moreover, median survival was 22.6 months and 5-year overall survival was 27 %. These results suggest the safety and feasibility of the RAMPS procedure and indicate the possibility that it could be performed without an increase in morbidity or mortality and that it might offer a survival benefit in comparison to standard DP.

Although postoperative complications occurred in 20 of the 49 patients (40.8 %), there were no postoperative or in-hospital deaths. Pancreatic fistula was the most frequently diagnosed complication, followed by abdominal abscess. The overall incidence of morbidity and mortality were similar to other RAMPS studies. Mitchem et al. [12] evaluated the long-term results of RAMPS among 47 patients who underwent anteroposterior RAMPS. They found that the overall in-hospital mortality rate

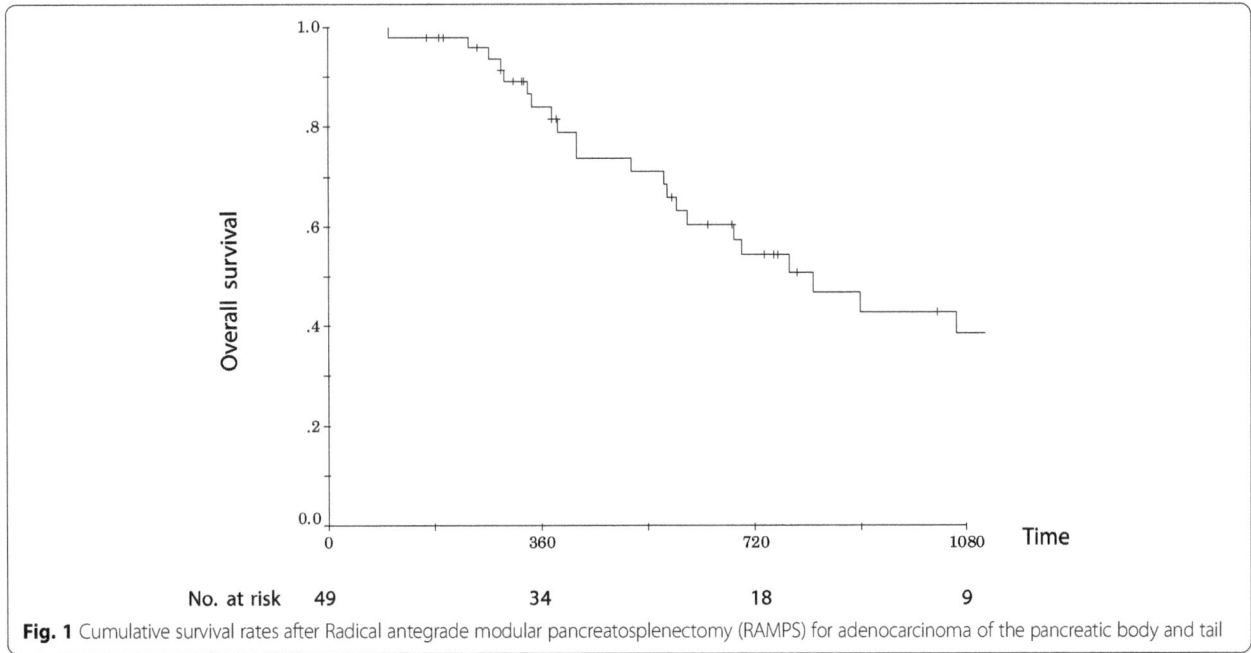

Fig. 1 Cumulative survival rates after Radical antegrade modular pancreatosplenectomy (RAMPS) for adenocarcinoma of the pancreatic body and tail

was 0 %, and that the morbidity rate was 39 % (18 patients). In addition, Chang et al. [13] evaluated the surgical outcome of RAMPS in 24 consecutive patients. They demonstrated that the overall in-hospital mortality rate was 0 % and that the morbidity rate was 37.5 % (9 patients). Previous studies have shown the incidence of the morbidity after conventional distal pancreatomy to be 23–58 % [14, 15]. These findings suggest the safety and feasibility of the RAMPS procedure and indicated that it is not associated with increased morbidity or mortality.

After the median follow-up period was 41.1 months, 1-year and 3-year overall survival rates were 84.1 and 38.6 %, respectively. Median overall survival was 22.6 months. Similar results were observed in the previous RAMPS studies. Table 2 showed the comparison of other published series of RAMPS and standard pancreatosplenectomy.

Mitchem et al. reported a median survival period of 26 months and a 5-year overall survival rate of 35 % in 47 patients who underwent anteroposterior RAMPS. In the same study, they reported that 23 patients who underwent RAMPS more than 5 years before the date of last follow-up, had a 5-year survival rate of 30.4 %. RAMPS appeared to offer superior survival in comparison to standard DP at high volume centers; the previously reported 5-year survival rates have ranged from 10–19 %. The first possible reason is that the negative margin rate was higher in the RAMPS procedures than in standard DP. When comparing with previous reports, the negative margin rate was 80–90 % in the previous RAMPS studies, while the negative margin was 70–80 % in the standard DP studies (Table 2). A second possibility is that different numbers of lymph nodes were harvested in the RAMPS and standard DP

Table 2 Comparison of published data of radical antegrade modular pancreatosplenectomy in other studies

Author (year)	Ref No.	Approach	Number of cases	Morbidity	Mortality	Harvest lymph nodes	Negative surgical margin	Median survival (months)	Five-year survival
Brennan (1996) [4]	4	Standard	34	23 %	0 %	13	68 %	12	14 %
Mitchem (2012) [12]	15	RAMPS	47	39 %	0 %	18.0	91.0 %	26	36 %
Chang (2012) [13]	16	RAMPS	24	37.5 %	0 %	20.9	91.7 %	18.2	NA
Latorre (2013) [17]	20	RAMPS	8	25 %	0 %	20.7	87.5 %	14	26 %
Trottman (2014) [16]	19	RAMPS	6	50 %	0 %	11.2	100 %	NA	NA
Kitagawa (2014) [5]	5	RAMPS	24	58 %	0 %	24	88 %	NA	53 %
Park (2014) [6]	6	Standard	54	22.2 %	0 %	9	85.1 %	NA	12.0 %
		RAMPS	38	18.4 %	0 %	14	89.5 %	NA	40.1 %
Our study (2015)	–	RAMPS	49	41 %	0 %	15	83.7 %	22.6	27 %

procedures. Trottman et al. [16] examined 26 cases in which RAMPS and standard resection was performed to identify differences in the clinicopathological outcomes of the patients. They demonstrated a significant difference in the mean number of lymph nodes that were removed in standard resection (4.3) and RAMPS (11.2) ($P = 0.03$). Moreover, La Torre et al. [17] compared the clinicopathological outcomes of 25 patients who underwent RAMPS or standard resection. They too demonstrated a significant difference in the mean number of lymph nodes that were removed in standard resection (16.2) and RAMPS (20.7) ($P = 0.04$).

The RAMPS procedure should be tested against standard DP in a randomized trial. According to Mitchem et al., a prospective randomized, controlled study should be performed to better determine the long-term outcomes. They calculated that in order to compare the two treatments with 5-year survival rates of 20 and 35 %, a total of 556 patients (228 patients per group) would be required to detect a difference at the 95 % CI. Such numbers would be difficult to obtain in a single institution because resections of adenocarcinoma of the pancreatic body and tail are uncommon in comparison to resections of the pancreatic head.

Special attention is required when interpreting the current results, because several potential limitations are associated with the present study. First, the present study was a retrospective analysis which was performed in a single institution. We cannot deny the possibility that our findings were observed by chance. Second, there was a selection bias in the patients in this series. Surgeons often avoid performing pancreatomy in the some patients, because pancreatectomy itself has a 1–1.5 % mortality rate and a 40–60 % morbidity rate. Thus, the fact that some of the patients in the present study received pancreatectomy could, in and of itself, be a potential bias. In addition, our hospital is a specialized cancer center. The third issue is the follow-up period. In our series, the median follow-up period was approximately 36 months. Our follow-up period may not have been sufficient to allow definite conclusions to be drawn. Considering these limitations, the current results should be validated in other series with a larger number of patients.

Conclusions

The results indicate that the RAMPS procedure might be safe feasible for the treatment of pancreatic cancer and that it might offer a survival benefit in comparison to standard DP.

Competing interests
The authors declare that they have no competing interests.

Authors' contributions
Our manuscript has 16 authors. Details of contributions by each author are as follows; M. Murakawa actively involved in this study especially in statistical design. Concept and clinical design were conducted by 2 surgeons (M. Murakawa and T. Aoyama). Acquisition of data was done by all physician. Interpretation of data, and drafting the article was done by M. Murakawa and T. Aoyama. Finally, this article was revised and approved by all 16 investigators. Thus, all 16 authors actively participated in this study.

Acknowledgements
We acknowledge Dr. Brian Quinn for revising English. No external funding was received for this manuscript.

Author details
[1]Department of Gastrointestinal Surgery, Kanagawa Cancer Center, 2 3 2 Nakao, Asahi-Ku, Yokohama 241-8515, Japan. [2]Department of Gastrointestinal medicine, Kanagawa Cancer Center, Yokohama, Japan. [3]Department of Surgery, Yokohama City University, Yokohama, Japan.

References
1. Raimondi S, Maisonneuve P, Lowenfels AB. Epidemiology of pancreatic cancer: an overview. Nat Rev Gastroenterol Hepatol. 2009;6(12):699–708.
2. Strasberg SM, Drebin JA, Linehan D. Radical antegrade modular pancreatosplenectomy. Surgery. 2003;133(5):521–7.
3. Strasberg SM, Linehan DC, Hawkins WG. Radical antegrade modular pancreatosplenectomy procedure for adenocarcinoma of the body and tail of the pancreas: ability to obtain negative tangential margins. J Am Coll Surg. 2007;204(2):244–9.
4. Brennan MF, Moccia RD, Klimstra D. Management of adenocarcinoma of the body and tail of the pancreas. Ann Surg. 1996;223(5):506–11. discussion 511–502.
5. Kitagawa H, Tajima H, Nakagawara H, Makino I, Miyashita T, Terakawa H, et al. A modification of radical antegrade modular pancreatosplenectomy for adenocarcinoma of the left pancreas: significance of en bloc resection including the anterior renal fascia. World J Surg. 2014;38(9):2448–54.
6. Park HJ, You DD, Choi DW, Heo JS, Choi SH. Role of radical antegrade modular pancreatosplenectomy for adenocarcinoma of the body and tail of the pancreas. World J Surg. 2014;38(1):186–93.
7. Scoazec JY, Sabourin JC. 2010: The seventh edition of the TNM classification. Ann Pathol. 2010;30(1):2–6.
8. Oettle H, Post S, Neuhaus P, Gellert K, Langrehr J, Ridwelski K, et al. Adjuvant chemotherapy with gemcitabine vs observation in patients undergoing curative-intent resection of pancreatic cancer: a randomized controlled trial. JAMA. 2007;297(3):267–77.
9. Maeda A, Boku N, Fukutomi A, Kondo S, Kinoshita T, Nagino M, et al. Randomized phase III trial of adjuvant chemotherapy with gemcitabine versus S-1 in patients with resected pancreatic cancer: Japan Adjuvant Study Group of Pancreatic Cancer (JASPAC-01). Jpn J Clin Oncol. 2008;38(3):227–9.
10. Clavien PA, Sanabria JR, Strasberg SM. Proposed classification of complications of surgery with examples of utility in cholecystectomy. Surgery. 1992;111(5):518–26.
11. Dindo D, Demartines N, Clavien PA. Classification of surgical complications: a new proposal with evaluation in a cohort of 6336 patients and results of a survey. Ann Surg. 2004;240(2):205–13.
12. Mitchem JB, Hamilton N, Gao F, Hawkins WG, Linehan DC, Strasberg SM. Long-term results of resection of adenocarcinoma of the body and tail of the pancreas using radical antegrade modular pancreatosplenectomy procedure. J Am Coll Surg. 2012;214(1):46–52.
13. Chang YR, Han SS, Park SJ, Lee SD, Yoo TS, Kim YK, et al. Surgical outcome of pancreatic cancer using radical antegrade modular pancreatosplenectomy procedure. World J Gastroenterol. 2012;18(39):5595–600.
14. Shoup M, Conlon KC, Klimstra D, Brennan MF. Is extended resection for adenocarcinoma of the body or tail of the pancreas justified? J Gastrointest Surg. 2003;7(8):946–52. discussion 952.

8

Pancreaticogastrostomy in pure laparoscopic pancreaticoduodenectomy—A novel pancreatic-gastric anastomosis technique

Masamichi Matsuda*, Shusuke Haruta, Hisashi Shinohara, Kazunari Sasaki and Goro Watanabe

Abstract

Background: Although many surgical procedures are now routinely performed laparoscopically, pure laparoscopic pancreaticoduodenectomy (LPD) is not commonly performed because of the technical difficulty of pancreatic resection and the associated reconstruction procedures. Several pancreatic-enteric anastomosis techniques for LPD have been reported, but most are adaptations of open procedures. To accomplish pure LPD, we consider it necessary to establish new pancreatic-enteric anastomosis techniques that are specifically developed for LPD and are safe and feasible to perform.

Results: One patient developed a postoperative pancreatic fistula (International Study Group of Pancreatic Fistula criteria, grade B) and subsequent postoperative delayed gastric emptying (International Study Group of Pancreatic Surgery criteria, grade C). No other major complications occurred. We developed a novel pancreatic-gastric anastomosis technique that enabled us to safely perform pure LPD. The main pancreatic duct was stented with a 4-Fr polyvinyl catheter during pancreatic resection. A small hole was created in the posterior wall of the stomach and was bluntly dilated. A 5-cm incision was made in the anterior stomach, and the pancreatic drainage tube was passed into the stomach through the hole in the posterior wall. The remnant pancreas was pulled into the stomach, and was easily positioned and secured in place with only four to six sutures between the pancreatic capsule and the gastric mucosa. We used this technique to perform pure LPD in five patients between December 2012 and July 2013.

Conclusions: Our new technique is technically easy and provides secure fixation between the gastric wall and the pancreas. This technique does not require main pancreatic duct dilatation, and the risk of intra-abdominal abscess formation due to postoperative pancreatic fistula may be minimized. Although this technique requires further investigation as it may increase the risk of delayed gastric emptying, it may be a useful method of performing pancreaticogastrostomy in pure LPD.

Keywords: Laparoscopy, Pancreaticoduodenectomy, Pancreatic surgery, Laparoscopic pancreaticoduodenectomy, Pancreaticogastrostomy, Pancreatic-enteric anastomosis

* Correspondence: eastcliff.on.sea@gmail.com
Department of Surgery, Toranomon Hospital, 2-2-2 Toranomon Minato-ku, Tokyo 105-8470, Japan

Background

Although many surgical procedures are now routinely performed laparoscopically, pure laparoscopic pancreaticoduodenectomy (LPD) is not widely performed because of the technical difficulty of pancreatic resection and the complexity of reconstruction procedures. As postoperative pancreatic anastomotic leakage carries an increased risk of intra-abdominal hemorrhage and a high mortality rate [1, 2], some surgeons avoid intracorporeal reconstruction, and use a hybrid laparoscopic-open approach to increase the safety and the feasibility of pancreatic anastomosis [3, 4]. Although a hybrid approach may reduce operative risk, it also results in loss of the potential advantages of minimally invasive surgery. Several reports have described techniques for laparoscopic pancreaticojejunostomy (PJ), but most are adaptations of open procedures [5–10]. Just as in open surgery, LPD carries an increased risk of postoperative pancreatic fistula formation in patients with soft pancreatic texture or a small pancreatic duct. This increased risk may be attributed to the technical difficulty of performing the traditional duct-to-mucosa anastomosis in the pancreatic-enteric reconstruction. Magnification laparoscopy can be useful for this duct-to-mucosa anastomosis, but the restricted range of motion of laparoscopic forceps sometimes makes it difficult to perform the anastomosis. There have been an increasing number of robotic PD which may facilitate execution of complex reconstruction, but robotic PD is feasible only for highly selected patients [11]. We therefore consider it necessary to establish novel pancreatic-enteric anastomosis techniques that are simple, feasible to perform, provide secure fixation between the enteric wall and the pancreas, and are specifically developed for LPD. We describe herein our novel pancreatic-gastric anastomosis technique (PG) in pure LPD.

Methods

From December 2012 to July 2013, we used our technique in five patients. Patients were eligible for this procedure if they were non-obese with no previous upper abdominal surgery. Three patients had intraductal papillary mucinous neoplasm, one had carcinoma of the papilla of Vater, and one had solid pseudopapillary neoplasm. Before surgery, the tumors were fully evaluated by abdominal computed tomography, magnetic resonance imaging, and endoscopic ultrasonography. All the tumors were restricted to the pancreatic head or periampullary region. The patients were three males and two females with a median age of 64 years (range, 47–76 years) and a median body mass index of 22.2 kg/m^2 (range, 17.4–25.5 kg/m^2). The patients were all East Asian and lived in the eastern part of Japan. The advantages, disadvantages, and potential risks of the surgical procedure were explained to patients and informed consent was obtained. Data recording and evaluation was approved by the ethics committee of Toranomon Hospital and was in accordance with the Declaration of Helsinki.

Technique

Surgery was performed under general anesthesia with the patient in the supine position with the legs apart. The first 12-mm umbilical trocar was inserted for an electrolaparoscope (LTF-VH, Olympus Medical Systems, Tokyo, Japan) using a mini-laparotomy technique, and a pneumoperitoneum was established with a CO_2 pressure of 10 mmHg. Three 12-mm trocars (left subcostal and bilateral supraumbilical pararectal) and one 5-mm trocar (right subcostal) were placed in the abdominal wall. The surgeon stood on the right side of the patient during reconstruction. After mobilization of the head of the pancreas, a tunnel was formed between the posterior aspect of the neck of the pancreas and the superior mesenteric and portal veins. If possible, the tunnel was extended 2–3 cm towards the body of the pancreas in preparation for easy reconstruction. The body of the pancreas was then slowly and gently dissected using laparoscopic coagulation shears (SonoSurg™, Olympus Medical Systems). The main pancreatic duct was identified, and was cut across half its width with scissors and then stented with a 4-Fr polyvinyl catheter (MD-41513 pancreatic duct tube, 65 cm; Sumitomo Bakelite, Tokyo, Japan). The tube was firmly attached to the distal pancreas in two places with 3–0 absorbable sutures (Vicril™ 3–0, Ethicon).

Reconstruction

After excision of the proximal portion of the pancreas, the specimen was removed via the umbilical trocar site, which was extended to 3 cm. The distal portion of the remnant pancreas was dissected from the splenic artery, splenic vein, and connecting tissues with laparoscopic coagulation shears, for up to 3 cm beyond the transection plane, in preparation for invagination into the stomach. Two anchoring sutures (Ti-Cron™ 3–0, Covidien) were placed in the remnant pancreas, 2 cm distal to the transection plane (Fig. 1 and Additional file 1). After deciding the site of the anastomosis (usually the posterior wall of the lower body of the stomach), a small hole was made in the gastric serosa at the planned anastomotic site by electrocautery, and the hole was bluntly dilated with forceps (Fig. 2 and Additional file 2). A 5-cm vertical incision was then made in the anterior wall of the stomach just ventral to the planned anastomotic site with laparoscopic coagulation shears (Fig. 3 and Additional file 3). The two anchoring sutures and the stenting tube were passed through the hole at the anastomotic site and pulled

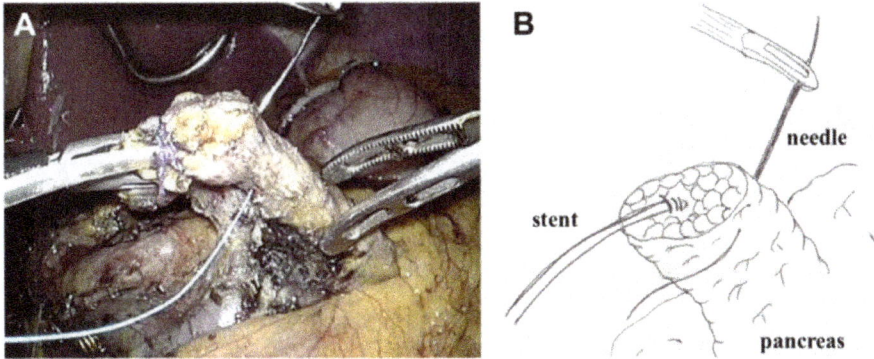

Fig. 1 Two anchoring sutures were placed in the remnant pancreas, 2 cm distal to the transection plane. The main pancreatic duct was already stented with a 4-Fr polyvinyl catheter. A: photo, B: illustration

into the stomach using forceps introduced through the gastric incision. The remnant pancreas was then pulled into the stomach through the hole at the anastomotic site and fixed in place with the anchoring sutures, taking care not to injure the pancreas (Fig. 4 and Additional file 4). After pulling the remnant pancreas 2–3 cm into the stomach, four to six interrupted sutures (Vicril™ 3–0, Ethicon) were placed between the pancreatic capsule and the gastric mucosa (Fig. 5 and Additional file 5). The stenting tube was passed through the incision in the anterior wall of the stomach, and the incision was closed with a continuous absorbable suture (PDS™ 4–0, Ethicon). The stenting tube was then passed through the abdominal wall (usually left subcostal) to form a gastrostomy (Fig. 6). Fibrin glue was placed around the PG site for protection. A prophylactic drainage tube (Multi-Channel™ Drainage Set 6.5 mm, Covidien) was placed at the pancreatic anastomosis.

Results

All the procedures were performed by the same surgeon (Table 1). The pancreatic texture was soft in all patients. The median estimated blood loss was 100 ml (range, 0–400 ml) and the median operative time was 492 min (range, 435–739 min). The median hospital stay was 35 days (range, 19–57 days). The external drainage tube was left in place for a median of 20 days after surgery (range, 18–22 days), and the drainage tube at the anastomotic site was left in place for a median of 24 days after surgery (range, 17–41 days). One patient developed a postoperative pancreatic fistula of International Study Group of Pancreatic Fistula (ISGPF) grade B [12] on postoperative day 7, and subsequently developed postoperative delayed gastric emptying of International Study Group of Pancreatic Surgery (ISGPS) grade C [13]. Both these complications resolved with conservative management. No major complications occurred in the other patients, and the postoperative follow-up period was uneventful (range, 7.7–15.5 months). All resection margins were tumor-free on frozen section examination.

Discussion

The incidence of postoperative pancreatic fistula ranges from 2 to more than 20 % after open pancreaticoduodenectomy [13], and from 1.8 to 20 % after LPD [6, 7, 9, 10]. It is important to achieve a good pancreatic-enteric anastomosis, because a postoperative pancreatic fistula may lead to major complications, prolonged hospital stay, and

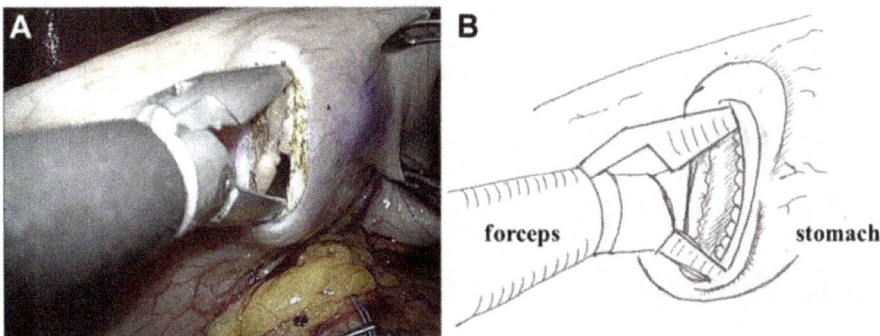

Fig. 2 A small hole was made in the gastric serosa at the planned anastomotic site, and was bluntly dilated with forceps. A: photo, B: illustration

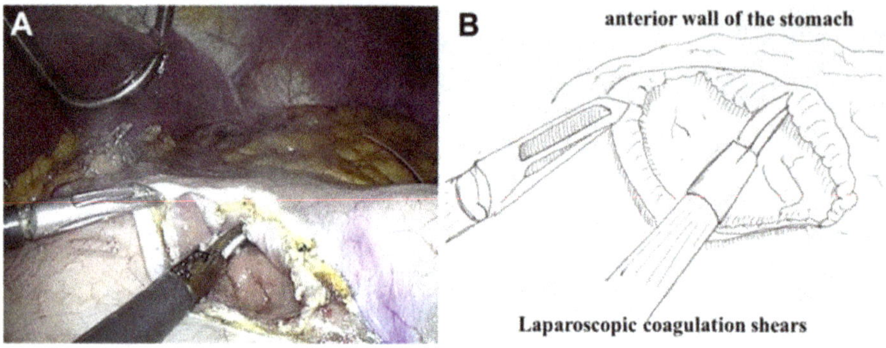

Fig. 3 A 5-cm vertical incision was made in the anterior wall of the stomach just ventral to the planned anastomotic site, using laparoscopic coagulation shears. A: photo, B: illustration

mortality [1, 2]. Minilaparotomy has been advised to ensure safe anastomosis. Although a hybrid laparoscopic-open technique may reduce operative risk, it also results in loss of the potential advantages of minimally invasive surgery. We developed a new PG technique to enable safe reconstruction in pure LPD.

Although PG has been considered an acceptable method of reconstruction after pancreaticoduodenectomy over the past 50 years, there is still controversy regarding the relative superiority of PG versus PJ in terms of outcomes. Wellner et al. reported that PG was superior to PJ in terms of postoperative pancreatic fistula formation judged according to the ISGPF criteria [14]. Also the recent meta-analysis done on PJ vs PG after PD revealed that PG seems to be superior to PJ in reducing the incidence of pancreatic fistula formation and intra-abdominal fluid collection [15–17].

The standard pancreatic-enteric anastomosis performed during LPD is PJ. Only one published case report has described reconstruction with PG in LPD [18]. In that case, the remnant pancreas was invaginated into the stomach and was fixed in place with two continuous purse-string sutures around the incision in the gastric wall using self-retaining monofilament sutures (V-Loc 180 3–0, Covidien). Our technique is relatively simpler to perform. We created a small hole in the posterior wall of the stomach and dilated it bluntly. The remnant pancreas was then pulled into the stomach, and easily positioned so that only a few sutures were required between the pancreatic capsule and gastric mucosa to hold it in place.

In LPD, reconstruction is usually performed by end-to-side PJ with duct-to-mucosa anastomosis [5–7]. Just as in open surgery, LPD carries an increased risk of pancreatic fistula formation in patients with a small pancreatic duct. This increased risk may be attributed to the technical difficulty of performing the duct-to-mucosa anastomotic portion of the pancreatic-enteric reconstruction. In such patients, magnification laparoscopy can be useful for performing duct-to-mucosa anastomosis, but the restricted range of motion of laparoscopic forceps sometimes makes this anastomosis difficult. Our technique does not require duct-to-mucosa anastomosis, and it can be easily used in patients with a small pancreatic duct.

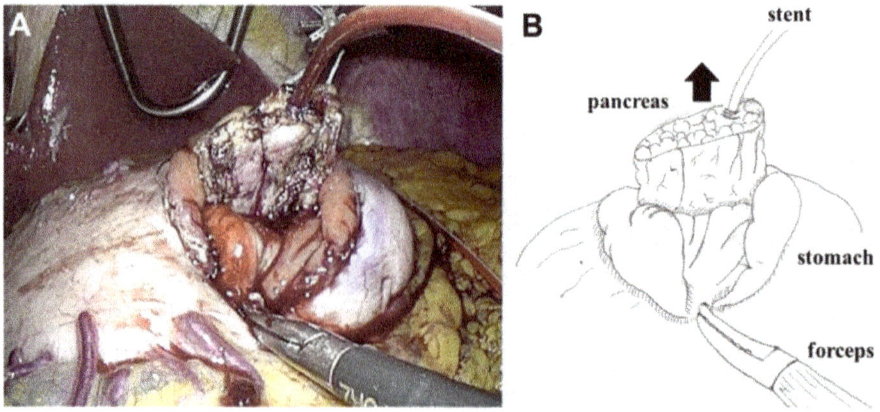

Fig. 4 The two anchoring sutures and the stenting tube were passed through the hole, and the remnant pancreas was then pulled into the stomach and fixed in place. A: photo, B: illustration

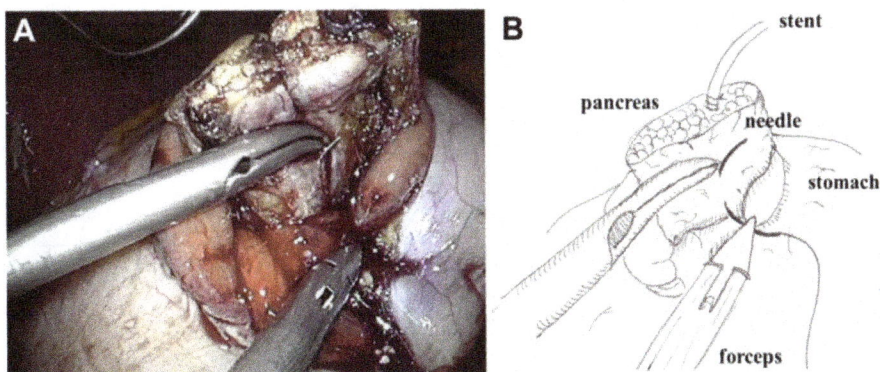

Fig. 5 After pulling the remnant pancreas 2–3 cm into the stomach, four to six interrupted sutures were placed between the pancreatic capsule and the gastric mucosa. A: photo, B: illustration

Our technique may also reduce the risk of intra-abdominal abscess formation due to minor leakage of pancreatic juice from the injured pancreatic capsule, because the sutures between the pancreas and the gastric wall are placed inside the stomach. As damage to the pancreatic capsule outside the stomach can be avoided, this technique may be safe in patients with a soft pancreatic texture.

One patient in our series developed a postoperative pancreatic fistula (ISGPF grade B). In this patient, only two sutures were placed between the pancreatic capsule and the gastric mucosa, which was probably inadequate and may have contributed to fistula formation. To reduce the risk of postoperative pancreatic fistula after PG, we suggest placement of a sufficient number of sutures between the pancreatic capsule and the gastric mucosa.

This patient also received only a short internal plastic stent across the PG site. A meta-analysis of randomized clinical trials found that placement of a stent in the pancreatic duct did not reduce the incidence of postoperative pancreatic fistula. However, subgroup analysis found that use of an external stent significantly reduced the incidence of postoperative pancreatic fistula [19]. Other randomized clinical trials found that external duct stenting after pancreaticoduodenectomy reduced the risk of clinically relevant postoperative pancreatic fistula formation [20, 21]. The majority of the selected patients of these studies used PJ for reconstruction, and subgroup analysis for external duct stenting in PG was not reported. Placement of an external stent across the PG anastomosis is not necessarily an essential part of PG, but could be used adjunct to reduce the risk of pancreatic fistula formation.

One of the disadvantages of our technique is that it may result in delayed gastric emptying, which is one of the most common postoperative complications after pancreatic surgery, occurring in 19–57 % of patients [13]. In patients with PG, gastric peristalsis is disturbed because the posterior wall of the stomach is held in place by the PG anastomosis. Additionally, incision of the anterior wall of the stomach increases the risk of delayed gastric emptying [22]. In our technique, the anterior wall of the stomach is incised, sutured, and attached to the abdominal wall by the gastrostomy, which may cause delayed gastric emptying.

The long-term oncologic and surgical outcomes after use of our procedure should be investigated, and future

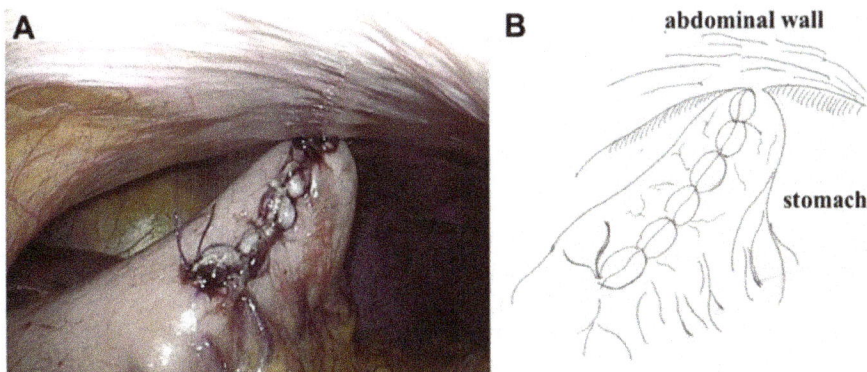

Fig. 6 The stenting tube was passed through the abdominal wall to form a gastrostomy. A: photo, B: illustration

Table 1 Patients demographics and surgical outcomes

Case	Diagnosis	ope time (min)	blood loss (ml)	stenting tube	PF (ISGPF)	DGE (ISGPS)	Length of stay (days)
1	Ampullary ca	492	0	internal	B	C	50
2	IPMN	739	350	external	0	A	57
3	IPMN	599	400	external	0	A	35
4	IPMN	435	100	external	0	A	29
5	SPN	450	100	external	0	0	19

Ampullary ca carcinoma of the ampulla of Vater, *IPMN* intraductal papillary mucinos neoplasm, *SPN* solid pseudo-papillary neoplasm, *PF* pacreatic fistula, *DGE* delayed gastric emptying

research should investigate whether LPD provides any significant advantages over other methods of performing pancreaticoduodenectomy. It is difficult to draw any sound conclusions about the safety or limitations of our technique with so little information about patient selection, but we consider our technique a relatively easy method for reconstruction in pure LPD. Our technique may also provide an alternative reconstruction method for use in a hybrid procedure. As reconstruction with PG in LPD is still a new technique, further clinical evaluation to compare outcomes between the use of PG and PJ in LPD is warranted.

Conclusions

We present a novel pancreatic-gastric anastomosis technique specifically developed for LPD. Our new technique is technically easy and provides excellent fixation between the gastric wall and pancreas. Main pancreatic duct dilatation is not required, and the risk of intra-abdominal abscess formation is minimized. Although further clinical evaluation is required, this technique is immediately clinically applicable and may serve as the basis for additional research.

Additional files

Additional file 1: Two anchoring sutures were placed in the remnant pancreas, 2 cm distal to the transection plane. The main pancreatic duct was already stented with a 4-Fr polyvinyl catheter.

Additional file 2: A small hole was made in the gastric serosa at the planned anastomotic site, and was bluntly dilated with forceps.

Additional file 3: A 5-cm vertical incision was made in the anterior wall of the stomach just ventral to the planned anastomotic site, using laparoscopic coagulation shears.

Additional file 4: The two anchoring sutures and the stenting tube were passed through the hole, and the remnant pancreas was then pulled into the stomach and fixed in place.

Additional file 5: After pulling the remnant pancreas 2–3 cm into the stomach, four to six interrupted sutures were placed between the pancreatic capsule and the gastric mucosa.

Abbreviations
LPD: Laparoscopic pancreaticoduodenectomy; PJ: Pancreaticojejunostomy; PG: Pancreaticogastrostomy; ISGPF: International Study Group of Pancreatic Fistula; ISGPS: International Study Group of Pancreatic Surgery.

Competing interests
The authors declare that they have no competing interests.

Authors' contributions
MM, SH, HS, and KS performed the surgical procedures. MM and KS collected the data, prepared the manuscript, and contributed to the analysis and interpretation of the results. GW contributed to the analysis and interpretation of the results. All authors read and approved the final manuscript.

References
1. Pratt WB, Calley MP, Vollmer Jr CM. The latent presentation of pancreatic fistulas. Br J Surg. 2009;96:641–9.
2. Fuks D, Piessen G, Huet E, Tavernier M, Zerbib P, Michot F, et al. Life-threatening postoperative pancreatic fistula (grade C) after pancreatcoduodenectomy: incidence, prognosis, and risk factors. Am J Surg. 2009;197:702–9.
3. Kimura Y, Hirata K, Mukaiya M, Mizuguchi T, Koito K, Katsuramaki T. Hand-assisted laparoscopic pylorus-preserving pancreaticoduodenectomy for pancreas head disease. Am J Surg. 2005;189:734–7.
4. Nakamura Y, Uchida E, Nomura T, Aimoto T, Matsumoto S, Tajiri T. Laparoscopic pancreatic resection: some benefits of evoluving surgical techniques. J Hepatobiliary Pancreat Surg. 2009;16:741–8.
5. Cho A, Yamamoto H, Nagata M, Nagata M, Takiguchi N, Shimada H, et al. A totally laparoscopic pylorus-preserving pancreaticoduodenectomy and reconstruction. Surg Today. 2009;39:359–62.
6. Palanivelu C, Rajan PS, Rangarajan M, Vaithiswaran V, Senthilnathan P, Parthasarathi R, et al. Evolution in techniques of laparoscopic pancreaticoduodenectomy: a decade long experience from a tertiary center. J Hepatobiliary Pancreat Surg. 2009;16:731–40.
7. Kendrick ML, Cusati D. Total laparoscopic pancreaticoduodenectomy. Arch Surg. 2010;145:19–23.
8. Gumbs AA, Gayet B, Hoffman JP. Laparoscopic whipple procedure with a two-layered pancreaticojejunostomy. Surg Endosc. 2011;25:3446–7.
9. Cho A, Yamamoto H, Kainuma O, Kainuma O, Muto Y, Park S, et al. Performing simple and safe dunking pancreaticojejunostomy using mattres sutures in pure laparoscopic pancreaticoduodenectomy. Surg Endosc. 2014;28:315–8.
10. Hughes SJ, Neichoy B, Behrns E. Laparoscopic intussuscepting pancreaticojejunostomy. J Gastrointest Surg. 2014;18:208–12.
11. Cirocchi R, Partelli S, Trastulli S, Coratti A, Parisi A. A systematic review on robotic pancreaticoduodenectomy. Surg Oncol. 2013;22:238–46.
12. Bassi C, Dervenis C, Butturini G, Fingerhut A, Yeo C, Izbicki J, et al. Postoperative pancreatic fistula: an International Study Group (ISGPF) definition. Surgery. 2005;138:8–13.
13. Wente MN, Bassi C, Dervenis C, Fingerhut A, Gouma DJ, Izbicki JR, et al. Delayed gastric emptying (DGE) after pancreatic surgery: a suggested definition by the International Study Group of Pancreas Surgery (ISGPS). Surgery. 2007;142:761–8.
14. Wellner U, Markowiec F, Fischer E, Hopt T, Keck T. Reduced postoperative pancreatic fistula rate after pancreatogastrostomy versus pancreaticojejunostomy. J Gastrointest Surg. 2009;13:745–51.
15. Chen Z, Song X, Yang D, Li Y, Xu K, He Y. Pancreaticogastrostomy versus pancreaticoduodenectomy: a meta-analysis of randomized control trials. Eur J Surg Oncol. 2014;40:1177–85.

16. Xiong JJ, Tan CL, Szatmary P, Huang W, Ke NW, Hu WM, et al. Meta-analysis of pancreaticogastrostomy versus pancreaticojejunostomy after pancreaticoduodenectoy. Br J Surg. 2014;101:1196–208.

17. Clerveus M, Moranderia-Rivas A, Picazo-Yeste J, Moreno-Sanz C. Pancreaticogastrostomy versus pancreaticojejunostomy after pancreaticoduodenectomy: a systemic review and meta-analysis of randomized controlled trials. J Gastrointest Surg. 2014;18:1693–704.

18. Keck T, Kusters S, Wellner UF, Hopt UT, Karcz KW. Total laparoscopic pancreatoduodenectomy and reconstruction via laparoscopic pancreatogastrostomy. Langenbecks Arch Surg. 2012;397:1009–12.

19. Xiong JJ, Altaf K, Mukherjee R, Huang W, Hu WM, Li A, et al. Systemic review and meta-analysis of outcomes. Br J Surg. 2012;99:1050–61.

20. Motoi F, Egawa S, Rikiyama Y, Katayose Y, Unnno M. Randomized clinical trial of external stent drainage of the pancreatic duct to reduce postoperative pancreatic fistula after pancreaticoduodenectomy. Br J Surg. 2012;99:524–31.

21. Pessaux P, Sauvanet A, Mariette C, Paye F, Muscari F, Cunha A, et al. External pancreatic duct stent decreases pancreatic fistula rate after pancreaticoduodenectomy: prospective multicenter randomized trial. Ann Surg. 2011;253:879–85.

22. Oida T, Mimatsu K, Kano H, Kawasaki A, Kuboi Y, Fukino N, et al. Horizontal vs. vertical incison on the anterior gastric wall in pancreaticogastrostomy. Hepatogastroenterology. 2012;59:2627–30.

9

The prognostic influence of intrapancreatic tumor location on survival after resection of pancreatic ductal adenocarcinoma

Dietrich A. Ruess[1], Frank Makowiec[1], Sophia Chikhladze[1], Olivia Sick[1], Hartwig Riediger[2], Ulrich T. Hopt[1] and Uwe A. Wittel[1*]

Abstract

Background: The prognosis of pancreatic ductal adenocarcinoma (PDAC) is worse when the tumor is located in the pancreatic body or tail, compared to being located in the pancreatic head. However, for localized, resectable tumors survival seems to be at least similar.

Methods: We analyzed and compared the outcome after pancreatoduodenectomy (PD) and distal pancreatectomy (DP) for PDAC at our institution. Clinical, pathological and survival data from patients undergoing pancreatic resection for PDAC 1994–2014 were explored retrospectively, accessing a prospective pancreatic database. Patients receiving primary total pancreatectomy were excluded.

Results: Four hundred and thirteen patients were treated for PDAC: 347 (84 %) underwent PD and 66 (16 %) DP. Tumors located in the pancreatic body and tail were significantly larger than their counterparts located in the head (30.6 mm vs. 41.2 mm; $p < 0.001$). However, distal tumors had significantly less nodal involvement (71 % vs. 57 %; $p = 0.03$). Portal-vein resection (PVR) was performed more often in PD, multivisceral resection (MVR) was more frequent in DP (37 % vs. 14 % and 4 % vs. 29 %; $p < 0.001$). Rates for negative resection margins and tumor grading were similar. Postoperative complication rates including morbidity, rates of re-operation and mortality were comparable. Long-term outcome revealed no significant difference between PD and DP with 5-year survival rates of 17.8 and 22 % respectively ($p = 0.284$). Multivariate analysis confirmed positive resection margin, positive nodal status, extended resection (PVR, MVR) and lack of adjuvant/additive chemotherapy as independent risk factors for poor survival after pancreatic resection.

Conclusion: Patients with resectable pancreatic ductal adenocarcinoma located in the body and tail of the pancreas display a similar postoperative oncological outcome despite larger tumors when compared to patients with resectable tumors located in the pancreatic head.

Keywords: Pancreatic cancer, Pancreatoduodenectomy, Distal pancreatectomy, Survival, Outcome

Background

Prognosis for pancreatic cancer (PC) has only slightly improved over the past decades and still is grim, with a current 5-year relative survival rate of about 6.9 % [1, 2]. Stratified by tumor site, mortality is even worse when the tumor is located in the pancreatic body and tail. A recent analysis based on SEER-data (*Surveillance, Epidemiology and End Results Program* by the National Cancer Institute, NCI, U.S.) revealed a significant difference in the 3-year survival rates of 3.9 % (body/tail) vs. 6.2 % (head) [3]. This observation is most likely due to delayed diagnosis in the case of tumor location in the pancreatic body and tail, since early symptoms are usually lacking. Therefore, a significantly higher percentage of patients is primarily diagnosed with advanced disease and stage IV PC (body/tail: 56–73 % vs. head: 26–39 %) [3, 4], where surgical therapy is not beneficial. Complete

---
* Correspondence: uwe.wittel@uniklinik-freiburg.de
[1]Department of Surgery, University of Freiburg, Freiburg, Germany
Full list of author information is available at the end of the article

resection at an early stage though, is the most important factor in multimodal treatment and the only chance for cure and long-term survival [5]. In combination with adjuvant chemotherapy, 5-year survival rates of up to 15–30 % can be achieved [6–9].

In the case of localized and resectable disease, some observational studies analyzing the outcome by tumor stage at diagnosis show superior survival for patients with cancer located in the pancreatic body/tail compared to patients with cancer located in the pancreatic head [3, 4]. A NCD-report (*National Cancer Database*, American College of Surgeons Commission on Cancer and American Cancer Society) pictures a 5-year survival-rate of 32 % (tail) vs. 11 % (head) for stage I disease (for stage II and stage III disease 12 % (tail) vs. 6 % (head) and 11 % (tail) vs. 7 % (head), respectively) [4]. However, when recently a surgical collective of patients after pancreatic resection for adenocarcinoma was examined, the survival benefit for patients with resectable disease located in the body and tail detected in these observational studies could yet not be confirmed [10]. In this and other studies, despite significantly larger size of tumors located in the body/tail, survival after proximal pancreatectomy and distal pancreatectomy was similar [6, 10–13].

To clarify these putative contradictions, our aim was to retrospectively examine our own single-institution collective regarding survival after resection for pancreatic ductal adenocarcinoma (PDAC). We intended to identify risk factors influencing survival in patients undergoing distal pancreatectomy (DP) or pancreatoduodenectomy (PD) for PDAC.

Methods
Patients
From July 1994 to December 2014, 413 patients with primary non-metastasized pancreatic adenocarcinoma were eligible for surgery (PD or DP) in our department (patients requiring total pancreatectomy were not included). 347 were treated by pancreatoduodenectomy and 66 by distal pancreatectomy.

Surgical technique and pathological analysis
Whenever possible, the pylorus was preserved during pancreatoduodenectomy. Complete lymphadenectomy was performed in the hepatic ligament, right of the celiac trunk and right of the mesenteric artery. Venous structures were resected whenever necessary to achieve complete resection. Intraoperative histopathologic evaluation was routinely performed at common bile duct and pancreatic resection margin. In recent years the mesopancreatic retroperitoneal margin was also examined. Other margins underwent frozen section analysis if intraoperatively indicated, such as in case of venous resection at both venous resection margins. In distal pancreatectomy with splenectomy, lymphadenectomy was performed left

of the celiac trunk and left of the mesenteric artery. Since 2005 resection was performed as described by Strasberg et al. [8, 14, 15] including the fascia of Gerota and when indicated the left adrenal gland. Intraoperative histopathologic evaluation was performed at the pancreatic resection margin. After formalin fixation, standard histopathological evaluation was performed on all operative specimens in which tumor size, lymph node status and resection margin were assessed. Negative resection margin was defined as tumor remote to the resection margin independent of the exact distance.

Since 2006 laparoscopic procedures for DP as well as PD increased in number. Pancreatic stump management (DP) and reconstruction (PD) were accomplished via mini-laparotomy.

Perioperative therapy
Neoadjuvant therapy was administered, in a few cases (n = 22) with locally advanced disease since year 2000, predominantly as radiochemotherapy. Postoperative adjuvant treatment was heterogeneous. In the early study phase adjuvant therapy was not routinely performed after curative resection. Since 2003 a few selected patients were included in studies. Later, due to evidence from randomized trials (*European Study Group for Pancreatic Cancer:* ESPAC-1 Trial) [16], adjuvant chemotherapy was regularly recommended and administered. In case of positive resection margins postoperative chemoradiation or additive chemotherapy was administered whenever applicable, preferentially in clinical trials.

Follow-up and statistical analysis
Perioperative data was collected prospectively in a SPSS database (IBM Corp. Released 2013. IBM SPSS Statistics for Windows, Version 22.0. Armonk, NY: IBM Corp.) The survival status was achieved from general practitioners or oncologists (until 2001) and regional cancer registries (since 2001). Data collection and analysis were performed in accordance with the Helsinki guidelines and approved by the local ethics committee (*Ethik-Kommission of the Albert-Ludwigs-Universtität Freiburg*), the need for individual verbal or written informed consent from participants or their next of kin was waived. Statistical analysis was performed with SPSS. In addition to descriptive statistics, inferential analysis (χ^2-test for categorical variables or Mann–Whitney-U-test for continuous variables) and Kaplan-Meier survival analyses with log-rank-test for the comparison of subgroups, multivariate analysis (Cox proportional hazards model) was performed to determine independent risk factors.

Results
Of the 413 resected patients nine (2.2 %) died due to postoperative complications, seven were lost to follow-

up. Therefore, 16 patients were excluded for survival analysis (11 patients from the PD-group and 5 patients from the DP-group). Survival was analyzed in the remaining 397 patients. Of those, 336 patients received PD while 61 patients were treated with DP. Median postoperative follow-up was 14 months (13 months for deceased patients; 16 months for censored patients).

Patient characteristics

In both groups patient characteristics were not significantly different in regard to gender, age and body mass index (Table 1).

Surgery

Regarding duration of surgery, a significant difference was detectable with PDs showing to be more time-consuming (PD: 440 (245–760) min vs. DP: 301 (140–717) min [median (range)]). If blood transfusions were necessary, the volume administered was significantly higher in the PD-group (PD: 423 ± 729 ml vs. DP: 192 ± 368 ml [mean $\pm$ SD]). The intraoperative involvement of the superior mesenteric vein or portal vein with a subsequent resection was higher in patients with tumors located in the pancreatic head (PD: 37 % vs. DP: 14 %). In contrast, multivisceral resections were performed more frequently in patients with tumors located in the

Table 1 Demographic, surgical, pathological and postoperative data from 413 patients undergoing pancreatic resection for pancreatic ductal adenocarcinoma (1994–2014)

	Pancreaticoduodenectomy	Distal pancreatectomy	p
N of resections	347	66	
Gender			0.755
Male	182 [52 %]	36 [55 %]	
Female	165 [48 %]	30 [45 %]	
Age in years median (range)	67.0 (31–89)	65.6 (35–88)	0.362
BMI in kg/m² median (range)	24.4 (7.6–38.8)	23.6 (18.2–35.4)	0.725
Operation time in min median (range)	440 (245–760)	301 (140–717)	<0.001
PRBC receivedif received, vol. in ml mean (±SD)	135 [39 %]	17 [27 %]	0.056
	423 (±729)	192 (±368)	0.024
Extended resection			
- none	204 [59 %]	38 [58 %]	<0.001
- portal vein	128 [37 %]	9 [14 %]	
- multivisceral	15 [4 %]	19 [29 %]	
Free resection margin	247 [71 %]	46 [73 %]	0.767
Grading[a]			
G1	11 [3 %]	5 [9 %]	0.229
G2	194 [57 %]	28 [51 %]	
G3	128 [38 %]	21 [38 %]	
G4	6 [2 %]	1 [2 %]	
Tumor size in mm median (range)	28 (1–130)	38 (5–110)	<0.001
Node positive	246 [71 %]	35 [57 %]	0.030
N of analyzed nodes median (range)	15 (2–47)	15 (2–32)	0.783
Any complication	181 [52 %]	32 [49 %]	0.584
Surgical complication	123 [35 %]	20 [30 %]	0.421
- POPF	48 [14 %]	25 [38 %]	<0.001
- IAA	25 [7 %]	8 [12 %]	0.177
- SSI	44 [13 %]	6 [9 %]	0.413
Re-operation	33 [10 %]	10 [15 %]	0.169
Mortality	7 [2 %]	2 [3 %]	0.605
Adjuvant/additive chemotherapy	188 [54 %]	35 [53 %]	0.864

BMI body mass index, *PRBC* packed red blood cells, *POPF* postoperative pancreatic fistula, *IAA* intraabdominal abscess, *SSI* surgical site infection
[a]Data for Tumor grading was not available for 19 patients (PD: 8 patients; DP: 11 patients)

pancreatic body and tail (PD: 4 % vs. DP: 29 %). Here atypical gastric resections and colon resections were mostly performed (data not shown). Resection of the left adrenal gland was considered as frequent part of the procedure for DP, therefore adrenalectomy was neglected when analyzing for multivisceral resections (Table 1).

Pathologic diagnosis

Tumors located in the pancreatic body and tail were significantly larger than tumors located in the pancreatic head (PD: 28 (1–130) mm vs. DP: 38 (5–110) mm [median (range)]. Despite larger tumors, margin negative (R0) resection was achieved with an equal rate (PD: 71 % vs. DP: 73 %). Histopathologic evaluation showed a comparable distribution of tumor grading. However, nodal involvement was less frequent when the tumor was located in the pancreatic body/tail (rate of N+: PD: 71 % vs. DP: 57 %, with similar median number of analyzed nodes) (Table 1).

Postoperative course

Postoperative complications of any kind and surgery related complications like pancreatic fistula, intraabdominal abscess, or wound infection were not significantly different between the two groups. However, evaluation by specific surgical complication revealed significance for a higher pancreatic fistula rate after distal resection. Necessity of re-operation and mortality (PD: 2 % vs. DP: 3 %) was similar (Table 1).

Adjuvant/additive therapy

Two-hundred and twenty-three patients received or were referred to oncologists to receive postoperative chemotherapy. Twenty-two of these had additionally been treated with neoadjuvant therapy for locally advanced, initially unresectable tumors; 62 had positive resection margins. The remaining group of 175 comprised patients who were either not treated in an adjuvant/additive manner (historical cohort or due to morbidity) or for whom this data was lacking. The rate of adjuvantly/additively treated patients did not differ between the PD- (54 %) and DP-group (53 %) (Table 1).

Survival

The entire group of 397 patients showed an overall 3- and 5-year survival after pancreatic resection of 29.5 and 18.3 % respectively with a median survival of 20.6 months (95 % CI: 17.4–23.8).

A trend to increased survival ($p = 0.284$) was observed in patients after surgery for tumors located in the pancreatic body and tail compared to those located in the pancreatic head. The 3- and 5-year survival rates of patients after pancreatoduodenectomy were 27.3 and 17.8 % compared to 45.5 and 22 % in patients treated with distal pancreatectomy. The median survival in patients after PD and DP was 20.4 months (95 % CI: 17.4–23.8) and 24.4 months (95 % CI: 2.9–45.8), respectively (Table 2 and Fig. 1).

In the subgroups with negative resection margin 3-year and 5-year survival rates were 33.7 and 21.1 % (PD) vs. 54.2 and 25.3 % (DP), respectively ($p = 0.212$). In the case of margin-positive resection, survival was considerably worse with 3-year and 5-year survival rates of 13 and 11.2 % after PD vs. 17.5 % vs. 0 % after DP ($p = 0.370$) (Fig. 2).

The *Strasberg*-approach for distal resection was performed since 2005 on 20 out of 61 patients with follow-up data. We could not detect a difference in survival between the historical and the *Strasberg*-cohort (data not shown).

Adjuvant/additive chemotherapy significantly improved oncological outcome after pancreatic surgery for PDAC. The group of patients who received or intended to receive adjuvant/additive therapy demonstrated a median survival of 25.8 months (95 % CI: 20.6–31.0). However, patients who did not receive adjuvant/additive therapy or for whom this information was lacking had a median survival of only 18 months (95 % CI: 14.9–21.1). 3-year and 5-year survival rates were 37.3 and 14.9 % (received/intended to receive) vs. 22 % and 15.7 % (not received/unknown), respectively ($p = 0.010$) (Table 2 and Fig. 3).

Risk factors for survival

In *univariate analysis* resection margin, nodal disease, extent of resection (portal vein and/or multivisceral), blood transfusion and adjuvant/additive chemotherapy showed significant impact on survival after pancreatic resection for PDAC. No effect was observed for patient gender, age and BMI. Furthermore, tumor size, tumor grading and the presence of postoperative complications also did not significantly affect survival (Table 2).

Multivariate survival analysis revealed resection margin, nodal disease, extended resection, and adjuvant/additive chemotherapy as independent risk factors for survival after pancreatic resection for PDAC (Table 3).

Discussion

Although stage-independent overall survival is worse for distally located pancreatic cancer, better long-term outcome for localized tumors of the pancreatic body/tail has been reported. This is probably due to surgical approaches. Delayed diagnosis of pancreatic cancer, when the tumor is located in the pancreatic body or tail, leads to a higher number of patients not being amenable to resection. Especially the lack of specific symptoms such as jaundice is responsible for that fact. Most likely, decreased survival is rather due to systemic spread and metastasis than to local unresectability. When located in the pancreatic body and tail, compared to the pancreatic

Table 2 Overall survival after resection for pancreatic ductal adenocarcinoma. Univariate survival analysis of 397 patients

Parameter	n	3-year-survival	5-year-survival	p
All	397	29.5 %	18.3 %	
Tumor location				
Head	336	27.3 %	17.8 %	
Distal	61	45.4 %	22.0 %	0.284
Gender				
Male	190	29.3 %	15.8 %	
Female	207	29.7 %	20.2 %	0.683
Age				
> 65 years	225	30.4 %	22.6 %	
< 65 years	172	28.3 %	13.8 %	0.493
BMI[a]				
> 25 kg/m^2	161	26.3 %	13.7 %	
< 25 kg/m^2	235	31.2 %	20.9 %	0.494
Tumor size[a]				
< 30 mm	223	28.8 %	18.4 %	
> 30 mm	157	30.4 %	16.9 %	0.860
Tumor grading[a]				
Grade 1 + 2	230	29.6 %	18.7 %	
Grade 3 + 4	151	26.5 %	15.3 %	0.191
Resection margin[a]				
R0	283	36.2 %	21.7 %	
R+	113	13.5 %	9.9 %	<0.001
Nodal status[a]				
Negative	121	41.1 %	27.7 %	
Positive	272	22.9 %	13.0 %	0.001
Extended resection				
None	233	35.9 %	26.1 %	
Portal Vein (PV)	133	21.5 %	7.9 %	
More than PV, multivisceral	31	12.8 %	0 %	<0.001
PRBC transfusion[a]				
Yes	143	22.4 %	15.6 %	
No	252	33.8 %	19.2 %	0.005
Any complication				
Yes	200	31.1 %	17.2 %	
No	197	27.8 %	18.7 %	0.916
Surgical complication				
Yes	133	37.0 %	18.1 %	
No	264	25.9 %	17.4 %	0.149
Adjuvant/additive chemotherapy				
Yes/Intended[b]	222	37.3 %	14.9 %	
No/Unknown	175	22.0 %	15.7 %	0.010

BMI body mass index, PRBC packed red blood cells
[a]Some parameters were not available for individual patients (BMI: 1 patient; Tumor size: 17 patients; Tumor grading: 16 patients; Resection margin: 1 patient; Nodal status: 4 patients; PRBC transfusion: 2 patients)
[b]Included are 22 patients with (additional) neoadjuvant therapy and 62 patients with additive therapy

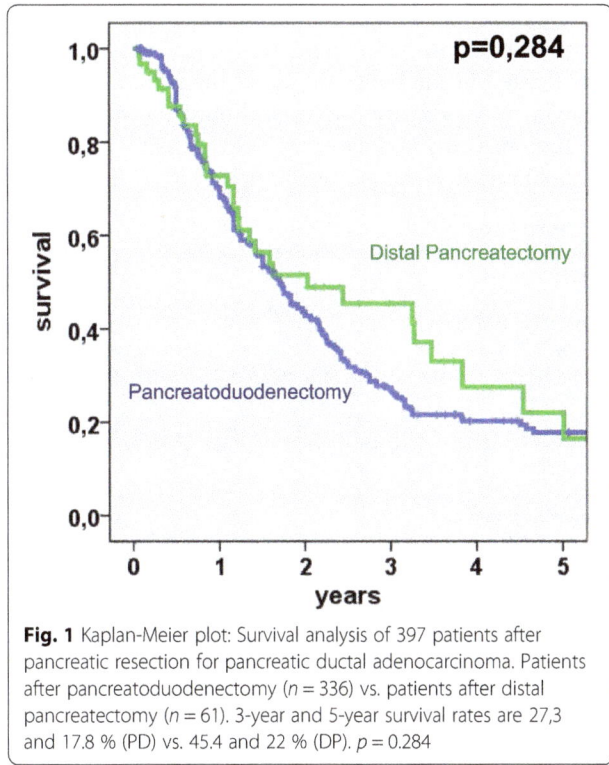

Fig. 1 Kaplan-Meier plot: Survival analysis of 397 patients after pancreatic resection for pancreatic ductal adenocarcinoma. Patients after pancreatoduodenectomy ($n = 336$) vs. patients after distal pancreatectomy ($n = 61$). 3-year and 5-year survival rates are 27,3 and 17.8 % (PD) vs. 45.4 and 22 % (DP). $p = 0.284$

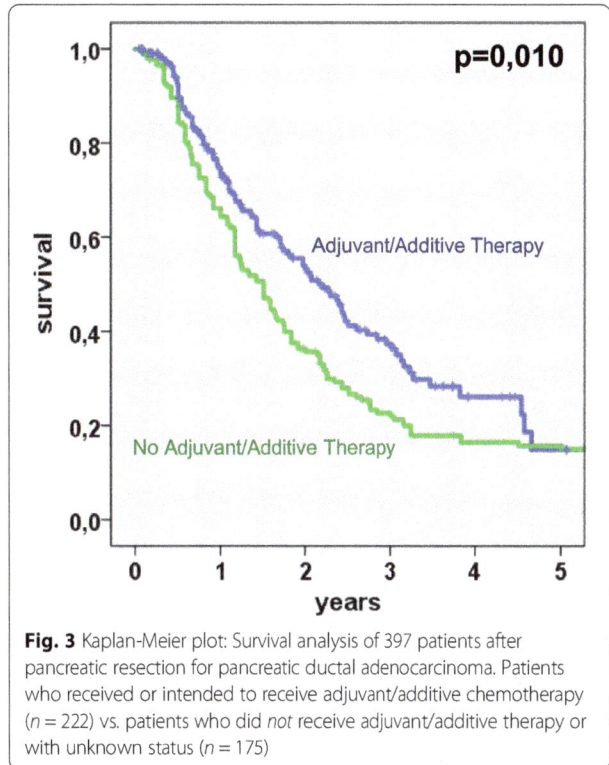

Fig. 3 Kaplan-Meier plot: Survival analysis of 397 patients after pancreatic resection for pancreatic ductal adenocarcinoma. Patients who received or intended to receive adjuvant/additive chemotherapy ($n = 222$) vs. patients who did *not* receive adjuvant/additive therapy or with unknown status ($n = 175$)

head, larger tumors can be resected more frequently and successfully, as measured by the rate of margin-free resections. In spite of larger tumor size, similar long-term outcome for DP and PD has been noted [6, 10–13].

One reason for this might be a favorable tumor biology of resectable PDAC of the pancreatic body/tail. Although the tumor grade usually increases with tumor size [6], this could not be demonstrated in our analysis. However, others have reported similar data with proximal tumors showing more dedifferentiation in spite of smaller size [17]. Similar to our study, nodal involvement seems to be less frequent in resectable distal tumors [6, 17]. Confirmed here as independent risk factor, nodal disease is well known to negatively correlate with survival [18–23].

Furthermore, technical advances in form of the radical antegrade modular pancreatosplenectomy, described by Strasberg et al. [14], may achieve higher rates of margin-free resection. This has probably contributed to improved survival-rates after DP in recent years [24]. Five-year-survival-rates of up to 30 % are reported [8, 21]. However, in our cohort we could not detect a survival benefit related to this procedure.

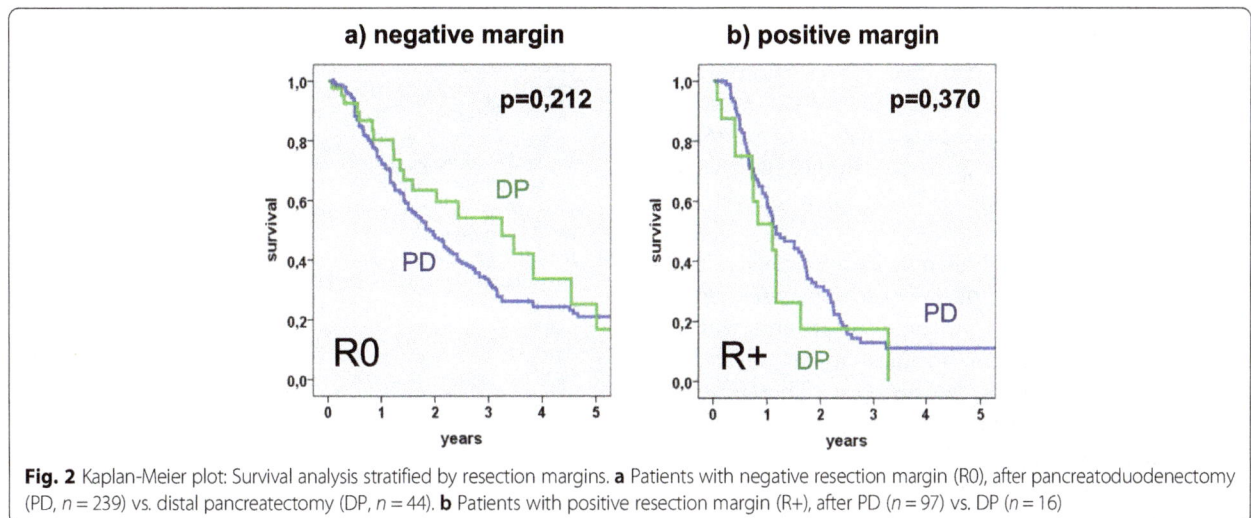

Fig. 2 Kaplan-Meier plot: Survival analysis stratified by resection margins. **a** Patients with negative resection margin (R0), after pancreatoduodenectomy (PD, $n = 239$) vs. distal pancreatectomy (DP, $n = 44$). **b** Patients with positive resection margin (R+), after PD ($n = 97$) vs. DP ($n = 16$)

Table 3 Multivariate analysis. Independent risk-factors for poor survival after pancreatic resection (pancreatoduodenectomies *and* distal pancreatectomies) for pancreatic ductal adenocarcinoma

	P-value	RR	95 %-CI
Positive resection margin	<0.001	1.7	1.3–2.2
Positive nodal status	<0.01	1.5	1.1–2.0
Extended resection			
- none	-	1	
- Portal Vein (PV)	<0.001	2.7	1.7–4.3
- more than PV (multivisceral)	<0.005	2.2	1.4–3.6
No adjuvant/additive chemotherapy (or unknown)	<0.05	1.4	1.1–1.8

Another factor is the possibility of resecting adjacent organs when involved in the tumor. Patients with tumors located in the pancreatic body and tail benefit from the fact that technically, distal pancreatectomies can be easily performed together with en bloc gastric or colon resections. Without the involvement of vital structures as in the case of the pancreatic head with its anatomical proximity to important vessels, this extended, or multivisceral resection is not only feasible but also safe and justified [25–27]. Our pooled data for PD and DP demonstrate that survival after portal vein (PVR) and especially multivisceral (MVR) resection is worse in contrast to the standard procedure. However, this observation may be biased by the skewed dataset in favor of PDs where MVR or extended resection for pancreatic head cancer is associated with increased perioperative risk and with worse oncological outcome [28]. In our study significantly more patients were able to undergo multivisceral resections when presenting with tumors of the pancreatic body/tail. Morbidity and mortality were not different between the two groups. Rates of margin-free resection were similar. As our data undermine (Table 2+3, Fig. 2), R0-resection is the mainstay of surgical therapy and one of the most important factors influencing long-term outcome [6, 17, 19, 29, 30]. However, it is to be completed by adjuvant chemotherapy (Table 2+3, Fig. 3) whenever possible [9].

Although this study is limited by its retrospective character, in summary our collective demonstrates similar postoperative oncological outcome for patients with resectable pancreatic ductal adenocarcinoma located in the body/tail or head of the pancreas. Therefore, the overall poorer survival in patients with tumors located in the pancreatic body or tail appears to be solely due to delayed diagnosis of disease with advanced stage and limited therapeutic options.

Conclusion

Patients with resectable pancreatic ductal adenocarcinoma located in the body and tail of the pancreas display a similar postoperative oncological outcome despite larger tumors when compared to patients with resectable tumors located in the pancreatic head.

Competing interests
No funding was received for this study. The authors declare no conflict of interest.

Authors' contributions
DAR interpreted data and drafted the manuscript. FM carried out data analysis, helped to interpret data and to draft the manuscript. OS performed data collection and administration. UAW conceived the study, participated in interpretation of data and assisted in drafting the manuscript. SC, HR and UTH revised critically and approved the final manuscript. All authors read and approved the final manuscript.

Acknowledgements
The article processing charge was funded by the German Research Foundation (DFG) and the Albert Ludwigs University Freiburg in the funding program *Open Access Publishing*.

Author details
[1]Department of Surgery, University of Freiburg, Freiburg, Germany.
[2]Department of Surgery, Vivantes-Humboldt-Clinic, Berlin, Germany.

References
1. Siegel RL, Miller KD, Jemal A. Cancer statistics, 2015. CA Cancer J Clin. 2015; 65:5–29.
2. Sun H, Ma H, Hong G, Sun H, Wang J. Survival improvement in patients with pancreatic cancer by decade: a period analysis of the SEER database, 1981–2010. Sci Rep. 2014;4:6747.
3. Lau MK, Davila JA, Shaib YH. Incidence and survival of pancreatic head and body and tail cancers: a population-based study in the United States. Pancreas. 2010;39:458–62.
4. Sener SF, Fremgen A, Menck HR, Winchester DP. Pancreatic cancer: a report of treatment and survival trends for 100,313 patients diagnosed from 1985–1995, using the National Cancer Database 1. J Am Coll Surg. 1999;189:1–7.
5. Wagner M, Redaelli C, Lietz M, Seiler CA, Friess H, Büchler MW. Curative resection is the single most important factor determining outcome in patients with pancreatic adenocarcinoma. Br J Surg. 2004;91:586–94.
6. Sohn TA, Yeo CJ, Cameron JL, Koniaris L, Kaushal S, Abrams RA, et al. Resected adenocarcinoma of the pancreas—616 patients: results, outcomes, and prognostic indicators. J Gastrointest Surg. 2000;4:567–79.
7. Franko J, Hugec V, Lopes TL, Goldman CD. Survival among pancreaticoduodenectomy patients treated for pancreatic head cancer <1 or 2 cm. Ann Surg Oncol. 2013;20:357–61.
8. Mitchem JB, Hamilton N, Gao F, Hawkins WG, Linehan DC, Strasberg SM. Long-term results of resection of adenocarcinoma of the body and tail of the pancreas using radical antegrade modular pancreatosplenectomy procedure. J Am Coll Surg. 2012;214:46–52.
9. Jones OP, Melling JD, Ghaneh P. Adjuvant therapy in pancreatic cancer. World J Gastroenterol. 2014;20:14733–46.
10. Toomey P, Hernandez J, Golkar F, Ross S, Luberice K, Rosemurgy A. Pancreatic adenocarcinoma: complete tumor extirpation improves survival benefit despite larger tumors for patients who undergo distal pancreatectomy and splenectomy. J Gastrointest Surg. 2012;16:376–81.
11. Dalton RR, Sarr MG, van Heerden JA, Colby TV. Carcinoma of the body and tail of the pancreas: is curative resection justified? Surgery. 1992;111:489–94.
12. Brennan MF, Moccia RD, Klimstra D. Management of adenocarcinoma of the body and tail of the pancreas. Ann Surg. 1996;223:506–11. discussion 511–512.
13. Sperti C, Pasquali C, Piccoli A, Pedrazzoli S. Survival after resection for ductal adenocarcinoma of the pancreas. Br J Surg. 1996;83:625–31.
14. Strasberg SM, Drebin JA, Linehan D. Radical antegrade modular pancreatosplenectomy. Surgery. 2003;133:521–7.

15. Strasberg SM, Linehan DC, Hawkins WG. Radical antegrade modular pancreatosplenectomy procedure for adenocarcinoma of the body and tail of the pancreas: ability to obtain negative tangential margins. J Am Coll Surg. 2007;204:244–9.

16. Neoptolemos JP, Stocken DD, Friess H, Bassi C, Dunn JA, Hickey H, et al. A randomized trial of chemoradiotherapy and chemotherapy after resection of pancreatic cancer. N Engl J Med. 2004;350:1200–10.

17. Moon HJ, An JY, Heo JS, Choi SH, Joh JW, Kim YI. Predicting survival after surgical resection for pancreatic ductal adenocarcinoma. Pancreas. 2006;32:37–43.

18. Shimada K, Sakamoto Y, Sano T, Kosuge T. Prognostic factors after distal pancreatectomy with extended lymphadenectomy for invasive pancreatic adenocarcinoma of the body and tail. Surgery. 2006;139:288–95.

19. Kooby DA, Hawkins WG, Schmidt CM, Weber SM, Bentrem DJ, Gillespie TW, et al. A multicenter analysis of distal pancreatectomy for adenocarcinoma: is laparoscopic resection appropriate? J Am Coll Surg. 2010;210:779–85. 786–787.

20. Fujita T, Nakagohri T, Gotohda N, Takahashi S, Konishi M, Kojima M, et al. Evaluation of the prognostic factors and significance of lymph node status in invasive ductal carcinoma of the body or tail of the pancreas. Pancreas. 2010;39:e48–54.

21. Paye F, Micelli Lupinacci R, Bachellier P, Boher J-M, Delpero J-R, French Surgical Association (AFC). Distal pancreatectomy for pancreatic carcinoma in the era of multimodal treatment. Br J Surg. 2015;102:229–36.

22. Riediger H, Keck T, Wellner U, Zur Hausen A, Adam U, Hopt UT, et al. The lymph node ratio is the strongest prognostic factor after resection of pancreatic cancer. J Gastrointest Surg Off J Soc Surg Aliment Tract. 2009;13:1337–44.

23. Ashfaq A, Pockaj BA, Gray RJ, Halfdanarson TR, Wasif N. Nodal counts and lymph node ratio impact survival after distal pancreatectomy for pancreatic adenocarcinoma. J Gastrointest Surg Off J Soc Surg Aliment Tract. 2014;18:1929–35.

24. Parikh PY, Lillemoe KD. Surgical management of pancreatic cancer-distal pancreatectomy. Semin Oncol. 2015;42:110–22.

25. Shoup M, Conlon KC, Klimstra D, Brennan MF. Is extended resection for adenocarcinoma of the body or tail of the pancreas justified? J Gastrointest Surg Off J Soc Surg Aliment Tract. 2003;7:946–52. discussion 952.

26. Christein JD, Kendrick ML, Iqbal CW, Nagorney DM, Farnell MB. Distal pancreatectomy for resectable adenocarcinoma of the body and tail of the pancreas. J Gastrointest Surg Off J Soc Surg Aliment Tract. 2005;9:922–7.

27. Roch AM, Singh H, Turner AP, Ceppa EP, House MG, Zyromski NJ, et al. Extended distal pancreatectomy for pancreatic adenocarcinoma with splenic vein thrombosis and/or adjacent organ invasion. Am J Surg. 2015; 209:564–9.

28. Kulemann B, Hoeppner J, Wittel U, Glatz T, Keck T, Wellner UF, et al. Perioperative and long-term outcome after standard pancreaticoduodenectomy, additional portal vein and multivisceral resection for pancreatic head cancer. J Gastrointest Surg Off J Soc Surg Aliment Tract. 2015;19:438–44.

29. Yamamoto J, Saiura A, Koga R, Seki M, Katori M, Kato Y, et al. Improved survival of left-sided pancreas cancer after surgery. Jpn J Clin Oncol. 2010;40:530–6.

30. Kang CM, Kim DH, Lee WJ. Ten years of experience with resection of left-sided pancreatic ductal adenocarcinoma: evolution and initial experience to a laparoscopic approach. Surg Endosc. 2010;24:1533–41.

10

Transumbilical single-incision laparoscopic distal pancreatectomy: preliminary experience and comparison to conventional multi-port laparoscopic surgery

Dianbo Yao[†], Shuodong Wu[*†], Yongnan Li, Yongsheng Chen, Xiaopeng Yu and Jinyan Han

Abstract

Background: Single-incision laparoscopic surgery (SILS), which has been demonstrated to be safely applied on kinds of surgeries, may represent an improvement over conventional multi-port laparoscopic surgery. However, there are still few clinical experiences of SILS in pancreatic surgery until now. In this study, we will summarize our experience of transumbilical single-incision laparoscopic distal pancreatectomy (TUSI-LDP), and compare its related parameters with conventional multi-port laparoscopic distal pancreatectomy (C-LDP).

Methods: A retrospective analysis was conducted for the patients who underwent C-LDP or TUSI-LDP in our department. The demographic data, operative parameters, and postoperative complications in the two groups were summarized and compared.

Results: Laparoscopic distal pancreatectomy was performed in a total of 21 cases, among which TUSI-LDP was performed in 14 cases. As far as the demographical results concerned, there were no significant differences between the two groups. The conversion to open surgery was conducted in one case in the TUSI-LDP group because of severe adhesion between pancreatic cyst and surrounding tissues, while in the C-LDP group the only one conversion was for the difficult detection of small lesion. The mean operating time and intraoperative blood loss in TUSI-LDP group was a little shorter (166.4 ± 57.4 versus 202.1 ± 122.5 minutes, $p > 0.05$, and 157.1 ± 162.4 versus 168.6 ± 157.4 ml, $p > 0.05$). The postoperative pain and post-operation lengths of hospital stay in the TUSI-LDP group were also less, though there was no significant statistical difference between the two groups. For the post-operation complications, in TUSI-LDP group the pancreatic leakage occurred in only one case, and ceased spontaneously with only a drain for 61 days. There were no other complications including postoperative hemorrhage, venous thrombosis, infections and so on in both groups.

Conclusion: For the experienced laparoscopic surgeons, in selected patients, TUSI-LDP is a feasible technique, with excellent cosmetic effect, less postoperative pain and post-operation lengths of hospital stay. With the experience accumulated, the operating time and intraoperative blood loss of TUSI-LDP could also gradually reduce.

Keywords: Single-incision laparoscopic surgery, Distal pancreatectomy, Minimally invasive surgery, Multi-incision laparoscopic surgery

* Correspondence: wushuodong1949@163.com
[†]Equal contributors
Department of General Surgery, Shengjing Hospital, China Medical University, Shenyang 110004, China

Background

Currently, the application of laparoscopic surgery for the distal pancreatectomy seems to become a trend in surgical technique, and might be considered as the first approach for distal pancreatectomy in the near future, possibly owing to its clear visual field, less injury, less postoperative pain, better cosmetic results, and faster recovery of patients [1-3]. Recently, for further minimizing surgical trauma by reducing the number of the port, many experienced laparoscopic surgeons have tried to develop a new minimally invasive technique called "single incision laparoscopic surgery" (SILS), which has been now successfully and widely applied in many fields of abdominal surgery [4,5]. However, The SILS performed on the pancreatic lesions has been reported only recently, and the experience is still limited now [6-13]. Therefore, more studies are still required to confirm the feasibility of transumbilical single-incision laparoscopic distal pancreatectomy (TUSI-LDP). In addition, there have been few comparisons with standard laparoscopic distal pancreatectomy in the literature until now.

In this study, we would report 14 cases in which TUSI-LDP was performed in the Shengjing Hospital of China Medical University, to summarize the clinical experiences, and the related data was also compared with that of conventional multi-port laparoscopic distal pancreatectomy (C-LDP).

Methods

Patient selection and data collection

The criteria for patient selection in our department for laparoscopic distal pancreatectomy are as follows: a benign lesion was found in preoperative examination, and distal pancreatectomy was intented to be performed. The diameter of the lesion should be less than 3.5 cm, and could be a little larger for a cystic lesion. The patient has strong preference for cosmetic appearance, with no contraindications for laparoscopic surgery. All the patients participating in this study gave informed consent, for SILS operations and the publication of their individual clinical details. The patient records were also granted by the hospital to be accessed. This study was approved by the ethical committee of Shengjing Hospital, China Medical University.

Since 2009, all the cases in which laparoscopic distal pancreatectomy was performed in our department in the Shengjing Hospital of China Medical University were retrospectively reviewed. Medical records were reviewed to collect relevant information in the perioperative period. Operation records were reviewed to obtain operation indications, incision length, operative time, estimated blood loss, intraoperative complications and so on. Pathology reports were reviewed to obtain final diagnosis. Medication records were reviewed to determine analgetica used during the hospital stay. Daily progress notes were reviewed to document length of stay and perioperative complications, and follow-up by telephone was for postoperative complications within 30 days.

Surgical technique

In the TUSI-LDP group, after the induction of general endotracheal anesthesia, the patient was placed in a supine position, with legs apart (Figure 1A). A transumbilical 3 cm superficial longitudinal incision was made. After the maintenance of pneumoperitoneum, a 10 mm trocar was inserted into the lower margin of the incision, for the lens, and another two trocars were inserted on the superior margin of incision, the left one, 5 mm for the grasper, and the right one, 12 mm in diameter for the plastic disposable trocar (Figure 1B, case 12). In the MPLDP group, the incision at the umbilicus was 10 mm for the lens, and three additional trocars were used, one in the midline between the xiphoid process and the umbilicus, one lateral to the right rectus muscle at the level of the umbilicus and the other one subcostally in the medioclavicular line.

The operative procedure was similar in the two groups. The operation began with the division of the gastrocolic ligament and the lower part of the gastrolienal ligament, to expose the body and tail of the pancreas and confirm the location and range of the mass or cyst (Figure 2A, case 12). Then, the serous membrane was dissected along the lower edge of pancreas on the right of the lesion. Loose connective tissue between the dorsal surface of the pancreas and the posterior abdominal wall was dissociated carefully, to not injure the splenic artery or splenic vein. When a tunnel would be built at the posterior surface of normal pancreatic body, the grasper was inserted into the tunnel and carried forward, to enlarge the visual fields behind the pancreas. The loose connective tissue was dissociated carefully by the ultrasonic scalpel towards the tail of the pancreas, and then the mass in the body of the pancreas was lifted and separated from posterior abdominal wall. When the body and tail of the pancreas from the normal pancreatic tissue on the right of the mass to the tail of pancreas near the hilum of spleen was completely separated, the pancreas would be divided with an endoscopic linear stapler device (Figure 2B).

If a splenectomy was to be simultaneously performed, the superior part of the gastrosplenic ligament, splenophrenic ligament, splenogastric ligament should be respectively dissected, and then the spleen was removed with the pancreas specimen. In the cases among which a spleen-preserving laparoscopic distal pancreatectomy was to be performed, the splenic vessels were mostly divided, with the short gastric vessels preserved to provide a blood supply. In some cases, the pancreatic branches

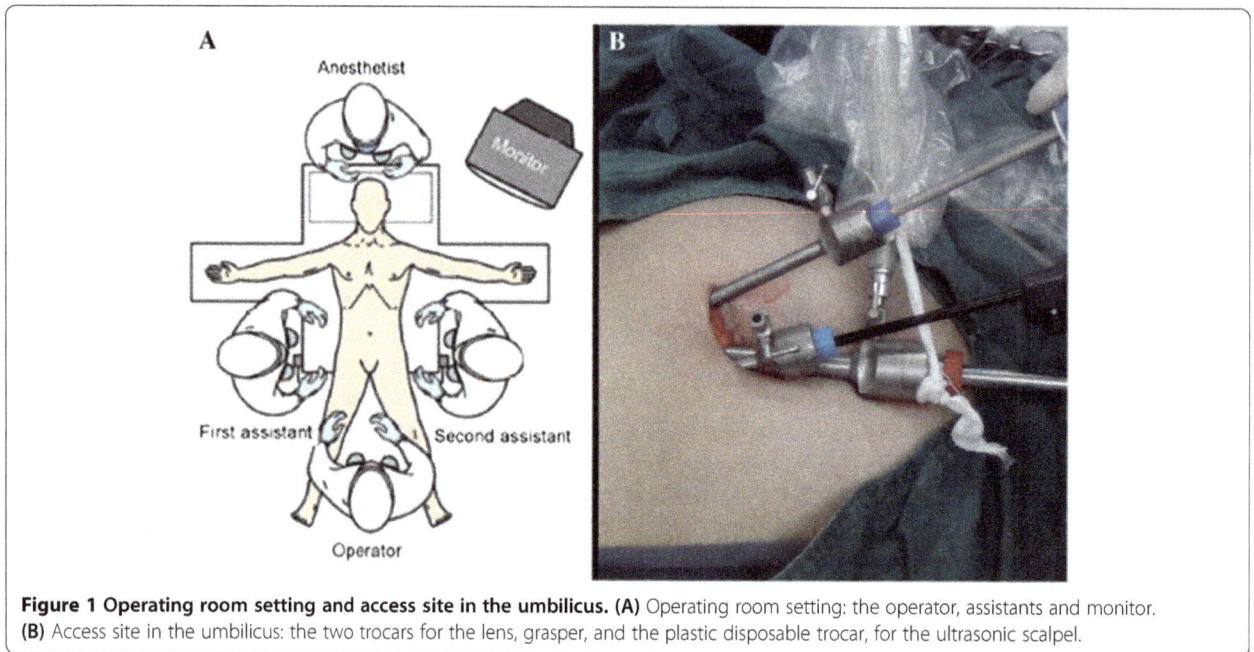

Figure 1 Operating room setting and access site in the umbilicus. (A) Operating room setting: the operator, assistants and monitor. **(B)** Access site in the umbilicus: the two trocars for the lens, grasper, and the plastic disposable trocar, for the ultrasonic scalpel.

of splenic vessels could be well dissected and divided, and the splenic vessels could also be separated from the pancreas and preserved.

A retrieval bag was placed through the plastic disposable trocar. The specimen was wrapped in the retrieval bag (Figure 2C) and extracted from the umbilical incision (Figure 2D). A closed drain was then placed near the stump of the pancreas, and brought out through the transumbilical incision (Figure 2E). A purse-string suture was beforehand reserved surrounding the drainage tube, and could be tensed to close the hole at the umbilicus when the intrabdominal drainage tube was pulled out.

Postoperative treatment
Patients were transferred to the recovery room after surgery. Nasogastric tube was removed after return of intestinal function, and oral feeding was mostly initiated immediately, usually on the fourth postoperative day. As a closed drainage was placed near the stump of the pancreas, the content and volume of pancreatic amylase, and bleeding, was closely monitored. For slight pancreatic leakage, the remaining drainage time was extended, and the regulation of food and use of somatostatin was utilized for healing. The drainage tube could be pulled out when the drainage volume was less than 10 ml in 24 hours and there were no biochemical or clinical signs of a pancreatic fistula. Patients were discharged when tolerating a soft diet and no signs of complication were identified, and a strict follow-up was still made.

Statistical analysis
Continuous data are presented as the mean ± standard deviation and the range. Categorical variables are expressed as numbers and percentages for each group. Continuous variables were compared between the two groups using an unpaired-sample student t test and Mann–Whitney test. Results were considered statistically significant for $p < 0.05$.

Results
Since 2009, laparoscopic distal pancreatectomy was performed in a total of 21 cases, among which TUSI-LDP was performed in 14 cases. In the TUSI-LDP group, the characteristics of patients are listed in Table 1. Only one patient of the 14 cases was male, and the age ranged from 20 to 73 years old, with the average of 40.2 years old. The average of body mass index (BMI) is 22.6 (18.4 ~ 27.0). Among the 14 cases, 6 cases were diagnosed as pancreatic mucinous cystadenoma, 3 cases were diagnosed as the pancreatic cyst, 2 cases were diagnosed as splenic artery aneurysm, and the other 3 cases were diagnosed as pancreatic serous cystadenoma (Figure 2F), islet cell tumor and abdominal cavity fibromatosis involving the tail of pancreas respectively. In the C-LDP group, only one patient of the 7 cases was male. The average age was 50.4 ± 11.3 years old (range, 35–65), and the average of BMI is 23.3 (21.3 ~ 25.2). The related parameters in the C-LDP group are evaluated as a control group.

Operative data are given in Table 2. The TUSI-LDP were successfully performed in the 13 cases, while in the other case the operation conversed to conventional open

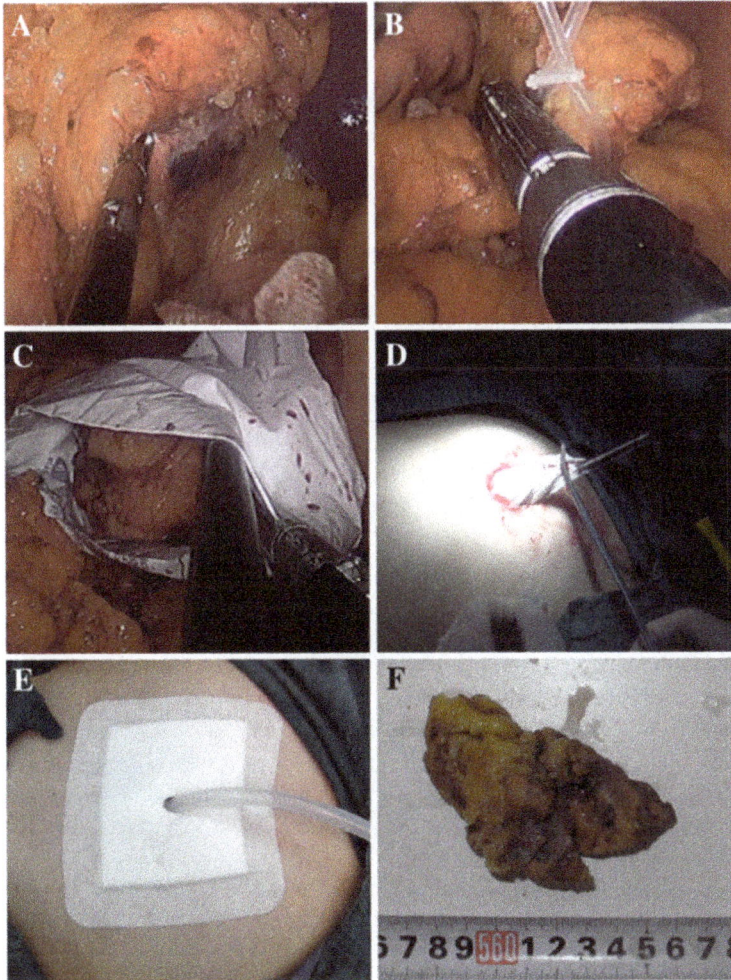

Figure 2 Operative procedure of laparoscopic distal pancreatectomy. (A) Exposure of pancreas. The lesion is seen at the right side of the picture. **(B)** The body to tail of the pancreas is mobilized and lifted from the retroperitoneum by a cloth tape, and pancreatic body is transected with an endoscopic linear stapler device. **(C)** The lesion was put into a retrieval bag. **(D)** The cyst contents were aspirated within the retrieval bag. **(E)** The closed drains brought out through the transumbilical incision. **(F)** The lesion, the serous cystadenoma in pathologic diagnosis.

surgery due to severe adhesion between pancreatic cyst and surrounding tissues. Among these 14 cases, laparoscopic distal pancreatectomy with splenectomy was performed in 7 cases (case 1, 3, 4, 5, 10, 11, 14), while spleen-preserving laparoscopic distal pancreatectomy was performed in the other 7 cases, including 2 cases in which the splenic vessels were successfully preserved (Table 2). The median operative time was (166.4 ± 57.4) min, with all procedures finished in <240 min in the 13 cases with successful TUSI-LDP, and the operative time in the case with conversion to open surgery was 300 min. The median estimated intraoperative blood loss was (157.1 ± 162.4) ml (10–500 ml), with none of the patients requiring perioperative transfusion of red blood cells. As for the postoperative complications, only in one case with the diagnosis of the pancreatic cyst, the pancreatic leakage occurred, and ceased spontaneously with

only a drain for 61 days. There were no other complications including postoperative hemorrhage, venous thrombosis, fever, infection and so on. Postoperative umbilical incision healed well, with no obvious scar, and cosmetic result was well. The patients were discharged from hospital in a mean of (7.6 ± 1.4) d (range, 5 to 10 d), with no mortality. All the patients resumed daily activities quickly.

For preoperative characteristics, there were no statistically significant differences between the two groups (Table 3). For the related data of operation (Table 4), the conversion to open surgery was conducted in one case in the TUSI-LDP group because of severe adhesion between pancreatic cyst and surrounding tissues, while in the C-LDP group the only one conversion was for the difficult detection of small lesion. The mean operative time was a little shorter in the single-incision laparoscopic

Table 1 General information of 14 cases

Patient number	Diagnosis	Tumor location	Age	Sex	BMI	Maximum diameter of lesion
1	Mucinous cystadenoma	body of pancreas	46	F	24.6	5
2	Fibromatosis	abdominal cavity	20	F	18.6	3.5
3	Serositic cyst	tail of pancreas	36	F	23.4	4.5
4	Pancreatic cyst	body of pancreas	42	F	22.2	4.5
5	Artery aneurysm	spleen	22	F	21.6	3.5
6	Mucinous cystadenoma and SPT	body and tail of pancreas	34	F	22.8	3.5
7	Pancreatic cyst	tail of pancreas	34	F	23.4	3.5
8	Mucinous cystadenoma	body and tail of pancreas	39	F	22.6	3
9	Islet cell tumor	tail of pancreas	73	F	26.2	1.2
10	Mucinous cystadenoma	body and tail of pancreas	27	F	22.2	4
11	Mucinous cystadenoma	tail of pancreas	45	F	21.8	6.2
12	Serous cystadenoma	tail of pancreas	50	F	21.5	3.2
13	Mucinous cystadenoma	tail of pancreas	37	F	18.4	11
14	Artery aneurysm	spleen	58	M	27.0	3.8

BMI body mass index; SPT solid-pseudopapillary tumor.

group (166.4 ± 57.4 versus 202.1 ± 122.5 min, $p > 0.05$), and the mean estimated blood loss in the single-incision group was also a little smaller (157.1 ± 162.4 versus 168.6 ± 157.4 ml, $p > 0.05$), though there was no significant difference between the two groups. There were no requiring blood transfusions in the two groups, and no deaths in either group. As for the postoperative complications, in only one case in the single-incision group the pancreatic leakage occurred, and ceased spontaneously with only a drain for 61 days. The use of in-hospital postoperative narcotics was evaluated in both groups of patients. While the patients in the TUSI-LDP group (0.7 ± 0.6 times) used a lower total dose of narcotic medication than that in the C-LDP group (1.1 ± 0.7 times), the difference was not significant, either. The mean length of stay in the two groups was 7.6 days and 9.0 days respectively.

Discussion

In recent years, the search for less morbidity and greater patient comfort has led surgeons to develop newer

Table 2 Operative parameters and postoperative recovery of patients

Cases	Operation time (min)	Intraoperative blood loss (ml)	Conversion to multi-incision surgery	Postoperative evacuating time (day)	Food intake time (day)	Drainage time (day)	Hospital stay (day)	Postoperative hemorrhage	Pancreatic leakage
1	300	500	yes	3	3	4	8	no	no
2*	240	500	no	4	4	7	9	no	no
3	150	10	no	3	3	>7	7	no	yes
4	125	100	no	4	5	7	8	no	no
5	170	10	no	3	3	4	6	no	no
6*	110	30	no	3	3	4	6	no	no
7*	115	50	no	2	3	7	8	no	no
8*	165	100	no	5	5	10	10	no	no
9#	170	50	no	3	4	7	8	no	no
10	155	200	no	4	5	7	7	no	no
11	95	200	no	3	4	5	5	no	no
12#	120	50	no	3	4	6	7	no	no
13*	185	200	no	3	4	7	9	no	no
14	230	200	no	5	5	8	9	no	no

*Splenic preservation; #Splenic and its vessels preservation.

Table 3 Demographical characteristics of the patients

	SILS (n =14)	Conventional (n = 7)	P
Age, mean ± SD [range]	40.2 ± 14.1 [20–73]	50.4 ± 11.3 [35–65]	0.66
Sex (% men)	7.1	14.3	0.61
Weight, mean ± SD [range]	59.6 ± 8.9 [45–80]	60.4 ± 5.1 [54–67]	0.21
BMI, mean ± SD [range], kg/m2	22.6 ± 2.4 [18.4–27.0]	23.3 ± 1.3 [21.3–25.2]	0.29
Size of lesion,, mean ± SD [range], cm	4.3 ± 2.2 [1.2–11]	3.7 ± 2.2 [0.7–6.0]	0.47
Lesion type (benign/malignant)	0/14	1/6	0.16

means of access to the abdominal cavity with less surgical trauma, such as natural-orifice transluminal endoscopic surgery and single-incision laparoscopic surgery. The scarce reproducibility and difficulty involved with the natural orifice technique made most surgeons opt for the single-incision technique, for its similarity with conventional laparoscopy and lower requirement of specific equipments. Since the first documented single incision laparoscopic procedure in 1997, SILS has already been applied dramatically in many surgical procedures, such as cholecystectomy [4], appendectomy [5,14], total extraperitoneal inguinal hernia repair [15], sleeve gastrectomy [16], gastrojejunostomy [17], splenectomy [18], nephrectomy [19], liver resection [20], and so on. However, TUSI-LDP has still been rarely reported, possibly because pancreatic surgery represents one of the most challenging areas in digestive surgery.

In 2010, Barbaros U et al. first reported the TUSI-LDP with splenectomy, and it was described that the overall procedures were similar to that performed in the conventional multi-port laparoscopic pancreatectomy [6]. The operation was successfully finished even though in the retroperitoneal region there was dense fibrosis caused by a previous left nephrectomy, confirming that TUSI-LDP could be performed technically. Since then, TUSI-LDP were reported a total of 26 cases, among which, the largest study was reported by us [11]. Recently, three more cases were performed in our department.

Table 4 Operative and postoperative results

	SILS (n =14)	Conventional (n = 7)	P
Operating time, mean ± SD, min	166.4 ± 57.4	202.1 ± 122.5	0.15
Estimated blood loss,mean ± SD, ml	157.1 ± 162.4	168.6 ± 157.4	0.66
Scale of pain, mean ± SD	0.7 ± 0.6	1.1 ± 0.7	0.90
Conversion to open surgery, %	1/14	1/7	0.61
Complications, %	1/14	0/7	0.48
Length of hospital stay, mean ± SD, d	7.6 ± 1.4	9.0 ± 3.0	0.17

Now, during the 29 cases, transumbilical single-incision laparoscopy spleen-preserving distal pancreatectomy in 16 cases and single-incision laparoscopy distal pancreatectomy without splenic preservation in 13 case were performed, and the patients' postoperative recoveries were all uneventful [6-13]. Now, these experiences well confirm the feasibility and safety of the TUSI-LDP in selected cases. However, for the pancreatic surgery, comparative studies are still needed, to compare the related parameters of the single-incision and conventional laparoscopic techniques, and lay down the foundation for the possible indications for this type of access.

As far as operating time concerned, some published studies for SILS reveal a longer operating time than conventional laparoscopy [21-23]. As in SILS all instruments are closely packed together, and the instruments, which are limited within a small range of motion, would interfere with each other, the operation of SILS is though to be more difficult. These would increase the difficulty of learning and practice, and also increase the operating time. However, as the SILS were performed, the operation could be more and more smoothly. One study [24], comparing colon resections for cancer using the 2 techniques, reported no differences and operating times were practically the same, although the size of the series was small. Now, in our study, we observed that in uncomplicated distal pancreatectomy with normal characteristics, operating times in SILS group would be similar or even shorter than that in conventional laparoscopy group, mainly because our experiences for LDP and SILS had accumulated much before TUSI-LDP began to be performed, making the operations in TUSI-LDP much more smoothly, just as our results for the gastric GIST [25]. Similarly in our study, the intraoperative blood loss in the single-incision laparoscopic group was also smaller than that in the conventional laparoscopic group, though the difference did not reach statistical significance. As our experiences of TUSI-LDP gradually accumulated, we could be more careful for the vessels during operation, and intraoperative blood loss could also be gradually well controlled. However, operating time or intraoperative blood loss might be much longer when there was severe adhesion between pancreatic cyst and surrounding tissues. In this study, one patient required even a conversion to open surgery because of severe adhesion.

Many studies have suggested that the single-incision laparoscopic surgery approach may have some advantages over conventional laparoscopic surgery: greater patient comfort, less postoperative pain, and a better cosmetic outcome due to a scareless procedure [26]. However, for the pancreatic surgery, the related reports were lacking. The less injury and less postoperative pain of SILS might be related with reducing the size of the skin incision and not perforating the aponeurosis or muscle. In some complex surgical procedures, such as colectomy, which requires a greater number of incisions or even minilaparotomy to complete the operation, postoperative pain may have important clinical repercussions in satisfaction, quality of life, and health state. Some previous prospective studies show no differences for the postoperative pain [21,22,27,28], but the results obtained in our study indicated that although there were no significant difference, the patients in the TUSI-LDP group indeed used a lower total dose of narcotic medication. Therefore, the controversy for the postoperative pain still exists, waiting for further confirmed.

For the postoperative complications, the well visual fields of operation provided by the laparoscope, and the rational utilization of sealing devices have made the complication in laparoscopic surgery rarely occur. It was found that compared with open distal pancreatectomy, LDP patients had significant fewer complications [29]. Cho CS et al. explored the risk factors for pancreatic fistula after distal pancreatectomy, and found that preoperative characteristics may identify cohorts of patients who will benefit more from LDP, and no patient cohorts had higher postoperative complication rates after LDP than open distal pancreatectomy, suggesting that LDP may be the better operative procedure of choice for less pancreatic fistula or other complications [30]. Now, for the TUSI-LDP, the pancreatic fistula occurred in only one case of our 14 cases and one case in the English literature [6], and conservative treatment was effective in the both cases. There were no other complications including postoperative hemorrhage, venous thrombosis, fever, infection and so on. These results suggest the patients with TUSI-LDP may also benefit much for less postoperative complications. Certainly, more definitive prospective and randomized comparisons are still needed for further confirmation.

As for the post-operation lengths of hospital stay, though no significant difference was found between the two groups, the mean lengths of hospital stay in the SILS group were also a little shorter. It may be related with the reduced postoperation pain, and early recovery of oral feeding. Certainly, we are beginning to try applying a relative fast-track protocol in one patient (case 11) with uncomplicated pancreatic cyst without increasing the number of complications, and the oral feeding initiation and the discharge time could still be futher earlier [31] in the near future.

Today, SILS is becoming popular, and its purpose is to cure the disease in a cosmetic method with minimal invasion. As these results suggest, the single incision approach could be applied successfully in the pancreatic surgery, providing high degree of satisfaction and well cosmetic advantages, though much more techniques are needed for the operator. It does not increase the rate of complications and represents a possible alternative to conventional laparoscopic distal pancreatectomy. With the related experience acquired, we believe that it could be applied more and more widely [32].

Conclusions
Our study suggests that for the experienced laparoscopic surgeons, TUSI-LDP is feasible and safe, with excellent cosmetic effect, and the single-incision technique is comparable to standard laparoscopic distal pancreatectomy in terms of operative time and perioperative outcomes. Certainly, the advantages and disadvantages of the TUSI-LDP compared with the conventional LDP still need further evaluated in prospective clinical researches.

Abbreviations
SILS: Single-incision laparoscopic surgery; TUSI-LDP: Transumbilical single-incision laparoscopic distal pancreatectomy; C-LDP: Conventional multi-port laparoscopic distal pancreatectomy; BMI: Body mass index.

Competing interests
The authors declare that they have no competing interests.

Authors' contributions
YD designed the study, collected and analyzed the data, and drafted the manuscript; YX and LY contributed to design of the study and participated in acquisition and analysis of data; CY and HJ participated in acquisition and analysis of data; WS contributed to conception and design of the study and edited the manuscript. All authors read and approved the final manuscript.

Acknowledgments
This work was not supported by any outside research funding.

References
1. Lee SY, Allen PJ, Sadot E, D'Angelica MI, DeMatteo RP, Fong Y, Jarnagin WR, Kingham TP: Distal Pancreatectomy: A Single Institution's Experience in Open, Laparoscopic, and Robotic Approaches. *J Am Coll Surg* 2014, doi:10.1016/j.jamcollsurg.2014.10.004.
2. Røsok BI, Marangos IP, Kazaryan AM, Rosseland AR, Buanes T, Mathisen O, Edwin B: Single-centre experience of laparoscopic pancreatic surgery. *Br J Surg* 2010, 97:902–909.
3. Kneuertz PJ, Patel SH, Chu CK, Fisher SB, Maithel SK, Sarmiento JM, Weber SM, Staley CA, Kooby DA: Laparoscopic distal pancreatectomy: trends and lessons learned through an 11-year experience. *J Am Coll Surg* 2012, 215:167–176.
4. Tranchart H, Ketoff S, Lainas P, Pourcher G, Di Giuro G, Tzanis D, Ferretti S, Dautruche A, Devaquet N, Dagher I: Single incision laparoscopic cholecystectomy: for what benefit? *HPB (Oxford)* 2013, 15:433–438.
5. Frutos MD, Abrisqueta J, Lujan J, Abellan I, Parrilla P: Randomized prospective study to compare laparoscopic appendectomy versus umbilical single-incision appendectomy. *Ann Surg* 2013, 257:413–418.
6. Barbaros U, Sümer A, Demirel T, Karakullukçu N, Batman B, Işcan Y, Sarıçam G, Serin K, Loh WL, Dinççağ A, Mercan S: Single incision laparoscopic pancreas resection for pancreatic metastasis of renal cell carcinoma. *JSLS* 2010, 14:566–570.

7. Kuroki T, Adachi T, Okamoto T, Kanematsu T: **Single-incision laparoscopic distal pancreatectomy.** *Hepatogastroenterology* 2011, **58**:1022–1024.

8. Chang SK, Lomanto D, Mayasari M: **Single-port laparoscopic spleen preserving distal pancreatectomy.** *Minim Invasive Surg* 2012, **2012**:197429.

9. Misawa T, Ito R, Futagawa Y, Fujiwara Y, Kitamura H, Tsutsui M, Shiba H, Wakiyama S, Ishida Y, Yanaga K: **Single-incision laparoscopic distal pancreatectomy with or without splenic preservation: how we do it.** *Asian J Endosc Surg* 2012, **5**:195–199.

10. Srikanth G, Shetty N, Dubey D: **Single incision laparoscopic distal pancreatectomy with splenectomy for neuroendocrine tumor of the tail of pancreas.** *J Minim Access Surg* 2013, **9**:132–135.

11. Yao D, Wu S, Tian Y, Fan Y, Kong J, Li Y: **Transumbilical Single-Incision Laparoscopic Distal Pancreatectomy: Primary Experience and Review of the English Literature.** *World J Surg* 2013, **38**:1196–1204.

12. Haugvik SP, Røsok BI, Waage A, Mathisen O, Edwin B: **Single-incision versus conventional laparoscopic distal pancreatectomy: a single-institution case–control study.** *Langenbecks Arch Surg* 2013, **398**:1091–1096.

13. Machado MA, Surjan RC, Makdissi FF: **First single-port laparoscopic pancreatectomy in Brazil.** *Arq Gastroenterol* 2013, **50**:310–312.

14. Hong TH, Kim HL, Lee YS, Kim JJ, Lee KH, You YK, Oh SJ, Park SM: **Transumbilical single-port laparoscopic appendectomy (TUSPLA): scarless intracorporeal appendectomy.** *J Laparoendosc Adv Surg Tech A* 2009, **19**:75–78.

15. Filipovic-Cugura J, Kirac I, Kulis T, Jankovic J, Bekavac-Beslin M: **Single-incision laparoscopic surgery (SILS) for totally extraperitoneal (TEP) inguinal hernia repair: first case.** *Surg Endosc* 2009, **4**:920–921.

16. Reavis KM, Hinojosa MW, Smith BR, Nguyen NT: **Single-laparoscopic incision transabdominal surgery sleeve gastrectomy.** *Obes Surg* 2008, **11**:1492–1494.

17. Bucher P, Pugin F, Morel P: **Transumbilical single-incision laparoscopic intracorporeal anastomosis for gastrojejunostomy: case report.** *Surg Endosc* 2009, **7**:1667–1670.

18. Barbaros U, Dinc¸c¸ag˘ A: **Single incision laparoscopic splenectomy: the first two cases.** *J Gastrointest Surg* 2009, **13**:1520–1523.

19. Raman JD, Bagrodia A, Cadeddu JA: **Single-incision, umbilical laparoscopic versus conventional laparoscopic nephrectomy: a comparison of perioperative outcomes and short-term measures of convalescence.** *Eur Urol* 2008, **5**:1198–1204.

20. Zhao G, Hu M, Liu R, Xu D, Ouyang C, Xu Y, Jiao H, Wang B, Gu X: **Laparoendoscopic single-site liver resection: a preliminary report of 12 cases.** *Surg Endosc* 2011, **25**:3286–3293.

21. Vidal O, Valentini M, Ginest'a C, Martí J, Espert JJ, Benarroch G, García-Valdecasas JC: **Laparoendoscopic single-site surgery appendectomy.** *Surg Endosc* 2010, **24**:686–691.

22. Lee J, Baek J, Kim W: **Laparoscopic transumbilical single-port appendectomy: initial experience and comparison with three-port appendectomy.** *Surg Laparosc Endosc Percutan Technol* 2010, **20**:100–103.

23. St Peter SD, Adibe OO, Juang D, Sharp SW, Garey CL, Laituri CA, Murphy JP, Andrews WS, Sharp RJ, Snyder CL, Holcomb GW 3rd, Ostlie DJ: **Single incision versus standard 3-port laparoscopic appendectomy: a prospective randomized trial.** *Ann Surg* 2011, **254**:586–590.

24. Papaconstantinou HT, Thomas JS: **Single-incision laparoscopic colectomy for cancer: assessment of oncologic resection and short-term outcomes in a case-matched comparison with standard laparoscopy.** *Surgery* 2011, **150**:820–827.

25. Kong J, Wu SD, Su Y, Fan Y: **Single incision versus conventional laparoscopic resection in gastrointestinal stromal tumors: a retrospective cohort analysis at a single tertiary care center.** *Onco Targets Ther* 2014, **7**:995–999.

26. Ahmed K, Wang TT, Patel VM, Nagpal K, Clark J, Ali M, Deeba S, Ashrafian H, Darzi A, Athanasiou T, Paraskeva P: **The role of single-incision laparoscopic surgery in abdominal and pelvic surgery: a systematic review.** *Surg Endosc* 2011, **25**:378–396.

27. Raakow R, Jacob DA: **Initial experience in laparoscopic single-port appendectomy: a pilot study.** *Dig Surg* 2011, **28**:74–79.

28. Teoh AY, Chiu PW, Wong TC, Wong SK, Lai PB, Ng EK: **A case-controlled comparison of singlesite access versus conventional three-port laparoscopic appendectomy.** *Surg Endosc* 2011, **25**:1415–1419.

29. Kooby DA, Gillespie T, Bentrem D, Nakeeb A, Schmidt MC, Merchant NB, Parikh AA, Martin RC 2nd, Scoggins CR, Ahmad S, Kim HJ, Park J, Johnston F, Strouch MJ, Menze A, Rymer J, McClaine R, Strasberg SM, Talamonti MS, Staley CA, McMasters KM, Lowy AM, Byrd-Sellers J, Wood WC, Hawkins WG: **Left-sided pancreatectomy: a multicenter comparison of laparoscopic and open approaches.** *Ann Surg* 2008, **248**:438–446.

30. Cho CS, Kooby DA, Schmidt CM, Nakeeb A, Bentrem DJ, Merchant NB, Parikh AA, Martin RC 2nd, Scoggins CR, Ahmad SA, Kim HJ, Hamilton N, Hawkins WG, Weber SM: **Laparoscopic versus open left pancreatectomy: can preoperative factors indicate the safer technique?** *Ann Surg* 2011, **253**:975–980.

31. Elola-Olaso AM, Allen A, Gagliardi RJ: **Laparoscopic distal pancreatectomy for solid and cystic pancreatic neoplasms: outpatient postoperative management.** *Surg Laparosc Endosc Percutan Tech* 2009, **19**:470–473.

32. Tsai AY, Selzer DJ: **Single-port laparoscopic surgery.** *Adv Surg* 2010, **44**:1–27.

11

Pancreato-jejunostomy versus hand-sewn closure of the pancreatic stump to prevent pancreatic fistula after distal pancreatectomy: a retrospective analysis

Roberto L Meniconi*, Roberto Caronna, Dario Borreca, Monica Schiratti and Piero Chirletti

Abstract

Background: Different methods of pancreatic stump closure after distal pancreatectomy (DP) have been described to decrease the incidence of pancreatic fistula (PF) which still represents one of the most common complications in pancreatic surgery. We retrospectively compared the pancreato-jejunostomy technique with the hand-sewn closure of the pancreatic stump after DP, and analyzed clinical outcomes between the two groups, focusing on PF rate.

Methods: Thirty-six patients undergoing open DP at our institution between May 2005 and December 2011 were included. They were divided in two groups depending on pancreatic remnant management: in 24 cases the stump was closed by hand-sewn suture (Group A), while in 12 earlier cases a pancreato-jejunostomy was performed (Group B). We analyzed postoperative data in terms of mortality, morbidity and length of hospital stay between the two groups.

Results: PF occurred in 7 of 24 (29.1%) cases of group A (control group) compared to zero fistula rate in group B (anastomosis group) (p=0.005). Operative time was significantly higher in the anastomosis group (p=0.024). Mortality rate was 0% in both groups. Other postoperative outcomes such as hemorrhages, infections, medical complications and length of hospital stay were not significant between the two groups.

Conclusion: Despite a higher operative time, the pancreato-jejunostomy after DP seems to be related to a lower incidence of PF compared to the hand-sewn closure of the pancreatic remnant.

Keywords: Distal Pancreatectomy, Pancreatic Fistula, Pancreato-jejunostomy, Roux-en-Y, Hand-sewn Closure

Background

Distal pancreatectomy (DP) is a surgical procedure performed mostly for benign, borderline or malignant tumors of the body and tail of the pancreas [1]. It is also indicated for the treatment of chronic pancreatitis [2]. Depending on the disease, it could be associated to splenectomy, lymphadenectomy or multivisceral resections. Despite this operation is performed with relatively low morbidity and mortality rates in high-volume centers, the leakage from pancreatic stump after DP remains a problem, determining a pancreatic fistula (PF) in 5-30% of cases according to recent papers [1,3,4] and contributing

to increased morbidity and overall costs. Different techniques of pancreatic stump closure have been described to reduce the incidence of PF, such as stapler transection, pancreatic duct occlusion by fibrin-glue sealant, serosal or artificial patches, ultrasonic scalpel or radiofrequency dissector [1,5-10], but none has proved to be the most effective in preventing PF. Up till now, few authors described the drainage of the pancreatic stump into a jejunal loop [5,11-13] and a recent study demonstrated a significant decrease of pancreatic leakage by performing a Roux-en-Y pancreato-jejunostomy [14]. The aim of this study is to confirm the efficacy of the pancreato-jejunostomy in reducing pancreatic fistula rate after DP, compared to simple hand-sewn closure of the pancreatic remnant.

* Correspondence: robmeni@tiscali.it

Department of Surgical Sciences, Sapienza University of Rome, Viale del Policlinico 155, Rome 00161, Italy

Methods

A total of 36 patients (14 males and 22 females) undergoing DP between May 2005 and December 2011 were included in this study and retrospectively analyzed. All patients were studied preoperatively by contrast-enhanced computed tomography or magnetic resonance imaging. Indications for surgery were benign, borderline or malignant tumors, chronic pancreatitis and pancreatic pseudocysts. Surgical operation consisted in an en-bloc resection of the pancreas tail, eventually extended to the body, associated with splenectomy or other organs resection if needed. In all cases an open approach was performed by a single surgeon. Most of pancreato-jejunostomies were performed not consecutively in the first period of this study, between May 2005 and October 2008, depending on the surgeon preference. From November 2008 all patients undergoing DP were enrolled in another survey in which the pancreatic stump was closed by direct suture with the technique described below. Then we retrospectively observed and analyzed different outcomes between the two techniques.

Patients were divided in two groups on the basis of pancreatic stump management. In the first group (Group A), after pancreatic resection, the stump closure was accomplished by ligating the main pancreatic duct with non-resorbable Z-shaped suture and the cut margin was over sewn a traumatically by U-shaped stitches using non-resorbable material (TiCron®, Covidien, Mansfield, MA, USA) supported by PTFE (Teflon) pledgets used as buttress for the suture (Figure 1). In the second group (Group B), the main pancreatic duct was closed with the same technique described above and the pancreatic stump was finally invaginated into a jejunal loop performing a Roux-en-Y end-to-end pancreato-jejunostomy. The anastomosis was completed by a capsule-to-seromuscular single layer suture with non-resorbable interrupted stitches (Figure 2).

A drain was placed intraoperatively in all cases near the anastomosis or the pancreatic stump. All patients received a short-term antibiotic prophylaxis.

Intravenous fluids, octreotide (3×0.1 mg s.c., daily for 5–7 days) and proton pump inhibitors (omeprazole, 40 mg i.v., daily) were administrated postoperatively. Oral feeding was generally resumed depending on gastrointestinal function. Drainage volume and amylase concentration of drained fluid were measured and registered in the 1st, 3rd, 5th and 7th postoperative day as well as blood tests.

Patient demographics, operation data, post-operative morbidity, mortality rate and length of hospital stay were analyzed and compared between the two groups. PF was defined as a drain output of any measurable volume of fluid on or after postoperative day 3 with an amylase content greater than 3 times the upper normal serum value, in accordance to the International Study Group of Pancreatic Fistula (ISGPF) [15]. PF was also classified into three grades (A,B,C) depending on clinical impact (none, moderate and severe, respectively), according to the ISGPF classification. The pancreatic texture was defined as "fibrotic" or "non-fibrotic" depending on histological findings of the specimens: presence of perilobular fibrosis, chronic inflammatory reactions with ductal dilatations, atrophy of the acinar cells. The main pancreatic duct (MPD) was also defined as "small" or "large" according to the diameter < or > 3 mm, respectively. Postoperative hemorrhage (PH) was defined and classified into three different grades (A,B,C), according to the International Study Group of Pancreatic Surgery definition (ISGPS) [16]. Mortality was considered as any death occurred intraoperatively or during the hospital stay.

Statistical analysis was performed using χ^2 test and Student's t-test. Differences were considered significant at p-value <0.05.

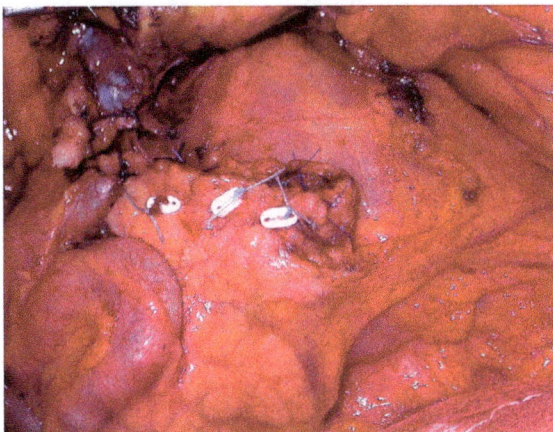

Figure 1 Hand-sewn closure of the pancreatic remnant.
The pancreatic remnant is closed using PTFE pledget-supported interrupted stitches of non-resorbable material.

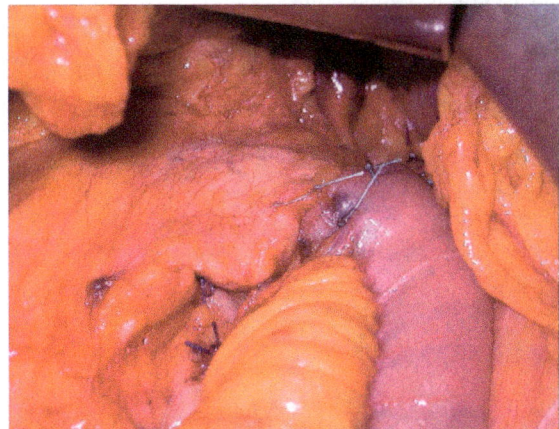

Figure 2 Roux-en-Y end-to-end pancreato-jejunostomy.
The pancreatic stump is invaginated into the jejunal loop and a capsule-to-seromuscular suture is performed using non-resorbable interrupted stitches.

The present study is a retrospective review of medical data and the human research ethics committee of our institution stated to exempt it from formal ethical review according to the ethical principles laid forth by the Helsinki Declaration. Written consent of patients was not sought. No identifying information was recorded by the authors.

Results

Between May 2005 and December 2011, thirty-six patients underwent DP at our institution. All patients were divided retrospectively in two groups depending on pancreatic stump management: Group A (control group) comprised 24 patients with a mean age of 53.6 years (range 25–75 years) in which the pancreatic remnant was closed by an hand-sewn technique; Group B (anastomosis group) comprised 12 patients with a mean age of 50.5 years (range 27–67 years) in which a pancreato-jejunostomy was performed. Patients demographics of two groups were compared and well-matched as reported in Table 1. Indications for surgical resection were pancreatic tumors in 30 patients (20 of group A, 10 of group B), chronic pancreatitis in 3 patients (2 of group A and 1 of group B), and pancreatic pseudocysts in 3 patients (2 of group A, 1 of group B). Splenectomy was performed in 22 cases (61,1%), while a cholecystectomy was carried out in 4 patients with gallstones; two cases required a left nephrectomy due to a locally advanced disease and in one case a portal vein resection with graft reconstruction was performed for suspicion of neoplastic venous infiltration. Mean operative time was significantly higher in the anastomosis group (192 min) compared to the control group (161 min) (p=0.024). 10 patients (83,6%) of the anastomosis group had a non-fibrotic pancreas compared to 18 patients (75%) of the control group (p=0.584); a small MPD was

found in 15 patients of group A and in 8 patents of group B (p=0.622). All operative data are summarized in Table 2.

Food oral intake depended on recovery of gastrointestinal motility and started generally from the third postoperative day. Abdominal drains were removed after a mean duration of 5 days.

PF rate was significantly higher in the group A (control) in which pancreatic leakage occurred in 7 patients (29.1%) compared to group B (anastomosis) where no patient had a PF (p=0.005). They were all pure fistulas, three of grade A and four of grade B, while no grade C fistula occurred. No correlation between PF development and histological findings of the specimens was found. All patients with a grade A fistula were treated conservatively by removing gradually the drain. Patients who had a grade B fistula received total parenteral nutrition (TPN), continuous intravenous somatostatin (6 mg, daily) and antibiotics. In two patients an amylase-rich intra-abdominal collection occurred and was drained by a percutaneous drainage with no severe clinical impact in both cases: this was the reason for classifying them as Grade B (rather than grade C) PF according to recent revisions of the ISGPF

Table 1 Patient demographics

Data	Group A (control; n=24)	Group B (anastomosis; n=12)	P-value
Age (years)	53.6 (25–72)	50.5 (27–67)	0.473
Gender			0.640
- Male	10	4	
- Female	14	8	
BMI	29.6 (24.1-40.5)	28.9 (22.5-35.4)	0.681
Tobacco use	11	5	0.819
Alcohol abuse	6	4	0.611
DM	8	5	0.635
HTN	11	5	0.819
COPD	1	1	0.619
CRF	1	0	0.487

All quantitative values are given as mean (range).
BMI Body Mass Index, DM diabetes mellitus, HTN arterial hypertension, COPD chronic obstructive pulmonary disease, CRF chronic renal failure.

Table 2 Operation data

Data	Group A (control; n=24)	Group B (anastomosis; n=12)	P-value
Histological findings:			0.836
-Adenocarcinoma	8	3	
- Mucinous cystic neoplasm	2	1	
- Serous cystic neoplasm	0	1	
- Chronic pancreatitis	2	1	
- Pancreatic pseudocyst	2	1	
- Neuroendocrine	10	5	
Pancreatic texture:			0.584
- Soft	18	10	
- Fibrous	6	2	
Main pancreatic duct size:			0.622
- Small	15	8	
- Larger	9	4	
Other surgical procedures:			
- Splenectomy	14	8	0.640
- Nephrectomy	2	0	0.162
- Cholecystectomy[a]	3	1	0.717
- Other procedures[b]	1	0	0.487
Operative time	161 (99–245 min)	192 (155–240 min)	0.024

Quantitative values are given as mean (range).
[a]All these patients had gallstones.
[b]In this case a vascular resection with graft reconstruction was performed.

classification [17]. These patients were discharged with drains in situ and observed in the outpatient setting. No patient was readmitted.

Other post-operative outcomes were not significant between the two groups as shown in Table 3.

Postoperative hemorrhage (PH) occurred in two patients of the control group. One patient with normal amylase values from the drain, had a grade C PH due to the rupture of a pseudoaneurysm of the splenic artery after a spleen-preserving DP, which required an angiographic embolization. In the other case the origin of the bleeding was from the retroperitoneal tissue in the spleen site after a DP associated to splenectomy: it was a grade B PH which was treated conservatively by fluids and blood transfusions.

The mean length of hospital stay was higher in group A compared to group B (9.5 vs 8.1 days, respectively), but it was not significant (p=0.077).

Mortality rate was zero in both groups.

Table 3 Post-operative outcomes

Data	Group A (control; n=24)	Group B (anastomosis; n=12)	P-value
Surgical morbidity:			
- Pancreatic fistula[a]	7 (29.1%)	0	0.002
Grade A	3		
Grade B	4		
Grade C	0		
- Hemorrhage[b]	1 (4.1%)	1 (8.3%)	0.162
Grade A	0	0	
Grade B	0	1	
Grade C	1	0	
- Intra-abdominal abscess	2	0	0.162
- Wound infection	1	0	0.424
Medical morbidity[c]:			
- Cardiac	4	1	0.509
- Pulmonary	1	0	0.487
- Renal	0	1	0.487
- Other	1	1	0.619
Length of hospital stay	9.5 (6–14 days)	8.1 (6–12 days)	0.077
Mortality	0	0	

Quantitative values are given as mean (range).
[a]According to the ISGPF classification [15].
[b]According to the ISGPS classification [16].
[c]Defined as non-surgical post-operative complications.

Discussion

DP is a surgical procedure performed with relatively low morbidity and mortality rates in high-volume centers. Surgical outcomes and long-term results have improved widely during the last two decades [18]. However, PF is still the most frequent complication after DP, with an incidence of 5-30% according to the literature [1,3-7], originating from the cut margin of the pancreatic remnant and contributing significantly to morbidity, length of hospital stay and overall costs.

Several approaches to pancreatic stump closure have been described in literature, but none has proved to be the most effective to prevent PF. In a large series by Ferrone et al. [6] different closure techniques were compared as hand-sewn closure, stapler with or without staple line reinforcement, use of free falciform patches and pancreatic duct ligation, but no significant difference in PF rate was found between groups. These data have been confirmed recently by the European multicentric DISPACT trial [7] in which two groups of patients were randomly assigned to stapler or hand-sewn closure of pancreatic remnant with no difference found in PF incidence. The use of artificial patches on the cut margin or the injection of fibrin-glue sealant into the pancreatic duct have also been described [8,9] with good results but larger series are required to demonstrate their efficacy. Recently a new method of stump closure by radiofrequency dissector has been reported with low PF rate, but further prospective studies are needed [10].

As shown in Table 4, few authors described retrospectively their experience of draining the pancreatic stump into a jejunal loop and small series are reported [5,11,12]. More recently, Wagner et al. [14], demonstrated the efficacy of this method comparing the hand-sewn closure to the Roux-en-Y end-to-side pancreato-jejunostomy: they found a zero PF rate in the anastomosis group compared to 20% of PF incidence without anastomosis. However, in that study PF was neither defined nor classified into three grades of severity according to the ISGPF classification [15]. We found same significant results in our series, but with two significant differences: we performed a different type of anastomosis (end-to-end pancreato-jejunostomy) and defined strictly the PF in accordance to the ISGPF classification. The rationale of these encouraging results is based on the assumption that after pancreatic resection the main pancreatic duct is usually visualized and ligated while secondary branches remain always patent owing to their small dimension and this may be a source of pancreatic leakage. This is confirmed by most Authors who reported unchanged PF rates despite they routinely ligated the main pancreatic duct [4,6]. For this reason we minimized the pancreatic secretion by closing the main pancreatic duct while secondary branches were drained by dunking the stump into a jejunal loop: in our opinion the

Table 4 Case series reporting pancreato-jejunostomy and other stump closure techniques after distal pancreatectomy

Authors	Study design	Variable	Sample size n (%)	PF rate (%)	P-value
Lillemoe et al. [1]	Retrospective	Pancreato-jejunostomy	10 (4%)	NA[a]	NA
		Hand-sewn closure	204 (87%)	NA	
		Stapled	11 (5%)	NA	
		Both	10 (4%)	NA	
Kleeff et al. [11]	Retrospective	Pancreatico-jejunostomy	24 (8%)	0	0.03
		Hand-sewn closure	97 (32.1%)	9.3	
		Stapled	145 (48%)	15.9	
		Serosal patches	36 (11.9%)	8.3	
Adam et al. [12]	Retrospective	Pancreatico-jejunostomy	27 (65.8%)	7	NS
		Hand-sewn closure	14 (34.2%)	29	
Wagner et al. [14]	Retrospective	Pancreato-jejunostomy	23 (53.5%)	0	0.04
		Hand-sewn closure	20 (46.5%)	20	

NA not available, NS not significant, PF pancreatic fistula.
[a]In this large series the authors reported a total PF rate of 5% with no comparison between methods of stump closure.

end-to-end anastomosis was the ideal method to achieve a complete drainage of pancreatic juice as the stump is entirely enveloped into the jejunum with this technique compared to the end-to-side anastomosis performed by Wagner et al. [14]. This may explain the low PF rate in our patients. On the other hand, it has to be considered that a pancreatic leakage following small bowel anastomosis could result in a clinically relevant PF (grade B/C PF) and in potentially more hazardous complications (e.g. activation of pancreatic enzymes, bacterial contamination) than leakage after hand-sewn closure of the pancreatic stump. In our series no patient experienced any complication related to the anastomosis, but the statistical power of this study is surely limited by the small sample size of patients, especially for the anastomosis group. For these reasons, at the end of this study, in our institution it currently depends on the surgeon preference to perform the pancreato-jejunostomy especially if it can be carried out safely in selected patients considering the higher operation time and the potential risks of this technique, as described above, despite of its promising results. Moreover there is a clear tendency to perform this operation with a laparoscopic approach, thus some surgeons would prefer anyhow the simple closure by laparoscopic stapler transection rather than open DP with pancreato-jejunostomy.

Besides different techniques of stump closure, other factors have been considered in PF development after DP: the texture of the pancreatic gland, the use of somatostatin and its analogues (octreotide) and the association with splenectomy. Some studies reported that a non-fibrotic (or soft) pancreas with a small MPD is related to an higher PF rate [19,20]: in our study most cases of both groups had a non-fibrotic pancreas and a small MPD but no PF occurred in the anastomosis groups. The role of somatostatin and its analogues in reducing PF rates after

pancreatic surgery is still debated and its use remains controversial [20-24]. Despite a recent Cochrane meta-analysis [22] concluded that the prophylactic use of somatostatin cannot be recommended, other surveys demonstrated its efficacy as consequence of pancreatic exocrine function inhibition after pancreatic surgery [23,24]. On the basis of these studies and in accordance to a more recent meta-analysis [25], we decided to administrate somatostatin analogues prophylactically to all patients, even if most studies cited about its efficacy involved patients undergoing proximal pancreatic resections. The impact of splenectomy on PF development after DP is still controversial [6,26] and we did not find any difference between patients undergoing DP with or without splenectomy.

The operative time was significantly different between the two groups with a mean difference of 31 min, but it was not related to PF development or other postoperative complications.

The length of hospital stay depended primarily on the presence of non-surgical complications.

Conclusion

In this study we observed the efficacy of the pancreato-jejunostomy to prevent PF after DP compared to the hand-sewn closure of the pancreatic remnant. Despite a higher operation time, it is a safe operation with low morbidity and no mortality rate. However, these are results of a retrospective non-randomized analysis of a small group of patients: larger series are required to confirm these data and several centers must be involved in prospective studies.

Competing interests
The authors declare that they have no competing interests.

Authors' contributions
RLM collected and analyzed clinical data, reviewed the literature and drafted the manuscript; RC, DB participated to the acquisition of data; MS, PC reviewed the manuscript for intellectual content. All authors read and approved the final manuscript.

Acknowledgements
This study did not involve any funding body.

References

1. Lillemoe KD, Kaushal S, Cameron JL, Sohn TA, Pitt HA, Yeo CJ: **Distal pancreatectomy: indications and outcomes in 235 patients.** *Ann Surg* 1999, **229**(5):693–698.
2. Schnelldorfer T, Mauldin PD, Lewin DN, Adams DB: **Distal pancreatectomy for chronic pancreatitis: risk factors for postoperative pancreatic fistula.** *J Gastrointest Surg* 2007, **11**(8):991–997.
3. Rodriguez JR, Germes SS, Pandharipande PV, Gazelle GS, Thayer SP, Warshaw AL, Fernandez-del Castillo C: **Implications and cost of pancreatic leak following distal pancreatic resection.** *Arch Surg* 2006, **141**(4):361–366.
4. Adam U, Makowiec F, Riediger H, Benz S, Liebe S, Hopt UT: **Pancreatic leakage after pancreas resection. An analysis of 345 operated patients.** *Chirurg* 2002, **73**(5):466–473.
5. Sheehan MK, Beck K, Creech S, Pickleman J, Aranha GV: **Distal pancreatectomy: does the method of closure influence fistula formation?** *Am Surg* 2002, **68**:264–267.
6. Ferrone CR, Warshaw AL, Rattner DW, Berger D, Zheng H, Rawal B, Rodriguez R, Thayer SP, Fernandez-del Castillo C: **Pancreatic fistula rates after 462 distal pancreatectomies. Stapler do not decrease fistula rates.** *J Gastrointest Surg* 2008, **12**:1691–1698.
7. Diener MK, Seiler CM, Rossion I, Kleeff J, Glanemann M, Butturini G, Tomazic A, Bruns CJ, Busch OR, Farkas S, Belyaev O, Neoptolemos JP, Halloran C, Keck T, Niedergethmann M, Gellert K, Witzigmann H, Kollmar O, Langer P, Steger U, Neudecker J, Berrevoet F, Ganzera S, Heiss MM, Luntz SP, Bruckner T, Kieser M, Büchler MW: **Efficacy of stapler versus hand-sewn closure after distal pancreatectomy (DISPACT): a randomised, controlled multicentre trial.** *Lancet* 2011, **377**(9776):1514–1522.
8. Konishi T, Hiraishi M, Kubota K, Bandai Y, Makuuchi M, Idezuki Y: **Segmental occlusion of the pancreatic duct with prolamine to prevent fistula formation after distal pancreatectomy.** *Ann Surg* 1995, **221**(2):165–170.
9. Ochiai T, Sonoyama T, Soga K, Inoue K, Ikoma H, Shiozaki A, Kuriu Y, Kubota T, Nakanishi M, Kikuchi S, Ichikawa D, Fujiwara H, Sakakura C, Okamoto K, Kokuba Y, Otsuji E: **Application of polyethylene glycolic acid felt with fibrin sealant to prevent postoperative pancreatic fistula in pancreatic surgery.** *J Gastrointest Surg* 2010, **14**(5):884–890.
10. Blansfield JA, Rapp MM, Chokshi RJ, Woll NL, Hunsinger MA, Sheldon DG, Shabahang MM: **Novel method of stump closure for distal pancreatectomy with a 75% reduction in pancreatic fistula rate.** *J Gastrointest Surg* 2012, **16**(3):524–528.
11. Kleeff J, Diener MK, Z'graggen K, Hinz U, Wagner M, Bachmann J, Zehetner J, Müller MW, Friess H, Büchler MW: **Distal pancreatectomy: risk factors for surgical failure in 302 consecutive cases.** *Ann Surg* 2007, **245**(4):573–582.
12. Adam U, Makowiec F, Riediger H, Trzeczak S, Benz S, Hopt UT: **Distal pancreatic resection - indications, techniques and complications.** *Zentralbl Chir* 2001, **126**(11):908–912.
13. Chirletti P, Peparini N, Caronna R, Fanello G, Delogu G, Meniconi RL: **Roux-en-Y end-to-end and end-to-side double pancreaticojejunostomy: application of the reconstructive method of the Beger procedure to central pancreatectomy.** *Langenbecks Arch Surg* 2010, **395**(1):89–93.
14. Wagner M, Gloor B, Ambühl M, Worni M, Lutz JA, Angst E, Candinas D: **Roux-en-Y drainage of the pancreatic stump decreases pancreatic fistula after distal pancreatic resection.** *J Gastrointest Surg* 2007, **11**(3):303–308.
15. Bassi C, Dervenis C, Butturini G, Fingerhut A, Yeo C, Izbicki J, Neoptolemos J, Sarr M, Traverso W, Buchler M: **Postoperative pancreatic fistula: an international study group (ISGPF) definition.** *Surgery* 2005, **138**(1):8–13.
16. Wente MN, Veit JA, Bassi C, Dervenis C, Fingerhut A, Gouma DJ, Izbicki JR, Neoptolemos JP, Padbury RT, Sarr MG, Yeo CJ, Büchler MW: **Postpancreatectomy hemorrhage (PPH): an International Study Group of Pancreatic Surgery (ISGPS) definition.** *Surgery* 2007, **142**(1):20–25.
17. Hashimoto Y, Traverso LW: **Incidence of pancreatic anastomotic failure and delayed gastric emptying after pancreatoduodenectomy in 507 consecutive patients: use of a web-based calculator to improve homogeneity of definition.** *Surgery* 2010, **147**(4):503–515.
18. Balcom JHIV, Rattner DW, Warshaw AL, Chang Y, Fernandez-del Castillo C: **Ten year experience with 733 pancreatic resections: changing indications, older patients and decreasing length of hospitalization.** *Arch Surg* 2001, **136**:391–398.
19. Hamanaka Y, Nishihara K, Hamasaki T, Kawabata A, Yamamoto S, Tsurumi M, Ueno T, Suzuki T: **Pancreatic juice output after pancreatoduodenectomy in relation to pancreatic consistency, duct size, and leakage.** *Surgery* 1996, **119**(3):281–287.
20. Yeo CJ, Cameron JL, Lillemoe KD, Sauter PK, Coleman J, Sohn TA, Campbell KA, Choti MA: **Does prophylactic octreotide decrease the rates of pancreatic fistula and other complications after pancreaticoduodenectomy? Results of a prospective randomized placebo-controlled trial.** *Ann Surg* 2000, **232**(3):419–429.
21. Lowy AM, Lee JE, Pisters PW, Davidson BS, Fenoglio CJ, Stanford P, Jinnah R, Evans DB: **Prospective, randomized trial of octreotide to prevent pancreatic fistula after pancreaticoduodenectomy for malignant disease.** *Ann Surg* 1997, **226**(5):632–641.
22. Gurusamy KS, Koti R, Fusai G, Davidson BR: **Somatostatin analogues for pancreatic surgery.** *Cochrane Database Syst Rev* 2010, **2**, CD008370.
23. Buchler M, Friess H, Kelmpa I, Hermanek P, Sulkowski U, Becker H, Schafmayer A, Baca I, Lorenz D, Meister R: **Role of octreotide in the prevention of postoperative complication following pancreatic resection.** *Am J Surg* 1992, **163**:125–131.
24. Montorsi M, Zago M, Mosca F, Capussotti L, Zotti E, Ribotta G, Fegiz G, Fissi S, Roviaro G, Peracchia A: **Efficacy of octreotide in the prevention of pancreatic fistula after elective pancreatic resections: a prospective, controlled, randomized trial.** *Surgery* 1995, **117**:26–31.
25. Connor S, Alexakis N, Garden OJ, Leandros E, Bramis J, Wigmore SJ: **Meta-analysis of the value of somatostatin and its analogues in reducing complications associated with pancreatic surgery.** *Br J Surg* 2005, **92**(9):1059–1067.
26. Goh BK, Tan YM, Chung YF, Cheow PC, Ong HS, Chan WH, Chow PK, Soo KC, Wong WK, Ooi LL: **Critical appraisal of 232 consecutive distal pancreatectomies with emphasis on risk factors, outcome, and management of the postoperative pancreatic fistula: a 21-year experience at a single institution.** *Arch Surg* 2008, **143**(10):956–965.

12

Extended resection in pancreatic metastases: feasibility, frequency, and long-term outcome: a retrospective analysis

Georg Wiltberger[1*], Julian Nikolaus Bucher[2], Felix Krenzien[3], Christian Benzing[3], Georgi Atanasov[3], Moritz Schmelzle[3], Hans-Michael Hau[1†] and Michael Bartels[1†]

Abstract

Background: Metastases to the pancreas are rare, accounting for less then 2 % of all pancreatic malignancies. However, both the benefit of extended tumor resection and the ideal oncological approach have not been established for such cases; therefore, we evaluated patients with metastasis to the pancreas who underwent pancreatic resection.

Methods: Between 1994 and 2012, 676 patients underwent pancreatic surgery in our institution. We retrospectively reviewed patients' medical records according to survival, and surgical and non-surgical complications. Student's t-test and the log-rank test were used for statistical analysis.

Results: Eighteen patients (2.7 %) received resection for pancreatic metastases (12 multivisceral resections and 6 standard resections). The pancreatic metastases originated from renal cell carcinoma ($n = 10$), malignant melanoma ($n = 2$), neuroendocrine tumor of the ileum ($n = 1$), sarcoma ($n = 1$), colon cancer ($n = 1$), gallbladder cancer ($n = 1$), gastrointestinal stromal tumor ($n = 1$), and non-small cell lung cancer ($n = 1$). The median time between primary malignancy resection to metastasectomy was 83 months (range, 0–228 months). Minor surgical complications (Grade I-IIIa) occurred in six patients (33.3 %) whereas major surgical complications (Grade IIIb-V) occurred in three patients (16.6 %). No patients died during hospitalization. The median follow-up was 76 months (range, 10–165 months). One-year, 3-year and 5-year survival for standard resection versus multivisceral resection was 83, 50, and 56 % versus 83, 66, and 50, respectively. Twelve patients died after a median of 26 months (range, 5–55 months).

Conclusions: A surgical approach with curative intent is justified in select patients suffering from metastases to the pancreas and offers good long-term survival. The resection of pancreatic metastases of different tumor types was associated with favorable morbidity and mortality when compared with resection of the primary pancreatic malignancies. Our findings also demonstrated that multivisceral resection was feasible, with acceptable long term outcomes, even though morbidity rates tended to be higher after multivisceral resection than after standard resection.

Keywords: Multivisceral resection, Metastases to the pancreas, Pancreaticoduodenectomy

* Correspondence: georg.wiltberger@medizin.uni-leipzig.de
†Equal contributors
[1]Department of Visceral, Transplantation, Thoracic, and Vascular Surgery, University Hospital Leipzig, 04103 Leipzig, Germany
Full list of author information is available at the end of the article

Background

Metastases to the pancreas are rare and account only for 1–2 % of all pancreatic malignancies [1]. Most primaries that spread to the pancreas are renal cell carcinomas (RCC), lung cancers, malignant melanomas, and malignancies of the gastrointestinal tract [2, 3]. However, at the time of diagnosis, patients often present with widespread systemic disease and therefore, no curative treatment is applicable. Several studies have demonstrated survival benefit and improved quality of life after complete metastasectomy for isolated lung or liver metastases [4, 5]. Therefore, extended surgical intervention is a well-established approach in a multidisciplinary concept for select patients suffering from colorectal or pulmonary metastases in the liver [6]. However, extended surgery for pancreatic metastasectomy is rare and remains debatable as there have been few studies on the procedure, all of which have reported controversial results [7–9]. Patients with localized extrapancreatic disease appear to be suitable for pancreatic resection but the ideal oncological approach has not been established and the benefit of multivisceral resection (MVR) remains undetermined. Our aim was to assess the frequency and feasibility of MVR for metastases to the pancreas. We also analyzed the influence of MVR on perioperative and long-term outcomes compared with standard resection.

Methods

We retrospectively analyzed the medical records of patients who underwent pancreatic resection at the Department of Visceral, Transplant, Thoracic, and Vascular Surgery, University Hospital Leipzig, Leipzig, Germany, between 1994 and 2012.

For this study ethical approval was obtained from the institutional local ethical committee (AZ 318-14-06102014, Ethical committee of the University Clinic Leipzig, Leipzig). Due to the retrospective design of the study and accordingly national guidelines, the local ethic committee confirmed, that informed consent was not necessary from participants.

All patients were operated on with curative intent. We included patients with extrapancreatic spread in this study only when extrapancreatic disease appeared to be resectable, and we excluded patients with primary tumors that had infiltrated the pancreas through direct extension.

We assessed the following patient characteristics: sex, age, body mass index, preoperative symptoms, comorbidities, type of resection, duration of operation, required units of fresh frozen plasma and/or packed red blood cells, median length of stay on the intensive care unit, total length of stay, time between surgery for the primary tumor and pancreatic resection, postoperative morbidity according to Clavien-Dindo classification [10], presence of pancreatic fistulae according to the International Study Group for Pancreatic Fistula criteria [11], hospital mortality defined as death within the first 60 days after resection, overall survival rate, disease-free survival, and histopathological data. Patients who died within the first 90 days after resection were excluded from further statistical analysis. MVR was defined as resection of one additional organ, excluding the spleen.

Statistics

Data are presented as median (range) unless otherwise specified. Statistical differences between groups were determined by Student's t-test. Student's t-test and the log-rank test were used to analyze continuous variables and overall survival excluding in-hospital mortality, respectively. All statistical analyses were performed with SPSS for Windows (version 12.0, SPSS Inc., Chicago, IL, USA).

Results

Patient characteristics and preoperative symptoms

Between 1994 and 2012, 676 patients were scheduled for pancreatic surgery, of which 18 (2.6 %) received resection for metastatic disease of the pancreas (Table 1). Eight of the patients were men and 10 were woman with a median age of 65 years (range, 22–75 years) and a median body mass index of 25.4 kg/m^2 (range, 18–31 kg/m^2). Four patients (22.2 %), had diabetes mellitus type II and 13 (72.2 %) patients received medication for high blood pressure (Table 2). At the time of diagnosis of pancreatic metastases, eight patients (44.4 %) had one or more tumor-related symptoms including weight loss ($n = 8$), abdominal pain ($n = 8$), decrease in general performance ($n = 5$), obstructive jaundice ($n = 2$), or absence of appetite ($n = 1$). Ten patients (55.5 %) had no specific symptoms and the diagnosis of pancreatic metastases was obtained through routine follow-up examinations.

Primary tumor characteristics

The majority of pancreatic metastases originated from renal cell carcinoma ($n = 10$; 55.5 %), malignant melanoma ($n = 2$), and neuroendocrine tumor of the ileum ($n = 1$). Other primaries included sarcoma ($n = 1$), colon cancer ($n = 1$), gallbladder cancer ($n = 1$), gastrointestinal stromal tumor ($n = 1$), and non-small cell lung cancer ($n = 1$). Metastases to the pancreas were located mainly in the pancreatic head ($n = 10$) followed by the total pancreas ($n = 3$) and the cauda region ($n = 3$). In two patients, metastases were simultaneously located in the corpus and cauda region. Eleven patients (61 %) had simultaneous metastases in other organs and seven of these patients underwent

Table 1 Patient characteristics

Case No.	Primary Malignancy	Location in the pancreas (sync./metac.)	Time interval (months)*	Type of Operation	further metastases at detection of pancreatic metastasis□	tumor recurrence/ survival status†
1	RCC	Head (sync.)	0	PPPD + Nephrectomy	no	no/alive
2	Lung-Cancer	Cauda (metac.)	83	DP + Gastrectomy + Splenectomy + vertebral body resection	Vertebral body (s)	no/TRD
3	RCC	Head (metac.)	142	PPPD	no	no/Non-TRD
4	RCC	Head (sync.)	0.8	PPPD	no	Local recurrence/alive
5	RCC	Head/Corpus/Cauda (metac.)	120	Enucleation in pancreatic head + DP + Splenectomy	Lung (s)	Thyroid/TRD
6	RCC	Head/Corpus/Cauda (metac.)	132	TP + Spleenectomy + distal Gastrectomy	Thyroid (s)	no/TRD
7	Gallblader-Cancer	Head (sync.)	0	PPPD + Liver resection (SII SIII)	Liver (a)	yes/TRD
8	RCC	Corpus/Cauda (sync.)	17	DP + Spleen + Colon +Jejunom	Pulmo (s)	no/TRD
9	GIST	Head (metac.)	34	PPPD + Hemicolectomy	Liver (a)	yes/alive
10	RCC	Head (metac.)	106	Whipple	no	Lung/TRD
11	Sarcoma	Head (sync.)	0	Whipple + Hemihepatectomy + Hemicolectomy	Liver (s)	Liver/TRD
12	RCC	Head/Corpus/Cauda (metac.)	66	TP + Spleen	no	Cerebral/TRD
13	Melanoma	Head/Corpus/Cauda (metac.)	90	TP + Segemental liver resection	Liver (a)	Liver/alive
14	RCC	Cauda (metac.)	123	DP	Pulmo (s)	Thyroid/TRD
15	Melanoma	Head (metac.)	228	PPPD + Hemihepatectomy	Liver (a)	Liver/TRD
16	RCC	Head (sync.)	0	DP + Spleen + Nephrctomy	no	no/alive
17	Colon-Cancer	Head (metac.)	29	PPPD + Liver resection (Lobus caudatus)	Liver (s)	no/alive
18	NET Ileum	Head (sync.)	78	PPPD + Jejunom	Jejunum (s)	no/alive

sync. indicates synchronous metastases to the pancreas; metac. indicates metachronous metastases to the pancreas; * interval from resection of primary tumor to resection of pancreatic metastasis; □ excluding pancreas (a, after; s, synchronous; p, prior); † at time of study; RCC indicates renal cell carcinoma; NET indicates neuroendocrine tumor; PPPD indicates pylorus-preserving pancreaticoduodenectomy; DP indicates distal pancreatectomy; TP indicates total pancreatectomy; TRD indicates tumor-related death

Table 2 Demographic data

Characteristics	Total (*n* = 18)	Standard Resection (*n* = 6)	Multivisceral resection (MVR; *n* = 12)	*p*-value*
Age (median; Range)	65 (22–75)	70 (49–75)	58 (22–72)	0.074
Gender (%)				
Female	10 (55.6)	4 (22.2)	6 (33.3)	0.548
Male	8 (44.4)	2 (11.1)	6 (33.3)	0.548
BMI (median; Range)	25.4 (18–31.1)	26 (21.7–30.4)	24.4 (18–31.1)	0.264
Comorbidities (%)				
Diabetes mellitus	4 (22.2)	2 (11.1)	2 (11.1)	0.932
Arterial hypertension	13 (72.2)	5 (33.3)	8 (44.4)	0.817
Metabolic syndrome	3 (16.7)	1 (5.6)	2 (11.1)	0.932
COPD*	2 (11.1)	0 (0)	2 (11.1)	0.104
CAD	5 (27.8)	1 (5.6)	4 (22.2)	0.374
Preoperative symptoms (%)				
Asymptomatic	10 (55.6)	4 (22.2)	6 (33.3)	0.548
Symptomatic				
Weight loss	8 (44.4)	3 (16.7)	5 (33.3)	0.984
Abdominal pain	7 (38.9)	3 (16.7)	4 (33.3)	0.682
obstructive jaundice	2 (11.1)	0 (0)	2 (11.1)	0.103
decrease in general performance	3 (16.7)	1 (5.6)	2 (11.1)	0.742
absence of appetite	1 (5.6)	1 (5.6)	0 (0)	0.170
Sleep hyperhidrosis	1 (5.6)	0 (0)	1 (5.6)	0.166
New onset of diabetes	1 (5.6)	0 (0)	1 (5.6)	0.166

COPD indicates chronic obstructive pulmonary disease; CAD indicates coronary artery disease

simultaneous resection of the extrapancreatic masses. The other four patients received a subsequent procedure (metastasectomy of the lungs in three cases and one thyroidectomy). In four patients, the diagnosis of pancreatic metastases coincided with that of the primary malignancy, which was RCC in all cases. In three of these patients, primary tumor and metastatic resection was performed as one procedure. In one patient, an intraoperative biopsy of the pancreatic head during tumor-nephrectomy confirmed metastatic disease and metastasectomy was performed four weeks later. In three patients (30 %) with RCC multifocal lesions in the resected specimens were detected.

Surgical procedures
The median time between resection of the primary malignancies to resection of the pancreatic metastases was 83 months (range, 0–228 months). The most frequently used surgical procedures were Whipple-procedure/pylorus-preserving pancreaticoduodenectomy (PPPD) in 10 patients and distal pancreatectomy (DP) in five patients. In four patients, DP was performed with and, in one patient, without splenectomy. In three patients, total pancreatectomy was performed, with simultaneous splenectomy in two cases. MVR was performed in 12

(66.6 %) patients. Five patients who received Whipple-procedure/PPPD or total pancreatectomy also required additional liver resection to remove synchronous extrapancreatic metastases. Two of these patients underwent additional bowel resection and three patients received additional gastric or bowel resection. In two patients who underwent PPPD or DP, simultaneous nephrectomy was performed and one patient received simultaneous vertebral body resection for solitary bone metastasis. The median operation time for all procedures was 322 min (range, 193–591 min). Ten patients received intraoperative fresh frozen plasma (median 3, range 0–18 units) and/or packed red blood cells (median 2, range, 0–10 units). Microscopically-free resection margins (R0) were achieved in 77.7 % of the patients.

Perioperative outcome
Length of stay in the intensive care unit and total length of stay were 2 days (range, 1–50 days) and 21.5 days (range, 12–55 days), respectively (Table 3). No patients died during hospitalization. Postoperative complications occurred in 11 patients (61.1 %), of which 81 % were surgical and 18 % were non-surgical complications. Minor surgical complications (Grade I-IIIa, *n* = 6) were: new onset of diabetes in two patients; wound infection

Table 3 Perioperative data

Data	Total (*n* = 18)	StandardResection (*n* = 6)	Multivisceral resection (*n* = 12)	*p*-Value
Operative Data				
Length of operation (min)	322 (193–591)	261 (193–462)	346 (216–591)	0.137
FFPs and/or pRBCs	3 (0–18) 2 (0–10)	3 (0– 3) 1 (0–8)	3 (0–18) 4 (1–10)	0.291/0.838
Perioperative Data				
LOS-ICU	2 (1–50)	1 (1–3)	3 (1–50)	0.205
T-LOS	21 (12–55)	20 (16– 2)	23 (12–55)	0.898
Time interval*	72 (0–228)	113 (0–142)	31.5 (0–228)	0.259
Follow-up	76 (10–165)	59 (28–95)	53 (10–165)	0.104
1-year/3-year/5-year survival	84/66/55	83/50/56	83/66/50	
Histopathological data				
RO/R1/R2	15/3/0 (83.3/16.7/0)	7/0/0 (38.9/0/0)	8/3/0 (44.4/16.7/0)	0.081
Negative/positive LN	13/5 (72.2/27.8)	6/1 (33.3/5.6)	7/4 (38.9/22.2)	0.278
Postoperative Complications (Clavien-Dindo classification)				
Non-Surgical related complications				
Minor (Grade I-IIIa)	0 (0)	0 (0)	0 (0)	0
Major (Grade IIIb – IV)	2 (11.1)	1 (5.6)	1 (5.6)	0.681
Surgical related complications				
Minor (Grade I-IIIa)	6 (33.3)	2 (11.1)	4 (22.2)	0.781
Major (Grade IIIb – IV)	3 (16.7)	1 (5.6)	2 (11.1)	0.932
Overall Morbidity				
Mortality (60 days)	0 (0)	0 (0)	0 (0)	0
Overall-Mortality				
Follow up				
Local recurrence	1 (5.6)	1 (5.6)	0 (0)	0.166
Extrapancreatic Recurrence	9 (50)	4 (22.2)	5 (33.3)	0.565
Further surgical interventions	6 (33.3)	2 (11.1)	4 (22.2)	0.781

FFP, fresh frozen plasma; pRBC, packed red blood cells; LOS-ICU, length of stay in intensive care unit; T-LOS; total length of stay

(*n* = 2), which was managed conservatively; and pancreatic fistula grade B with prolonged use of abdominal drainage (*n* = 2). Major surgical complications (Grade IIIb-V, *n* = 3) were: leakage from the hepaticojejunostomy site with the need for relaparotomy, bowel perforation with the need for relaparotomy, biliary leakage after combined liver and pancreas resection that had to be treated with an interventional drain, and a wound infection that required re-operation under general anesthesia, with each complication occurring in one case. Major non-surgical complications (Grade IIIb-V, *n* = 2) occurred in two patients and both developed pneumonia requiring readmission to the intensive care unit.

Follow-up and survival

No patient was lost to follow-up and the median follow-up time was 76 months (range, 10–165 months) with 12 patients dying after a median of 26 months (range, 5–55 months). Death was tumor-related in 11 cases and non-

tumor-related in one case. During follow-up, nine patients suffered from extrapancreatic recurrence. Five patients received further surgical treatment including thyroidectomy, liver resection, or metastasectomy of the lungs. In one patient, cerebral metastasis was treated by stereotactic irradiation. Local recurrence of pancreatic disease was seen in one patient and was successfully controlled by total resection of the pancreatic remnant.

In our sample, the time interval between resection of the primary malignancy and detection of metastatic disease did not correlate significantly with overall survival after resection of the pancreatic metastases. Kaplan-Meier curve for survival with standard resection versus MVR are shown in Fig. 1. One-, 3- and 5-year survival for standard resection versus MVR was 83, 50, and 56 %, versus 83, 66, and 50 %, respectively.

Discussion

Surgical interventions for metastatic disease have increased over the last decade, concurrent with considerable

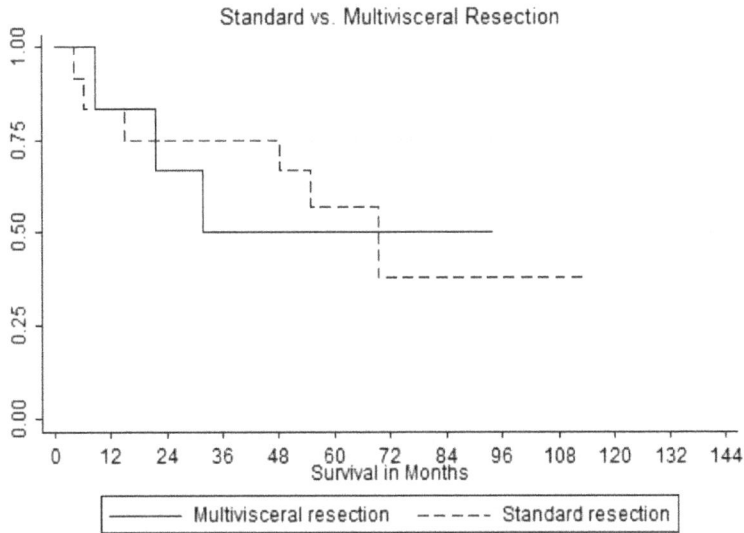

Fig. 1 Kaplan–Meier survival curve showing survival for patients who underwent standard resection (solid line) versus multivisceral resection (dotted line) (in months)

improvement in quality of life and long-term survival of up to 10 years following resection for the most common (liver or lung) metastases [12, 13]. As a result, surgical resection of metastases is now an integral part of a multidisciplinary oncological approach [6]. In contrast, metastases to the pancreas are uncommon and the majority of patients present with no specific symptoms [14] and with non-resectable widespread disease at the time of diagnosis. However, in cases of isolated disease, surgical intervention may be beneficial in terms of overall survival, even in patients with localized extrapancreatic metastases, and in terms of the need for MVR to obtain complete tumor-free resection margins.

Based on our experience, surgical intervention is justified in select patients diagnosed with metastases to the pancreas. Our data showed that surgical resection for pancreatic metastases is feasible and provides good long term results, even in patients undergoing MVR. Perioperative morbidity and in-hospital mortality were comparable to studies evaluating standard pancreatic resection for primary malignancies [15]. In our study, morbidity after MVR tended to be higher than after standard resection. However, MVR for pancreatic metastases should not be considered an absolute contraindication for surgery, because our results indicated equivalent overall survival in the MVR group.

The limitations of our study are the small cohort and the absence of a control group treated by other therapeutic strategies. Therefore, general recommendations cannot be made based on our data, even though complete resection (R0) is generally considered a good prognostic marker for patients' overall survival [16]. For instance, long-term survival of 10 years can be seen after

complete resection of colorectal liver metastases, which emphasizes the importance of this therapeutic option [12]. In our study, the rate of microscopically-free resection margins (77.7 %) did not differ from other studies reporting positive resection margins for pancreatic cancer of 17–30 % [17–19].

Because of the high incidence of metastatic disease originating from RCC, the most valid conclusions can be provided for this tumor type. Consequently, most reported data refer to RCC and are comparable with our results in terms of incidence and overall survival [1, 8, 20]. In our study, 10 patients (55.5 %) had pancreatic metastases from RCC and the overall survival of this subgroup was 60 %. In a recently published review, Tanis et al. reported a 5-year survival rate of 72.6 % in 311 cases following pancreatic surgery for RCC metastases [21]. In this context, time of metastatic onset is discussed as a prognostic marker for long-term survival. A small number of studies have observed a trend to better overall survival in patients with long disease-free interval when evaluating primary tumor resection and onset of metastases to the pancreas. We did not see a similar effect in our patients because overall survival did not differ significantly between patients with longer disease-free interval. These findings are supported by the results of a meta-analysis which identified 15 studies addressing pancreatic metastasectomy for RCC [1]. In the univariate analysis, time from resection of the primary tumor did not affect overall survival.

Many changes have been made, regarding the oncological treatment for metastatic RCC. Individualized immunotherapy based on immunoreactive cytokines and/ or antiangiogenetic agents (e.g. bevacizumab, sunitinib,

and sorafenib) have showed encouraging results. Therefore, surgical resection should not be considered as the
only therapeutic option: An interdisciplinary approach
including visceral surgeons, urologists and oncologists
should be performed for the treatment against pancreatic metastases to obtain sufficient synergistic antitumor
effects. However, the best way to combine surgery with
oncological treatment has to be evaluated addressed by
future studies.

Pancreatic metastases can occur after a long disease-
free interval, with a median time between resection of
the primary tumor and detection of pancreatic metastases of 72 months (range, 0–228 months). This biological
tumor behavior reflects the importance of a prudent
long-term follow-up in these patients, even if specific
symptoms are missing. This point is supported by our
findings, which revealed that only 44.4 % of the patients
had specific symptoms. We recommend that regular
follow-up including radiological imaging should be performed even after a long disease-free interval.

Very few data are available regarding the potential impact of MVR for pancreatic metastases on morbidity and
mortality because of the low proportion of patients with
MVR in most of the published studies [20]. However, in
our study, the majority of patients (66.6 %) were treated
by a multivisceral approach. In a retrospective analysis,
Strobel et al. compared patients who received either
standard resection or MVR for pancreatic metastases of
different tumor types [22]. The authors reported no significant difference for morbidity and mortality between
groups, although morbidity in the MVR group tended to
be higher. Also, the majority of complications were surgical, with one patient dying in each group. These results
are comparable to our results where the majority of
postoperative complications were also surgical. We also
saw that major surgical complications occurred more
frequently in the MVR group, although this result was
not statistically significant. Because of its potentially
beneficial impact on long-term survival, we do not consider that MVR is an absolute contraindication but that
the increased operative risk should be considered in the
decision making process. The overall morbidity in our
study was not increased compared with the reported
morbidity rate for resection of primary pancreatic malignancies of up to 58.5 %, even though major surgical
complications occurred more frequently in our study
[15]. This might be attributable to the high proportion
of patients who underwent MVR.

During our study follow-up, only one patient suffered from tumor recurrence in the pancreas and this
was successfully treated by resection of the pancreatic
remnant without further tumor recurrence. This might be
interpreted as a sign of good local tumor control and is
supported by other studies [22].

In total, nine of our patients (50 %) developed extrapancreatic recurrence, of which five (33.3 %) had undergone previous MVR. Four patients received primarily
combined liver and pancreas resection for metastases of
sarcoma or gallbladder cancer (n = 1 for each cancer)
and for metastases of malignant melanoma in two cases.
In the latter patients, hepatic recurrence occurred and
further surgical intervention was performed in one patient, who is still alive. These results are consistent with
other reports showing a survival rate of 50 % after liver
resection for malignant melanoma [23]. Therefore, the
type of the primary tumor should also be considered
when deciding on surgery and the patient should be informed of the risk of recurrence.

Conclusions
A surgical approach with curative intent is justified in
select patients suffering from metastases to the pancreas and offers good long-term survival. Our results
showed that resection of pancreatic metastases of different tumor types was associated with favorable morbidity and mortality when compared with resection of
the primary pancreatic malignancies. Our findings also
demonstrated that MVR was feasible, with acceptable
long term outcomes, even though morbidity tended to
be higher than with standard resection.

Abbreviations
DP: distal pancreatectomy; MVR: multivisceral resection; PPPD: pylorus-preserving
pancreaticoduodenectomy; RCC: renal cell carcinoma.

Competing interests
The authors declare that they have no competing interests.

Authors' contributions
GW, JB, HMH and MB were responsible for the study conception and design;
GW, CB, JB, FK, GA, and HMH were responsible for data acquisition; GW, JB,
HMH, and MB analyzed and interpreted the data; GW, JB, and HMH drafted
the manuscript; and FK, JB, CB, MS, HMH and MB critically revised the
manuscript. All authors read and approved the final manuscript.

Acknowledgements
The authors declare that no funding was received for the study.

Author details
[1]Department of Visceral, Transplantation, Thoracic, and Vascular Surgery,
University Hospital Leipzig, 04103 Leipzig, Germany. [2]Department of Surgery,
University Hospital Großhadern (LMU), Munich, Germany. [3]Department of
General, Visceral, and Transplant Surgery, Charité - Universitätsmedizin Berlin,
Campus Virchow Klinikum, Augustenburger Platz 1, 13353 Berlin, Germany.

References
1. Reddy S, Wolfgang CL. The role of surgery in the management of isolated
    metastases to the pancreas. Lancet Oncol. 2009;10:287–93.
2. Eidt S, Jergas M, Schmidt R, Siedek M. Metastasis to the pancreas–an
    indication for pancreatic resection? Langenbecks Arch Surg. 2007;392:
    539–42.
3. Sellner F, Tykalsky N, De Santis M, Pont J, Klimpfinger M. Solitary and
    multiple isolated metastases of clear cell renal carcinoma to the pancreas:
    an indication for pancreatic surgery. Ann Surg Oncol. 2006;13(1):75–85.

4. Quiros RM, Scott WJ. Surgical treatment of metastatic disease to the lung. Semin Oncol. 2008;35(2):134–46.
5. Choti MA, Sitzmann JV, Tiburi MF, Sumetchotimetha W, Rangsin R, Schulick RD, et al. Trends in long-term survival following liver resection for hepatic colorectal metastases. Ann Surg. 2002;235(6):759–66.
6. Garden OJ, Rees M, Poston GJ, Mirza D, Saunders M, Ledermann J, et al. Guidelines for resection of colorectal cancer liver metastases. Gut. 2006;55 Suppl 3:iii1–8.
7. Hiotis SP, Klimstra DS, Conlon KC, Brennan MF. Results after pancreatic resection for metastatic lesions. Ann Surg Oncol. 2002;9(7):675–9.
8. Zerbi A, Ortolano E, Balzano G, Borri A, Beneduce AA, Di Carlo V. Pancreatic metastasis from renal cell carcinoma: which patients benefit from surgical resection? Ann Surg Oncol. 2008;15(4):1161–8.
9. Bahra M, Jacob D, Langrehr JM, Glanemann M, Schumacher G, Lopez-Hanninen E, et al. Metastatic lesions to the pancreas. When is resection reasonable? Chirurg. 2008;79(3):241–8.
10. DeOliveira ML, Winter JM, Schafer M, Cunningham SC, Cameron JL, Yeo CJ, et al. Assessment of complications after pancreatic surgery: A novel grading system applied to 633 patients undergoing pancreaticoduodenectomy. Ann Surg. 2006;244(6):931–7. discussion 937–939.
11. Bassi C, Dervenis C, Butturini G, Fingerhut A, Yeo C, Izbicki J, et al. Postoperative pancreatic fistula: an international study group (ISGPF) definition. Surgery. 2005;138(1):8–13.
12. Tomlinson JS, Jarnagin WR, DeMatteo RP, Fong Y, Kornprat P, Gonen M, et al. Actual 10-year survival after resection of colorectal liver metastases defines cure. J Clin Oncol. 2007;25(29):4575–80.
13. Marudanayagam R, Ramkumar K, Shanmugam V, Langman G, Rajesh P, Coldham C, et al. Long-term outcome after sequential resections of liver and lung metastases from colorectal carcinoma. HPB (Oxford). 2009;11(8):671–6.
14. Konstantinidis IT, Dursun A, Zheng H, Wargo JA, Thayer SP, Fernandez-del Castillo C, et al. Metastatic tumors in the pancreas in the modern era. J Am Coll Surg. 2010;211(6):749–53.
15. Addeo P, Delpero JR, Paye F, Oussoultzoglou E, Fuchshuber PR, Sauvanet A, et al. Pancreatic fistula after a pancreaticoduodenectomy for ductal adenocarcinoma and its association with morbidity: a multicentre study of the French Surgical Association. HPB (Oxford). 2014;16(1):46–55.
16. Rau BM, Moritz K, Schuschan S, Alsfasser G, Prall F, Klar E. R1 resection in pancreatic cancer has significant impact on long-term outcome in standardized pathology modified for routine use. Surgery. 2012;152(3 Suppl 1):S103–11.
17. Sohn TA, Yeo CJ, Cameron JL, Koniaris L, Kaushal S, Abrams RA, et al. Resected adenocarcinoma of the pancreas-616 patients: results, outcomes, and prognostic indicators. J Gastrointest Surg. 2000;4(6):567–79.
18. Howard TJ, Krug JE, Yu J, Zyromski NJ, Schmidt CM, Jacobson LE, et al. A margin-negative R0 resection accomplished with minimal postoperative complications is the surgeon's contribution to long-term survival in pancreatic cancer. J Gastrointest Surg. 2006;10(10):1338–45. discussion 1345–1336.
19. Butturini G, Stocken DD, Wente MN, Jeekel H, Klinkenbijl JH, Bakkevold KE, et al. Influence of resection margins and treatment on survival in patients with pancreatic cancer: meta-analysis of randomized controlled trials. Arch Surg. 2008;143(1):75–83. discussion 83.
20. Niess H, Conrad C, Kleespies A, Haas F, Bao Q, Jauch KW, et al. Surgery for metastasis to the pancreas: is it safe and effective? J Surg Oncol. 2013;107(8):859–64.
21. Tanis PJ, van der Gaag NA, Busch OR, van Gulik TM, Gouma DJ. Systematic review of pancreatic surgery for metastatic renal cell carcinoma. Br J Surg. 2009;96(6):579–92.
22. Strobel O, Hackert T, Hartwig W, Bergmann F, Hinz U, Wente MN, et al. Survival data justifies resection for pancreatic metastases. Ann Surg Oncol. 2009;16(12):3340–9.
23. Ryu SW, Saw R, Scolyer RA, Crawford M, Thompson JF, Sandroussi C. Liver resection for metastatic melanoma: equivalent survival for cutaneous and ocular primaries. J Surg Oncol. 2013;108(2):129–35.

13

Large retroperitoneal isolated fibrous cyst in absence of preceding trauma or acute pancreatitis

Julie Ahn[1], Manju D Chandrasegaram[1,2], Khaled Alsaleh[2], Benjamin L Woodham[1,2], Adrian Teo[2], Amithaba Das[2], Neil D Merrett[1,2]* and Christos Apostolou[2]

Abstract

Background: Isolated retroperitoneal cystic masses are uncommon with an estimated incidence of 1/5750 to 1/250,000. The majority present with size related symptoms, complications, or a mass. Approximately a third of patients are asymptomatic and are diagnosed incidentally.

Aetiologies of retroperitoneal cystic masses (RPC) include mesenteric, omental, splenic and enteric duplication cysts. Neoplastic RPCs can be divided into epithelial (mucinous or serous cystadenoma), mesothelial (mesothelioma), germ cell (cystic teratoma) and cystic changes in a solid neoplasm (paraganglioma, neurilemmoma, sarcoma).

Case presentation: A 53 year-old man presented to us with abdominal pain related to a large mass in his left upper quadrant with associated anorexia and weight loss. He gave no history of previous trauma and denied having symptoms or a history of pancreatitis. He said he had felt this mass increasing in size over the course of several years.

Clinical examination of his abdomen revealed a large firm left sided mass extending to his left upper quadrant. Imaging with computed tomography (CT) and magnetic resonance imaging cholangio-pancreatogram (MRCP) revealed a 13.7 cm × 12.2 cm × 10.9 cm cystic lesion in the retroperitoneum which was separate from the kidney, pancreas, spleen and bowel. At laparotomy, this mass was easily dissected from the surrounding viscera and was excised completely intact.

Histopathological assessment found the mass to be a large fibrous pseudocyst with no epithelial lining.

Conclusion: We present a rare case of an isolated large retroperitoneal fibrous pseudocyst unrelated to previous pancreatitis which was successfully managed with surgery.

Keywords: Retroperitoneal cyst, Fibrous cyst, Retroperitoneal mass, Pseudocyst, Cystic mass

Background

Retroperitoneal cystic masses, which are isolated and separate from surrounding major organs are uncommon, with an estimated incidence of 1/5750 to 1/250,000 [1]. Approximately one third of patients with a retroperitoneal cyst (RPC) are asymptomatic and are diagnosed as an incidental finding [1,2]. Two thirds present with symptoms relating to size and complications, and this most often is from a noticeable abdominal mass [3].

The most common cause of retroperitoneal cystic masses are pseudocysts related to pancreatitis which occur more frequently with acute-on chronic pancreatitis [4]. Other causes of retroperitoneal cysts include cysts that develop from surrounding structures such as mesenteric, omental, splenic and enteric duplication cysts. Neoplastic causes included cystadenomas, mesotheliomas, and cystic degeneration that can arise from solid neoplasms [2]. Non-neoplastic causes include haematomas, urinomas, lymphoceles, pancreatic and non-pancreatic pseudocysts [2].

We report a case of a patient presenting with a large isolated retroperitoneal cystic mass in the absence of preceding trauma or pancreatitis.

* Correspondence: neil.merrett@sswahs.nsw.gov.au
[1]Division of Surgery, University of Western Sydney, Sydney, Australia
[2]Upper Gastrointestinal Unit, Bankstown Hospital, Sydney, Australia

Case presentation

A 53-year-old man presented with a four-week history of worsening abdominal pain, anorexia and weight loss. This was on a background of a known large left sided cystic mass, which was discovered on imaging while he resided overseas nine months ago. He described his symptoms up until this presentation as mild but now complained of post-prandial abdominal pain, occasional vomiting and diarrhea. His impression was that the mass had been increasing in size for the past month. His past medical history included hepatitis C and diverticulosis. He gave no history of previous trauma and denied having symptoms or a history of pancreatitis in the past. There was no history of gallstones and no evidence of gallstones on prior or current imaging. His alcohol intake approximated 20 standard drinks a week. He also gave a 30 pack-year smoking history in addition to smoking marijuana daily.

On clinical examination, he had a grossly visible mass in his left upper quadrant, which could be appreciated at the end of the bed. This mass was firm and mildly tender. His blood examination revealed haemoglobin 124 g/L (Reference range: 130–180 g/L), l white cell count of 6.4 x10^9/L (Reference range: 4–11 x10^9/L) and CRP of 11.3 mg/L (Reference range: <5 mg/L). Renal function and liver enzymes were normal. His CEA was elevated at 9.5 µg/L (Reference range: <2.5 µg/L). CA 19.9 and AFP tumour marker were normal.

Computed tomography (CT) scan of the abdomen and magnetic resonance cholangio-pancreatogram (MRCP) revealed a large retroperitoneal cystic lesion in the left flank with no septations or enhancement, measuring 13.7 cm craniocaudally, 12.2 cm transversely and 10.9 cm anteroposteriorly. It appeared to be isolated and separate from the adjacent organs including the pancreas, stomach, spleen and left kidney (Figure 1). There were two small simple cysts in the spleen. There was mild to moderate dilation of the left renal pelvis, calyces and proximal left ureter. This was likely due to partial mechanical distortion from the mass, which displaced the left ureter laterally. The right kidney was normal.

After discussion with the patient, the decision was made to resect the cyst due to his increasing symptoms of abdominal pain and for diagnostic certainty. At operation, the cyst was isolated from the pancreas and dissected from the left ureter, left kidney, renal vessels and aorta and did not communicate with any of these structures (Figures 2 and 3). The spleen was preserved. His recovery post-operatively was uneventful. His post-prandial pain and vomiting resolved and he was able to eat better post-operatively.

Histopathological assessment of the resected cyst revealed no epithelial lining to this cyst, and it was in fact a large fibrous pseudocyst.

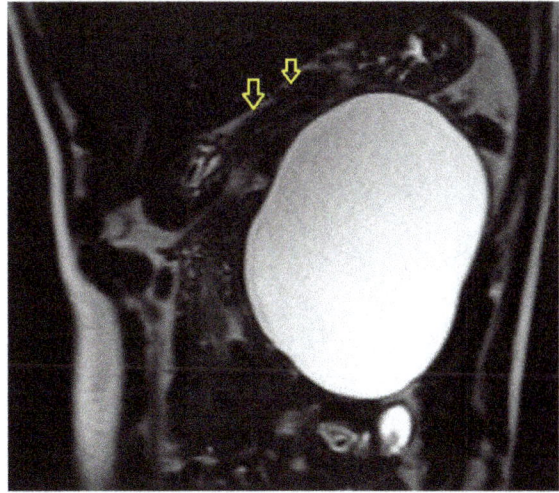

Figure 1 Coronal MRI (T2 phase) showing large retroperitoneal cyst with no septations. The retroperitoneal cyst is separate to the pancreas (Pancreas – yellow arrow).

As the cyst was delivered intact for pathological assessment, the fluid was not tested for amylase, or lipase.

Discussion

Our patient had a large pseudocyst in the retroperitoneum, which developed in the absence of a history of pancreatitis. Non-pancreatic pseudocysts are rare lesions which often arise from the mesentery or omentum [2]. They characteristically have a thick, fibrous wall lacking an epithelial lining, and contain haemorrhage, pus or serous fluid, which unlike pancreatic pseudocysts is not associated with high levels of amylase and lipase. On imaging they present as unilocular or multilocular cystic masses with thick walls [3]. They can develop secondary to trauma or infection and are thought to be the

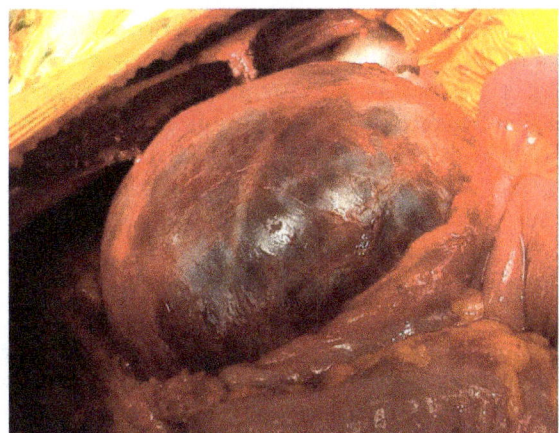

Figure 2 Operative image of retroperitoneal cyst.

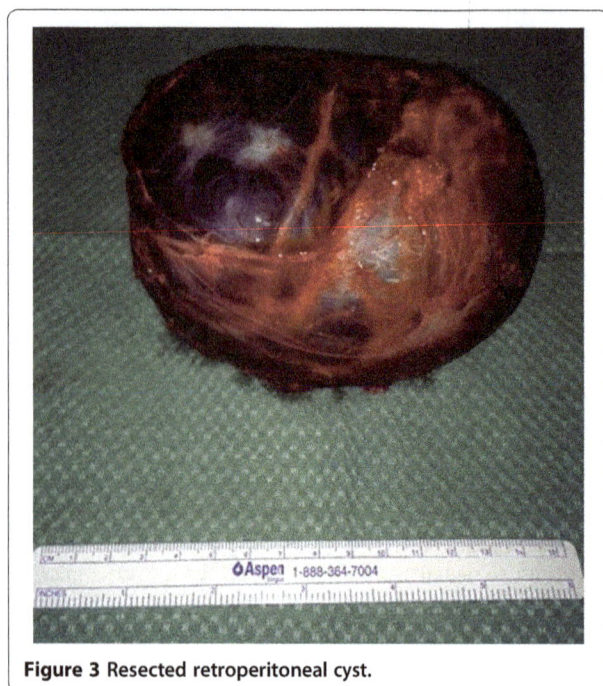

Figure 3 Resected retroperitoneal cyst.

sequelae of a mesenteric or omental haematoma or an abscess which was not resorbed [5,6].

A RPC includes a wide differential such as mesenteric, omental, splenic and enteric duplication cysts [2]. Neoplastic RPCs can be divided into epithelial (mucinous or serous cystadenoma), mesothelial (mesothelioma), germ cell (cystic teratoma) and cystic changes in a solid neoplasm (paraganglioma, neurilemmoma, sarcoma) [2]. Other rare cysts such as lymphangioma (1 % of all retroperitoneal neoplasms [7]), mullerian cyst, epidermoid cyst, tailgut cyst, bronchogenic cyst, pseudomyxoma retroperitonei, perianal mucinous cystadenoma have been described. Non-neoplastic causes include haematoma, urinoma, lymphocele, pancreatic pseudocyst and nonpancreatic pseudocyst [7].

Diagnostic work-up should include a thorough history, laboratory investigations including tumour markers and imaging. Assessment of the retroperitoneum with a CT will allow characterisation of the cystic mass and its relationship with surrounding organs. Magnetic resonance imaging (MRI) was used in this instance, as MRI has superior contrast resolution enabling soft-tissue delineation and is useful in characterising cysts by depicting septae, ductal communications, wall thickening and enhancement [2,8].

Many cystic lesions cannot be accurately diagnosed as clearly benign without operative and pathological evaluation. The decision to proceed to surgery is determined by the presence of symptoms, risk of complications without intervention (infection, rupture,

possibility of malignant change) and diagnostic uncertainty [9].

In this case we were unable to assess the cyst fluid for amylase, as the cyst was sent for pathological assessment intact, and a pancreatic pseudocyst was low in our differentials, given the patient gave no history of pancreatitis and there was no communication with the pancreas.

Pseudocysts can be complicated by infection, haemorrhage and mass effects [9,10]. Management options include simple drainage and complete excision by laparotomy, an extraperitoneal approach, transperitoneal flank approach or laparoscopic excision. Complete excision is preferred to avoid potential for recurrence [2,11].

Conclusions
We present a rare case of an isolated large retroperitoneal fibrous pseudocyst unrelated to previous pancreatitis which was successfully managed with surgery.

Competing interests
The authors declare that they have no competing interests.

Authors' contributions
JA was involved in the conception of the case report, drafted the manuscript and subsequent revisions while critically reviewing the literature. MD, KA, BW, AT, AD, NM, and CA were involved in the conception and design of the case report and ongoing critical revisions of the manuscript. All authors gave final approval of the version to be published.

Acknowledgement
We have no sources of funding to declare.

References
1. Izaraa A, Mousa H, Dickens P, Allen J, Benhamida A. Idiopathic benign retroperitoneal cyst: a case report. J Med Case Rep. 2008;2:43.
2. Yang DM, Jung DH, Kim H, Kang JH, Kim SH, Kim JH, et al. Retroperitoneal cystic masses: CT, clinical and pathological findings and literature review. Radiographics. 2004;24:353–65.
3. Rajiah P, Sinha R, Cuevas C, Dubinsky T, Bush W, Kolokythas O. Imaging of uncommon retroperitoneal masses. Radiographics. 2011;31:949–76.
4. Kim KO, Kim TN. Acute pancreatic pseudocyst: incidence, risk factors and clinical outcomes. Pancreas. 2012;41:577–81.
5. Cizginer S, Tatli S, Snyder E, Goldberg J, Silverman S. CT and MRI imaging features of a non-pancreatic pseudocyst of the mesentery. European J Gen Med. 2009;6:49–51.
6. Stoupis C, Ros P, Abbitt P, Burton S, Gauger J. Bubbles in the belly: imaging of cystic mesenteric or omental masses. Radiographics. 1994;14:729–37.
7. Nishino M, Hayakawa K, Minami M, Yamamoto A, Ueda H, Takasu K. Primary retroperitoneal neoplasms: CT and MR findings with anatomic and pathologic diagnostic clues. Radiographics. 2003;23:45–57.
8. Renzulli P, Candidas D. Symptomatic retroperitoneal cyst: a diagnostic challenge. Ann R Coll Surg Engl. 2009;91:9–11.
9. Tanaka M, Castillo C, Adsay V, Chari S, Falconi M, Jang JY, et al. International consensus guidelines 2012 for the management of IPMN and MCN of the pancreas. Pancreatology. 2012;12:183–97.
10. Oray-Schrom P, Martin D, Bartelloni P, Amoateng-Adjepong Y. Giant nonpancreatic pseudocyst causing acute anuria. J Clin Gastroenterol. 2002;34:160–3.
11. Geng JH, Huang CH, Wu WJ, Huang SP, Chen YT. Huge retroperitoneal nonpancreatic pseudocyst. Urological Sci. 2012;23:61–3.

14

Chronic pancreatitis of the pancreatic remnant is an independent risk factor for pancreatic fistula after distal pancreatectomy

Marius Distler[1]*, Stephan Kersting[1], Felix Rückert[2], Peggy Kross[1], Hans-Detlev Saeger[1], Jürgen Weitz[1] and Robert Grützmann[1]

Abstract

Background: There is an ongoing debate about the best closure technique after distal pancreatectomy (DP). The aim of the closure is to prevent the formation of a clinically relevant post-operative pancreatic fistula (POPF). Stapler technique seems to be equal compared with hand-sewn closure of the remnant. For both techniques, a fistula rate of approximately 30% has been reported.

Methods: We retrospectively analyzed our DPs between 01/2000 and 12/2010. In all cases, the pancreatic duct was over sewn with a separately stitched ligation of the pancreatic duct (5*0 PDS) followed by a single-stitched hand-sewn closure of the residual pancreatic gland. The POPF was classified according to the criteria of the International Study Group for Pancreatic Fistula (ISGPF). Univariate and multivariate analyses of potential risk factors for the formation of POPF were performed. Indications for operations included cystic tumors (n = 53), neuroendocrine tumors (n = 27), adenocarcinoma (n = 22), chronic pancreatitis (n = 9), metastasis (n = 6), and others (n = 7).

Results: During the period, we performed 124 DPs (♀ = 74, ♂ = 50). The mean age was 57.5 years (18–82). The POPF rates according to the ISGPF criteria were: no fistula, 54.8% (n = 68); grade A, 24.2% (n = 30); grade B, 19.3% (n = 24); and grade C, 1.7% (n = 2). Therefore, in 21.0% (n = 26) of the cases, a clinically relevant pancreatic fistula occurred. The mean postoperative stay was significantly higher after grade B/C fistula (26.3 days) compared with no fistula/grade A fistula (13.7 days) (p < 0.05). The uni- and multivariate analyses showed chronic pancreatitis of the pancreatic remnant to be an independent risk factor for the development of POPF (p = 0.004 OR 7.09).

Conclusion: By using a standardized hand-sewn closure technique of the pancreatic remnant after DP with separately stitched ligation of the pancreatic duct, a comparably low fistula rate can be achieved. Signs of chronic pancreatitis of the pancreatic remnant may represent a risk factor for the development of a pancreatic fistula after DP and therefore an anastomosis of the remnant to the intestine should be considered.

Keywords: Distal pancreatectomy, Pancreatic fistula, Chronic pancreatitis, Pancreas surgery

Background

A pancreatic resection left of the superior mesenteric artery (SMA) is termed left resection or distal pancreatectomy (DP). This pancreatic resection technique can be performed, according to the indication of the operation, as a spleen-preserving resection, or it can be combined with a splenectomy. There are various indications for a distal pancreatectomy. The most common indications are patients with malignant diseases, cystic or neuroendocrine tumors or even chronic pancreatitis [1]. A major cause of postoperative morbidity is the development of a pancreatic fistula (POPF). A pancreatic fistula after DP can lead to hemorrhages, abscesses, sepsis or wound infections [2]. A variety of procedures have been recommended to reduce the frequency of pancreatic fistula [2,3]. In particular, the stapler transection and the hand-sewn closure technique have been widely analyzed. For both techniques, a fistula rate of approximately 30% has been reported [4,5].

* Correspondence: marius.distler@uniklinikum-dresden.de
[1]Department of General, Thoracic and Vascular Surgery, University Hospital Carl Gustav Carus, TU, Dresden, Germany
Full list of author information is available at the end of the article

The present analysis demonstrates our experience with the hand-sewn closure technique (including separately stitched ligation of the pancreatic duct) at a single German pancreatic center. The primary outcome of our study was the formation of a pancreatic fistula. Furthermore, we analyzed our data regarding the risk factors for the development of a POPF.

Methods

Patients

Between January 2000 and December 2010 we performed a total of 872 pancreatic resections in the Department for General, Thoracic and Vascular Surgery in the Carl Gustav Carus University Hospital, Dresden. Eight pancreatobiliary surgeons performed 124 consecutive DPs in this period. Indications for operations were cystic tumors (mainly IPMN) or suspicion of a malignant pancreatic tumor (or proven malignant tumor) or metastasis. Postoperative histological diagnosis after pancreatic left resections were IPMN (n = 53), neuroendocrine tumors (n = 27), adenocarcinoma (n = 22), chronic pancreatitis (n = 9), metastasis (n = 6), and others (n = 7). The patient characteristics are summarized in Table 1.

Data collection

The medical records from a prospective database of patients who underwent DP were analyzed retrospectively for each case. Multivisceral resections had not been included into this cohort to obtain a homogenous group. In accordance with the guidelines for human subject research, approval was obtained from the ethics committee at the Carl Gustav Carus University Hospital. The survey data were complemented by the clinical notes of the patients' physicians and surgeons. Furthermore, the histological diagnostic findings of each case were reviewed. In particular, pathology reports of each patient were screened for histological signs of chronic pancreatitis in the frozen section of the pancreatic remnant, independently from the major pathological finding (indication for operation). Information for possibly deceased patients was obtained from family members or from the general practitioner. The median postoperative follow up of all patients was 27 months. The clinical data and demographics of our cohort are shown in Table 1.

For the statistical analysis, we used the following parameters: sex, age, intraoperative blood loss, OR time, diagnosis, ASA scores, nicotine abuse, alcohol abuse, hypertension, pre- and/or postoperative diabetes, insulin use, weight loss, histologically proven chronic pancreatitis of the pancreatic remnant and UICC stage (if available) (Table 2). The postoperative events and clinical outcomes were also recorded prospectively and analyzed retrospectively (Table 1).

Table 1 Demographic and clinical data from our patient cohort (n = 124)

	Distal pancreatectomies (n = 124)
Sex (m/f)	n = 74 (59.7%)/n = 50 (40.3%)
Age y (±SD)	57.5 (±14.2) 95% CI 55.0-60.1
BMI (m/kg^2)	25.8 (±5.1) 95% CI 24.9-26.8
ASA scores	
1	n = 14 (11.3%)
2	n = 75 (60.5%)
3	n = 35 (28.2%)
Nicotine abuse (yes/no)	n = 27 (21.8%)/n = 97 (78.2%)
Alcohol abuse (yes/no)	n = 35 (28.2%)/n = 89 (71.8%)
Hypertension (yes/no)	n = 56 (45.2%)/n = 68 (54.8%)
Weight loss (yes/no)	n = 38 (30.6%)/n = 86 (69.4%)
Preoperative Diabetes (Total)	n = 32 (25.8%)
Oral	n = 22 (17.7%)
IDDM	n = 10 (8.0%)
Diagnosis	
Adenocarcinomas	n = 22 (17.7%)
IPMN	n = 53 (42.7%)
Chronic pancreatitis	n = 9 (7.3%)
Metastasis	n = 6 (4.8%)
NET	n = 27 (21.9%)
Others	n = 7 (5.6%)
Postoperative Pancreatic Fistula (POPF)	
Grade A	n = 30 (24.2%)
Grade B	n = 24 (19.3%)
Grade C	n = 2 (1.7%)
OP-time (min) (±SD)	282.2 (±106.8) 95% CI 263.2-301.2
Intraop. blood loss (ml) (±SD)	834 (±787.1) 95% CI 694.6-1217.4

Hand-sewn closure technique of the pancreatic remnant

All resections were performed as open operations. In all cases with malignancy, a concomitant splenectomy was performed. In benign cases, the operation was performed as a spleen-preserving operation, if possible. The pancreatic gland was cut wedge-shaped to facilitate a fish-mouth closure of the stump.

In all cases, the pancreatic duct was thoroughly identified and over sewn with a separately stitched figure-of-eight ligation (5*0 PDS) (Figures 1 and 2). Then, a simple single-stitched hand-sewn closure of the fish-mouth was accomplished. In Figures 1,2,3 our technique is shown in detail. No additional treatment (e.g. octreotide) or covering of the pancreatic remnant was performed. Every patient received one intraabdominal drain, and the enzyme parameter (amylase) was determined daily in the fluid collected from the drain after the operation.

Table 2 Univariate analysis of independent risk factors for the development of a clinically relevant POPF after DP (Type 0/A versus B/C)

	POPF 0/A n = 98	POPF B/C n = 26	P-value
Sex (m/f)	n = 59/ n = 39	n = 15/ n = 11	0.816*
Age	95% CI 0.952-1.009		0.179** (OR 0.98)
Blood loss (intraoperative)	95% CI 1.000-1.001		0.007** (OR 1.001)
OR time	95% CI 1.000-1.007		0.082** (OR 1.003)
Diagnosis			0.072*
PDAC	n = 16	n = 6	
IPMN	n = 42	n = 11	
Chronic pancreatitis	n = 8	n = 1	
Metastasis	n = 4	n = 2	
NET	n = 25	n = 2	
Others	n = 3	n = 4	
ASA score			0.335*
1	n = 9	n = 5	
2	n = 60	n = 15	
3	n = 29	n = 6	
Nicotine			
Yes/No	n = 20/n = 78	n = 7/n = 19	0.474*
Alcohol abuse			
Yes/No	n = 26/n = 72	n = 9/n = 17	0.416*
Hypertension			
Yes/No	n = 48/n = 50	n = 8/n = 18	0.097*
Preoperative diabetes			
Yes/No	n = 28/n = 70	n = 4/n = 22	0.172*
Postoperative diabetes			
Yes/No	n = 29/n = 69	n = 4/n = 22	0.145*
Preoperative IDDM			
Yes/No	n = 10/n = 88	n = 0/n = 26	0.089*
Chronic pancreatitis in remnant			
Yes/No	n = 12/n = 86	n = 9/n = 17	0.007*
Preoperative weight loss			
Yes/No	n = 31/n = 67	n = 7/n = 19	0.643*
UICC Stage (any malignant tumor)			
0	n = 69	n = 16	
Ia	n = 3	n = 0	
Ib	n = 6	n = 1	0.512*
IIa	n = 4	n = 2	

Table 2 Univariate analysis of independent risk factors for the development of a clinically relevant POPF after DP (Type 0/A versus B/C) *(Continued)*

IIb		n = 12	n = 6
III		n = 1	n = 1
IV		n = 3	n = 0

*χ2-test , **binary logistic regression analysis; p < 0.05 statistically significant.

Definitions

Postoperative Pancreatic Fistula (POPF) was defined analogous to the ISGPF criteria. By examination of the fluid collected from the intraoperatively placed drain, a POPF was defined as amylase content greater than three times the upper normal serum level after postoperative day three. The POPF was stratified into grades A, B and C [6].

Management of the persistent pancreatic fistula

We did not use any standard treatment protocol for POPF. In general, the drains were left in place, or in cases with drain removal, the drains were re-placed interventionally. In some cases, octreotide was also used. Usually, oral food intake was not stopped. Therefore, the basic principle of therapy was adequate drainage and patience.

Statistical analysis

The statistical analysis was performed using SPSS for Windows, version 19.0 (SPSS, Inc., Chicago, IL). All clinical and pathological characteristics were grouped to build categorical or nominal variables. The cutoff points used for categorizations were based on previously described cutoff points in the literature and/or recursive partitioning as previously described [7]. Continuous data are presented as 95% confidence intervals (95% CI) and SDs. Univariate examination of the relationship between the assessed criteria and POPF was performed with a

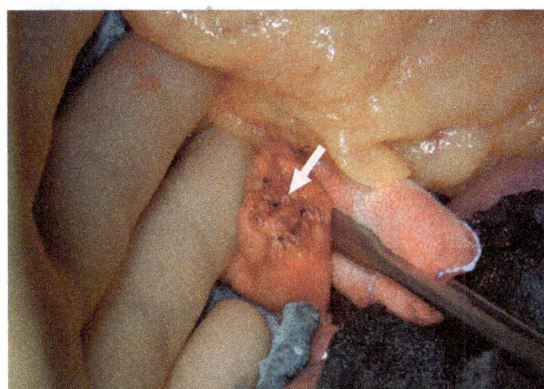

Figure 1 Pancreatic remnant after transection with a scalpel and stitch ligation (5*0 Vicryl) of small vessels. Arrow: pancreatic duct.

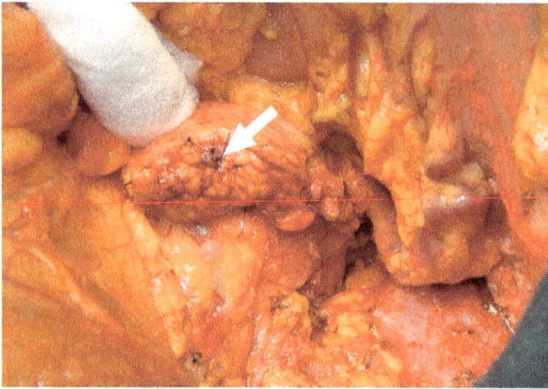

Figure 2 Arrow: Figure-of-eight stitch ligation of the pancreatic duct (5*0 PDS).

χ2-test and by binary logistic regression analysis. For multivariate analysis a logistic regression model of the preoperative parameters with stepwise backwards elimination based on likelihood ratios was employed to test for independent predictors of POPF. However the odds ratios of the parameters OR time, age and blood loss were close to 1 and therefore they rendered the model unstable, these parameters were not included into the multivariate analysis. A two-sided p-value <0.05 was considered statistically significant.

Results

Patient demographics and preoperative parameters

From 2000 to 2010, we performed 124 DPs. The mean age of the patients undergoing DP was 57.5 years, with a range of 18 to 82 years, and there were 74 female and 50 male patients. The indications for the operation are shown in Table 1. Approximately 60% of the patients had an ASA II status, and the mean BMI was 28.5. The most frequent concomitant diagnoses at the time of presentation were hypertension (45.2%), diabetes (25.8%), nicotine abuse (18.1%) and alcohol abuse (28.2%). The

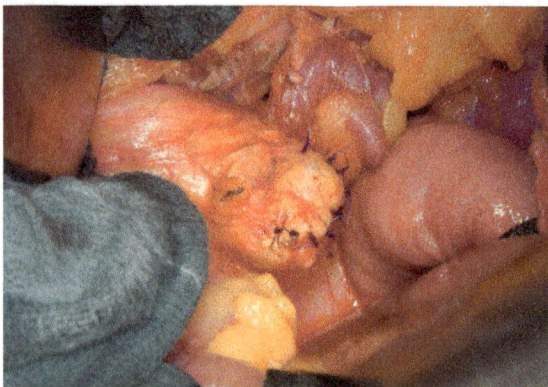

Figure 3 Simple, single-stich suture fish-mouth closure of the pancreatic remnant (4*0 PDS).

mean operation time was 282 minutes (range 100–640), and the mean intraoperative blood loss was 834 ml (range 0–2500) (Table 1).

Postoperative pancreatic fistula (POPF)

By using the ISGPF grading system, we identified a total of 56 POPFs (45.2%). We recognized 30 (24.2%) grade A fistulas and 24 (19.3%) grade B fistulas, and 2 (1.7%) patients developed a grade C fistula (Table 1). Thus in 21% of the cases, a clinically relevant POPF (grade B/C) occurred. Repeat operations were performed on both patients with grade C fistulas. In one case, an intraabdominal abscess was drained, and an additional drain was placed. In the second patient, the pancreatic remnant was closed by a pancreatojejunostomy (end-to-side). Two patients (1.6%) died during the hospital stay, but none of them died due to a POPF. One patient died after bleeding of esophageal varicose, and the other died due to a complication after pleural drainage. The mean postoperative stay was significantly higher after grade B/C fistulas (26.3 days) compared with no fistula/grade A fistulas (13.7 days) (p < 0.001). In addition, there were no differences between the eight pancreatic surgeons performing DP.

Univariate and multivariate analysis of risk factors for POPF

The above mentioned perioperative parameters and patient demographics were used for univariate analysis regarding the development of a clinically relevant POPF (B/C). Univariate analysis showed that histologically proven chronic pancreatitis of the pancreatic remnant (p = 0.007) and intraoperative blood loss (p = 0.007, OR 1.0) are a risk factor for the development of a POPF (Table 2). The diagnosis alone (p = 0.072), preoperative IDDM (p = 0.089), OR time (P = 0.082) and the presence of hypertension (p = 0.097) appear to be marginally significant factors (Table 2). A multivariate analysis with backward elimination confirmed the results of the univariate analysis. Chronic pancreatitis of the pancreatic remnant is an independent risk factor for the development of a clinically relevant POPF (grade B/C) (p = 0.004, OR 7.09). Furthermore, the presence of hypertension was detected as a significant factor for POPF (p = 0.05, OR 2.80) (Table 3).

Discussion

The technique of stump closure after DP has been widely debated. Different approaches have been tested in various studies, and in a comparative analysis, no significant advantage for any specific method was detected [8]. Recent publications, such as the DISPACT trial, have compared the stapler and the hand-sewn closure techniques. No difference between these techniques was shown in regard to POPF [4]. Moreover a current randomized controlled trial

Table 3 Multivariate analysis of risk factors for the development of a clinically relevant POPF

	OR	95% confidence interval OR		P-value
		Lower	Upper	
Step 1				
Sex	0.60	0.131	2.802	0.520
PDAC	0.50	0.084	2.984	0.447
IPMN	0.04	0.002	1.003	0.050
Chronic pancreatitis	1.38	0.113	16.939	0.798
Metastasis	0.28	0.031	2.540	0.259
NET	4.68	0.423	51.818	0.208
ASA	0.85	0.302	2.421	0.768
Nicotine	2.34	0.525	10.446	0.265
Alcohol	1.82	0.504	6.572	0.361
Hypertension	2.32	0.609	8.854	0.218
Preoperative Diabetes	0.93	0.160	5.490	0.943
Postoperative Diabetes	0.33	0.054	2.077	0.240
Chronic pancreatitis in remnant	6.51	1.390	30.545	0.017
Preoperative Weight loss	0.40	0.101	1.648	0.208
Step 13				
Hypertension	2.80	0.980	8.033	0.050
Chronic pancreatitis in remnant	7.09	1.867	26.994	0.004

by Carter et al. evaluated the additional effect of fibrin glue or autologous falciform patch after stapler or hand-sewn closure of the pancreatic remnant [5]. They found no benefit for this additional measure regarding POPF. Finally, various studies evaluated the use of somatostatin analogues perioperatively or postoperatively. However, a meta-analysis by Koti et al. found a decrease of morbidity only in selected patients [9]. Thus, POPF remains a major source of morbidity and is therefore a relevant clinical problem after DP even though it does not lead to a high postoperative mortality. Considering this background, we present our experiences with the hand-sewn closure technique in the current report.

In our study, we specifically focused on factors contributing to pancreatic fistula. In the present series, all DPs were performed during open laparotomy using the same technique of selective ligation of the pancreatic duct. Currently, there is a tendency to perform this operation laparoscopically. This approach, however, presents the same complications as those associated with open resection and stapler closure; safe closure of the pancreatic remnant is therefore an important issue for laparoscopic distal pancreatectomy [10].

During the follow up, nearly half of the patients (45%) showed a POPF after PD. However, a clinically relevant POPF (grade B/C) was evaluated in only 21% of the

cases. These results are consistent with the published data [5, 11, 12,]. The recently published DISPACT trial showed comparable results related to POPF (approximately 20-21%) for the stapler transection and the hand-sewn closure technique [4]. By using a standardized closure technique, we could reproduce the published results for development of a clinically relevant POPF in our cohort. Although it should be noted that the present study is a retrospective analysis.

We support the importance of the selective ligation of the pancreatic duct. A previous study by Pannegeon et al. [11] confirmed the findings of a multivariate analysis by Bilimoria et al. [12] indicating that specific ligation of the main pancreatic duct is an independent protective factor for POPF. Other authors have noted that an inability to find the main pancreatic duct for ligation is a major factor related to the occurrence of postoperative fistula [13].

In our study, chronic pancreatitis of the pancreatic remnant was identified as an independent risk factor for POPF in the univariate (p = 0.007) and multivariate analyses (OR 7.09) (Table 2 and 3). Similarly to other authors, we believe that this is due to downstream stenosis of the main pancreatic duct, most likely in the pancreatic head region, due to chronic inflammation. Preoperative diabetes was not detected as a significant risk factor for POPF in our analysis, but it is important to note that in most cases, diabetes is concomitant with chronic pancreatitis and therefore could be a preoperative indicator [14]. We infer from our data that in cases with a potential obstruction of the pancreatic duct in the pancreatic head/periampullary region (e.g. due to chronic pancreatitis), and therefore an increased likelihood of POPF, the pancreatic remnant should be anastomosed. This seems especially important in patients with preoperatively or intraoperatively detected dilatation of the pancreatic duct. Pancreatic anastomosis seems to be a safe method of closure in these cases after DP. However, one could speculate that pancreatic leakage following small bowel anastomosis could result in potentially more serious complications than leakage without anastomosis (e.g. activation of pancreatic enzymes, bacterial contamination). Therefore, a pancreatic anastomosis following DP should only be performed if it can be carried out safely [15].

Hypertension has also been noted as a risk factor for the development of POPF in our analyses. This might be due to the pathophysiological effect of hypertension, which causes generalized atherosclerosis and thereby limits the microcirculation of the tissue. Perfusion is a particularly important factor for wound healing. By compromising the healing process, hypertension could negatively affect the postoperative course. This negative effect of hypertension has been reported previously [16]. Moreover, hypertension is also a parameter of the POSSUM score, which accurately predicts morbidity in various operation procedures [17,18].

In addition, our analysis confirms that patients with a clinically relevant pancreatic fistula had a mean extension of their hospital stay (B/C fistula (26.3 days) vs. no fistula/grade A fistula (13.7 days)) (p < 0.001). This tendency was also recently reported by the DISPACT trial [4].

Conclusion

Our data support the assumption that DP can now be performed without significant mortality (i.e., 1.6% in our analysis) [4,11,18]. However, the morbidity after DP is still high due to the occurrence of POPF. By selective stitched ligation of the pancreatic duct and fish-mouth closure of the pancreatic remnant, a low POPF rate comparable to the results in the literature could be achieved. Chronic inflammation of the pancreatic remnant should be considered a risk factor for POPF during the intraoperative decision process for stump closure, and maybe an anastomosis of the remnant to the small intestine, e.g. using a jejunal limb, should be considered in these cases.

Abbreviations

POPF: Postoperative pancreatic fistula; DP: Distal pancreatectomy; ISGPF: International Study Group for Pancreatic Fistula; IDDM: Insulin depending diabetes mellitus.

Competing interests

The authors declare no competing interests. This research received no specific grant from any funding agency in public, commercial, or not-for-profit sectors.

Authors' contributions

DM wrote the manuscript, collected the data, interpreted the results and statistically analyzed the data, RF and KS analyzed the data statistically, interpreted the results and critically revised the manuscript, KP collected the data and wrote parts of the manuscript, SHD and JW designed the concept of the manuscript operations and critically revised the manuscript, and GR designed the study, collected data, and drafted the manuscript. All authors read and approved the final manuscript.

Acknowledgments

We acknowledge the service of the "American Journal Experts" (Durham, US) editing the paper.

Author details

[1]Department of General, Thoracic and Vascular Surgery, University Hospital Carl Gustav Carus, TU, Dresden, Germany. [2]Department of Surgery, University Hospital Mannheim, Mannheim, Germany.

References

1. Lillemoe KD, Kaushal S, Cameron JL, Sohn TA, Pitt HA, Yeo CJ: **Distal pancreatectomy: indications and outcomes in 235 patients.** *Ann Surg* 1999, **229**(5):693–698. discussion 698–700.
2. Knaebel HP, Diener MK, Wente MN, Büchler MW, Seiler CM: **Systematic review and meta-analysis of technique for closure of the pancreatic remnant after distal pancreatectomy.** *Br J Surg* 2005, **92**(5):539–546.
3. Blansfield JA, Rapp MM, Chokshi RJ, Woll NL, Hunsinger MA, Sheldon DG, Shabahang MM: **Novel method of stump closure for distal pancreatectomy with a 75% reduction in pancreatic fistula rate.** *J Gastrointest Surg* 2012, **16**(3):524–528.
4. Diener MK, Seiler CM, Rossion I, Kleeff J, Glanemann M, Butturini G, Tomazic A, Bruns CJ, Busch OR, Farkas S, Belyaev O, Neoptolemos JP, Halloran C, Keck T, Niedergethmann M, Gellert K, Witzigmann H, Kollmar O, Langer P, Steger U, Neudecker J, Berrevoet F, Ganzera S, Heiss MM, Luntz SP, Bruckner T, Kieser M, Büchler MW: **Efficacy of stapler versus hand-sewn closure after distal pancreatectomy (DISPACT): a randomised, controlled multicentre trial.** *Lancet* 2011, **377**(9776):1514–1522.
5. Carter TI, Fong ZV, Hyslop T, Lavu H, Tan WP, Hardacre J, Sauter PK, Kennedy EP, Yeo CJ, Rosato EL: **A Dual-Institution Randomized Controlled Trial of Remnant Closure after Distal Pancreatectomy: Does the Addition of a Falciform Patch and Fibrin Glue Improve Outcomes?** *J Gastrointest Surg* 2012. Jul 14. [Epub ahead of print].
6. Bassi C, Dervenis C, Butturini G, Fingerhut A, Yeo C, Izbicki J, Neoptolemos J, Sarr M, Traverso W, Buchler M: **International Study Group on Pancreatic Fistula Definition. Postoperative pancreatic fistula: an international study group (ISGPF) definition.** *Surgery* 2005, **138**(1):8–13.
7. Rueckert F, Distler M, Hoffmann S, Hoffmann D, Pilarsky C, Dobrowolski F, Saeger HD, Gruetzmann R: **Quality of life in patients after pancreaticoduodenectomy for chronic pancreatitis.** *J Gastrointest Surg* 2011, **15**(7):1143–1150.
8. Ferrone CR, Warshaw AL, Rattner DW, Berger D, Zheng H, Rawal B, Rodriguez R, Thayer SP, Fernandez-del CC: **Pancreatic fistula rates after 462 distal pancreatectomies: staplers do not decrease fistula rates.** *J Gastrointest Surg* 2008, **12**(10):1691–1697. discussion 1697–8.
9. Gurusamy KS, Koti R, Fusai G, Davidson BR: **Somatostatin analogues for pancreatic surgery.** *Cochrane Database Syst Rev* 2012. Jun 13;6:CD008370.].
10. Fernández-Cruz L, Martínez I, Gilabert R, Cesar-Borges G, Astudillo E, Navarro S: **Laparoscopic distal pancreatectomy combined with preservation of the spleen for cystic neoplasms of the pancreas.** *J Gastrointest Surg* 2004, **8**(4):493–501.
11. Pannegeon V, Pessaux P, Sauvanet A, Vullierme MP, Kianmanesh R, Belghiti J: **Pancreatic fistula after distal pancreatectomy: predictive risk factors and value of conservative treatment.** *Arch Surg* 2006, **141**(11):1071–1076. discussion 1076.
12. Bilimoria MM, Cormier JN, Mun Y, Lee JE, Evans DB, Pisters PW: **Pancreatic leak after left pancreatectomy is reduced following main pancreatic duct ligation.** *Br J Surg* 2003, **90**(2):190–196.
13. Howard TJ, Stonerock CE, Sarkar J, Lehman GA, Sherman S, Wiebke EA, Madura JA, Broadie TA: **Contemporary treatment strategies for external pancreatic fistulas.** *Surgery* 1998, **124**(4):627–632. discussion 632–3.
14. Rückert F, Kersting S, Fiedler D, Distler M, Dobrowolski F, Pilarsky C, Saeger HD, Grützmann R: **Chronic pancreatitis: early results of pancreatoduodenectomy and analysis of risk factors.** *Pancreas* 2011, **40**(6):925–930.
15. Kleeff J, Diener MK, Z'graggen K, Hinz U, Wagner M, Bachmann J, Zehetner J, Müller MW, Friess H, Büchler MW: **Distal pancreatectomy: risk factors for surgical failure in 302 consecutive cases.** *Ann Surg* 2007, **245**(4):573–582.
16. Henry SL, Crawford JL, Puckett CL: **Risk factors and complications in reduction mammaplasty: novel associations and preoperative assessment.** *Plast Reconstr Surg* 2009, **124**(4):1040–1046.
17. Jones DR, Copeland GP, de Cossart L: **Comparison of POSSUM with APACHE II for prediction of outcome from a surgical high-dependency unit.** *Br J Surg* 1992, **79**(12):1293–1296.
18. Sheehan MK, Beck K, Creech S, Pickleman J, Aranha GV: **Distal pancreatectomy: does the method of closure influence fistula formation?** *Am Surg* 2002, **68**(3):264–267. discussion 267–8.

15

Outcomes of resections for pancreatic adenocarcinoma with suspected venous involvement: a single center experience

Christoph W. Michalski[1,4], Bo Kong[1], Carsten Jäger[1], Silke Kloe[1], Barbara Beier[1], Rickmer Braren[2], Irene Esposito[3,5], Mert Erkan[1,6], Helmut Friess[1†] and Jorg Kleeff[1*†]

Abstract

Background: Pancreatic ductal adenocarcinoma (PDAC) patients frequently present with borderline resectable disease, which can be due to invasion of the portal/superior mesenteric vein (PV/SMV). Here, we analyzed this group of patients, with emphasis on short and long-term outcomes.

Methods: 156 patients who underwent a resection for PDAC were included in the analysis and sub-stratified into a cohort of patients with PV/SMV resection ($n = 54$) versus those with standard surgeries ($n = 102$).

Results: While venous resections could be performed safely, there was a trend towards shorter median survival in the PV/SMV resection group (22.7 vs. 15.8 months, $p = 0.157$). These tumors were significantly larger (3.5 vs 4.3 cm; $p = 0.026$) and margin-positivity was more frequent (30.4 % vs 44.4 %, $p = 0.046$).

Conclusion: Venous resection was associated with a higher rate of margin positivity and a trend towards shorter survival. However, compared to non-surgical treatment, resection offers the best chance for long term survival.

Keywords: Pancreatic cancer, Venous invasion, Upfront surgery, Prognosis

Background

The extension of the resectability criteria for pancreatic adenocarcinoma (PDAC) has been intensively discussed in the last decade. It has been shown that arterial resections significantly increase mortality [1] but that resections for presumed invasion of the superior mesenteric/portal vein axis (PV/SMV, "venous resections") can be carried out safely without increased morbidity/mortality. In addition, taken all patients together, venous resections are not associated with an inferior survival than standard resections [2]. However, some groups have argued that true (in contrast to suspected) venous infiltration was associated with significantly shorter survival [3–6] while others have not reproduced these results [7–9]. Nonetheless the data on venous resections, especially those on perioperative

outcome, have changed clinical practice in that these resections have become the standard for such tumors. Despite these technical improvements and the wide-spread introduction of adjuvant (and neoadjuvant) chemotherapy, prognosis has not much changed [10, 11].

At the same time, outcome prediction remains challenging because a considerable subgroup of patients probably does not benefit from surgery. This is because it is difficult to predict pre-/intraoperative undetectable ("subclinical") metastatic disease and in line with this it is currently impossible to predict the biological behaviour of the tumors. Thus, there is currently a gap between our knowledge of the biology of PDAC and the technical/surgical advances. This is also underscored by a recent hypothesis that tumor size (and thus likelihood of vascular infiltration) and the time of metastasis are closely linked. Here, an exponential probability for metastatic spread was calculated depending on the size of the primary tumor [12]. Thus, many tumors deemed resectable will probably already have metastasized, though clinically not detectable [12]. In this study, we analysed our cohort of resected PDAC patients with special

* Correspondence: kleeff@tum.de
†Equal contributors
[1]Department of Surgery, Technische Universität München, Ismaningerstrasse 22, 81675 Munich, Germany
Full list of author information is available at the end of the article

Table 1 Patients characteristics, venous resection vs. no venous resection

	Venous resection (VR) (n = 54)		No venous resection (NVR) (n = 102)		p-value[1]
Sex					0.24
M	27	(50.0 %)	61	(59.8 %)	
F	27	(50.0 %)	41	(40.2 %)	
Age, mean (STD). yrs	67.8	(10.7)	67.2	(11)	0.95
Preoperative performance status					
ASA					0.86
1	3	(5.6 %)	8	(7.8 %)	
2	31	(57.4 %)	58	(56.9 %)	
3	20	(37.0 %)	36	(35.3 %)	
Diabetes mellitus	16	(29.6 %)	27	(26.5 %)	0.67
Bile duct stent	18	(33.3 %)	39	(38.2 %)	0.54
Pancreatitis	2	(3.7 %)	12	(11.8 %)	0.09
Neoadjuvant treatment	4	(7.4 %)	6	(5.9 %)	0.43
Type of Surgery					0.001
pp-Whipple	25	(46.3 %)	63	(61.7 %)	
cl-Whipple	8	(14.8 %)	6	(5.9 %)	
TP	16	(29.6 %)	9	(8.8 %)	
DP	5	(9.3 %)	22	(21.7 %)	
DPH	0		2	(1.9 %)	
Vein resection technique					
End-to-End-Anastomosis	33	(61.1 %)			
Wedge-Resection	15	(27.8 %)			
goretex™ graft	6	(11.1 %)			
Operative time, mean (STD), min.	378	(103)	317	(85)	<0.001[2]
Blood transfusion	9	(16,7 %)	4	(4,0 %)	0.012
Adjuvant chemotherapy	46	(85.2 %)	87	(85.3 %)	0.97
Pathological findings					
Tumor grade of differentiation					0.28
G1	1	(1.8 %)	8	(7.8 %)	
G2	25	(46.3 %)	41	(40.2 %)	
G3	28	(51.9 %)	53	(52.0 %)	
T-stage					0.36
T1	1	(1.8 %)	4	(3.9 %)	
T2	3	(5.6 %)	7	(6.9 %)	
T3	41	(75.9 %)	83	(81.4 %)	
T4	9	(16.7 %)	8	(7.8 %)	
Tumor size in cm (median, min-max)	4.3	1.5-12	3.5	1.2-8.5	0.026[3]

Table 1 Patients characteristics, venous resection vs. no venous resection (Continued)

Nodal status					0.82
0	16	(29.6 %)	32	(31.4 %)	
1	38	(70.4 %)	70	(68.6 %)	
Number of lymph nodes (median, min-max)	21	(5–62)	20	(7–54)	0.92
Resection margins					0.046[4]
R0	22	(40.8 %)	60	(58.8 %)	
R1	24	(44.4 %)	31	(30.4 %)	
R2	0		1	(1.0 %)	
Rx	8	(14.8 %)	10	(9.8 %)	
Pathology report: venous infiltration					
no	8	(14.8 %)			
yes	19	(35.2 %)			
unkown	27	(50.0 %)			

[1]X^2-test; [2]Student's t-test; [3]Mann–Whitney-U-test; [4]X^2-test: R0 vs. R1
Abbreviations: pp-Whipple pylorus-preserving Whipple (=pp-partial pancreaticoduodenectomy), cl-Whipple "classical" Whipple, TP total pancreatectomy, DP distal pancreatectomy, DPH DP plus partial pancreatic head resection, STD standard deviation

emphasis on venous resection/involvement and tumor biology/outcome.

Methods

The Institutional Review Board (Ethikkommission der Medizinischen Fakultät der Technischen Universität München, Munich, Germany) approved prospective and retrospective data collection as well as tissue collection (1926/07 and 5893/13). Written informed consent was obtained from all patients. Analysis was conducted on an anonymized data set.

Database and recorded parameters

In July 2007, we established a prospective database for the assessment of patients who underwent surgery for pancreatic diseases. The following parameters were recorded: tumor entity, age, gender, pre-operative weight loss, the following preoperative blood parameters: GPT/ALAT, GOT/ASAT, bilirubin, AP, gamma-GT and CA19-9, comorbidities (pre-operative presence of diabetes mellitus, previous or concomitant cancer diagnoses other than PDAC, a history of (acute/chronic) pancreatitis, medical co-morbidities as reflected by the ASA score), presence of preoperative jaundice and/or ERCP/bile duct/pancreatic duct stenting, treatment (e.g. surgical technique, (neo-)adjuvant therapy), intraoperative blood transfusion(s), duration of operation, resection (and reconstruction) of the portal/superior mesenteric vein, histologically confirmed presence of venous invasion, size of the tumor (T), lymph node status (N), resection margin (R), grading (G), UICC-classification, postoperative complications (according to the Clavien-Dindo classification [13]). The characteristics of the patients in the different cohorts are depicted in Table 1. Resectability criteria were defined according to the NCCN [14]. Locally advanced unresectable tumors were treated with neoadjuvant treatment protocols as decided in a multidisciplinary tumor board. Occasionally, patients were referred to our hospital after neoadjuvant or palliative intended therapy for borderline or locally advanced tumors. Lymph node dissection was standardized for all cases as described in the recent ISGP definition [15]. Venous resection was not considered a contraindication for surgery. The described approach did not change during the study period.

Inclusion and exclusion criteria

We retrospectively identified 209 patients who underwent an elective pancreatic resection with a final histopathological diagnosis of PDAC between 07/2007 and 07/2011

(Fig. 1). The following patients were excluded from the analysis: UICC stage IV disease ($n = 19$), patients who were resected for local tumor recurrence ($n = 3$), patients on whom arterial resections were performed ($n = 6$), patients with a history of another cancer disease ($n = 17$) and patients who died because of surgery-related complications within 4 months from surgery (extension as suggested by Strasberg et al. [16], $n = 6$); three patients were lost to follow-up. Due to the relatively small patient cohort and considering the 2:1 ratio of the non-vein resected to the vein resected group, we opted for the inclusion of all patients and against a matched case analysis.

At the time of analysis, 17 out of 54 patients in the group of vein-resected patients and 34 out of 102 patients in the standard resection group were alive. Median follow-up for all patients was 20.8 months (3.3-69.8 months) and median follow-up for patients alive was 37.7 months (21.0-69.6 months). Patient charts were reviewed for

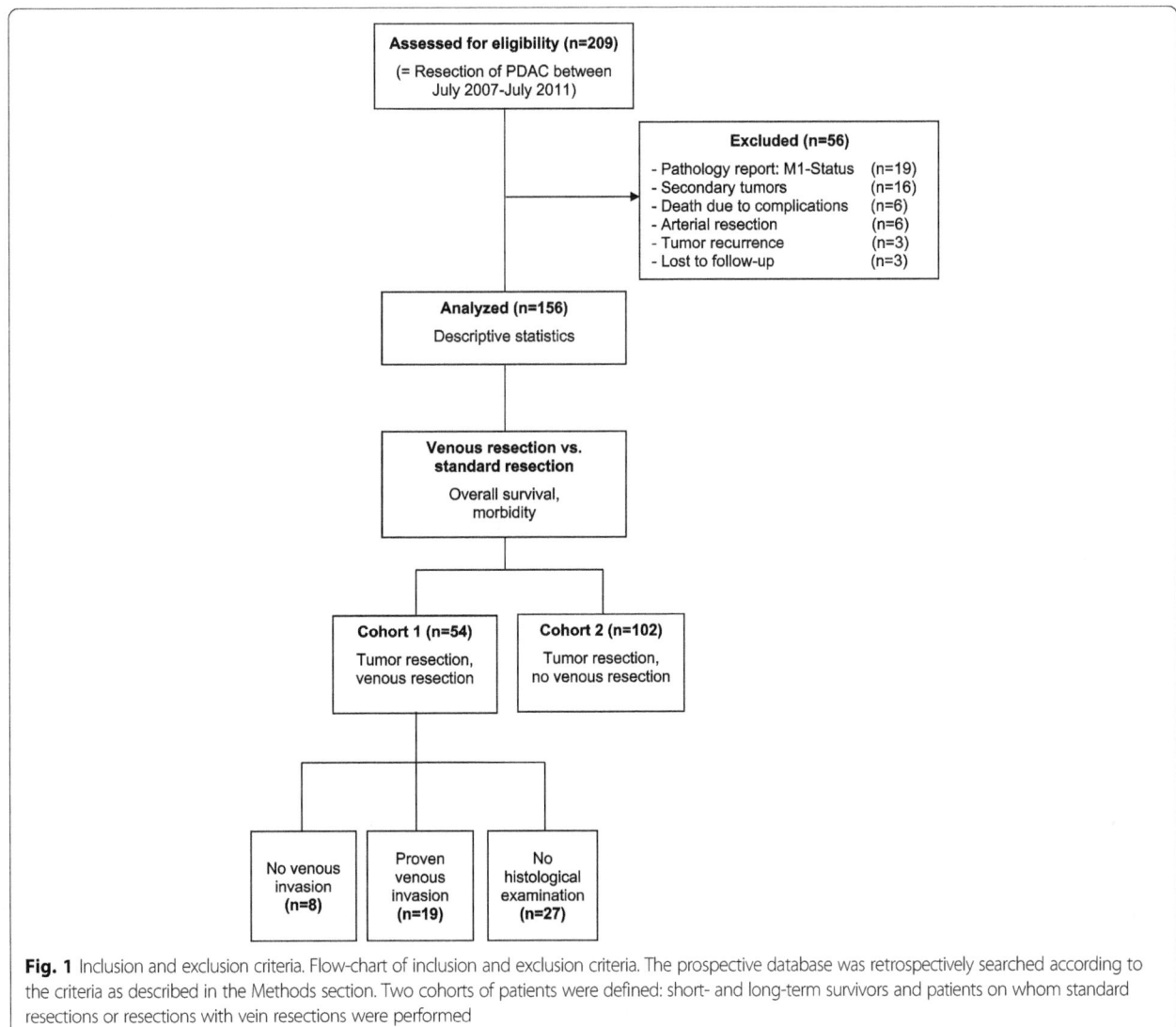

Fig. 1 Inclusion and exclusion criteria. Flow-chart of inclusion and exclusion criteria. The prospective database was retrospectively searched according to the criteria as described in the Methods section. Two cohorts of patients were defined: short- and long-term survivors and patients on whom standard resections or resections with vein resections were performed

whether or not a resection of the PV/SMV (wedge resection, complete resection with end-to-end anastomosis or interposition of a goretex™ graft) had been performed. In this cohort of patients, preoperative imaging (computed tomography of the abdomen or magnetic resonance imaging/magnetic resonance cholangiopancreaticography (MRI/MRCP)) was evaluated to estimate sensitivity and specificity in regard to defining the presence of true venous invasion (versus an inflammatory/desmoplastic reaction at the PV/SMV).

Statistics

Continuous variables are reported as means ± SD or median (min.-max./95 %-CI), and were compared using a Student's t-test or a Mann–Whitney-U-test, as appropriate. Categorical variables are summarized as frequency counts and percentages and were compared using Fischer's exact test or Pearsons's chi-square test, as appropriate. Overall survival was defined as time from resection until death or until last follow-up.

Survival analysis was performed using the Kaplan-Meier method; differences were evaluated with the log rank test. A two-sided P value of <0.05 was considered as significant. All statistical analyses were performed using IBM SPSS, v20 for Windows (IBM Inc., USA).

Results
Analysis of venous resection

The cohort of patients on whom venous resections have been performed was compared with the cohort of patients on whom standard pancreatic resections have been performed (Table 1). Except for late portal vein thrombosis (7 cases in the venous resection cohort versus one case in standard resection group), postoperative complications and (early and late) mortality were comparable in both groups (Table 2). These findings are in line with published data [2, 7, 17, 18], demonstrating that venous resections can be performed safely. Interestingly however, significantly more resections were margin-positive (i.e. R1; 44.4 % vs. 30.4 %, $p = 0.046$) in the venous resection cohort of patients. This might be a reflection of

Table 2 Postoperative complications (30-days), venous resection vs. no venous resection

		Venous resection VR ($n = 54$)		No venous resection NVR ($n = 102$)	p-value[1]
Postoperative complications[2]					0.38
Grade I	12	22.2 %	15	14.71 %	0.19
Grade II[3]	19	35.2 %	38	37.3 %	0.86
Grade III	8	14.8 %	9	8.8 %	0.28
Grade IV	1	1.8 %	1	1.0 %	1.00
120 day mortality[4]	3	5.3 %	3	2.9 %	0.37
Portal vein thrombosis					
30 days	1	1.8 %	1	1.0 %	0.69
total	7	13.0 %	1	1.0 %	0.001
Pancreatic fistula, grade C	2	3.7 %	4	3.9 %	
Lymph fistula	2	3.7 %	3	2.9 %	
Delayed gastric emptying	6	11.1 %	4	3.9 %	0.09
Diarrhea	4	7.4 %	4	3.9 %	
Intraabdominalabscess	2	3.7 %	5	4.9 %	
Cholangitis	3	5.6 %	15	14.7 %	0.11
Wound infection	3	5.6 %	8	7.8 %	
Liver ischemia	1	1.8 %	0	0.0 %	
Bleeding	2	3.7 %	0	0.0 %	
Re-operation	2	3.7 %	3	2.9 %	
Pneumonia	0	0.0 %	1	1.0 %	
Urinary tract infection	2	3.7 %	2	2.0 %	
Cardiac dysfunction	1	1.8 %	3	2.9 %	

[1]χ^2-test
[2]Clavien-Dindo-Classification
[3]VR: 9 patients (47.4 %) only blood transfusion. 6 patients (31.5 %) antibiotics. 1 patient (5.3 %) blood transfusion and antibiotics; without VR: 4 patients (10.5 %) only blood transfusion. 21 patients (55.3 %) only antibiotics; 4 patients (10.5 %) blood transfusion and antibiotics
[4]VR ($n = 57$) vs. NVR ($n = 105$)

Table 3 Characteristics of 27 patients with vein resection and confirmed pathology report

	No venous invasion ($n = 8$)		Venous invasion ($n = 19$)		p-value[1]
Sex					0.33
M	5	(62.3 %)	8	(42.1 %)	
F	3	(37.4 %)	11	(57.9 %)	
Age, mean (STD), yrs	61.7	(13.2)	65.0	(10.3)	0.48
Preoperative performance status					
ASA					0.23
1/2	4	(50.0 %)	14	(73.7 %)	
3	4	(50.0 %)	5	(26.3 %)	
Diabetes mellitus	1	(12.5 %)	6	(31.6 %)	0.41
Bile duct stent	2	(25.0 %)	11	(57.9 %)	0.23
Type of surgery					0.55
ppWhipple/cl-Whipple	6	(75.0 %)	12	(63.2 %)	
TP	2	(25.0 %)	7	(36.8 %)	
Vein resection technique					0.19
End-to-End anastomosis	6	(75.0 %)	15	(78.9 %)	
Wedge- Resection	2	(25.0 %)	1	(5.3 %)	
goretex™ graft	0		3	(15.8 %)	
Operative time, mean (STD), min.	416	(42)	379	(85)	0.222[2]
c[3]					0.52
Grade I/II	4	(50.0 %)	11	(57.9 %)	
Grade III/IV	2	(25.0 %)	4	(21.1 %)	
Pathological findings					
Tumor grade of differentiation					0.47
G1/G2	6	(75.0 %)	9	(47.4 %)	
G3	2	(25.0 %)	10	(52.6 %)	
T-stage					0.001
T1/T2	4	(50.0 %)	0		
T3/T4	4	(50.0 %)	19	(100.0 %)	
Nodal status					0.038
N0	6	(75.0 %)	6	(31.6 %)	
N1	2	(25.0 %)	13	(68.4 %)	
Resection margins					0.36
R0	4	(50.0 %)	6	(31.6 %)	
R1 (incl. RX)	4	(50.0 %)	13	(68.5 %)	
Localization of tumor					0.099
Pancreatic head	7	(87.5 %)	14	(73.7 %)	
Multifocal	1	(12.5 %)	5	(26.3 %)	
Pre-operative prediction venous infiltration					
CT/MRT+	5		11		Sensitivity: 0.69
CT/MRT-	2		5		Specificity: 0.29

[1]X^2-test; [2]Student's t-test; [3]Clavien-Dindo-Classification
Abbreviations: *pp-Whipple* pylorus-preserving Whipple (=pp-partial pancreaticoduodenectomy), *cl-Whipple* "classical" Whipple, *TP* total pancreatectomy, *STD* standard deviation

larger tumors in the patients with venous resections
(4.3 cm vs. 3.5 cm, $p = 0.026$, Table 1). While some groups
demonstrated that true tumor cell invasion of the PV/
SMV negatively impacted on prognosis [3–6, 19], others
have denied such an association [7–9]. We thus re-
assessed the histo-pathology reports on invasion/no-
invasion of the vein (Table 1). In those cases were data
on vein invasion was available, 30 % were tumor cell-
negative whereas in 70 %, tumor cell invasion of the
vein was seen. We then analyzed the patients with
confirmed invasion of the vein vs. no-invasion; here,
no significant differences in regard to preoperative
markers, operative time or surgical technique were
found (Table 3). Comparable to the whole cohort of
venous resection patients, postoperative complications
(including late surgical related mortality) occurred at
similar frequencies in both groups. Further analysis
however demonstrated that the tumors in the true
venous invasion group of patients were significantly
more advanced (T3/4 tumors in the no-venous invasion vs. venous invasion groups: 4/8 vs. 19/19, $p =
0.001$, Table 3). In line with these findings that

implicated more advanced tumors in the true invasion
group, significantly more patients had lymph node
metastases when the vein was truly infiltrated
(Table 3). CT or MRI scans were available in our
digital imaging system from 23 of 27 patients. Radiological assessment of these scans revealed that CT or MRI
predicted true invasion of the vein only at a sensitivity of
69 % and a specificity of 29 % (Table 3). Though the patient number is low, these data demonstrate the difficulties
in preoperative prediction of the presence/extent of PV/
SMV invasion.

Survival following venous resections

To determine the extent of selection bias in the venous
resection cohort of patients, we stratified these according
to the UICC classification and plotted the subgroups following Kaplan-Meier survival analysis (Fig. 2a). This analysis demonstrates that the general prognosis of this
cohort of patients is accurately predicted by the UICC.
Thus, we assumed that selection bias was not overly
strong in our cohort of patients and considered that the
following analyses were statistically justified.

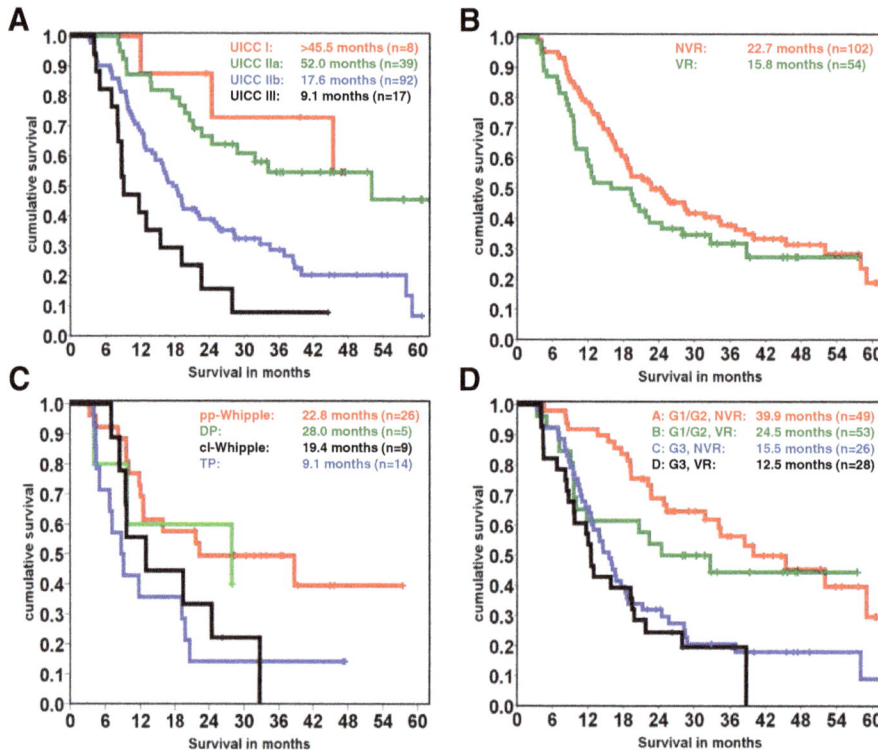

Fig. 2 Survival analysis. **a**, Survival according to the UICC stages was assessed using the Kaplan-Meier method and the log rank test. The overall *p*-value is
0.001. **b**, Survival in the patient groups with standard (no venous resection, NVR) and with venous resection (VR) was compared using Kaplan-Meier curves
and the log rank test; *p* = 0.157. **c**, Survival according to different operative techniques was assessed using Kaplan-Meier curves and the log rank test. TP:
total pancreatectomy; DP: distal pancreatectomy; pp-Whipple: partial, pylorus-preserving pancreaticoduodenectomy; cl-Whipple: "classical" Whipple, partial
pancreaticoduodenectomy. **d**, Comparisons between the following groups were done using the Kaplan-Meier method and log rank testing: G1/2 without
vein resection (**a**), G1/2 with vein resection (**b**), G3 without vein resection (**c**), G3 vein resection (**d**). The overall *p*-value is <0.001. **a** vs **c**: *p* < 0.001; **b** vs
d: *p* = 0.023

Though there was a trend towards shorter survival of patients in whom venous resections had to be performed, this was not statistically significant (median survival 22.7 vs. 15.8 months, Fig. 2b; $p = 0.157$). Pathologically confirmed invasion of the vein was not relevant for prognosis. In addition, patients on whom a total pancreatectomy had to be performed lived shorter than those with pancreaticoduodenectomy or distal pancreatectomy (9.1 months versus 19.4 - 28 months, Fig. 2c).

Next, we analyzed tumor grade as a surrogate marker for tumor biology. Patients with well- and moderately differentiated PDACs lived significantly longer than those with poorly differentiated tumors (overall $p < 0.001$, median survival 39.9 vs. 15.5 months, $p < 0.001$; Fig. 2d), and this stratification was also significant in the venous resection cohort (median survival 24.5 vs. 12.5 months, $p = 0.023$).

Discussion

The data presented in this paper confirm previously published results on portal vein resections during surgery for pancreatic adenocarcinoma, i.e. that it can be performed safely without increased morbidity and (early and late) mortality. There was a trend towards shorter survival and more frequent margin-positivity in the group of patients in whom venous resections had been performed. However, this was mainly a result of the outcomes after combined total pancreatectomy and portal vein resection. Such operations were only performed if a pancreaticoduodenectomy or a distal pancreatectomy were technically impossible or not sufficient to achieve macroscopic tumor clearance. This is also reflected in the finding that outcomes were worse in larger tumors. For partial pancreaticoduodenectomy and distal pancreatectomy with venous resections, there were no considerable differences compared to the respective standard resections. Thus, our data are in line with previous publications and support the concept that partial resection of the PV/SMV is justified to achieve negative margins and thereby better local control [20, 21]. However, as patients undergoing total pancreatectomy plus PV/SMV resection had worse outcomes, it might be argued that this group of patients with centrally located, large tumors, for whom total pancreatectomy is anticipated/likely, should not be operated upfront, but might be better candidates for neoadjuvant treatment.

Our study also highlights the prognostic importance of tumor biology, using grading as a surrogate marker. Obviously, tumor biology rather than tumor location (and vascular abutment/invasion) is a stronger prognostic factor. This is also supported by recent data on long term survival after PDAC resections. Here, tumor biology was identified as the most important factor, with a significant number of long term survivors having a positive margin status and lymph node metastasis

[11]. Further studies are required to better predict and understand tumor biology and stratify patients that benefit most from extensive surgical procedures.

There are some drawbacks of the present study. Although standardized histopathological reporting with special emphasis on resection margins had been introduced in our center in 2007 [22–24], venous involvement had not been assessed in all cases. Thus, data regarding preoperative diagnostic accuracy and true venous infiltration have to be interpreted cautiously.

Conclusion

In summary, our data support the current clinical practice of operating on patients with suspected involvement of the PV/SMV, and to perform (partial) resection of the PV/SMV if necessary to achieve tumor-free margins.

Competing interests
All authors declare that there is no potential or actual conflict of interest.

Authors' contributions
CWM, ME, JK designed the study. CJ, SK, BB, RB, IE contributed to data acquisition. BK, RB, IE contributed to data analysis and interpretation. CWM, ME, JK drafted the manuscript. BK, CJ, SK, BB, RB, IE, HF revised the manuscript critically for important intellectual content. All authors approved the final version of the manuscript.

Acknowledgement
The study was funded by the Technische Universität München, Munich Germany (institutional funding). There was no role of the funding body in design, in the collection, analysis, and interpretation of data; in the writing of the manuscript; and in the decision to submit the manuscript for publication.

Author details
[1]Department of Surgery, Technische Universität München, Ismaningerstrasse 22, 81675 Munich, Germany. [2]Institute of Radiology, Technische Universität München, Munich, Germany. [3]Institute of Pathology, Technische Universität München, Munich, Germany. [4]Current address: Department of Surgery, University of Heidelberg, Heidelberg, Germany. [5]Current address: Institute of Pathology, Heinrich Heine University Düsseldorf, Düsseldorf, Germany. [6]Current address: Department of Surgery, Koc University School of Medicine, Istanbul, Turkey.

References
1. Mollberg N, Rahbari NN, Koch M, Hartwig W, Hoeger Y, Buchler MW, et al. Arterial resection during pancreatectomy for pancreatic cancer: a systematic review and meta-analysis. Ann Surg. 2011;254(6):882–93.
2. Zhou Y, Zhang Z, Liu Y, Li B, Xu D. Pancreatectomy combined with superior mesenteric vein-portal vein resection for pancreatic cancer: a meta-analysis. World J Surg. 2012;36(4):884–91.
3. Shibata C, Kobari M, Tsuchiya T, Arai K, Anzai R, Takahashi M, et al. Pancreatectomy combined with superior mesenteric-portal vein resection for adenocarcinoma in pancreas. World J Surg. 2001;25(8):1002–5.
4. Boggi U, Del Chiaro M, Croce C, Vistoli F, Signori S, Moretto C, et al. Prognostic implications of tumor invasion or adhesion to peripancreatic vessels in resected pancreatic cancer. Surgery. 2009;146(5):869–81.
5. Wang J, Estrella JS, Peng L, Rashid A, Varadhachary GR, Wang H, et al. Histologic tumor involvement of superior mesenteric vein/portal vein predicts poor prognosis in patients with stage II pancreatic adenocarcinoma treated with neoadjuvant chemoradiation. Cancer. 2012;118(15):3801–11.
6. Nakao A, Kanzaki A, Fujii T, Kodera Y, Yamada S, Sugimoto H, et al. Correlation between radiographic classification and pathological grade of

portal vein wall invasion in pancreatic head cancer. Annals of surgery. 2012;255(1):103–8.

7. Shimada K, Sano T, Sakamoto Y, Kosuge T. Clinical implications of combined portal vein resection as a palliative procedure in patients undergoing pancreaticoduodenectomy for pancreatic head carcinoma. Ann Surg Oncol. 2006;13(12):1569–78.

8. Carrere N, Sauvanet A, Goere D, Kianmanesh R, Vullierme MP, Couvelard A, et al. Pancreaticoduodenectomy with mesentericoportal vein resection for adenocarcinoma of the pancreatic head. World J Surg. 2006;30(8):1526–35.

9. Yekebas EF, Bogoevski D, Cataldegirmen G, Kunze C, Marx A, Vashist YK, et al. En bloc vascular resection for locally advanced pancreatic malignancies infiltrating major blood vessels: perioperative outcome and long-term survival in 136 patients. Ann Surg. 2008;247(2):300–9.

10. Winter JM, Brennan MF, Tang LH, D'Angelica MI, Dematteo RP, Fong Y, et al. Survival after resection of pancreatic adenocarcinoma: results from a single institution over three decades. Annals of surgical oncology. 2012;19(1):169–75.

11. Ferrone CR, Pieretti-Vanmarcke R, Bloom JP, Zheng H, Szymonifka J, Wargo JA, et al. Pancreatic ductal adenocarcinoma: long-term survival does not equal cure. Surgery. 2012;152(3 Suppl 1):S43–9.

12. Haeno H, Gonen M, Davis MB, Herman JM, Iacobuzio-Donahue CA, Michor F. Computational modeling of pancreatic cancer reveals kinetics of metastasis suggesting optimum treatment strategies. Cell. 2012;148(1–2):362–75.

13. Dindo D, Demartines N, Clavien PA. Classification of surgical complications: a new proposal with evaluation in a cohort of 6336 patients and results of a survey. Ann Surg. 2004;240(2):205–13.

14. Tempero MA, Malafa MP, Behrman SW, Benson 3rd AB, Casper ES, Chiorean EG, et al. Pancreatic adenocarcinoma, version 2.2014: featured updates to the NCCN guidelines. Journal of the National Comprehensive Cancer Network : JNCCN. 2014;12(8):1083–93.

15. Tol JA, Gouma DJ, Bassi C, Dervenis C, Montorsi M, Adham M, et al. Definition of a standard lymphadenectomy in surgery for pancreatic ductal adenocarcinoma: a consensus statement by the International Study Group on Pancreatic Surgery (ISGPS). Surgery. 2014;156(3):591–600.

16. Strasberg SM, Linehan DC, Hawkins WG. The accordion severity grading system of surgical complications. Ann Surg. 2009;250(2):177–86.

17. Riediger H, Keck T, Wellner U, zur Hausen A, Adam U, Hopt UT, et al. The lymph node ratio is the strongest prognostic factor after resection of pancreatic cancer. J Gastrointest Surg. 2009;13(7):1337–44.

18. Harrison LE, Klimstra DS, Brennan MF. Isolated portal vein involvement in pancreatic adenocarcinoma. A contraindication for resection? Ann Surg. 1996;224(3):342–7. discussion 347–349.

19. Fukuda S, Oussoultzoglou E, Bachellier P, Rosso E, Nakano H, Audet M, et al. Significance of the depth of portal vein wall invasion after curative resection for pancreatic adenocarcinoma. Archives of surgery. 2007;142(2):172–9. discussion 180.

20. Wagner M, Redaelli C, Lietz M, Seiler CA, Friess H, Buchler MW. Curative resection is the single most important factor determining outcome in patients with pancreatic adenocarcinoma. Br J Surg. 2004;91(5):586–94.

21. Buchler MW, Werner J, Weitz J. R0 in pancreatic cancer surgery: surgery, pathology, biology, or definition matters? Ann Surg. 2010;251(6):1011–2.

22. Esposito I, Kleeff J, Bergmann F, Reiser C, Herpel E, Friess H, et al. Most pancreatic cancer resections are R1 resections. Ann Surg Oncol. 2008;15(6):1651–60.

23. Schlitter AM, Esposito I. Definition of microscopic tumor clearance (r0) in pancreatic cancer resections. Cancers. 2010;2(4):2001–10.

24. Seufferlein T, Porzner M, Becker T, Budach V, Ceyhan G, Esposito I, et al. S3-guideline exocrine pancreatic cancer. Zeitschrift fur Gastroenterologie. 2013;51(12):1395–440.

16

Predictors for resectability and survival in locally advanced pancreatic cancer after gemcitabine-based neoadjuvant therapy

Ying-Jui Chao[1], Edgar D Sy[1], Hui-Ping Hsu[1] and Yan-Shen Shan[1,2]*

Abstract

Background: To evaluate the predictors for resectability and survival of patients with locally advanced pancreatic cancer (LAPC) treated with gemcitabine-based neoadjuvant therapy (GBNAT).

Methods: Between May 2003 and Dec 2009, 41 tissue-proved LAPC were treated with GBNAT. The location of pancreatic cancer in the head, body and tail was 17, 18 and 6 patients respectively. The treatment response was evaluated by RECIST criteria. Surgical exploration was based on the response and the clear plan between tumor and celiac artery/superior mesentery artery. Kaplan–Meier analysis and Cox Model were used to calculate the resectability and survival rates.

Results: Finally, 25 patients received chemotherapy (CT) and 16 patients received concurrent chemoradiation therapy (CRT). The response rate was 51% (21 patients), 2 CR (1 in CT and 1 in CRT) and 19 PR (10 in CT and 9 in CRT). 20 patients (48.8%) were assessed as surgically resectable, in which 17 (41.5%) underwent successful resection with a 17.6% positive-margin rate and 3 failed explorations were pancreatic head cancer for dense adhesion. Two pancreatic neck cancer turned fibrosis only. Patients with surgical intervention had significant actuarial overall survival. Tumor location and post-GBNAT CA199 < 152 were predictors for resectability. Post-GBNAT CA-199 < 152 and post-GBNAT CA-125 < 32.8 were predictors for longer disease progression-free survival. Pre-GBNAT CA-199 < 294, post-GBNAT CA-125 < 32.8, and post-op CEA < 6 were predictors for longer overall survival.

Conclusion: Tumor location and post-GBNAT CA199 < 152 are predictors for resectability while pre-GBNAT CA-199 < 294, post-GBNAT CA-125 < 32.8, post-GBNAT CA-199 < 152 and post-op CEA < 6 are survival predictors in LAPC patients with GBNAT.

Keywords: Locally advanced pancreatic cancer (LAPC), Neoadjuvant therapy, Concurrent chemoradiation therapy (CCRT)

Background

Pancreatic cancer is the most formidable malignancy with annual mortality nearly equal to its annual incidence and the 5-year survival rate was less than 5%. Surgical resection is the only potentially curative treatment. However, less than 20% cases are eligible for resection at presentation with a 5-year survival rate of 20% [1]. Locally advanced pancreatic cancer (LAPC) is defined as surgically unresectable pancreatic cancer involving the celiac artery or the superior mesentery artery without

evidence of distant metastasis [2]. It accounts for 26% of newly diagnosed pancreatic cancer with a 5-year survival rate of 8.7% [3]. With amelioration of the resectability of LAPC, the overall survival of pancreatic cancer can be improved.

Several randomized trials have been performed to increase the resectability of LAPC. The 5-fluorouracil (5-FU) based chemoradiotherapy has been supported as the most acceptable treatment [4-6]. In the recent decade, gemcitabine has been considered as the standard agent for advanced pancreatic cancer and also act as a radiosensitizer during radiotherapy [7-9]. In year 2003, an algorithm for management of LAPC with intends of improving the survival rate and quality of life of patients

* Correspondence: ysshan@mail.ncku.edu.tw
[1]Division of General Surgery, Department of Surgery, National Cheng Kung University Hospital, Tainan, Taiwan
[2]Institute of Clinical Medicine, College of Medicine, National Cheng Kung University, Tainan, Taiwan

was set up using gemcitabine-based neoadjuvant therapy in National Cheng Kung University Hospital. In this study, the effect on surgical resection, survival rate and predictors for resectability of patients with LAPC after neoadjuvant therapy with gemcitabine-based chemotherapy or gemcitabine-based concurrent chemoradiation therapy is presented.

Methods

Patients and treatments

From January 2003 to Dec 2009, patients with LAPC were enrolled for gemcitabine-based chemotherapy or gemcitabine-based concurrent chemoradiation therapy. The diagnosis of LAPC was based on thin sliced enhanced multi-detected computed tomography (MDCT) [10] with inclusion criteria of 1) abutment or encasement of celiac artery or superior mesentery artery (cT4) [2]; 2) the involvement of portal vein at the confluence superior mesentery vein and splenic vein [11]; 3) severe extra-pancreatic soft tissue involvement. All patients underwent CT-guide core-biopsy and proved to have pancreatic ductal adenocarcinoma. Patients, who had previous surgical exploration with proved pancreatic ductal adenocarcinoma was also enrolled. The treatment plan was based on the algorithm treatment of LAPC in the National Cheng Kung University Hospital. This study was approved by the Institutioal Review Board of National Cheng Kung University Hospital, ER-98-023. The informed consent for participation in the study was obtained from participants.

Three GBNAT were used for LAPC patients: 1) the first regimen was institutional phase II trial of chemotherapy (CT). The regimen was combined intravenous infusion of gemcitabine 1000 mg/m^2 for 100 minutes and oxaliplatin 70 mg/m^2 for 2 hours on day 1, and fluorouracil (5-FU) 1000 mg/m^2 for 24 hours on day 2, and followed by oral thalidomide 100 mg per day after intravenous infusion therapy every 2 week for 6 cycles. 2) the second regimen was intravenous infusion of gemcitabine 1000 mg/m^2 for 100 minutes and oxaliplatin 70 mg/m^2 for 2 hours on day 1, and fluorouracil (5-FU) 1000 mg/m^2 for 24 hours on day 2and followed by oral Sunitinib 12.5 mg per day after intravenous infusion therapy, every 2 week for 6 cycle. 3) the third regimen was gemcitabine-based concurrent chemoradiation therapy (CRT). In this regimen, patients received three-dimensional conformal radiotherapy at the target area, pancreatic lesion and nodal area, with a total dose of 50.4 Gy (1.8 Gy/day). The chemotherapy included concurrent 30-minute intravenous infusion of gemcitabine at a dose of 400 mg/m^2 every week during radiation and 60-minute intravenous infusion of gemcitabine at a dose of 1000 mg/m ^{2} for three continuous weeks after radiation. The choice of gemcitabine-based CT or gemcitabine-based CRT was dependent on

patient's preference following explanation of the side effects of different regimens.

Assessment of response and indications for operation

The response to treatment after GBNAT was restaged by MDCT scan of the abdomen at 8 weeks routinely. The response of downing size of the tumor was determined by the RECIST criteria. Surgical exploration was done in patients with evidence of downsizing of the tumor mass and the clear plan between tumor and celiac artery/superior mesentery artery after treatment. In patients with a stable disease, reevaluation of tumor response was performed at 12 weeks after GBNAT, and surgical exploration is performed only if there is evidence of downsizing of the mass or stable disease without increasing tumor markers. Tumor markers; CA199, CA125, and CEA were determined at pre-GBNAT, post-GBNAT and 1 months post-resection. During exploration, pancreatic resection (conventional Whipple's procedure, pylorus-preserving pancreaticoduodenectomy, central pancreatectomy or distal pancreatectomy) with regional lymphadenectomy was determined by surgeon according to preoperative evaluation from MDCT, patients' co-morbidities, and preoperative nutrition status. Pathologic stage was defined according to the American International Union against Cancer (AJCC) [2]. Resection margin were examined for defined radicality (including proximal and peripancreatic margins). Postoperative follow-up included routine chest X-ray, and MDCT of the abdomen every 3 months and every 6 months during the first and second postoperative year respectively or if patients had suspicious sign of recurrence. Routine bone scan was done every 6 months or when suspicious symptom of bone metastasis is present. Tumor markers were evaluated every 3 months during the first two postoperative years. Additional tests, cytologic examination of ascites and pleural effusion and brain CT, were performed when a recurrence or distant metastasis was suspected. In those patients with disease progression or distant metastasis, further chemotherapy, pain control, or best supportive care were arranged according to patient's clinical condition based on our LAPC management algorithm.

Statistical analysis

Continuous variables were expressed as mean ± S.D. and compared with a two-tailed *t-test*. Categoric variables were compared with Fisher's exact test. Univariate and multivariate analyses for predictors of resectability rate were performed using Cox stepwise regression. Univariatee analysis for survival was calculated as the interval from registration until death using Kaplan-Meier method and the difference in survival between groups was compared using log-rank test. A univariate $p \leq 0.05$ in each of these analyses were considered for entry into multivariate analyses Cox model calculation. Results were considered significant for value of p ≤ 0.05. All analyses were performed using SPSS statistical software (version 13th, SPSS, Inc., Chicago, IL).

Results

Between May 2003 and Dec 2009, 41 tissue-proved LAPC patients, 27 male and 14 female, with mean age of 63.5 years were treated with GBNAT. There were 25 patients received gemcitabine-based CT and 16 patients received gemcitabine-based CRT in the National Cheng Kung University Hospital. 9 patients had previous failed surgical resection before enrollment and 32 patients were naïve patients with MDCT unresectable LAPC. The location of LAPC in the head, body and tail was 17, 18 and 6 patients respectively. The pre-GBNAT serum of tumor markers level were CEA 24.9 ± 28.6, CA199 1641 ± 3697, and CA125 51.1 ± 51.9. After treatment, the response rate was 51.2%, 2 CR and 19 PR. There were 10 PR and 1 CR in the 25 (44%) patients received gemcitabine-based CT, and 9 PR and 1 CR in the 16 (62.5%) patients received gemcitabine-based CRT. There were 20 patients received exploration by response rate and MDCT evaluation but 17 patients had successful tumor resection (14 R0, 2 R1 and 1 R2), in which 6, 5 and 6 patients received Whipple's operation, central pancreatectomy, and distal pancreatectomy respectively. In these resectable cases, two pancreatic neck cancer patients received central pancreatectomy and pathology revealed fibrotic change only. The harvested and positive node number was lower. The positive surgical margin rate was 17.6% (3 of 17 patients). Three patients had failed surgical resection due to severe dense adhesion around the retroperitoneal region and SMA/SMV area. Those patients with R2 resection and failed surgical resection were all pancreatic head cancer with uncinate process extension (Table 1).

After GBNAT, the level of tumor markers CEA, CA199 and CA125 were 20.3 ± 51.2, 1820 ± 4780, and 82.3 ± 135.5 respectively. The median progression-free survival was 9.0 (18.4 ± 3.0) months, patients with surgical exploration had significant longer progression-free survival than those without surgical exploration; 15.0 (32.1 ± 6.0) months versus 4.0 (6.7 ± 2.0) months. The 5-year progression-free survival rate was 12.5%, 28.5% in those patients with surgical exploration versus 0% in those patients without surgical exploration. In those patients only had 4.8% 2-year progression-free survival rate, P < 0.0001 (Figure 1). The median overall survival was 12.5 (20.8 ± 4.0) months, patients with surgical exploration had longer overall survival than those without surgical exploration; 21.0 (33.1 ± 7.0) months versus 9.0 (10.5 ± 2.0) months. The 5-year overall survival rate was

Table 1 Demographics of patients with locally advanced pancreatic cancer received gemcitabine-based neoadjuvant therapy (GBNAT) and surgical resection

Characteristics	Number of patients, n = 41
Sex (M:F)	27:14
Age (years), mean (range)	63.5 (39–80)
Location: Head: body: tail	17:18: 6
Naïve: failed exploration	32:9
Chemotherapy(CT)[#]: chemoradiation therapy (CRT)*	25:16
Response rate	21 (51.2%)
CR: PR	2:19
Surgery: non-surgery	20:21
Successful resection	17 (41.5%)
Surgical procedure	
Whipple: central pancreatectomy: distal pancreatectomy	6: 5: 6
Surgical margin	
R0: R1: R2	14: 2:1
Pre-GBNAT tumor marker level	
CEA	24.9 ± 28.6
CA199	1641 ± 3697
CA125	51.1 ± 51.9
Post-GBNAT tumor marker level	
CEA	20.3 ± 51.2
CA199	1820 ± 4780
CA125	82.3 ± 135.5
Progression-free survival, median (mean ± SD), months	9.0 (18.4 ± 3.0)
Surgery vs non-surgery	15.0 (32.1 ± 6.0) vs 4.0 (6.7 ± 2.0)
Overall survival, median (mean ± SD), months	12.5 (20.8 ± 4.0)
Surgery vs non-surgery	21.0 (33.1 ± 7.0) vs 9.0 (10.5 ± 2.0)

[#]17 patients received phase I/II GOFT, 8 patients with GOFS, *7 patients received CCRT Tainan program, 9 patients received gemcitabine induction chemotherapy and reduced dose gemcitabine with R/T.

7.7%, 17.9% in those patients with surgical exploration compared to 4.8% in those patients without surgical exploration, P = 0.0001 (Figure 2). The progression-free survival and overall survival of LAPC with surgical exploration after GBNAT were similar to those of patients with initial primary resectable pancreatic cancer.

There were 20 patients received planned surgical exploration after evaluation. However, only 17 patients received successful resection (Table 1). Comparison of patients without exploration or failed exploration, tumor location (tail vs head and body), post-GBNAT serum CA199 (<152 vs ≥152), a decrease of CA199 and CA125 before surgery (post-GBNAT) was significant predictors

Progression-free Survival

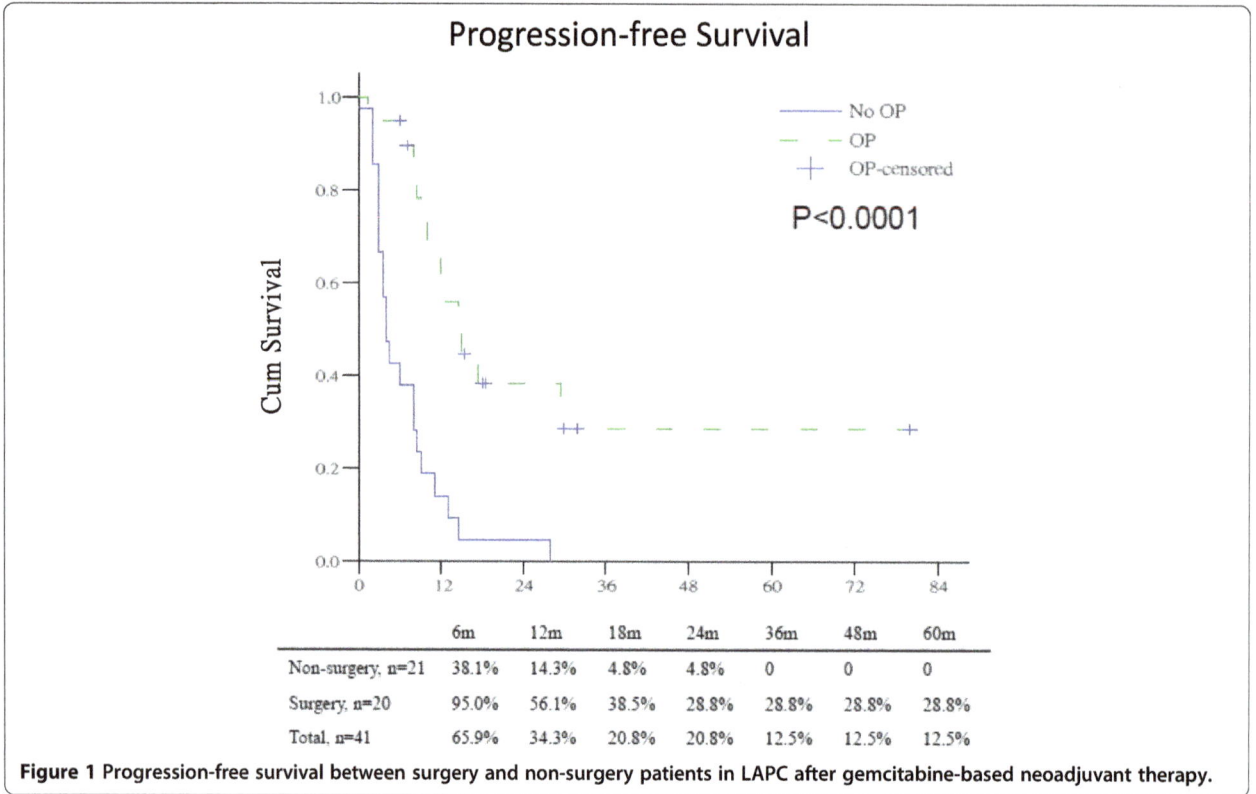

	6m	12m	18m	24m	36m	48m	60m
Non-surgery, n=21	38.1%	14.3%	4.8%	4.8%	0	0	0
Surgery, n=20	95.0%	56.1%	38.5%	28.8%	28.8%	28.8%	28.8%
Total, n=41	65.9%	34.3%	20.8%	20.8%	12.5%	12.5%	12.5%

Figure 1 Progression-free survival between surgery and non-surgery patients in LAPC after gemcitabine-based neoadjuvant therapy.

Overall Survival

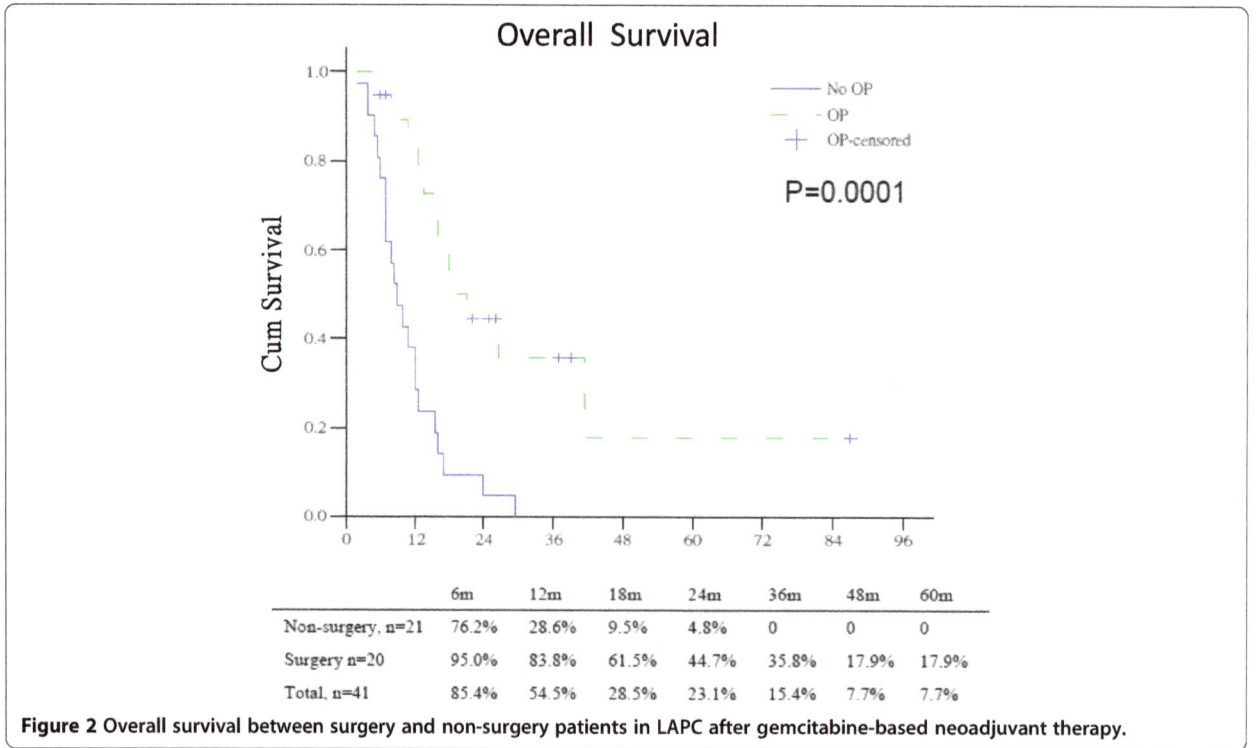

	6m	12m	18m	24m	36m	48m	60m
Non-surgery, n=21	76.2%	28.6%	9.5%	4.8%	0	0	0
Surgery n=20	95.0%	83.8%	61.5%	44.7%	35.8%	17.9%	17.9%
Total, n=41	85.4%	54.5%	28.5%	23.1%	15.4%	7.7%	7.7%

Figure 2 Overall survival between surgery and non-surgery patients in LAPC after gemcitabine-based neoadjuvant therapy.

for resectability in the univariate analysis. However, after using multivariate analysis, tumor location (OR: 50, CI: 1.218~ > 100. P = 0.039) and post-GBNAT CA199 < 152 (OR: 14.686, CI: 1.114 ~ 193.6, P = 0.041) were significant predictors for resection after GBNAT (Table 2).

Table 3 showed the predictors for progression-free survival of LAPC patients following GBNAT. In univariate analysis, several factors were identified as predictors for progression-free survival, such as tumor location, pre-GBNAT CA-199 < 294, post-GBNAT CA-199 < 152, post-op CA-199 < 82, post-GBNAT CA125 < 32.8, and post-op CEA <6. However, after using multivariate analysis, **post-GBNAT CA-199 < 152 (OR 26.32, CI 3.300 ~ 200, P = 0.002) and post-GBNAT CA-125 < 32.8 (OR 55.56, CI 6.759 ~ 500, P < 0.001)** were significant predictors for patients with longer disease progression-free survival.

The predictors for overall survival following GBNAT were shown in Table 4. Using univariate analysis, tumor location, resectable operation, post-op CEA < 6, pre-GBNAT CA-199 < 294, post-GBNAT CA-199 < 152, post-op CA-199 < 82, and post-GBNAT CA-125 < 32.8 were significance. Using multivariate analysis, **post-op CEA < 6 (OR 0.054, CI 0.005 ~ 0.0631, P = 0.020), pre-GBNAT CA-199 < 294 (0.033, CI 0.002 ~ 0.522, P = 0.015), and post-GBNAT CA-125 < 32.8 (OR = 0.034, CI 0.003 ~ 0.372, P = 0.006)** were significant predictors for patients with longer overall survival.

After GBNAT and surgical intervention, the metastatic/recurrent patterns were different in groups of patients with or without surgical exploration. Based on MDCT during the follow up period, 1/17 (6%) cases had loco-regional recurrence after surgical resection. The ratio of liver metastasis and peritoneal metastasis were improved in patients with surgical exploration compared to those without surgical exploration, 40% versus 100% and 30% versus 57.1%. However, the ratio of other distant metastasis was similar (Table 5).

Discussion

Surgery is the mainstay of treatment that offers significant survival in patients with pancreatic cancer, however, the overall survival is still poor due to low resectability. The challenging milestone for the improvement of outcome in LAPC is to increase the chance of surgical resection of patients either using chemotherapy or radiotherapy or combination [12-17]. Those patients who can benefit from neoadjuvant therapy and have the chance of surgical resection are still uncertain. In 2003, we set an algorithm for management of LAPC using GBNAT and responsive patients underwent surgical exploration at National Cheng Kung University Hospital. Following GBNAT, our study showed 17 of the 41 (41.5%) LAPC patients can be resected with a lower positive margin rate 17.6% (3 of 17 patients). Tumor

Table 2 Univariate and multivariate analysis of parameters associated with resectability after GBNAT

Parameters		Non-resectable	Resectable	Univariate	Multivariate		
		N = 24	N = 17	P	OR	95% CI	P
Age	≥60y/o	18	12	0.735	0.939	0.876-1.00	0.075
	<60y/o	6	5				
CCRT	Yes	6	7	0.273			
	Nil	18	10				
Tumor location	Tail	0	6	**<0.001**	50	**1.218- >100**	**0.039**
	Head/body	24	11				
CEA(post-GBNAT)	<4.9	13	7	0.280			
	≥4.9	11	10				
CEA decrease (post-GBNAT)	Yes	10	8	0.821			
	Nil	14	9				
CA199 (post-GBNAT)	<152	9	13	**0.007**	14.686	**1.114-193.6**	**0.041**
	≥152	15	4				
CA199 decrease (post-GBNAT)	Yes	11	14	**0.008**	66.67	0.416- >100	0.105
	Nil	13	3				
CA125(post-GBNAT)	<32.8	12	9	0.790			
	≥32.8	12	8				
CA125 decrease (post-GBNAT)	Yes	14	4	**0.026**	8.547	0.138- >100	0.308
	Nil	10	13				

Bold letter means the p-values less than 0.05.

Table 3 Univariate and Multivariate analysis of risk factors for progression-free survival following GBNAT and surgical resection

Parameter	Univariate	Multivariate		
	P	OR	95% CI	P
Age	0.362	0.990	0.914-1.072	0.806
Tumor location: tail vs head or body	0.004	2.048	0.495-8.474	0.323
CA 199: pre-GBNAT <294 vs ≥294	0.003	1.776	0.357-8.850	0.483
CA 199: post-GBNAT <152 vs ≥152	0.000	**26.32**	**3.300-200**	**0.002**
CA 199: post-op <82 vs ≥82	0.007	2.137	0.524-8.696	0.290
CEA: post-op <6 vs ≥6	0.04	2.604	0.749-9.091	0.132
CA 125: post-GBNAT <32.8 vs ≥32.8	0.035	**55.56**	**6.579-500**	**<0.001**

Abbreviations: OR odds ratio, 95% CI 95% confidence interval. Bold letter means the p-values less than 0.05.

location and post-GBNAT CA19-9 < 152 can be used as predictors for surgical resection. Post-GBNAT CA19-9 < 152 and post-GBNAT CA-125 < 32.8 are both predictors for longer disease progression-free survival. Patient with pre-GBNAT CA19-9 < 294, post-GBNAT CA-125 < 32.8 and post-op CEA < 6 had significant longer overall survival.

There were three major points of concern in the management of LAPC prior surgery. Firstly, what is the effective preoperative neoadjuvant regimen for LAPC? From the report of Gastrointestinal Tumor Study Group (GITSG), 5-fluorouracil (5-Fu) based chemoradiation can increase survival of pancreatic cancer patients [4]. Several studies used 5-Fu based chemoradiation to treat LAPC and the improvement of resection rate varies [4-6,18]. Kim HJ et al. found that in spite of the use of various chemoradiation protocols, it was impossible to downsize the tumor to obtain resectability and only one of 87 patients could be resected in that study [18]. However, Wanebo et al., using 5-Fu based chemoradiation, reported a resection rate up to 65% in 14 patients with LAPC [6]. Over the past 10 years, gemcitabine has become the standard of chemotherapy in advanced pancreatic cancer, and is also noted to be a potent radiosensitizer of epithelial cancer. Heinemann et al. reported that gemcitabine-based combination chemotherapy applied in

advanced pancreatic cancer could show survival benefit, especially in those pancreatic cancer patients with a good performance status [8]. Many phase I and II studies demonstrated the feasibility of combining radiation with low dose gemcitabine weekly followed sequential full-dose gemcitabine [9]. These neoadjuvant treatments with gemcitabine-based CT or CRT was able to increase the resectability rate with clear margin and improved the prognosis of curative cases with comparable survival as initially resectable pancreatic cancer. Gillen et al. reported one-third unresectable tumor patients could be resected after neoadjunvant therapy [19]. A meta-analysis of 20 phase 3 trials by Bria E et al. concluded that gemcitabine-based chemotherapy could improve progression free survival in selected patients with inoperable pancreatic cancer [7]. In our series, 41.5% of LAPC patients could be resected; 55.6% (5 of 9) in previous failed exploration (borderline resectable) patients and 37.5% (12 of 32) in LAPC patient with long-term comparable outcome as initial resectable pancreatic cancer. Though different regimens were used in these patients, our results confirmed the efficacy of gemcitabine-based combination CT or CRT in our protocol.

The second concern is the definition of locally advanced pancreatic cancer. In the 6th edition AJCC

Table 4 Univarite and multivariate analysis of risk factors for overall survival following GBNAT and surgical resection

Parameter	Univariate	Multivariate		
	P	OR	95% CI	P
Age	0.308	0.982	0.891-1.082	0.709
Tumor location: head or body vs tail	0.003	4.689	0.048-458.2	0.509
Resectable operation: resectable vs non-resectable	0.001	5.492	0.122-246.7	0.380
CEA: post-op <6 vs >6	0.059	**0.054**	**0.005-0.631**	**0.020**
CA 199: pre-GBNAT <294 vs >294	0.011	**0.033**	**0.002-0.522**	**0.015**
CA 199: post-GBNAT <152 vs >152	0.008	0.464	0.041-5.672	0.536
CA 199: post-op <82 vs >82	0.000	0.201	0.015-2.652	0.223
CA125: post-GBNAT <32.8 vs >32.8	0.018	**0.034**	**0.003-0.372**	**0.006**

Abbreviations: OR odds ratio, 95% CI 95% confidence interval. Bold letter means the p-values less than 0.05.

Table 5 Patterns of failure after gemcitabine-based neoadjuvant therapy in locally advanced pancreatic cancer

Metastatic/Recurrent Sites	Surgery n = 20 (%)	Non-surgery/ n = 21 (%)
Liver	8 (40%)	21 (100%)
Peritoneum	6 (30%)	12 (57.1%)
Others (bone, lung, soft tissue, brain)	5 (25%)	5 (23.8%)
Loco-regional recurrence in resectable cases*	1 (6%)	0
Disease free	3 (15%)	0

*One of the 17 resectable cases.

staging of pancreatic cancer, the pancreatic tumor with involvement of SMA or celiac plexus was rendered unresectable [2]. Occlusion of the confluence of portal vein (PV) and superior mesentery vein (SMV) was also considered unresectable according to the definition of resectable pancreatic cancer [11]. In 2006, a new category of borderline resectable pancreatic cancer was proposed by Varadhachary based on the extent of artery involvement and technical capability of reconstructing the vein [20]. The Fox Chase Cancer Center also suggested that tumor-induced unilateral shift or narrowing of the SPMV confluence as one of criteria of borderline resectable [21]. In resectable pancreatic cancer, the reported positive margin rate (R1 + R2) ranged from 19% to 68% and the positive margin strongly predicts the short survival and early recurrence rate [20]. Thus, patients with borderline resectable pancreatic head cancer are at higher risk for a margin-positive resection. The consensus of the Fox Chase group and the American-Hepato-Pancreato-Biliary Association (AHPBA)-Society of Surgical Oncology (SSO)-Society for Surgery of the Alimentary Tract (SSAT) suggested that borderline resectable pancreatic cancer should be treated with induction therapy before surgery [22]. In our study, the inclusion criteria were according to the 6th edition of AJCC, tumor involving the confluence of portal vein and superior mesentery veins, tumor with severe extra-pancreatic soft tissue invasion, and previous failed exploration. Our recruited patients were 32 unresectable locally advanced pancreatic cancer and 9 patients with failed prior surgical exploration were borderline resectable pancreatic cancer. It is compatible with the definition of LAPC by 6th edition AJCC staging of pancreatic cancer.

The third concern is the predictors for resectability and survival after GBNAT. The response of pancreatic cancer for GBNAT was based on the MDCT image findings. The criteria of exploration after GBNAT are downsizing of lesion and the clear plan between tumor and celiac artery/superior mesentery artery from the followed up MDCT [10]. Though the advancement in MDCT improved the accuracy of diagnosing tumor invasion in the area of SMA and celiac trunk, it is still unable to

distinguish neoplastic reaction and fibrosis tissue, and can result in high unresectable rate even when considered as a resectable. Kim reported that neoadjuvant therapy could reduce the accuracy in tumor restaging [23], a possible reason for failure in exploration after neoadjuvant therapy. Massucco et al. reported that the interventions were more technically demanding [14] which reflect the difficulty in resection of LAPC after neoadjuvant therapy. Chao et al. reported that only minority of patients with unresectable tumor might become resectable after neoadjuvant treatment, and some of these resectable cases required portal venorrhaphy and hepatic artery reconstruction [13]. The absence of reliable biological or radiological predictor for exploration, a more aggressive policy, to explore all patients without disease progression, in order to improve the resection rate was suggested by Massucco et al. [14]. From our results, the surgical resection rate was 85% (17 of 20) and all the 3 failed re-explored patients were pancreatic head cancer with severe dense fibrosis between the retroperitoneal region and mesentery root area. The 6 tail patients could be resected after treatment because there was no hindrance in multi-organs resection for pancreatic surgeon. The multivariate analysis of clinicopathological factors showed that tumor location and post-GBNAT CA19-9 < 152 could be used as predictors for resection after GBNAT. Recently, based on this study, we have applied the predictors as criteria for exploration and SMA approach with portal vein reconstruction for uncinated process pancreatic cancer to increase resection rate. Now, the resected LAPC has increased to 30 cases in our hospital.

Surgery alone is not a good option for LAPC because of the high probability of incomplete surgical resection with residual cancer at the surgical margin or in draining lymph nodes. Multidisciplinary approach using CT or CRT is required to improve the survival rate of LAPC. Previous reports have showed that one-third of the selective borderline resectable pancreatic cancer or LAPC can achieve longer disease free survival [19]. In comparison, the positive lymph node and the positive margin rate was lower than the previous report and might be one of the reasons for better outcome in our study. Massucco et al. agreed that R0 resection give the chance of longer survival [14]. Takahashi et al. identified CA19-9 that substantially decreased after preoperative CRT was an indicator for therapeutic selection and survival [24]. In this study, we also found that patients with decreased preoperative CA19-9 and decreased preoperative CA125 were predictors for resectability in univariate analysis, but the significance vanished under multivariate analysis. However, our analysis proved that post-GBNAT CA-199 < 152 and post-GBNAT CA-125 < 32.8 were both predictors for patients with longer disease progression-free survival, and post-op CEA < 6, pre-GBNAT CA-199 < 294, and post-GBNAT CA-125 < 32.8 had significant longer overall survival.

Conclusion

In conclusion, treatment of LAPC is challenging and requires multidisciplinary approach. With the advancement in neoadjuvant therapy and surgical techniques, we can improve the local and distant tumor control. Patients with resected LAPC following GBNAT can be expected to have comparable survival with initial resectable pancreatic cancer. Tumor location at pancreatic tail, post-GBNAT CA19-9 < 152, and post-GBNAT CA-125 < 32.8 could be used as predictors for resectability, disease-free survival, and overall survival of LAPC after GBNAT.

Competing interests
The authors declare that they have no competing interests.

Authors' contributions
In this study, the surgery was performed by YJC and YSS, treatments were performed by YSS. YJC and EDS written the manuscript and revised the manuscript initially and final revision was done by YSS. The biostatistic was performed by HPH. All the study was performed under the supervision of YSS. All authors read and approved the final manuscript.

Acknowledgement
This study is partly funded from the Department of Health (DOH101-TD-C-111-003) and the National Science Council (98-2314-B-006-052-MY3), Executive Yuan, Taiwan.

References
1. Li D, Xie K, Wolff R, Abbruzzese JL: Pancreatic cancer. *Lancet* 2004, 363(9414):1049–1057.
2. *AJCC Cancer Staging Manual.* 6th edition. Chicago, Ill: Springer; 2002.
3. Homer CG, Ries LAG, Krapcho M: In *SEER Cancer Statistics Review, 1975–2006.* Bethesda, MD: Bethesda, MD; [http://seer.cancer.gov/archive/csr/1975_2006/index.html]
4. Moertel CG, Frytak S, Hahn RG, O'Connell MJ, Reitemeier RJ, Rubin J, Schutt AJ, Weiland LH, Childs DS, Holbrook MA, Lavin PT, Livstone E, Spiro H, Knowlton A, Kalser M, Barkin J, Lessner H, Mann-Kaplan R, Ramming K, Douglas HO Jr, Thomas P, Nave H, Bateman J, Lokich J, Brooks J, Chaffey J, Corson JM, Zamcheck N, Novak JW: Therapy of locally unresectable pancreatic cancer: a randomized comparison of high dose (6000 rads) radiation alone, moderate dose radiation (4000 rads + 5-fluorouracil), and high dose radiation + 5-fluorouracil: the gastrointestinal tumor study group. *Cancer* 1981, 48(8):1705–1710.
5. Cohen SJ, Dobelbower R Jr, Lipsitz S, Catalano PJ, Sischy B, Smith TJ, Haller DG: A randomized phase III study of radiotherapy alone or with 5-fluorouracil and mitomycin-C in patients with locally advanced adenocarcinoma of the pancreas: eastern cooperative oncology group study E8282. *Int J Radiat Oncol Bio Phys* 2005, 62(5):1345–1350.
6. Wanebo HJ, Glicksman AS, Vezeridis MP, Clark J, Tibbetts L, Koness RJ, Levy A: Preoperative chemotherapy, radiotherapy, and surgical resection of locally advanced pancreatic cancer. *Arch Surg* 2000, 135(1):81–87. discussion 88.
7. Bria E, Milella M, Gelibter A, Cuppone F, Pino MS, Ruggeri EM, Carlini P, Nistico C, Terzoli E, Cognetti F, Giannarelli D: Gemcitabine-based combinations for inoperable pancreatic cancer: have we made real progress? *Cancer* 2007, 110(3):525–533.
8. Heinemann V, Boeck S, Hinke A, Labianca R, Louvet C: Meta-analysis of randomized trials: evaluation of benefit from gemcitabine-based combination chemotherapy applied in advanced pancreatic cancer. *BMC Cancer* 2008, 8:82.
9. Xie DR, Liang HL, Wang Y, Guo SS, Yang Q: Meta-analysis on inoperable pancreatic cancer: a comparison between gemcitabine-based combination therapy and gemcitabine alone. *World J Gastroenterol* 2006, 12(43):6973–6981.
10. Tamm EP, Silveman PM, Chamsangavej C, Evans DB: Diagnosis, staging, and surveillance of pancreatic cancer. *Am J Roentgenol* 2003, 180(5):1311–1323.
11. Tseng JF, Raut CP, Lee JE, Pisters PW, Vauthey JN, Abdalla EK, Gomez HF, Sun CC, Crane CH, Wolff RA, Evans DB: Pancreaticoduodenectomy with vascular resection: margin status and survival duration. *J Gastrointest Surg* 2004, 8(8):935–950. discussion 949-950.
12. Pliarchopoulou K, Pectasides D: Pancreatic cancer: current and future treatment strategies. *Cancer Treat Rev* 2009, 35:431–436.
13. Chao C, Hoffman JP, Rose EA, Torosian MH, Eisenberg BL: Pancreatic carcinoma deemed unresectable at exploration may be resected for cure: an institutional experience. *Am Surg* 2000, 66(4):378–385.
14. Massucco P, Capussotti L, Magnino A, Sperti E, Gatti M, Muratore A, Sgotto E, Gabriele P, Aglietta M: Pancreatic resections after chemoradiotherapy for locally advanced ductal adenocarcinoma: analysis of perioperative outcome and survival. *Ann Surg Oncol* 2006, 13(9):1201–1208.
15. Satol S, Yanagimoto H, Toyokawa H, Takahashi K, Matsui Y, Kitade H, Mergental H, Tanigawa N, Takai S, Kwon AH: Surgical results after preoperative chemoradiation therapy for patients with pancreatic cancer. *Pancreas* 2009, 38(3):282–288.
16. Golcher H, Brunner T, Grabenbauer G, Merkel S, Papadopoulos T, Hohenberger W, Meyer T: Preoperative chemoradiation in adenocarcinoma of the pancreas. A single centre experience advocating a new treatment strategy. *Eur J Surg Oncol* 2008, 34(7):756–764.
17. Brown KM, Siripurapu V, Davidson M, Cohen SJ, Konski A, Watson JC, Li TN, Ciocca V, Cooper H, Hoffman JP: Chemoradiation followed by chemotherapy before resection for borderline pancreatic cancer. *Am J Surg* 2008, 195(3):318–321.
18. Kim HJ, Czischke K, Brennan MF, Conlon KC: Does neoadjuvant chemoradiation downstage locally advanced pancreatic cancer? *J Gastrointest Surg* 2002, 6:763–769.
19. Gillen S, Schuster T, Büschenfelde CMZ, Friess H, Kleeff J: Preoperative/ neoadjuvant therapy in pancreatic cancer: a systematic review and meta-analysis of response and resection percentages. *PLoS Med* 2010, 7(4):e1000267.
20. Varadhachary GR, Tamm EP, Abbruzzese JL, Xiong HQ, Crane CH, Wang H, Lee JE, Pisters PW, Evans DB, Wolff RA: Borderline resectable pancreatic cancer: definitions, management, and role of preoperative therapy. *Ann Surg Oncol* 2006, 13(8):1035–1046.
21. Chun YS, Milestone BN, Watson LC, Cohen SJ, Burtness B, Engstrom PF, Haluszka O, Tokar JL, Hall MJ, Denlinger CS, Astsaturov I, Hoffman JP: Defining venous involvement in borderline resectable pancreatic cancer. *Ann Surg Oncol* 2010, 17(11):2832–2838.
22. Callery MP, Chang KJ, Fishman EK, Talamonti MS, William Traverso L, Linehan DC: Pretreatment assessment of resectable and borderline resectable pancreatic cancer. Expert consensus statement. *Ann Surg Oncol* 2009, 16(7):1727–1733.
23. Kim YE, Park MS, Hong HS, Kang CM, Choi JY, Lim JS, Lee WJ, Kim MJ, Kim KW: Effects of neoadjuvant combined chemotherapy and radiation therapy on the CT evaluation of resectablity and staging in patients with pancreatic head cancer. *Radiology* 2009, 250(3):758–765.
24. Takahashi H, Ohigashi H, Ishikawa O, Eguchi H, Gotoh K, Yamada T, Nakaizumi A, Uehara H, Tomita Y, Nishiyama K, Yano M: Serum CA19-9 alterations during preoperative gemcitabine-based chemoradiation therapy for resectable invasive ductal carcinoma of the pancreas as indicator for therapeutic selection and survival. *Ann Surg* 2010, 251(3):461–469.

17

Invasive treatment of pain associated with pancreatic cancer on different levels of WHO analgesic ladder

Łukasz Dobosz[*], Tomasz Stefaniak, Małgorzata Dobrzycka, Jagoda Wieczorek, Paula Franczak, Dominika Ptaszyńska, Katarzyna Zasada and Peter Kanyion

Abstract

Background: Pancreatic cancer is a malignant neoplasm with a high mortality rate, often associated with a delayed diagnosis, the early occurrence of metastasis and an overall, poor response to chemotherapy and radiotherapy. Pain management in pancreatic cancer consists mainly of pharmacological treatment according to the WHO analgesic ladder. Surgical treatment for pain relief, such as splanchnicectomy, is considered amongst the final step of pain management. It has been proven that splanchnicectomy is a safe procedure with a small percentage of complications, nevertheless, it is often used as a last resort, which can significantly decrease its effectiveness. Performance of thoracoscopic splanchnicectomy along the first step of the analgesic ladder may lead to long-lasting protection against the presence and severity of pain.

Methods/Design: A prospective, open label, 1:1 randomized, controlled trial, conducted at a single institution to determine the effectiveness of invasive treatment of pain via splanchnicectomy, in patients with advanced pancreatic cancer. The size of tested group will consist of 26 participants in each arm of the trial, to evaluate the level of pain relief and its impact on quality of life. To evaluate the influence on patients' rate of overall survival, a sample size of 105 patients is necessary, in each trial arm. Assessments will not only include the usage of analgesic pharmacotherapy throughout the course of disease, and overall patient survival, but also subjective pain perception at rest, in movement, and after meals (measured by NRS score questionnaire), the patient's quality of life (measured using the QLQ-C30 and FACIT questionnaires), and any pain-related suffering (measured with the PRISM projection test). The primary endpoint will consist of pain intensity. Questionnaires will be obtained upon the initial visit, the day of surgery, the day after surgery, as well as during long-term follow-up visits, held every two weeks thereafter.

Discussion: Earlier implementation of invasive treatment, such as thoracoscopic splanchnicectomy, can provide a higher efficacy of pain management, prevent deterioration in the patient's quality of life, and lengthen their overall survival.

Keywords: Splanchnicectomy, Pancreatic cancer, Pain

* Correspondence: lukaszdobosz@gumed.edu.pl
Department of General, Endocrine and Transplant Surgery, Medical University of Gdansk, ul. Smoluchowskiego 17, 80-214 Gdansk, Poland

Background

Difficulties in the treatment of pancreatic cancer are frequently connected to the fact that the diagnosis is often made in the late stages of the disease. Total resection of the lesion is the treatment of choice, but is possible only in less than 20 % of cases [1]. The course of the disease in pancreatic cancer is extremely dramatic, with only 16 % of patients still alive 1 year after diagnosis. The average 5-year survival rate in patients with pancreatic cancer drastically decreases to a mere 5 % [2, 3]. Patients often suffer from intense chronic pain which leaves them severely debilitated, leading to a significant deterioration in their quality of life [4].

One of the available methods for the treatment of pain associated with pancreatic cancer, is thoracoscopic splanchnicectomy. It has been proven that splanchnicectomy is a safe procedure, with only a small amount of complications [5, 6], nevertheless, it is often used as a last resort in pain management, which can significantly decrease its effectiveness [7]. In a review of the current literature, there are many trials evaluating the safety and efficacy of splanchnicectomy in both patients with chronic pancreatitis and late-stage pancreatic cancer; however, there are no similar randomized trials about the effectiveness of this treatment in the early stages of pancreatic cancer, for patients with little to no complaints of pain.

Hypothesis

The use of invasive treatment, such as thoracoscopic splanchnicectomy, as part of the first step of the analgesic ladder, can lead to long-lasting protection against the presence and severity of pain, help maintain a satisfactory quality of life despite disease progression, or may even extend the patient's total survival time due to a reduction in the use and thus decrease in the adverse side effects of analgesic pharmacotherapy, such as the immunosuppressive effect of opioids and common postprandial ailments leading to decreased nutrient intake.

Methods and design

Trial design

This trial is a prospective, open label, 1:1 randomized, controlled trial, conducted at a single institution. The aim of this study is to determine the effectiveness of invasive treatment of pain via splanchnicectomy, in patients with advanced pancreatic cancer. Assessments will

not only include the usage of analgesic pharmacotherapy throughout the course of disease, and overall patient survival, but also subjective pain perception at rest, in movement, and after meals (measured by NRS score questionnaire), the patient's quality of life (measured using the QLQ-C30 and FACIT questionnaires) [8, 9], and any pain-related suffering (measured with the PRISM projection test) [10, 11]. In addition, we intend to ascertain if earlier qualification for splanchnicectomy (upon lower steps of the WHO analgesic ladder) allows for a better therapeutic effect with this type of pain management.

A flow diagram of the trial is depicted in Fig. 1.

Ethics and permissions

The final protocol was approved by the independent ethics committee of the Medical University of Gdansk (approval number NKBBN/216/2014). Informed consent will be obtained from the patient in both oral and written form prior to inclusion in the clinical trial.

Patient evaluation and selection

Patients of both sexes with unresectable pancreatic cancer (determined upon intraoperative findings of local lesions or distant metastases, radiological advancement, or recurrence of local lesion and/or distant metastases) will be considered for inclusion in the study. All tumors of the pancreas will be confirmed histologically. Patients after prior surgical treatment of pancreatic cancer with radical intent will also be allowed to join the study. Patients will be enrolled in the study despite their incidence of pain symptoms and/or the intensity of pain therapy used, according to the WHO analgesic ladder steps 1, 2, or 3.

In Poland, according to the National Cancer Registry, about 3,000 patients are diagnosed with pancreatic cancer each year. In our Clinic, we treat about 50 patients per year with this type of carcinoma. We assume that a time period of 24 months will be sufficient enough to enroll a statistically significant group of patients in our trial.

Inclusion criteria

- Patients with diagnosed pancreatic cancer: both non-operative tumor (intraoperative statement of organ and/or vessel infiltration, with local or distant

Table 1 Plan of proceedings

Group	Initial visit: NRS, QLQ-C30, FACIT, PRISM	Surgery	The measurement of pain intensity: 0 day after surgery	The measurement of pain intensity: 1 day after surgery	Follow up (every 2 weeks): NRS, QLQ-C30, FACIT, PRISM	Patient survival
Splanchnicectomy	+	+	+	+	+	+
NIPC	+			+	+	+

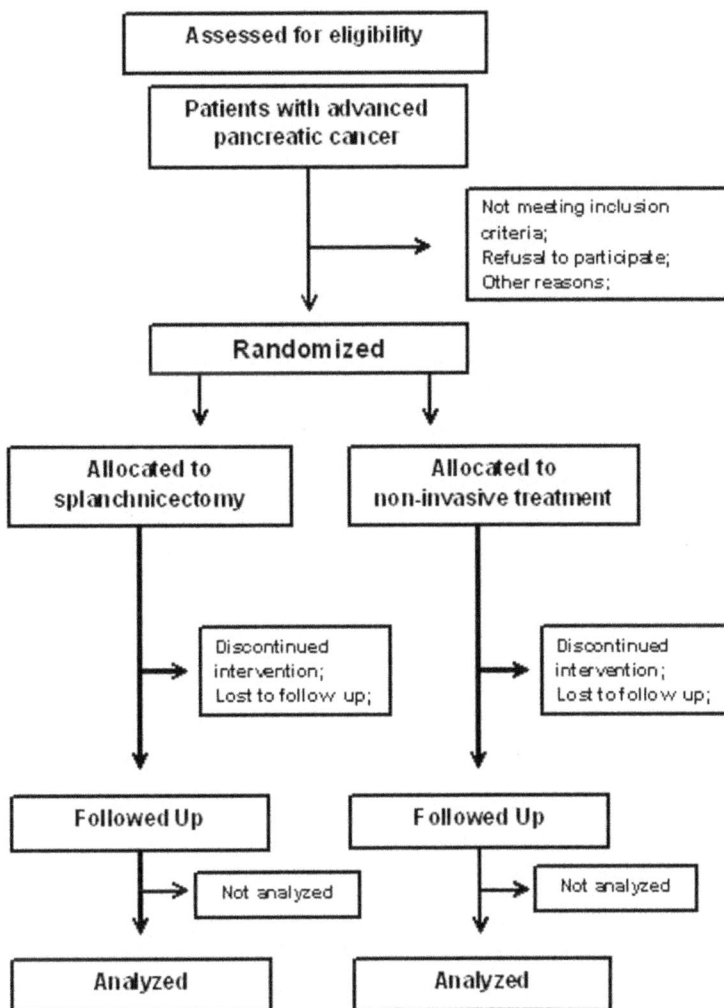

Fig. 1 Flow diagram

metastases, radiological statement of progression, or local recurrence of tumor and/or distant metastases) and/or after prior surgical treatment.

- Age over 18 years.
- Signed informed consent to participate in the study.

Exclusion criteria

- Age under 18 years.
- Intellectual inadequacy to complete necessary questionnaires.
- Coexistence of a disease or disease state in which there is significant chronic pain, which has been identified before the onset of pancreatic cancer.

Setting

The setting of the study is the Department of General, Endocrine and Transplantation Surgery within the Medical University of Gdansk, Poland.

Study design
Registration and randomization procedure

Prior to participation in the trial, patients determined as potential candidates will be informed about the purpose of the study and its implementation. In addition, each person will receive detailed information about the trial in writing. Patients will be allowed to review the methodology of the project and discuss any possible questions with their doctor, before they decide to take part in the trial. During their initial visit at the Clinic, participants will again go over the principles of the study. Upon agreement of both the doctor and patient for inclusion in the clinical trial, the patient must then state their intent to enroll in the study, both verbally and with a written consent form. If the patient is currently taking any analgesic pharmacotherapy, a grade according to the WHO analgesic ladder will be assigned to them [12]. Patients will then be randomly assigned to one of two groups. 1:1 Randomization will be generated for all strata by computer (Urbaniak, G. C., & Plous, S. (2013). Research Randomizer (Version 4.0) [Computer software]. Retrieved on June 22, 2013, from http://www.randomizer.org/). The first group will be offered the invasive treatment of pain with splanchnicectomy through a thoracoscopic approach, while the second group will be offered non-invasive conservative treatment, with the most appropriate available non-invasive pain control (NIPC). At each stage of the clinical trial, patients will be able to convert from the non-invasive intervention group to that of the group with invasive treatment (splanchnicectomy). However, these patients will then be excluded from participation in the clinical trial.

Interventions
Surgical treatment
Each patient in the invasive intervention group will undergo a thoracoscopic splanchnicectomy. Prior to surgery, all electrolyte disturbances and fluid balance are corrected. A 1000 mg dose of Cefazolin is given as a single dose, thirty minutes prior to surgical incision as antibiotic prophylaxis. The surgery is performed under general anesthesia with endotracheal ventilation. The patient is placed in the flank thoracotomy position, with the initial procedure done on the patient's left side. The skin and subcutaneous tissue is anesthetized locally with the injection of 0.5 % Bupivacine and then, by the use of two 5 mm ports, access to the left pleural cavity is obtained after lung collapse. Block of T6, T7, and T8 intercostal nerves is performed. The pleural cavity is insufflated with carbon dioxide and maintained at 8 mmHg throughout the procedure. The greater splanchnic nerve is identified at its origin in the sympathetic trunk, then isolated along with its lateral branches to the level of diaphragm and resected. Additional splanchnic nerves may be incised or excised if they are found connected to the greater splanchnic nerve. A pleural drain is inserted for a short period of time during desufflation, and is then removed. The incision points of the ports are closed with single sutures placed on the skin. The same procedure is performed on the patient's right side. There is no histopathological examination of the excised tissue. Patients are given routine postoperative pain management. The procedure is recorded for future assessment. Patients are allowed to leave the hospital and return home on the first postoperative day.

Bilateral thoracoscopic splanchnicectomy has been shown to be a safe and effective procedure with a minimal mortality rate. It ensures precise visualisation of the splachnic nerves endoscopically without the need for a thoracotomy, which minimises blood loss during the procedure. Among the complications that can occur after this procedure, intercostal neuralgia is the most common, and occurs in about 25 % of cases. Less than 2 % of patients can suffer from other complications such as pulmonary atelectasis, chylothorax and orthostatic hypotension.

Conservative treatment
Patients in the non-invasive, conservative treatment group are treated with the most appropriate available non-invasive pain control (NIPC). The therapy is conducted according to WHO and IASP (International Association for Study of Pain) guidelines. Pharmacotherapy is administered in accordance with the WHO analgesic ladder. The first step medications include non-opioid analgesics: paracetamol, ibuprofen, diclofenac, indometacine, and naproxen. In the second step, drugs from first step are still used, along with mild opioids such as codeine, and tramadol. Finally, the third step includes drugs from second step as well as strong opioids: morphine, fentanyl, oxycodon, and pethidine. Oral or percutaneous administration is the preferred route of administration as opposed to intravenous, subcutaneous or intramuscular administration. The analgesics are given in time-contingent basis. The patient is transferred to next step of the pain management ladder if their pain is stronger than a 6 in the NRS scale and/or if it continues for more than 5 days.

Follow-up
Measurements of pain score (collected using the NRS - Numeric Rating Scale and the BPI - Brief Pain Inventory [13]) will be obtained upon the patient's initial visit to the clinic and for the first group of patients (invasive treatment), prior to surgery, during the early postoperative period and on the first day after surgery, both in the primary location of pain (upper abdomen, epigastrium) and in the incision sites of the trocars.

After the initiation of treatment for both the invasive and non-invasive groups, the severity of pain will be measured in each group at two-week intervals during the patient's follow-up visits in the clinic, or at the patient's home, if there constitutes a physical or organization impediment to the patient's abilities to participate in follow-up care. These visits will continue indefinitely, or until the patient's death. All the measurement points are shown in Table 1.

End points
Primary end points

- Pain intensity (NRS score questionnaire).

Secondary end points

- Pain impact on quality of life (QLQ-C30 and FACIT questionnaire).

- Perception of the illness, suffering (PRISM questionnaire).
- Total need of analgesics.
- Total lifespan, overall survival time.
- The effectiveness of splanchnicectomy performed on early stages of pancreatic cancer.
- Postoperative complications.

Sample size calculation (power of the study)

Analyzing the power of the study, we estimate that a test group of 26 participants in each arm of the trial will be required to be able to evaluate the level of pain relief and its impact on quality of life. To evaluate the influence on the patients' rate of overall survive, a sample size of 105 patients is necessary, in each trial arm.

Statistical analysis

Continuous data will be presented as the mean ± standard deviation and the range. Continuous variables will be compared between the two groups using an unpaired-sample student t test and Mann–Whitney test. Parametric variables will be analyzed using ANOVA and non-parametric variables will be analyzed with chi-square test. Statistical analysis will be performed using Statistica 11 PL licensed to the Medical University of Gdansk, in Poland. Results will be considered statistically significant for $p < 0.05$. An interim analysis will be performed after 52 patients have been randomized and treated.

Discussion

Pancreatic cancer is a malignant neoplasm with a high mortality rate, often associated with a delayed diagnosis, the early occurrence of metastasis and an overall, poor response to chemotherapy and radiotherapy [2, 14]. A majority of patients are diagnosed with pancreatic cancer already in the advanced stages, where tumor resection is not a possible method of treatment. The average survival in unresectable tumors is currently 5.8 months and for those patients with resectable lesions, the average survival extends to about 12–15.9 months from the time of initial diagnosis [14].

Pancreatic cancer is a disease associated with severe chronic pain that leads to a dramatic worsening of the patient's quality of life [15]. Upon initial diagnosis, already 75 % of patients admit to experiencing pain, and during the further progression of the disease, that percentage grows to over 90 % of patients with pancreatic cancer [16]. It has been established that a patient's perception of pain intensity correlates with their overall survival, thus proving that pain management can be a remarkable challenge and demands an interdisciplinary approach [17]. The origin of pain caused by pancreatic cancer can be somatic, visceral or neuropathic. It can be induced by damage to healthy tissues mediated by the cancer cells, or due to the organism's inflammatory response to the disease, even obstruction of the pancreatic duct, or by infiltration of the neoplasm into the surrounding tissues, especially that of the nerves and ganglia. Splanchnic pain impulses are transmitted by the sympathetic nerves to the splanchnic plexus and the sympathetic ganglions (Th12-L2). These nerve impulses are conveyed to the posterior cornua (T5-T12), and then continue their conduction to specific pain perception areas in the central nervous system [18].

The main basis for the treatment of chronic pain in pancreatic cancer is the WHO analgesic ladder, which is divided into three stages of intensity, depending on the pharmacotherapy used by the patient [12]. The medications used in the first step include non-opioid analgesics: paracetamol, ibuprofen, diclofenac, indometacine, and naproxen. In the second step, drugs from first step are still used, along with mild opioids such as codeine, and tramadol. Finally, the third step includes drugs from second step as well as strong opioids: morphine, fentanyl, oxycodon, and pethidine. However, it has been established that conservative treatment with analgesics, in many cases, does not allow for adequate analgesia. In addition, is often associated not only with tolerance, but also with the emergence of numerous adverse events such as pruritus, constipation, drowsiness, and impaired social interactions [18, 19]. Experimental data has demonstrated the superiority of pain prevention (preemptive analgesia) rather than that of reactive treatment of pain, due to the fact that prolonged activation of nociceptive pathways can lead to an activity-dependent plasticity, resulting in an increased response to the stimuli of pain and thus, the ineffectiveness of treatment [20, 21].

The fourth stage of the analgesic ladder proposes surgical treatment for the management of pain. It is possible to interrupt the conduction of pain impulses along the pain tract at the level of the celiac plexus (celiac plexus block) or splanchnic nerves (splanchnicectomy) [16].

However, present surgical methods such as celiac plexus block or thoracoscopic splanchnicectomy are considered to be reserved only for cases refractory to pharmacological analgesic treatment up to the third level of the analgesic ladder [22]. It has been demonstrated in the literature, that thoracoscopic splanchnicectomy is associated with a similar morbidity and mortality rate as performing a celiac plexus block. Splanchnicectomy has also been correlated with a longer-lasting analgesic effect, leading to a successful reduction in pain sensation and thus improvement of the patient's quality of life, both in patients with chronic pancreatitis and those with pancreatic cancer [23–26]. Moreover, it appears that undergoing splanchnicectomy before the onset of pain, can in turn, offer a higher efficacy of future pain management therapies and even prolong a patient's overall survival [7]. Therefore, it should be strongly emphasized that earlier implementation of thoracoscopic splanchnicectomy requires further thorough investigation as a modality for initial pain management.

Abbreviations

NIPC: most appropriate available, Non-Invasive Pain Control; NRS: Numeric Rating Scale.

Competing interests

The authors declare that they have no competing interests.

Authors' contributions

All authors have made substantial contributions to the conception and design of this study. DŁ, ST, DM, WJ, FP, PD, ZK have been involved in drafting the manuscript or revising it critically for important intellectual content. DŁ, ST, KP have made contributions to the design of this study. All authors read and approved the final manuscript.

References

1. Bilimoria KY, Bentrem DJ, Ko CY, Ritchey J, Stewart AK, Winchester DP, Talamonti MS. Validation of the 6th edition AJCC pancreatic cancer staging system. Cancer. 2007;110(4):738–44.
2. Siegel R, Ma J, Zou Z, Jemal A. Cancer statistics 2014. CA Cancer J Clin. 2014;64(1):9–29.
3. Nienhuijs SW, van den Akker SA, de Vries E, de Hingh IH, Visser O, Lemmens VE. Nationwide improvement of only short-term survival after resection for pancreatic cancer in the Netherlands. Pancreas. 2012;41(7):1063–6.
4. Müller-Nordhorn J, Roll S, Böhmig M, Nocon M, Reich A, Braun C, Noesselt L, Wiedenmann B, Willich SN, Brüggenjürgen B. Health-related quality of life in patients with pancreatic cancer. Digestion. 2006;74(2):118–25.
5. Smigielski J, Piskorz L, Wawrzycki M, Kutwin L, Misiak P, Brocki M. Assessment of quality of life in patients with non-operated pancreatic cancer after videothoracoscopic splanchnicectomy. Videosurgery and other miniinvasive techniques. 2011;6(3):132–7.
6. Baghdadi S, Abbas MH, Albouz F, Ammori BJ. Systematic review of the role of thoracoscopic splanchnicectomy in palliating the pain of patients with chronic pancreatitis. Surg Endosc. 2008;22(3):580–8.
7. Johnson CD, Berry DP, Harris S, Pickering RM, Davis C, George S, Imrie CW, Neoptolemos JP, Sutton R. An open randomized comparison of clinical effectiveness of protocol-driven opioid analgesia, celiac plexus block or thoracoscopic splanchnicectomy for pain management in patients with pancreatic and other abdominal malignancies. Pancreatology. 2009;9(6):755–63.
8. Smith AB, Cocks K, Taylor M, Parry D. Most domains of the european organisation for research and treatment of cancer quality of life questionnaire C30 are reliable. J Clin Epidemiol. 2014;67(8):952–7.
9. Webster K, Cella D, Yost K. The Functional Assessment of Chronic Illness Therapy (FACIT) Measurement System: properties, applications, and interpretation. Health Qual Life Outcomes. 2003;1:79.
10. Klis S, Vingerhoets AJ, de Wit M, Zandbelt N, Snoek FJ. Pictorial Representation of Illness and Self Measure Revised II (PRISM-RII) – a novel method to assess perceived burden of illness in diabetes patients. Health Qual Life Outcomes. 2008;6:104.
11. Krikorian A, Limonero JT, Vargas JJ, Palacio C. Assessing suffering in advanced cancer patients using Pictorial Representation of Illness and Self-Measure (PRISM), preliminary validation of the Spanish version in a Latin American population. Support Care Cancer. 2013;21(12):3327–36.
12. World Health Organization. Cancer pain relief: with a guide to opioid availability. 2nd ed. Geneva: Switzerland, WHO; 1996.
13. Atkinson TM, Halabi S, Bennett AV, Rogak L, Sit L, Li Y, Kaplan E, Basch E. Cancer and leukemia group B. Measurement of affective and activity pain interference using the brief pain inventory (BPI): cancer and leukemia group B 70903. Pain Med. 2012;13(11):1417–24.
14. Shoup M, Conlon KC, Klimstra D, Brennan MF. Is extended resection for adenocarcinoma of the body and tail of the pancreas justified? J Gastrointest Surg. 2003;7:946–52.
15. Stefaniak T, Basinski A, Vingerhoets A, Makarewicz W, Connor S, Kaska L, Stanek A, Kwiecinska B, Lachinski AJ, Sledzinski Z. A comparison of two invasive techniques in the management of intractable pain due to inoperable pancreatic cancer: neurolytic celiac plexus block and videothoracoscopic splanchnicectomy. Eur J Surg Oncol. 2005;31:768–73.
16. Yan BM, Myers RP. Neurolytic celiac plexus block for pain control in unresectable pancreatic cancer. Am J Gastroenterol. 2007;102:430–8.
17. Wong GY, Schroeder DR, Carns PE, Wilson JL, Martin DP, Kinney MO, Mantilla CB, Warner DO. Effect of neurolytic celiac plexus block on pain relief, quality of life, and survival in patients with unresectable pancreatic cancer. A randomized controlled trial. JAMA. 2004;291(9):1092–9.
18. Lebovits AH, Lefkowitz M. Pain management of pancreatic carcinoma: a review. Pain. 1989;36.1–11.
19. Vargas-Schaffer G. Is the WHO analgesic ladder still valid? Twenty-four years of experience. Can Fam Physician. 2010;56(6):514–7. e202–5.
20. Woolf CJ, Salter MW. Neuronal plasticity: increasing the gain in pain. Science. 2000;288(5472):1765–9.
21. Dahl JB, Møiniche S. Pre-emptive analgesia. Br Med Bull. 2004;71:13–27.
22. Zhong W, Yu Z, Zeng JX, Lin Y, Yu T, Min XH, Yuan YH, Chen QK. Celiac plexus block for treatment of pain associated with pancreatic cancer: a meta-analysis. Pain Pract. 2014;14(1):43–51.
23. Basinski A, Stefaniak T, Vingerhoets A, Makarewicz W, Kaska L, Stanek A, Lachinski AJ, Sledzinski Z. Effect of NCPB and VSPL on pain and quality of life in chronic pancreatitis patients. World J Gastroenterol. 2005;11(32):5010–4.
24. Buscher HC, Jansen JB, van Dongen R, Bleichrodt RP, van Goor H. Long-term results of bilateral thoracoscopic splanchnicectomy in patients with chronic pancreatitis. Br J Surg. 2002;89(2):158–62.
25. Tomulescu V, Grigoroiu M, Stǎnescu C, Kosa A, Merlusca G, Vasilescu C, Ionescu M, Popescu I. Thoracoscopic splanchnicectomy - a method of pain palliation in non-resectable pancreatic cancer and chronic pancreatitis. Chirurgia (Bucur). 2005;100(6):535–40.
26. Lică I, Jinescu G, Pavelescu C, Beuran M. Thoracoscopic left splanchnicectomy - role in pain control in unresectable pancreatic cancer. Initial experience. Chirurgia (Bucur). 2014;109(3):313–7.

18

Neoadjuvant chemotherapy versus surgery first for resectable pancreatic cancer (Norwegian Pancreatic Cancer Trial - 1 (NorPACT-1)) – study protocol for a national multicentre randomized controlled trial

Knut Jørgen Labori[1*], Kristoffer Lassen[1], Dag Hoem[2], Jon Erik Grønbech[3,4], Jon Arne Søreide[5,6], Kim Mortensen[7], Rune Smaaland[8], Halfdan Sorbye[9,10], Caroline Verbeke[11,12] and Svein Dueland[13]

Abstract

Background: Pancreatic cancer is the fourth leading cause of cancer-related death. While surgical resection remains the foundation for potentially curative treatment, survival benefit is achieved with adjuvant oncological treatment. Thus, completion of multimodality treatment (surgical resection and (neo)adjuvant chemotherapy) to all patients and early treatment of micrometastatic disease is the ideal goal. NorPACT–1 aims to test the hypothesis that overall mortality at one year after allocation of treatment can be reduced with neoadjuvant chemotherapy in surgically treated patients with resectable pancreatic cancer.

Methods/Design: The NorPACT– 1 is a multicentre, randomized controlled phase III trial organized by the Norwegian Gastrointestinal Cancer Group for Hepato-Pancreato-Biliary cancer. Patients with resectable adenocarcinoma of the pancreatic head are randomized to receive either surgery first (Group 1: SF/control) or neoadjuvant chemotherapy (Group 2: NT/intervention) with four cycles FOLFIRINOX followed by resection. Both groups receive adjuvant chemotherapy with gemcitabine and capecitabine (six cycles in Group 1, four cycles in Group 2). In total 90 patients will be randomized in all the five Norwegian university hospitals performing pancreatic surgery. Primary endpoint is overall mortality at one year following commencement of treatment for those who ultimately undergo resection. Secondary endpoints are overall survival after date of randomization (intention to treat), overall survival after resection, disease-free survival, histopathological response, complication rates after surgery, feasibility of neoadjuvant and adjuvant chemotherapy, completion rates of all parts of multimodal treatment, and quality-of-life. Bolt-on to the study is a translational research program that aims at identifying factors that are predictive of response to NT, the risk of distant cancer spread, and patient outcome.

Discussion: NorPACT– 1 is designed to investigate the additional benefit of NT compared to standard treatment only (surgery + adjuvant chemotherapy) for resectable cancer of the pancreatic head to decrease early mortality (within one year) in resected patients.

Keywords: Resectable pancreatic cancer, Neoadjuvant chemotherapy, Overall survival

* Correspondence: uxknab@ous-hf.no
[1]Department of Hepato-Pancreato-Biliary Surgery, Oslo University Hospital, Oslo, Norway
Full list of author information is available at the end of the article

Background

Pancreatic cancer is the fourth leading cause of cancer-related death in Europe and the United States [1, 2]. Surgical resection remains the only potentially curative treatment. However, the median survival of patients undergoing pancreatic resection alone is 16–23 months, with a 5-year overall survival between 10 and 20% [3–6]. Adjuvant chemotherapy improves the median and 5-year overall survival [4, 7]. Thus, completion of multimodality treatment is the ideal goal and standard of care for treatment of pancreatic ductal adenocarcinoma (PDAC). It is well known that initiation and completion of adjuvant chemotherapy can be precluded by perioperative complications [6, 8, 9]. Complications following pancreatoduodenectomy are encountered in 40–50% of patients, with a perioperative mortality rate of 2–4% [10–12]. The technical complexity of the operation and the frailty and co-morbidity of the patient population contribute to the high rate of complications. A significant proportion of patients undergoing pancreatectomy for PDAC develops recurrent disease within 2 years after surgery, and about 20% of the patients have early disease progression within six months after resection [6, 13]. Likely, patients with early distant recurrence had occult metastasis at the time of operation, and may thus have been inadequately selected for surgery. However, useful clinical criteria for accurate prediction of patients suspectable to suffer an early distant or loco-regional recurrence are not available.

Currently, the surgery-first (SF) strategy is the most universally accepted approach (and the standard of care in Norway) to the treatment of resectable PDAC. Still, the optimal sequence of surgery and chemotherapy remains unclear [14, 15]. In three European well-designed randomized controlled trials that accrued patients with good performance status and following stringent tumour biology criteria (such as low CA 19–9 levels), the initiation rate of adjuvant therapy was 83–90% [4, 5, 7]. However, only 50–62% completed multimodal treatment in these highly selected patients. Given the significant survival benefit of adjuvant chemotherapy, the completion rates reported in the literature remain too low. Some centres advocate neoadjuvant chemotherapy (NT) as an alternative to the SF approach [16, 17]. Proponents of the NT strategy suggest that the negative impact of early cancer progression and postoperative complications upon completion of multimodality treatment is reduced by delivery of NT prior to pancreatoduodenectomy [8]. However, the scheduled resection has to be cancelled in up to 20% of patients receiving NT due to early metastases, reduced performance-status or comorbidities during NT, but very rarely due to local tumour progression alone [17]. Chemotherapy employed upfront (before surgery) in patients with resectable pancreatic cancer could potentially increase the proportion of patients who eventually received both treatment modalities, and thus, may benefit from a combined effect.

To date, there are no prospective data proving the superiority of one sequence strategy over the other. Recent studies have shown promising results using NT with FOLFIRINOX for locally advanced and borderline resectable pancreatic cancer, and for the palliative treatment of metastatic pancreatic cancer [18, 19]. Available data on early distant recurrence after pancreatoduodenectomy or during NT support the concept of pancreatic cancer as a systemic disease, even in early-stage settings [20]. Currently, by comparing multi-agent regimens to single-agent approaches efforts are made to bring systemic therapy upfront to study the effect of aggressive chemotherapy regimens in well-designed clinical trials. To circumvent patient selection bias, only a randomized comparison can objectively show benefit of one strategy over the other. The purpose of this study is to further investigate the benefit of adding NT in comparison to standard treatment only for resectable cancer of the pancreatic head (surgery followed by adjuvant chemotherapy).

Methods/Design
Design

The Norwegian Pancreatic Cancer Trial (NorPACT) - 1 is a multicentre, randomized controlled phase III trial organized by the Norwegian Gastrointestinal Cancer Group (NGICG) for Hepato-Pancreato-Biliary (HPB) cancer. Eligible patients are randomized in non-equal groups (3:2) to either receive NT followed by resection or standard treatment ((pancreatoduodenectomy) followed by adjuvant chemotherapy) (Fig. 1). The aim of this study is to evaluate the additional benefit of NT to the standard treatment (surgery + adjuvant chemotherapy) to decrease early mortality (within one year) in resected patients with resectable cancer of the pancreatic head.

Primary end points:

☐ overall mortality at one year following commencement of treatment (NT or SF) for those patients who undergo resection (i.e. only resected patients are included in the analysis)

Secondary end points:

☐ overall survival after date of randomization (intention to treat)
☐ overall survival following resection
☐ overall survival after 3 and 5 years
☐ disease-free survival
☐ histopathological tumour stage ((y)pTN), R0 rate, grade of tumour regression

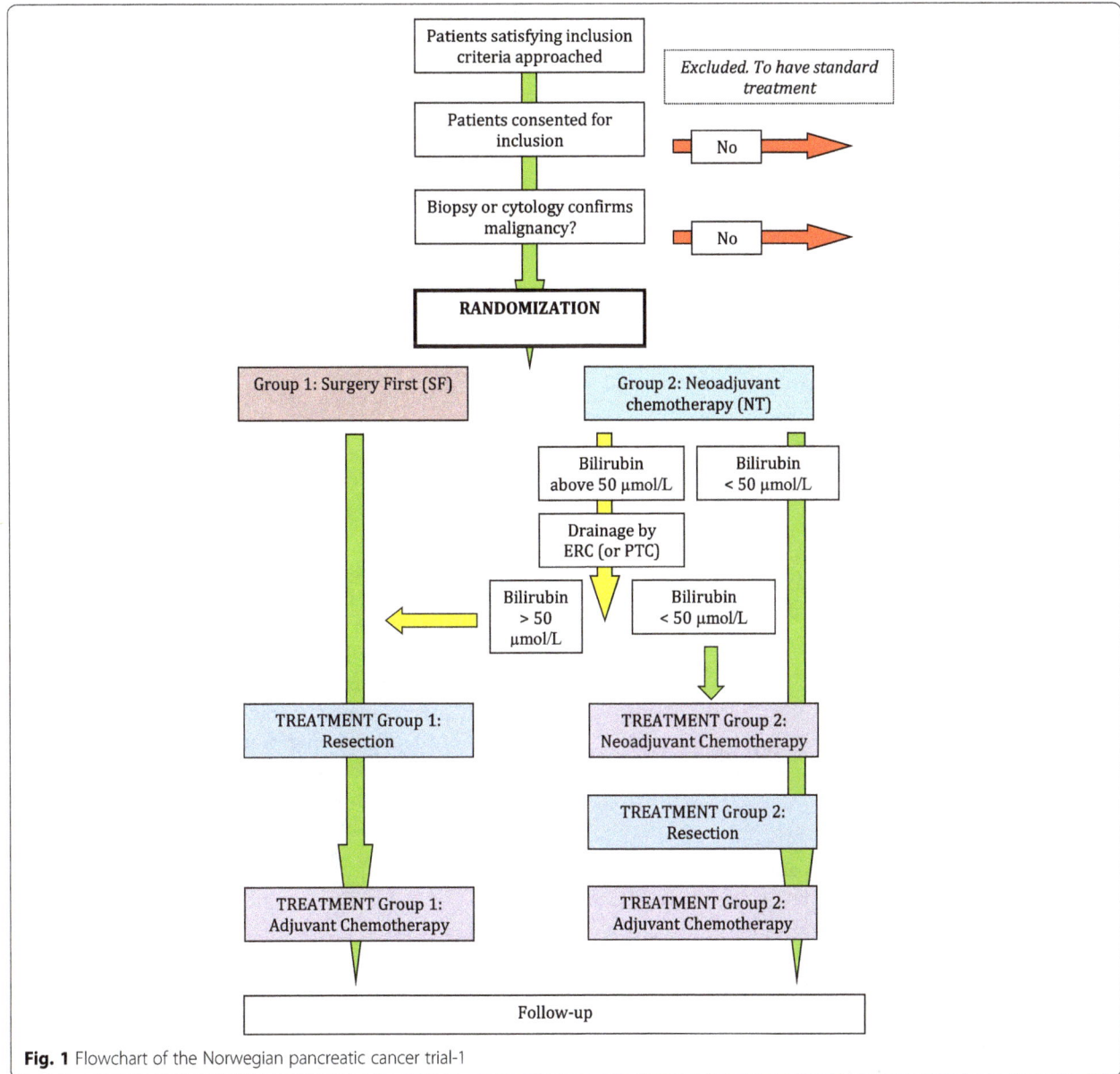

Fig. 1 Flowchart of the Norwegian pancreatic cancer trial-1

☐ complication rates after surgery (30 and 90 days, Dindo-Clavien and International Study Group of Pancreatic Surgery (ISGPS) classification systems) [21–25]
☐ feasibility of neoadjuvant and adjuvant chemotherapy (Common Terminology Criteria for Adverse Events, grade 3–5, dose reduction, dose delay)
☐ completion rates of all parts of multimodal treatment
☐ quality of life (EORTC QLQ-30)
☐ performance status (ECOG) compared to baseline values
☐ exploratory translational research

Study population

Patients meeting the National Comprehensive Cancer Network criteria for resectable pancreatic adenocarcinoma in the pancreatic head are eligible [14]. This implies: 1) no tumour contact with the superior mesenteric vein or portal vein or ≤180 ° contact without vein contour irregularity, 2) no arterial tumour contact (coeliac axis, common hepatic artery or superior mesenteric artery), 3) no distant metastasis.

Inclusion criteria (all of the following):

☐ resectable ductal adenocarcinoma of the pancreatic head

☐ T1–3, Nx, M0 (UICC 7th edition, 2010)
☐ cytological or histological confirmation or strong suspicion of adenocarcinoma
☐ age > 18 year and considered fit for major surgery
☐ written informed consent
☐ considered able to receive the study-specific chemotherapy

Exclusion criteria (one or more of the following):

☐ co-morbidity precluding pancreatoduodenectomy
☐ histological type other than ductal adenocarcinoma
☐ chronic neuropathy ≥ grade 2
☐ World Health Organization performance score > 2
☐ granulocyte count <1500 per cubic millimetre
☐ platelet count <100,000 per cubic millimetre
☐ serum creatinine >1.5 UNL (upper limit normal range)
☐ albumin <2.5 g/dl
☐ female patients in child-bearing age not using adequate contraception, pregnant or lactating women
☐ mental or physical disorders that could interfere with treatment or the provision of informed consent
☐ other malignancy within the past 5 years, except curatively treated non-melanomatous skin or non-invasive cervical cancer
☐ percutaneous tumour biopsy
☐ any reason why, in the opinion of the investigator, the patient should not participate

Locations
Surgery for malignancies of the pancreatic head is currently performed only at five university hospitals in Norway. These departments have all agreed to participate in this trial.

Participating centres are: Oslo University Hospital, Haukeland University Hospital (Bergen), Stavanger University Hospital, St. Olav University Hospital (Trondheim), and the University Hospital Northern Norway in Tromsø. Each centre has a main investigator who liaises with the central study board.

Time frame
In Norway, annually 60–70 patients are expected to have primary resectable pancreatic adenocarcinoma in the pancreatic head. Patients will be recruited into the trial between 1st of January 2017 and 31st of December 2019 (36 months).

Randomization
After the patient has given oral and written consent, computer-generated randomization will be performed. Randomization is to either

☐ GROUP 1 (control): Surgery First

☐ GROUP 2 (intervention): Neoadjuvant Chemotherapy

There will be an overweight of Group 2 allocations by a ratio of 3:2 to ensure equal groups at primary endpoint (cfr. below). Randomization is stratified for each centre and will be generated in blocks with unknown and varying size (4–6 patients per block) to ensure that groups are balanced at all centres, irrespective of the final number of patients recruited.

Sample-size calculation
Based on available data, we assume a one-year overall mortality rate of 25% in the SF arm (Group 1) [5, 6, 26]. Based on highly selected patient series, a suggested one-year mortality rate of 5% is estimated in patients who receive NT and eventually a pancreatoduodenectomy (Group 2) [16, 17]. We aim to evaluate if this improvement is achievable in a randomized controlled trial. To show a reduction in one-year mortality rate from 25 to 5% in a two-armed, parallel-group design with alpha (significance level) 0.05 and beta (power) of 0.79, a sample of 34 patients per group is needed.

An estimated one-third of the NT group will not reach resection and thus not be available for evaluation with regard to the primary endpoint. Furthermore, we estimate that two patients per study group will have their scheduled surgery aborted because of unexpected intraoperative findings. To correct for these patients, a 3:2 randomization is designed, with 36 patients randomized to SF (Group 1) and 54 patients to NT (Group 2), yielding a total of 90 patients.

Handling cross-over, drop-outs and exclusion
Post-randomisation exclusion is to be avoided at "all costs". While patients are offered to withdraw without giving any reason, this is not considered very likely as both groups provide standard treatment of today, albeit at reversed sequence for some (Group 2). Patients who for some reason cannot fulfil neoadjuvant chemotherapy (Group 2) but are still considered candidates for resection will be offered resection according to standard criteria. The reasons for this might be:

• Inability to achieve adequate reduction of bilirubin levels by drainage within 4 weeks
• Massive adverse reactions to first cycle chemotherapy

These patients are considered cross-over provided no single cycle was completed, but remain under analysis by intention-to-treat. They are not excluded from the trial. Patients who suffer other incidents post-randomisation but prior to any treatment are still analysed under intention-to-treat.

Treatment

Chemotherapy

Neoadjuvant group (Group 2) Neoadjuvant chemotherapy consists of 4 cycles (2 months) of FOLFIRINOX (oxaliplatin 85 mg/m^2, irinotecan 180 mg/m^2, leucovorin 400 mg/m^2, and 5-fluorouracil (400 mg/m^2 bolus then 2400 mg/m^2 over 46 h)) [18, 19]. Patients who undergo surgical resection will receive adjuvant chemotherapy with 4 cycles (4 months) Gemicitabine 1000 mg/m^2 over 30 min at day 1, 8, 15 of each 28-day cycle and capecitabine 830 mg/m^2 ×2 daily for 3 weeks and one week rest of each 28-day cycle [27]. Adjuvant chemotherapy must be started within 12 weeks after resection [28]. Dose reduction or dose delays are acted upon according to local clinical practice at each centre.

Surgery-first group (Group 1) Following pancreatic resection, all patients receive adjuvant chemotherapy with 6 cycles (6 months) Gemicitabine 1000 mg/m^2 over 30 min at day 1, 8, 15 of each 28-day cycle and capecitabine 830 mg/m^2 ×2 daily for 3 weeks and one week rest of each 28-day cycle [27]. Adjuvant chemotherapy must be started within 12 weeks after resection [28].

Side effects of chemotherapy are graded by the "Common Terminology Criteria for Adverse Events" version 4 https://evs.nci.nih.gov/ftp1/CTCAE/About.html. Grade 3–5 are reported. At each study visit, laboratory parameters are determined for dose adjustments. Dose reduction or dose delays are acted upon according to local clinical practice at each centre.

Surgery

Surgery is scheduled within 4 weeks in the control arm, and also within 4 weeks after the last neoadjuvant infusion in the treatment arm. Resection of the pancreatic head will be performed as a standard or pylorus-preserving pancreatoduodenectomy with standard lymphadenectomy [29]. The reconstruction is done by a retrocolic end-to-side pancreatico-jejunostomy and an end-to-side hepatico-jejunostomy. In addition, an end-to-side duodeno- or gastrojejunostomy is performed on a jejunal alpha-loop. Otherwise, each centre may use its standard perioperative management for pancreatoduodenectomies. Surgical morbidity is assessed by the Dindo/Clavien classification [21, 30]. Pancreatic fistulas, biliary leakages, delayed gastric emptying and postoperative haemorrhage are reported according to the definitions of the ISGPS [22–25].

Pathology examination

The resection specimen will be evaluated according to a detailed standardized pathology examination protocol [31, 32]. At the discretion of the local team, the anterior and posterior surfaces of the pancreas, as well as the superior mesenteric vein groove and surface towards the superior mesenteric artery may be inked by the surgeon according to an agreed colour code. The histopathological response of the tumor to the neoadjuvant treatment will be assessed according to an established tumour regression grading system [33].

Follow-up

Follow-up is based on physical examination, blood samples (hemoglobim, white blood cell count, differential blood count, platelets, creatinin, bilirubin, aspartate aminotransferase, alanine aminotransferase, lactate dehydrogenase, gamma-glutamyl transpeptidase, prothrombin time, albumin, sodium, potassium, CA19–9 and carcinoembryonic antigen) and CT scans of chest and abdomen at 6, 9, 12, 15 months after surgery and every six months thereafter until disease recurrence or, in patients without relapse, at 5-years following surgery. Any newly appearing lesion with histological documentation of cancer defines recurrent disease. Also, any newly appearing lesion(s) suspicious for malignancy without histological documentation but increasing in size upon repeated follow-up exams, especially in the context of progressive symptoms (pain, weight loss) or increasing tumor marker (CA 19–9) levels, are considered recurrent disease, either distant, regionally or in the former surgical bed. The date of recurrence is defined as the date of radiological or histological evidence of relapse. The study ends when the last randomized patient has been followed for 5 years after surgery.

Quality of life

Quality of life will be assessed by the QLQ-30 of the European Organization for Research and Treatment of Cancer at study inclusion, before randomization, before surgery in the neoadjuvant arm, and at 4 weeks after surgery, as well as at any follow-up visit.

Translational research

Blood samples and tumour tissue will be stored to enable further translational research.

Safety

Suspected Unexpected Serious Adverse Reactions will be reported to the Competent Authority and Ethics Committee according to national regulation. The sponsor will ensure that all relevant information about suspected serious unexpected adverse reactions that are fatal or life-threatening is recorded and reported as soon as possible to the Competent Authority and Ethics Committee after knowledge by the sponsor of such a case, and that relevant follow-up information is subsequently communicated. All other suspected serious unexpected adverse reactions will be reported to the Competent Authority concerned and to the Ethics Committee concerned as soon as of first knowledge by the sponsor. A Data Monitoring Committee will be established with specialists in gastroenterological surgery and medical oncology. The study will be closed if 50% or more of the patients randomized to NT do not receive the planned surgery or if the reason for not receiving surgery is reduced performance status or side effects due to neoadjuvant chemotherapy in more than 30% of the randomized patients.

Ethics

The study protocol was approved by the Regional Committee for Medical and Health Research Ethics (2015/610/REK Nord) and The Norwegian Medicines Agency (15/05308–8). Patients must provide written consent before entering the trial. All data will be handled with strict confidentiality, and study reports or presentations will maintain the anonymity of patients.

Discussion

The NorPACT-1 study investigates the benefit of NT to the standard treatment (surgery + adjuvant chemotherapy) for resectable cancer of the pancreatic head as a means of avoiding early mortality (within one year) in resected patients. The study results will show which of the two treatment strategies is superior with respect to survival and quality of life in patients undergoing surgery for resectable pancreatic cancer. Non-randomized data have provided some support for NT, but these observations may be biased by patient selection bias. Hence, only a randomized comparison can objectively show benefit of one strategy over the other. The main rationale for NT in this patient group is twofold. First, upfront chemotherapy enable early treatment of micrometastases. Second, postoperative complications often preclude initiation or completion of adjuvant chemotherapy and thereby annul the benefits of multimodal treatment. By delivering NT prior to surgical resection, the chance of receiving both modalities is increased. Furthermore, NT is likely to result in improved patient selection for surgery, as individuals with rapidly progressive disease under NT can be spared from major surgery, which is unlikely to be beneficial and associated with significant morbidity risk. Systemic therapy in NorPACT-1 is given with chemotherapy combinations that have shown promising results in two recent randomized controlled trials [19, 27]. The multicentre design with participation of the five centres that perform pancreatic surgery in Norway ensures that any eligible patient has the opportunity to participate in the clinical trial at the centre closest to his/her home. Bolt-on to the proposed study is a translational research program that aims at identifying factors that are predictive of response to NT, the risk of distant cancer spread and patient outcome. These potential biomarkers will allow better patient selection for surgery and/or NT.

Abbreviations

CA19–9: Cancer antigen 19–9; CT: Computer tomography; ECOG: Eastern cooperative oncology group; EORTC QLQ: European organization for research and treatment of cancer quality of life questionnaire; FOLFIRINOX: Oxaliplatin, irinotecan, fluorouracil, and leucovorin; ISGPS: International Study Group of Pancreatic Surgery; NGICG-HPB: Norwegian Gastrointestinal Cancer Group for Hepato-Pancreato-Biliary cancer; NorPACT-1: Norwegian Pancreatic Cancer Trial-1; NT: Neoadjuvant chemotherapy; PDAC: Pancreatic ductal adenocarcinoma; SF: Surgery first; TNM: Tumor, node metastasis staging system

Acknowledgements

Not applicable.

Funding

No external funding was received.

Availability of data and materials

Not applicable.

Authors' contributions

KJL, KL and SD drafted the manuscript. DH, JEG, JAS, KM, RS, HS and CV co-authored the writing of the manuscript. KJL, KL and SD designed the study. All authors participated in the final design during several meetings. All authors edited the manuscript and approved the final version of the manuscript.

Competing interests

The authors declare that they have no competing interests.

Author details

[1]Department of Hepato-Pancreato-Biliary Surgery, Oslo University Hospital, Oslo, Norway. [2]Department of Acute and Digestive Surgery, Haukeland University Hospital, Bergen, Norway. [3]Department of Gastrointestinal Surgery, St. Olavs Hospital, Trondheim University Hospital, Trondheim, Norway. [4]Department of Clinical and Molecular Medicine, Norwegian University of Science and Technology, Trondheim, Norway. [5]Department of Gastrointestinal Surgery, Stavanger University Hospital, Stavanger, Norway. [6]Department of Clinical Medicine, University of Bergen, Bergen, Norway. [7]Department of Gastrointestinal and Hepatobiliary Surgery, University Hospital of Northern Norway, Tromsø, Norway. [8]Department of Haematology and Oncology, Stavanger University Hospital, Stavanger, Norway. [9]Department of Oncology, Haukeland University Hospital, Bergen, Norway. [10]Department of Clinical Science, Haukeland University Hospital, University of Bergen, Bergen, Norway. [11]Department of Pathology, Oslo University Hospital, Oslo, Norway. [12]Institute of Clinical Medicine, University of Oslo, Oslo, Norway. [13]Department of Oncology, Oslo University Hospital, Oslo, Norway.

References

1. Malvezzi M, Arfe A, Bertuccio P, Levi F, La VC, Negri E. European cancer mortality predictions for the year 2011. Ann Oncol. 2011;22(4):947–56.
2. Siegel R, Ma J, Zou Z, Jemal A. Cancer statistics, 2014. CA Cancer J Clin. 2014;64(1):9–29.

3. Winter JM, Brennan MF, Tang LH, D'Angelica MI, DeMatteo RP, Fong Y, et al. Survival after resection of pancreatic adenocarcinoma: results from a single institution over three decades. Ann Surg Oncol. 2012;19(1):169–75.

4. Neoptolemos JP, Stocken DD, Friess H, Bassi C, Dunn JA, Hickey H, et al. A randomized trial of chemoradiotherapy and chemotherapy after resection of pancreatic cancer. N Engl J Med. 2004;350(12):1200–10.

5. Neoptolemos JP, Stocken DD, Bassi C, Ghaneh P, Cunningham D, Goldstein D, et al. Adjuvant chemotherapy with fluorouracil plus folinic acid vs gemcitabine following pancreatic cancer resection: a randomized controlled trial. JAMA. 2010;304(10):1073–81.

6. Labori KJ, Katz MH, Tzeng CW, Bjornbeth BA, Cvancarova M, Edwin B, et al. Impact of early disease progression and surgical complications on adjuvant chemotherapy completion rates and survival in patients undergoing the surgery first approach for resectable pancreatic ductal adenocarcinoma - a population-based cohort study. Acta Oncol. 2016;55(3):265–77.

7. Oettle H, Post S, Neuhaus P, Gellert K, Langrehr J, Ridwelski K, et al. Adjuvant chemotherapy with gemcitabine vs observation in patients undergoing curative-intent resection of pancreatic cancer: a randomized controlled trial. JAMA. 2007;297(3):267–77.

8. Tzeng CW, Tran Cao HS, Lee JE, Pisters PW, Varadhachary GR, Wolff RA, et al. Treatment sequencing for resectable pancreatic cancer: influence of early metastases and surgical complications on multimodality therapy completion and survival. J Gastrointest Surg. 2014;18(1):16–25.

9. Merkow RP, Bilimoria KY, Tomlinson JS, Paruch JL, Fleming JB, Talamonti MS, et al. Postoperative complications reduce adjuvant chemotherapy use in resectable pancreatic cancer. Ann Surg. 2014;260(2):372–7.

10. Ziegler KM, Nakeeb A, Pitt HA, Schmidt CM, Bishop SN, Moreno J, et al. Pancreatic surgery: evolution at a high-volume center. Surgery. 2010;148(4):702–9.

11. Winter JM, Cameron JL, Campbell KA, Arnold MA, Chang DC, Coleman J, et al. 1423 pancreaticoduodenectomies for pancreatic cancer: a single-institution experience. J Gastrointest Surg. 2006;10(9):1199–210.

12. Gouma DJ, van Geenen RC, van Gulik TM, de Haan RJ, de Wit LT, Busch OR, et al. Rates of complications and death after pancreaticoduodenectomy: risk factors and the impact of hospital volume. Ann Surg. 2000;232(6):786–95.

13. Groot VP, Rezaee N, Wu W, Cameron JL, Fishman EK, Hruban RH, et al. Patterns, timing, and predictors of recurrence following pancreatectomy for pancreatic ductal adenocarcinoma. Ann Surg. 2017. [Epub ahead of print].

14. National Comprehensive Cancer Network Clinical Practice Guidelines in Oncology: Pancreatic adenocarcinoma v2.2015. 2015. Accessed 31 Dec 2016.

15. Ducreux M, Cuhna AS, Caramella C, Hollebecque A, Burtin P, Goere D, et al. Cancer of the pancreas: ESMO clinical practice guidelines for diagnosis, treatment and follow-up. Ann Oncol. 2015;26(Suppl 5):v56–68.

16. Christians KK, Heimler JW, George B, Ritch PS, Erickson BA, Johnston F, et al. Survival of patients with resectable pancreatic cancer who received neoadjuvant therapy. Surgery. 2016;159(3):893–900.

17. Tzeng CW, Fleming JB, Lee JE, Xiao L, Pisters PW, Vauthey JN, et al. Defined clinical classifications are associated with outcome of patients with anatomically resectable pancreatic adenocarcinoma treated with neoadjuvant therapy. Ann Surg Oncol. 2012;19(6):2045–53.

18. Ferrone CR, Marchegiani G, Hong TS, Ryan DP, Deshpande V, McDonnell EI, et al. Radiological and surgical implications of neoadjuvant treatment with FOLFIRINOX for locally advanced and borderline resectable pancreatic cancer. Ann Surg. 2015;261(1):12–7.

19. Conroy T, Desseigne F, Ychou M, Bouche O, Guimbaud R, Becouarn Y, et al. FOLFIRINOX versus gemcitabine for metastatic pancreatic cancer. N Engl J Med. 2011;364(19):1817–25.

20. Sohal DP, Walsh RM, Ramanathan RK, Khorana AA. Pancreatic adenocarcinoma: treating a systemic disease with systemic therapy. J Natl Cancer Inst. 2014;106(3):dju011.

21. Dindo D, Demartines N, Clavien PA. Classification of surgical complications: a new proposal with evaluation in a cohort of 6336 patients and results of a survey. Ann Surg. 2004;240(2):205–13.

22. Bassi C, Dervenis C, Butturini G, Fingerhut A, Yeo C, Izbicki J, et al. Postoperative pancreatic fistula: an international study group (ISGPF) definition. Surgery. 2005;138(1):8–13.

23. Wente MN, Bassi C, Dervenis C, Fingerhut A, Gouma DJ, Izbicki JR, et al. Delayed gastric emptying (DGE) after pancreatic surgery: a suggested definition by the international study Group of Pancreatic Surgery (ISGPS). Surgery. 2007;142(5):761–8.

24. Wente MN, Veit JA, Bassi C, Dervenis C, Fingerhut A, Gouma DJ, et al. Postpancreatectomy hemorrhage (PPH): an international study Group of Pancreatic Surgery (ISGPS) definition. Surgery. 2007;142(1):20–5.

25. Koch M, Garden OJ, Padbury R, Rahbari NN, Adam R, Capussotti L, et al. Bile leakage after hepatobiliary and pancreatic surgery: a definition and grading of severity by the international study Group of Liver Surgery. Surgery. 2011; 149(5):680–8.

26. Hoem D, Viste A. Improving survival following surgery for pancreatic ductal adenocarcinoma–a ten-year experience. Eur J Surg Oncol. 2012;38(3):245–51.

27. Neoptolemos JP, Palmer DH, Ghaneh P, Psarelli EE, Valle JW, Halloran CM, et al. Comparison of adjuvant gemcitabine and capecitabine with gemcitabine monotherapy in patients with resected pancreatic cancer (ESPAC-4): a multicentre, open-label, randomised, phase 3 trial. Lancet. 2017;389(10073): 1011–24.

28. Valle JW, Palmer D, Jackson R, Cox T, Neoptolemos JP, Ghaneh P, et al. Optimal duration and timing of adjuvant chemotherapy after definitive surgery for ductal adenocarcinoma of the pancreas: ongoing lessons from the ESPAC-3 study. J Clin Oncol. 2014;32(6):504–12.

29. Tol JA, Gouma DJ, Bassi C, Dervenis C, Montorsi M, Adham M, et al. Definition of a standard lymphadenectomy in surgery for pancreatic ductal adenocarcinoma: a consensus statement by the international study group on pancreatic surgery (ISGPS). Surgery. 2014;156(3):591–600.

30. Clavien PA, Barkun J, de Oliveira ML, Vauthey JN, Dindo D, Schulick RD, et al. The Clavien-Dindo classification of surgical complications: five-year experience. Ann Surg. 2009;250(2):187–96.

31. Verbeke CS, Gladhaug IP. Dissection of pancreatic resection specimens. Surg Pathol Clin. 2016;9(4):523–38.

32. Verbeke C, Lohr M, Karlsson JS, Del Chiaro M. Pathology reporting of pancreatic cancer following neoadjuvant therapy: challenges and uncertainties. Cancer Treat Rev. 2015;41(1):17–26.

33. Washington K, Berlin J, Branton P, Burgart LJ, Carter DK, Compton CC, et al.: Protocol for the examination of specimens from patients with carcinoma of the pancreas. 2016. Accessed 30 Apr 2017.

19

Acute pancreatitis after thoracic duct ligation for iatrogenic chylothorax

Benoît Bédat*, Cosimo Riccardo Scarpa, Samira Mercedes Sadowski, Frédéric Triponez and Wolfram Karenovics

Abstract

Background: To report the association between thoracic duct ligation and acute pancreatitis. The association between sudden stop of lymphatic flow and pancreatitis has been established in experimental models.

Case presentation: *A 57-year-old woman operated for thymoma presented a iatrogenic chylothorax. After thoracic duct ligation, she presented an acute pancreatitis which resolved after conservative treatment. The chylothorax disappeared within 4 days of thoracic duct ligation.*

Conclusions: This is the first report of acute pancreatitis following thoracic duct ligation. The pancreas and digestive tract should be assessed in symptomatic patients after thoracic duct ligation.

Keywords: Case report, Thoracic surgery, Thoracic duct ligation, Acute pancreatitis, Iatrogenic chylothorax, Thymoma

Background

Chylothorax is a rare disease defined as a leakage of chyle into the pleural space, and can be classified as traumatic or non traumatic. Esophageal surgery is the major cause of traumatic iatrogenic chylothorax. Other iatrogenic causes include lymph node dissection, lung resection and mediastinal tumor resection [1, 2]. A large leak flow of chyle may cause dehydration, nutrient loss and immunodeficiency. However, there is no consensus in the management of chylothorax. Depending on etiology, duration and flow output, therapy may either be conservative or surgical. Low-output chyle flow (<1000 mL/day) can generally be managed conservatively. Failure of conservative treatment on the other hand, typically in situations of high-output chyle flow (>1000 mL/day), requires intervention, such as thoracic duct ligation. This procedure has a high success rate of up to 95% [3]. Thoracic duct ligation has shown to have a 38% rate of comorbidities linked to procedure, such as atrial fibrillation and need of prolonged ventilation [2]. To our knowledge, there have been no abdominal complications reported or associated with ligation of the thoracic duct. In experimental models, some studies demonstrated that the sudden stop of lymphatic flow may induce intestinal and pancreatic edema with the presence of an inflammatory infiltrate [4, 5].

We report herein the first case of an abdominal complication associated with thoracic duct ligation, such as acute pancreatitis.

Case presentation

A 57-year-old woman with a history of back pain underwent a thoracic CT-scan in 2016 with the incidental discovery of an anterior mediastinal mass. The mass had a size of 4x3cm, was round and was well delimited, compatible with a teratoma or a thymoma. The patient had no symptom or clinical manifestations of myasthenia gravis, with a Quantitative Myasthenic Gravis Score grade 0. A thymomectomy was performed using a right single-port video-assisted thoracoscopic surgery (VATS). A chest drain was left after the procedure. Histopathology confirmed a thymoma, type B1, Masaoka-Koga stage 1. Two days after surgery, the patient developed a high output chylothorax (>1000 mL/day), without any signs of infection or inflammation in the blood tests. We introduced a low-fat diet for 6 days and then she was fasting for two more days. However, the chyle continued to flow with an output of 750 mL/day without other complications. No somatostatin or analog was introduced.

---
* Correspondence: benoit.bedat@hcuge.ch
Thoracic and Endocrine Surgery, University Hospitals of Geneva, 1211 Geneva, Switzerland

A lymphangio-magnetic resonance imaging (MRI) didn't show aberrant thoracic duct anatomy nor chyle-leak (Fig. 1). At day 10, the patient was taken to the operating room for a right VATS. The thoracic duct was visualized and the thoracic duct was clipped just above the diaphragm (Fig. 2). Two days later, the chylothorax reappeared and the patient developed increasing pain in the left hemi-abdomen, with sign of peritonitis and abdominal distention. Her blood test showed absence of leucocytosis, a C-reactive protein (CRP) of 230 mg/L, and normal lipid, electrolytes, hepatic and pancreatic levels (see Additional file 1). A CT-scan demonstrated pancreatic edema and a peri-pancreatic infiltration that extended to the bilateral kidney fasciae, compatible with an acute pancreatitis (Fig. 3). Etiologies of acute pancreatitis such as gallstone migration, alcohol, medications, hypotension during the perioperative period, lipidic and IgG4 disease were excluded (see Additional file 1). There was no hypotension during the perioperative periode. After medical supportive management the abdominal pain resolved within 2 days and CRP decreased. The chylothorax was treated with restricted low-fat diet, resolved 4 days after the thoracic duct ligation, and the chest tube was removed 16 days after the initial thymomectomy. Six months later, the patient is healthy and has had no recurrence of chylothorax.

This case presentation was conducted in accordance with the CARE guidelines and methodology.

Conclusions

The occurrence of chylothorax after thymomectomy is a rare complication and usually associated with extensive

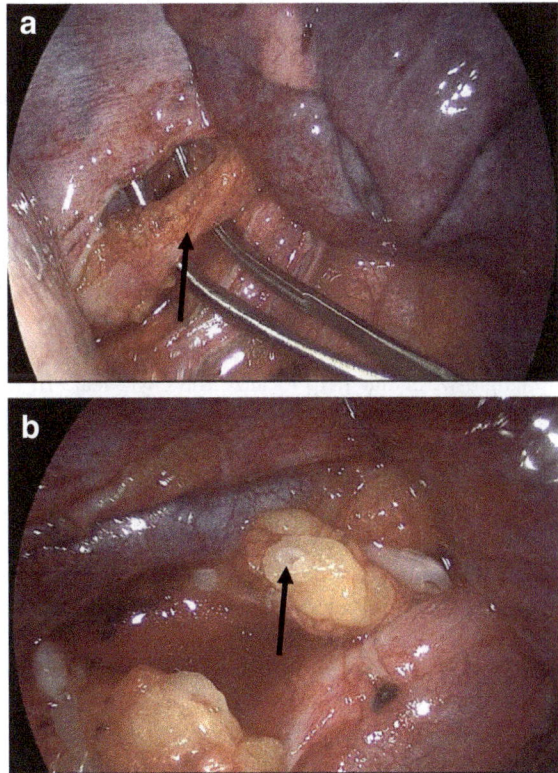

Fig. 2 Dissection (**a**), clipping and section (**b**) of the thoracic duct (black arrow)

dissection [6]. In this case, the resection was localized, without radical thymectomy.

For chyle leak of traumatic iatrogenic etiology, such as mediastinal tumor resection, management is debated and to date no consensus exists. Initial conservative treatment involving chest drainage and a low-fat diet except for the medium-chain triglycerides or fasting with

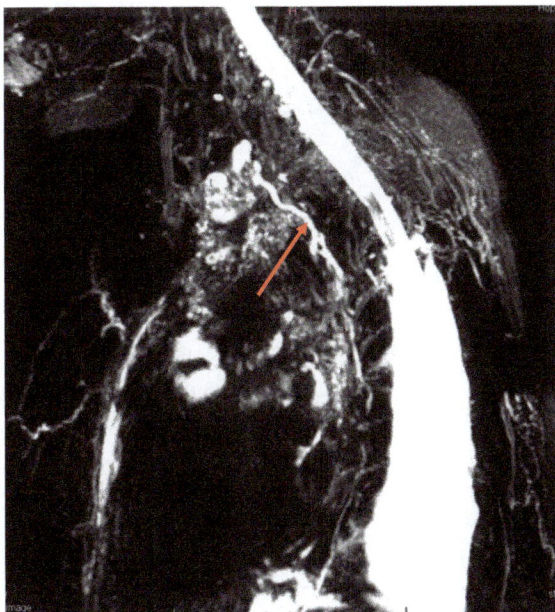

Fig. 1 Axial MRI T2 showing the thoracic duct (red arrow)

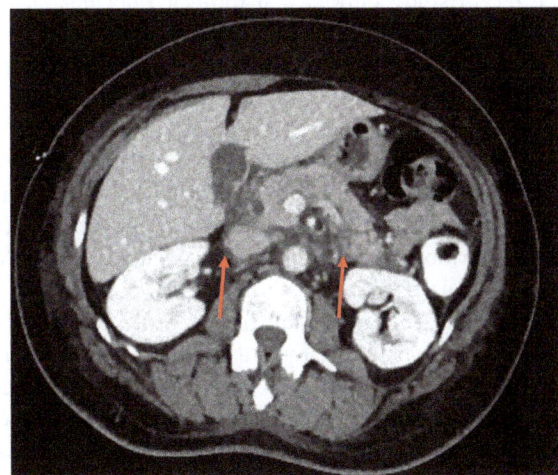

Fig. 3 Arterial phase contrast CT showing an acute pancreatitis with edema around the pancreas (red arrows)

parenteral nutrition has shown excellent outcome. Octreotide or somatostatin therapy can be efficient for the medical approach [7]. However, the level of evidence about the efficacy of these treatments remains low. Furthermore, octreotide is a class II medication associated with acute pancreatitis, and its use should be cautious [8]. For patients who fail conservative management, surgical repair with ligation using VATS is shown to be highly successful and is considered a safe procedure [3]. The difficulty lies in the visualization of the thoracic duct injury during the surgery and its anatomic variations. A lymphangiography, lymphoscintigraphy and lymphangio-MRI may help localize the chyle-leak. In this case, the leak site was not found on lympangio-MRI nor during surgery. An intraoperatively administration of oral cream via a stomach probe can be more easily identify the duct and other accessory lymphatic channels [9]. In this situation, the upstream clipping of the thoracic duct just above the diaphragm appears favorable for better result than a mass ligation of the tissue in the presumed course.

The consequences of sudden disturbed lymph drainage of the abdominal viscera, which constitutes 80% of the lymphatic flow in the thoracic duct, are not known. It is assumed that with time collateral lymphatic vessels overcome the thoracic duct obstruction. Reports in literature show that thoracic duct ligation is safe and has no known associated abdominal or lymphatic complications, except two cases of leg edema associated with thoracic duct embolization [10]. However, the role of mesenteric lymph drainage in acute illness such as pancreatitis, burns and hemorrhagic shock is well established in experimental models [11]. The impact of thoracic duct ligation on the pancreas is known since 1958 by Papp et al. and was more investigated by Müller et al. in 1988 with thoracic duct ligation in rats [4, 12]. Their results demonstrated a long-lasting pancreatic edema. A more recent study showed that thoracic duct ligation in rats with acute hemorrhagic necrotizing pancreatitis reduced lung injury by a decreased neutrophil infiltration and TNF-alpha release, but increased pancreas injury [13]. In the intestine and the pancreas, the myeloperoxidase activity, a marker of neutrophils infiltration, was increased without any change of serum amylase and diamine oxidase level. In another study, lymphatic obstruction in dogs caused an intestinal mucosal atrophy similar to malabsorption syndrome [14].

In our case, common etiologies of acute pancreatitis were excluded, including hypotension and medications. Auto-immune-like pancreatitis was previously described in a patient with myasthenia gravis and autoantibodies [15]. However, our patient had no symptom or clinical manifestations of myasthenia gravis with a Quantitative Myasthenic Gravis Score grade 0. Therefore an immune etiology seemed unlikely. The diagnosis of pancreatitis is only based on the CT-scan. Otherwise, acute pancreatitis with normoamylasemia and lipasemia is not uncommon, and is a known entity [16]. Another explanation could be a pancreatic edema caused by a congestive lymphatic vessels with similar symptoms. The comparison of the experimental studies with our case is clearly limited by their experimental design. However, the impact of a sudden lymphatic obstruction on the pancreas and digestive tract can be easily understood.

The recurrence of chylothorax 2 days after surgery evokes aberrant collateral thoracic duct, which has not been seen on MRI nor during surgery. Probably this duct was small with a low chyle flow that could explain a rapid healing after a conservative treatment and a persistant disturbed lymph drainage of the abdominal viscera with abdominal pain.

In conclusion, this is the first report of a patient developing acute pancreatitis after thoracic duct clipping. Although our knowledge relies on experimental models, edema of the abdominal viscera should be assessed in symptomatic patients with a CT-scan and a pancreatic enzymes analysis.

Abbreviations
CRP: C-reactive protein; MRI: Magnetic resonance imaging; VATS: Video-assisted thoracoscopic surgery

Acknowledgements
Not applicable.

Funding
No funding.

Authors' contributions
BB, CRS and WK designed the report; WK performed the surgery; BB, CRS and SMS collected the data; BB, FT and WK analyzed the data; BB and CRS drafted the article; SMS, FT and WK revised the paper and gave the final approval of the definitive version of the article. All authors read and approved the final manuscript.

Competing interests
The authors declare that they have no competing interests.

References
1. Dougenis D, Walker WS, Cameron EW, Walbaum PR. Management of chylothorax complicating extensive esophageal resection. Surg Gynecol Obstet. 1992;17:501–6.
2. Cerfolio RJ, Allen MS, Deschamps C, Trastek VF, Pairolero PC. Postoperative chylothorax. J Thorac Cardiovasc Surg. 1996;112:1361–5.
3. Paul S, Altorki NK, Port JL, Stiles BM, Lee PC. Surgical management of chylothorax. Thorac Cardiov Surg. 2009;57:226–8.
4. Müller M, Putzke HP, Siegmund E, Dummler W. Significance of disturbed lymph flow for the pathogenesis of pancreatitis. I. Ligature of the ductus thoracicus in the rat. Exp Pathol. 1988;33(2):95–101.
5. Putzke HP, Müller M, Siegmund E, Dummler W. Lymph drainage disorder as a pathogenetic co-factor in acute pancreatitis? Gastroenterol J. 1990;50(3):149–52.
6. Huang CS, Hsu HS, Kao KP, Hsieh CC, Wu YC, Hsu WH, et al. Chylothorax following extended thymectomy for myasthenia gravis. Thorac Cardiovasc Surg. 2007;55(4):274.

7. Ohkura Y, Ueno M, Iizuka T, Haruta S, Tanaka T, Udagawa H. New combined medical treatment with etilefrine and octreotide for chylothorax after esophagectomy: A case report and review of the literature. Medicine (Baltimore). 2015;94:49.

8. Trivedi CD, Pitchumoni CS. Drug-induced pancreatitis : An update. J Clin Gastroenterol. 2005;39:709–16.

9. Shackcloth MJ, Poullis M, Lu J, Page RD. Preventing of chylothorax after oesophagectomy by routine pre-operative administration of oral cream. Eur J Cardiotharac Surg. 2001;20:1035.

10. Itkin M, Kucharczuk JC, Kwak A, Trerotola SO, Kaiser LR. Nonoperative thoracic duct embolization for traumatic thoracic duct leak: Experience in 109 patients. J Thorac Cardiovasc Surg. 2010;139:584–90.

11. Fanous MY, Phillips AJ, Windsor JA. Mesenteric lymph: the bridge to future management of critical illness. JOP. 2007;8(4):374–99.

12. Papp JL, Nemeth E, Feuer I, Fodor I. Effect of an impairment of lymph flow on experimental acute "pancreatitis". Acta Med Acad Sci Hung. 1958;11:203–8.

13. Peng H, Zhi-fen W, Su-mei J, Yun-zhen G, Yan L, Li-ping C. Blocking abdominal lymphatic flow attenuates acute hemorrhagic necrotizing pancreatitis -associated lung injury in rats. J Inflamm. 2013;10:9.

14. Fish JC, McNeel L, Holaday WJ. Lymphatic obstruction in the pathogenesis of intestinal mucosal atrophy. Ann Surg. 1969;169:316–25.

15. Colaut F, Toniolo L, Sperti C, Pozzobon M, Scapinello A, Sartori CA. Autoimmune-like pancreatitis in thymoma with myasthenia gravis. Chir Ital. 2002;54(1):91.

16. Clavien PA, Robert J, Meyer P, Borst F, Hauser H, Herrmann F, et al. Acute pancreatitis and normoamylasemia. Not an uncommon combination. Ann Surg. 1989;210(5):614.

20

Does intraoperative closed-suction drainage influence the rate of pancreatic fistula after pancreaticoduodenectomy?

Ophélie Aumont[1], Aurélien Dupré[2], Adeline Abjean[1], Bruno Pereira[3], Julie Veziant[1], Bertrand Le Roy[1], Denis Pezet[1,4], Emmanuel Buc[1,4] and Johan Gagnière[1,4*]

Abstract

Background: Although drainage of pancreatic anastomoses after pancreaticoduodenectomy (PD) is still debated, it remains recommended, especially in patients with a high risk of post-operative pancreatic fistula (POPF). Modalities of drainage of pancreatic anastomoses, especially the use of passive (PAD) or closed-suction (CSD) drains, and their impact on surgical outcomes, have been poorly studied. The aim was to compare CSD versus PAD on surgical outcomes after PD.

Methods: Retrospective analysis of 197 consecutive patients who underwent a standardized PD at two tertiary centers between March 2012 and April 2015. Patients with PAD ($n = 132$) or CSD ($n = 65$) were compared.

Results: There was no significant difference in terms of 30-day overall and severe post-operative morbidity, post-operative hemorrhage, post-operative intra-abdominal fluid collections, 90-day post-operative mortality and mean length of hospital stay. The rate of POPF was significantly increased in the CSD group (47.7% vs. 32.6%; $p = 0.04$). CSD was associated with an increase of grade A POPF (21.5% vs. 8.3%; $p = 0.03$), while clinically relevant POPF were not impacted. In patients with grade A POPF, the rate of undrained intra-abdominal fluid collections was increased in the PAD group (46.1% vs. 21.4%; $p = 0.18$). After multivariate analysis, CSD was an independent factor associated with an increased rate of POPF (OR = 2.43; $p = 0.012$).

Conclusions: There was no strongly relevant difference in terms of surgical outcomes between PAD or CSD of pancreatic anastomoses after PD, but CSD may help to decrease the rate of undrained post-operative intra-abdominal collections in some patients. Further randomized, multi-institutional studies are needed.

Keywords: Pancreaticoduodenectomy, Drainage, Pancreatic Fistula, Morbidity, Complications

Background

Despite recent improvements in surgical techniques and peri-operative management, the post-operative morbidity after pancreaticoduodenectomy (PD) remains high, ranging from 16 to 77% [1–12]. Post-operative pancreatic fistula (POPF) is the most frequent and feared complication after PD, reported in 5 to 48% of patients [2–5, 7, 9, 10, 12, 13] and is responsible for a high post-operative mortality that could reach 12% after PD [2–5, 7, 9]. POPF is also linked to other post-operative complications, such as delayed gastric emptying and hemorrhage, which can extend the length of hospital stay, increase the readmission rate and raise health care costs. Moreover, POPF could be responsible for delayed adjuvant chemotherapy administration that could alter the prognosis of patients treated for pancreatic cancer [7, 14–19]. Preventive strategies such as main pancreatic duct (MPD) drainage, the use of somatostatin analogs or biological sealants, and the optimization of pancreatic anastomosis techniques have failed to decrease significantly the rate of POPF after PD.

Drainage of the pancreatic anastomosis is routinely used after PD to allow earlier diagnosis of POPF and to prevent/diagnose its related complications, especially

* Correspondence: jgagniere@chu-clermontferrand.fr
[1]Department of Digestive and Hepatobiliary Surgery, Estaing University Hospital, 1, place Lucie et Raymond Aubrac, 63000 Clermont-Ferrand, France
[4]UMR 1071 INSERM / Clermont Auvergne University, Clermont-Ferrand, France
Full list of author information is available at the end of the article

hemorrhages. However, drainage of the operative site could be responsible of a specific post-operative morbidity, particularly infectious complications, post-operative pain and increased lengths of hospital stay [20–24]. Although prophylactic drainage in hepatic and colorectal surgery has shown no clear benefit on post-operative morbidity [25–28], the problematic is highly different in pancreatic surgery due to the high risk of non-diagnosed and undrained POPF, with high risk of post-operative hemorrhage and death. On the other hand, drain can increase post-operative morbidity through the increase of surgical site infection. Routine drainage in pancreatic surgery remains controversial [11, 24, 29–34], but several studies have reported a significant increase of both morbidity and mortality in the absence of drainage [11, 30, 35]. Thus, regarding the current literature, drainage of pancreatic anastomoses after PD remains still recommended, especially in patients with a high risk of POPF [36], and should therefore be optimized. Indeed, modalities of drainage of pancreatic anastomoses, especially the use of passive (PAD) or closed-suction (CSD) drains, strongly vary among surgical teams, and their impact on surgical outcomes has been poorly studied. The aim of our study was to compare the use of CSD versus PAD on surgical outcomes after PD at two tertiary centers.

Methods

Study population and data collection

We retrospectively analyzed data from all patients who underwent a PD for benign or malignant tumors of the head of the pancreas or peri-ampullary area at two tertiary centers between March 2012 and April 2015. The recorded data included the patient demographics, co-morbidities, ASA score, need for pre-operative biliary drainage, administration of a neoadjuvant treatment, intra-operative blood loss, blood transfusions, operative time, intra-operative MPD diameter and pancreatic gland texture, need for vascular resection, type of pancreatic anastomosis, pylorus preservation, modality of drainage of the pancreatic anastomosis and/or the MPD, amylase levels on operatively placed drains, use of somatostatin analogs, type and severity of post-operative complications, length of hospital stay and histopathological data.

Treatment and follow-up

Therapeutic management for all patients was systematically discussed in digestive cancer board meetings at our institutions. A standardized classical Whipple procedure was usually performed. Reconstruction with duct-to-mucosa pancreaticojejunostomy or pancreaticogastrostomy was at the surgeon's discretion, with routine use of external drainage of the MPD. Sealants were not used. At the end of the procedure, one PAD

or CSD (Shirley drain) was systematically placed near the pancreatic anastomosis at surgeon's discretion in both centers.

All of the patients were treated by a standardized post-operative care pathway for pancreatic resection used at our institutions. Patients were systematically transferred to an intensive care unit post-operatively. Somatostatin analogs were used at the operating surgeon's discretion. Drain outputs were recorded, and amylase levels were measured at post-operative day 1, 3 and 5. Abdominal drains were removed at post-operative day 5, except in case of POPF or biliary leak. A computed tomography (CT)-scan was systematically performed at post-operative day 5, to detect undrained intra-abdominal collections that were systematically drained with percutaneous CT-guided and/or endoscopic trans-gastric and/or surgical approaches. Amylase levels in post-operatively drained intra-abdominal collections were also systematically measured to detect POPF. Additional management methods for suspected POPF included the administration of antibiotics and supplemental parenteral or enteral nutrition support. Every post-operative complications occurring during the first 90 post-operative days were recorded.

Endpoints and definitions

Endpoints included both rate and severity of POPF (according to the ISGPF definition and classification [37]), post-operative hemorrhage and intra-abdominal fluid collections rates, 30-day overall post-operative morbidity rate and severity (according to the Dindo and Clavien classification [38]), 90-day post-operative mortality and the mean length of hospital stay.

Statistical analysis

All analyses were performed using Stata software (version 13; StataCorp, College Station, TX) and were performed for a two-sided type I error of $\alpha = 5\%$. Baseline characteristics were presented as the mean ± standard deviation for continuous data (Shapiro-Wilk test was used to assess normality), and as the number of patients and associated percentages for categorical parameters. Comparisons of the patient's characteristics between groups were carried out using the chi-squared test for categorical variables, and Student's t-test or the Mann-Whitney test when assumptions of the t-test were not met (normality and homoscedasticity studied using Fisher-Snedecor test) for quantitative variables. Next, a generalized linear regression model (logistic for dichotomous dependent outcome) was considered to study the effect of predictive factors in multivariate analysis by backward and forward stepwise regression of the factors considered significant in univariate analysis and according to clinically relevant parameters. The results were expressed as odds ratios (OR) and

95% confidence intervals. The final model was analyzed by a two-step bootstrapping process.

Results

One hundred and ninety-seven consecutive patients underwent PD for benign or malignant tumors involving the head of the pancreas or the peri-ampullary area at two tertiary centers between March 2012 and April 2015. The clinicopathological and therapeutic features are detailed in Table 1.

Patients with PAD (n = 132) or CSD (n = 65) were compared (Table 1). Pylorus-preserving PD (80.3% vs. 55.4%; p = 0.001), venous resections (24.2% vs. 9.2%; p = 0.012), pancreaticogastrostomies (60.3% vs. 28.1%; p = 0.001) and adenocarcinomas (73.5% vs. 56.9%; p = 0.008) were preferentially reported in patients with PAD. Both groups were

comparable regarding BMI (p = 0.21), chronic pancreatitis rates (p = 0.46), operative time (p = 0.16), intraoperative blood loss (p = 0.89), pancreas texture (p = 0.66), drainage of the MPD (p = 0.79), and use of somatostatin analogs (p = 0.65).

There was no significant difference between the two groups in terms of 30-day overall (71.2% vs. 70.8% (n = 46); p = 0.93) and severe (grade $\geq$ III) (37.9% vs. 40%; p = 0.93) post-operative morbidity, post-operative hemorrhage (9.0% vs. 9.2%; p = 0.97), 90-day post-operative mortality (15.2% vs. 12.3%; p = 0.59) and mean length of hospital stay (28 ± 18 days vs. 31 ± 48 days; p = 0.17) (Table 2).

The rate of POPF was significantly increased in the CSD group (47.7% vs. 32.6%; p = 0.04). Considering the grade of POPF according to the ISGPF classification,

Table 1 Clinicopathological and therapeutic features of patients who underwent duodenopancreatectomy

Characteristics	Study population (n = 197)		Passive drainage (n = 132)		Closed-suction drainage (n = 65)		
	No./mean ± SD[a]	(%)	No./mean ± SD[a]	(%)	No./mean ± SD[a]	(%)	p
Age (years)	66.2 ± 11.8	-	64.8 ± 11.3	-	68.5 ± 11.8	-	0.08
Male	108	(54.8)	70	(53.0)	38	(58.5)	0.47
Body mass index (kg/m^2)	25.0 ± 4.3	-	24.7 ± 4.1	-	25.5 ± 4.4	-	0.21
ASA[b] score							0.31
1	44	(22.3)	34	(25.0)	10	(15.4)	
2	114	(57.9)	75	(56.8)	39	(60.0)	
3	39	(18.3)	23	(17.4)	16	(24.6)	
Chronic pancreatitis	30	(19.8)	19	(14.4)	12	(18.5)	0.46
Pathology							<0.01
Adenocarcinoma	134	(68.0)	97	(73.5)	37	(56.9)	
Cholangiocarcinoma	7	(3.6)	6	(4.5)	1	(1.5)	
Ampullocarcinoma	6	(3.0)	5	(3.8)	1	(1.5)	
Other	50	(25.4)	24	(18.2)	26	(40.1)	
Neoadjuvant treatment	22	(11.2)	13	(9.8)	9	(13.8)	0.40
Pre-operative biliary drainage	93	(47.2)	66	(50.0)	27	(41.5)	0.26
Artery resection	1	(0.5)	1	(0.8)	0	(0)	1.00
Vein resection	38	(19.3)	32	(24.2)	6	(9.2)	0.01
Pylorus preservation	142	(72.1)	106	(80.3)	36	(55.4)	<0.01
Type of pancreatic anastomosis							<0.01
Pancreaticogastrostomy	97	(49.2)	79	(60.3)	18	(28.1)	
Pancreaticojejunostomy	98	(49.8)	52	(39.7)	46	(71.9)	
Soft pancreatic gland texture	28	(14.2)	18	(13.6)	10	(15.4)	0.66
Main pancreatic duct diameter	4.93 ± 2.45	-	5.0 ± 2.3	-	5.1 ± 2.7	-	0.79
Intra-operative blood loss (mL)	685 ± 588	-	664 ± 519	-	728 ± 719	-	0.89
Blood transfusion	44	(22.3)	28	(22.8)	16	(24.6)	0.78
Operative time (minutes)	388 ± 125	-	339 ± 136	-	377 ± 95	-	0.16
Somatostatin analogs	89	45.2	61	47.3	28	43.7	0.65

[a]Standard deviation
[b]American Society of Anesthesiology

Table 2 Studied endpoints of patients who underwent duodenopancreatectomy

Endpoints	Study population (n = 197)		Passive drainage (n = 132)		Closed-suction drainage (n = 65)		
	No./mean ± SD[a]	(%)	No./mean ± SD[a]	(%)	No./mean ± SD[a]	(%)	p
30-day post-operative morbidity							0.93
Overall	140	(71.0)	94	(71.2)	46	(70.8)	
Grade I-II	64	(32.5)	44	(33.3)	20	(30.8)	
Grade ≥ III	76	(38.6)	50	(37.9)	26	(40.0)	
POPF[b]							
Overall	75	(38.1)	43	(32.6)	32	(47.7)	0.04
Grade A	25	(12.7)	11	(8.3)	14	(21.5)	0.03
Grade B	22	(11.2)	14	(10.6)	8	(12.3)	0.74
Grade C	27	(13.7)	18	(13.6)	9	(13.8)	0.91
Intra-abdominal fluid collection	45	(22.9)	28	(21.1)	17	(26.1)	0.44
Post-operative hemorrhage	18	(9.1)	12	(9.0)	6	(9.2)	0.97
90-day post-operative mortality	28	(14.2)	20	(15.2)	8	(12.3)	0.59
Length of hospital stay (days)	30 ± 33	-	28 ± 18	-	31 ± 48	-	0.17

[a]Standard deviation
[b]Post-operative pancreatic fistula

CSD was associated with an increase of grade A POPF (21.5% vs. 8.3%; p = 0.03), while clinically relevant grade B/C POPF were not influenced by the modality of drainage (Table 2).

Given the fact that the higher rate of grade A POPF in the CSD group could be explained by a more accurate diagnosis of latent POPF, we investigated the rate of un-drained post-operative intra-abdominal fluid collections between the two groups. This rate was not significantly different between the two groups (21.1% in the CSD group vs. 26.1% in the PAD group; p = 0.44) (Table 2). In patients with grade A POPF (n = 27), the rate of un-drained intra-abdominal fluid collections was increased in the PAD group (46.1% vs. 21.4%) but this difference was not significant (p = 0.18). In patients with clinically relevant grade B/C POPF (n = 51), this rate was comparable between the two studied groups (47.0% vs. 58.8%; p = 0.43) (Table 2).

After multivariate analysis, only CSD was an independent factor associated with an increased rate of POPF after PD (OR = 2.43, 95% CI [1.21–4.87]; p = 0.012).

Discussion

Systematic drainage after PD is still debated [11, 24, 29–35] but remains still recommended in patients with a high risk of POPF [36]. Optimization of the drainage modalities is a major concern, with the aim to improve detection of POPF and to prevent/diagnose related complications, especially hemorrhages. We present herein a study which has compared the efficacy of closed-suction drainage versus passive drainage of pancreatic anastomoses on surgical outcomes after PD. We reported that the rate of POPF, especially regarding grade A POPF, was significantly increased in patients with CSD, but there was no impact on clinically relevant grade B/C POPF, post-operative morbidity and length of hospital stay. Nevertheless, it remains unclear whether CSD allows better detection of grade A POPF or could directly favor it. Patients in the PAD group with grade A POPF had more undrained peri-anastomotic intra-abdominal fluid collections. This could be explained by undiagnosed POPF according to the ISGPF definition [37] and a higher efficacy of CSD. However, as grade A POPF do not imply any specific therapeutic changes, and as grade B/C POPF were similar in both groups, we can conclude that there was no strongly relevant difference in terms of surgical outcomes between PAD and CSD, but that CSD could probably help to decrease rate of undrained post-operative intra-abdominal collections in some patients.

As mentioned above, the relation between the modalities of intra-operative drainage and the postoperative complications after PD has been poorly studied. The use of single or multiple drains in pancreatic surgery has failed to show any relevant interest in a single center retrospective study [39]. In the same topic as our study, a chinese randomized trial from Jiang et al. has reported a decrease of both grade C POPF rate and length of hospital stay with CSD [40]. However, even randomized, this study cannot provide adequate conclusions due to the presence of major biases. Firstly, the sample size was calculated based on the overall post-operative morbidity as primary endpoint, and did not thus allow making formal conclusions on secondary endpoints such as the rate of POPF. Secondly, no systematic post-operative CT-scan was performed, that could thus have underestimated both POPF (especially grade A POPF) and intra-abdominal fluid collections rates. And most importantly, the unusual use of CSD that were systematically irrigated with 3 l normal saline every day for the first 3 post-operative days and kept with intermittent suction for the following 2 days has to be highlighted. It is important to note that most of the studies that have investigated the role of drainage in pancreatic surgery reported the use of CSD [24, 29, 31–33]. Even if CSD were not compared to PAD in these studies, some reported no benefit of CSD over no drain [24, 33], while others reported less intra-abdominal undrained fluid collections with CSD [31]. Further specific studies are thus needed, such as the DRAPA trial [41].

Our study demonstrated a benefit of CSD over PAD, but only to detect grade A POPF, with no clinical relevance. However, this was limited by its retrospective nature and by imbalanced compared groups. Indeed, patients in the CSD group were older ($p = 0.08$), had significantly less adenocarcinomas ($p < 0.01$), and high operative time (+38 min; $p = 0.16$), which are known risks of relevant POPF. Furthermore, type of pancreatic anastomosis was different between the two groups, which could have introduced a bias. Thus, this work could constitute a basis for further controlled randomized, multi-institutional studies to validate these conclusions. Regarding emerging concepts of enhanced recovery which favors the absence or early removal of drains, these studies should especially include patients with high risk of POPF [42–44], who would probably benefit from the drainage of pancreatic anastomoses [36, 45].

Conclusions

The rate of grade A POPF after PD was significantly increased in patients with CSD, but that modality of drainage did not impact clinically relevant grade B/C POPF, post-operative morbidity, mortality and length of hospital stay. The rate of undrained peri-anastomotic intra-abdominal fluid collections in patients carrying a PAD and presenting with grade A POPF was also increased. Regarding the fact that grade A POPF do not imply any specific therapeutic changes we can conclude that, if performed, there was no strongly relevant difference in terms of surgical outcomes between PAD or CSD after PD, but that CSD could probably help to decrease the rate of undrained post-operative intra-abdominal collections in some patients. Further randomized, multi-institutional studies are needed to validate these conclusions.

Acknowledgments
Not applicable.

Funding
None to declare.

Authors' contributions
JG, AD, DP and EB participated to both the conception and the design of the study. OA, JG, AA, AD, BP, JV and BLR participated to both the analysis and the interpretation of the data. OA, JG, EB, AD, JV and BLR drafted the article. BP, AA, JG, DP and EB critically revised the article. All authors read and approved the final manuscript.

Competing interests
The authors declare that they have no competing interests.

Author details
[1]Department of Digestive and Hepatobiliary Surgery, Estaing University Hospital, 1, place Lucie et Raymond Aubrac, 63000 Clermont-Ferrand, France. [2]Department of Surgical Oncology, Léon Bérard Cancer Center, Lyon, France. [3]Biostatistics, Délégation à la Recherche Clinique et à l'Innovation, University Hospital of Clermont-Ferrand, Clermont-Ferrand, France. [4]UMR 1071 INSERM / Clermont Auvergne University, Clermont-Ferrand, France.

References
1. Aroori S, Puneet P, Bramhall SR, Muiesan P, Mayer AD, Mirza DF, Buckels JC, Isaac J. Outcomes comparing a pancreaticogastrostomy (PG) and a pancreaticojejunostomy (PJ) after a pancreaticoduodenectomy (PD). HPB (Oxford). 2011;13(10):723–31.
2. Bassi C, Falconi M, Molinari E, Salvia R, Butturini G, Sartori N, Mantovani W, Pederzoli P. Reconstruction by pancreaticojejunostomy versus pancreaticogastrostomy following pancreatectomy: results of a comparative study. Ann Surg. 2005;242(6):767–71. discussion 771-763
3. Duffas JP, Suc B, Msika S, Fourtanier G, Muscari F, Hay JM, Fingerhut A, Millat B, Radovanowic A, Fagniez PL, et al. A controlled randomized multicenter trial of pancreatogastrostomy or pancreatojejunostomy after pancreatoduodenectomy. Am J Surg. 2005;189(6):720–9.
4. Fernandez-Cruz L, Cosa R, Blanco L, Lopez-Boado MA, Astudillo E. Pancreatogastrostomy with gastric partition after pylorus-preserving pancreatoduodenectomy versus conventional pancreatojejunostomy: a prospective randomized study. Ann Surg. 2008;248(6):930–8.
5. Figueras J, Sabater L, Planellas P, Munoz-Forner E, Lopez-Ben S, Falgueras L, Sala-Palau C, Albiol M, Ortega-Serrano J, Castro-Gutierrez E. Randomized clinical trial of pancreaticogastrostomy versus pancreaticojejunostomy on the rate and severity of pancreatic fistula after pancreaticoduodenectomy. Br J Surg. 2013;100(12):1597–605.
6. McPhee JT, Hill JS, Whalen GF, Zayaruzny M, Litwin DE, Sullivan ME, Anderson FA, Tseng JF. Perioperative mortality for pancreatectomy: a national perspective. Ann Surg. 2007;246(2):246–53.
7. Muscari F, Suc B, Kirzin S, Hay JM, Fourtanier G, Fingerhut A, Sastre B, Chipponi J, Fagniez PL, Radovanovic A, et al. Risk factors for mortality and intra-abdominal complications after pancreatoduodenectomy: multivariate analysis in 300 patients. Surgery. 2006;139(5):591–8.
8. Schmidt CM, Turrini O, Parikh P, House MG, Zyromski NJ, Nakeeb A, Howard TJ, Pitt HA, Lillemoe KD. Effect of hospital volume, surgeon experience, and surgeon volume on patient outcomes after pancreaticoduodenectomy: a single-institution experience. Arch Surg. 2010;145(7):634–40.
9. Topal B, Fieuws S, Aerts R, Weerts J, Feryn T, Roeyen G, Bertrand C, Hubert C, Janssens M, Closset J, et al. Pancreaticojejunostomy versus pancreaticogastrostomy reconstruction after pancreaticoduodenectomy for pancreatic or periampullary tumours: a multicentre randomised trial. Lancet Oncol. 2013;14(7):655–62.
10. Yeo CJ, Cameron JL, Maher MM, Sauter PK, Zahurak ML, Talamini MA, Lillemoe KD, Pitt HA. A prospective randomized trial of pancreaticogastrostomy versus pancreaticojejunostomy after pancreaticoduodenectomy. Ann Surg. 1995;222(4):580–8. discussion 588-592
11. Van Buren G, 2nd, Bloomston M, Hughes SJ, Winter J, Behrman SW, Zyromski NJ, Vollmer C, Velanovich V, Riall T, Muscarella P et al. A randomized prospective multicenter trial of pancreaticoduodenectomy with and without routine intraperitoneal drainage. Ann Surg 2014, 259(4):605-612.

12. Perinel J, Mariette C, Dousset B, Sielezneff I, Gainant A, Mabrut JY, Bin-Dorel S, Bechwaty ME, Delaunay D, Bernard L, et al. Early enteral versus total parenteral nutrition in patients undergoing pancreaticoduodenectomy: a randomized multicenter controlled trial (Nutri-DPC). Ann Surg. 2016;264(5):731-7.

13. Kajiwara T, Sakamoto Y, Morofuji N, Nara S, Esaki M, Shimada K, Kosuge T. An analysis of risk factors for pancreatic fistula after pancreaticoduodenectomy: clinical impact of bile juice infection on day 1. Langenbeck's Arch Surg. 2010;395(6):707-12.

14. Aloia TA, Lee JE, Vauthey JN, Abdalla EK, Wolff RA, Varadhachary GR, Abbruzzese JL, Crane CH, Evans DB, Pisters PW. Delayed recovery after pancreaticoduodenectomy: a major factor impairing the delivery of adjuvant therapy? J Am Coll Surg. 2007;204(3):347-55.

15. Gouma DJ, van Geenen RC, van Gulik TM, de Haan RJ, de Wit LT, Busch OR, Obertop H. Rates of complications and death after pancreaticoduodenectomy: risk factors and the impact of hospital volume. Ann Surg. 2000;232(6):786-95.

16. Kent TS, Sachs TE, Callery MP, Vollmer CM Jr. Readmission after major pancreatic resection: a necessary evil? J Am Coll Surg. 2011;213(4):515-23.

17. Niedergethmann M, Farag Soliman M, Post S. Postoperative complications of pancreatic cancer surgery. Minerva Chir. 2004;59(2):175-83.

18. Sohn TA, Yeo CJ, Cameron JL, Pitt HA, Lillemoe KD. Do preoperative biliary stents increase postpancreaticoduodenectomy complications? J Gastrointest Surg. 2000;4(3):258-67. discussion 267-258

19. Vollmer CM Jr, Sanchez N, Gondek S, McAuliffe J, Kent TS, Christein JD, Callery MP, Pancreatic Surgery Mortality Study G. A root-cause analysis of mortality following major pancreatectomy. J Gastrointest Surg. 2012;16(1):89-102. discussion 102-103

20. Jesus EC, Karliczek A, Matos D, Castro AA, Atallah AN. Prophylactic anastomotic drainage for colorectal surgery. Cochrane Database Syst Rev. 2004;4:CD002100.

21. Nora PF, Vanecko RM, Bransfield JJ. Prophylactic abdominal drains. Arch Surg. 1972;105(2):173-6.

22. Raves JJ, Slifkin M, Diamond DL. A bacteriologic study comparing closed suction and simple conduit drainage. Am J Surg. 1984;148(5):618-20.

23. Urbach DR, Kennedy ED, Cohen MM. Colon and rectal anastomoses do not require routine drainage: a systematic review and meta-analysis. Ann Surg. 1999;229(2):174-80.

24. Conlon KC, Labow D, Leung D, Smith A, Jarnagin W, Coit DG, Merchant N, Brennan MF. Prospective randomized clinical trial of the value of intraperitoneal drainage after pancreatic resection. Ann Surg. 2001;234(4):487-93. discussion 493-484

25. Brauer DG, Nywening TM, Jaques DP, Doyle MB, Chapman WC, Fields RC, Hawkins WG. Operative site drainage after hepatectomy: a propensity score matched analysis using the American College of surgeons NSQIP targeted hepatectomy database. J Am Coll Surg. 2016;223(6):774-83. e772

26. Denost Q, Rouanet P, Faucheron JL, Panis Y, Meunier B, Cotte E, Meurette G, Kirzin S, Sabbagh C, Loriau J, et al. To Drain or Not to Drain Infraperitoneal Anastomosis After Rectal Excision for Cancer: The GRECCAR 5 Randomized Trial. Ann Surg. 2016;265(3):474-480.

27. Gavriilidis P, Hidalgo E, de'Angelis N, Lodge P, Azoulay D. Re-appraisal of prophylactic drainage in uncomplicated liver resections: a systematic review and meta-analysis. HPB (Oxford). 2016;19(1):16-20.

28. Petrowsky H, Demartines N, Rousson V, Clavien PA. Evidence-based value of prophylactic drainage in gastrointestinal surgery: a systematic review and meta-analyses. Ann Surg. 2004;240(6):1074-84. discussion 1084-1075

29. Correa-Gallego C, Brennan MF, D'Angelica M, Fong Y, Dematteo RP, Kingham TP, Jarnagin WR, Allen PJ. Operative drainage following pancreatic resection: analysis of 1122 patients resected over 5 years at a single institution. Ann Surg. 2013;258(6):1051-8.

30. Dou CW, Liu ZK, Jia YL, Zheng X, Tu KS, Yao YM, Liu QG. Systematic review and meta-analysis of prophylactic abdominal drainage after pancreatic resection. World J Gastroenterol: WJG. 2015;21(18):5719-34.

31. Fisher WE, Hodges SE, Silberfein EJ, Artinyan A, Ahern CH, Jo E, Brunicardi FC. Pancreatic resection without routine intraperitoneal drainage. HPB (Oxford). 2011;13(7):503-10.

32. Heslin MJ, Harrison LE, Brooks AD, Hochwald SN, Coit DG, Brennan MF. Is intra-abdominal drainage necessary after pancreaticoduodenectomy? J Gastrointest Surg. 1998;2(4):373-8.

33. Mehta VV, Fisher SB, Maithel SK, Sarmiento JM, Staley CA, Kooby DA. Is it time to abandon routine operative drain use? A single institution assessment of 709 consecutive pancreaticoduodenectomies. J Am Coll Surg. 2013;216(4):635-42. discussion 642-634

34. Wang Q, Jiang YJ, Li J, Yang F, Di Y, Yao L, Jin C, Fu DL. Is routine drainage necessary after pancreaticoduodenectomy? World J Gastroenterol: WJG. 2014;20(25):8110-8.

35. Wang YC, Szatmary P, Zhu JQ, Xiong JJ, Huang W, Gomatos I, Nunes QM, Sutton R, Liu XB. Prophylactic intra-peritoneal drain placement following pancreaticoduodenectomy: a systematic review and meta-analysis. World J Gastroenterol: WJG. 2015;21(8):2510-21.

36. McMillan MT, Malleo G, Bassi C, Butturini G, Salvia R, Roses RE, Lee MK, Fraker DL, Drebin JA, Vollmer CM Jr. Drain management after pancreatoduodenectomy: reappraisal of a prospective randomized trial using risk stratification. J Am Coll Surg. 2015;221(4):798-809.

37. Bassi C, Marchegiani G, Dervenis C, Sarr M, Abu Hilal M, Adham M, Allen P, Andersson R, Asbun HJ, Besselink MG, et al. The 2016 update of the International Study Group (ISGPS) definition and grading of postoperative pancreatic fistula: 11 Years After. Surgery. 2017;161(3):584-91.

38. Dindo D, Demartines N, Clavien PA. Classification of surgical complications: a new proposal with evaluation in a cohort of 6336 patients and results of a survey. Ann Surg. 2004;240(2):205-13.

39. Shrikhande SV, Barreto SG, Shetty G, Suradkar K, Bodhankar YD, Shah SB, Goel M. Post-operative abdominal drainage following major upper gastrointestinal surgery: single drain versus two drains. J Cancer Res Ther. 2013;9(2):267-71.

40. Jiang H, Liu N, Zhang M, Lu L, Dou R, Qu L. A Randomized Trial on the Efficacy of Prophylactic Active Drainage in Prevention of Complications after Pancreaticoduodenectomy. Scand J Surg. 2016. [Epub ahead of print].

41. Cecka F, Lovecek M, Jon B, Skalicky P, Subrt Z, Ferko A. DRAPA trial–closed-suction drains versus closed gravity drains in pancreatic surgery: study protocol for a randomized controlled trial. Trials. 2015;16:207.

42. Callery MP, Pratt WB, Kent TS, Chaikof EL, Vollmer CM Jr. A prospectively validated clinical risk score accurately predicts pancreatic fistula after pancreatoduodenectomy. J Am Coll Surg. 2013;216(1):1-14.

43. Roberts KJ, Hodson J, Mehrzad H, Marudanayagam R, Sutcliffe RP, Muiesan P, Isaac J, Bramhall SR, Mirza DF. A preoperative predictive score of pancreatic fistula following pancreatoduodenectomy. HPB (Oxford). 2014;16(7):620-8.

44. Yamamoto Y, Sakamoto Y, Nara S, Esaki M, Shimada K, Kosuge T. A preoperative predictive scoring system for postoperative pancreatic fistula after pancreaticoduodenectomy. World J Surg. 2011;35(12):2747-55.

45. McMillan MT, Malleo G, Bassi C, Allegrini V, Casetti L, Drebin JA, Esposito A, Landoni L, Lee MK, Pulvirenti A, et al. Multicenter, Prospective Trial of Selective Drain Management for Pancreatoduodenectomy Using Risk Stratification. Ann Surg. 2016;265(6):1209-1218.

21

Radiographic sarcopenia predicts postoperative infectious complications in patients undergoing pancreaticoduodenectomy

Kosei Takagi, Ryuichi Yoshida*⍟, Takahito Yagi, Yuzo Umeda, Daisuke Nobuoka, Takashi Kuise and Toshiyoshi Fujiwara

Abstract

Background: Recently, skeletal muscle depletion (sarcopenia) has been reported to influence postoperative outcomes after certain procedures. This study investigated the impact of sarcopenia on postoperative outcomes following pancreaticoduodenectomy (PD).

Methods: We performed a retrospective study of consecutive patients ($n = 219$) who underwent PD at our institution between January 2007 and May 2013. Sarcopenia was evaluated using preoperative computed tomography. We evaluated postoperative outcomes and the influence of sarcopenia on short-term outcomes, especially infectious complications. Subsequently, multivariate analysis was used to assess the impact of prognostic factors (including sarcopenia) on postoperative infections.

Results: The mortality, major complication, and infectious complication rates for all patients were 1.4%, 16.4%, and 47.0%, respectively. Fifty-five patients met the criteria for sarcopenia. Sarcopenia was significantly associated with a higher incidence of in-hospital mortality ($P = 0.004$) and infectious complications ($P < 0.001$). In multivariate analyses, sarcopenia (odds ratio = 3.43; $P < 0.001$), preoperative biliary drainage (odds ratio = 2.20; $P = 0.014$), blood loss (odds ratio = 1.92; $P = 0.048$), and soft pancreatic texture (odds ratio = 3.71; $P < 0.001$) were independent predictors of postoperative infections.

Conclusions: Sarcopenia is an independent preoperative predictor of infectious complications after PD. Clinical assessment combined with sarcopenia may be helpful for understanding the risk of postoperative outcomes and determining perioperative management strategies.

Keywords: Sarcopenia, Complication, Infection, Pancreaticoduodenectomy

Background

Pancreaticoduodenectomy (PD) is one of the most complicated procedures in the field of gastroenterological surgery. As a result, the postoperative mortality and morbidity rates after PD remain high (2.8–3.5% and 40%, respectively) according to nationwide surveys performed in Japan [1, 2]. Furthermore, infectious complications after pancreatic surgery are common during the postoperative

course, and can lead to fatal outcomes [3]. High morbidity rates are associated with the need for further treatment and extended hospital stays. Thus, a precise method of predicting postoperative complications is urgently required to ensure patient safety following PD.

Recent studies have shown that computed tomography (CT)-assessed sarcopenia (radiographic sarcopenia), which is characterized by skeletal muscle depletion and is an objective predictor of frailty, is associated with poor outcomes in gastrointestinal and hepatopancreatobiliary malignancies [4]. Previous studies have also shown that sarcopenia is associated with short-term outcomes, and

* Correspondence: r9232001@yahoo.co.jp
Department of Gastroenterological Surgery, Okayama University Graduate School of Medicine, Dentistry, and Pharmaceutical Sciences, 2-5-1 Shikata-cho, Kita-ku, Okayama 700-8558, Japan

especially with postoperative pancreatic fistula (POPF), in patients undergoing PD. [5–8] However, the influence of sarcopenia in terms of postoperative infectious complications has not been assessed in detail. We hypothesized that sarcopenia is associated with postoperative infections in patients undergoing PD.

With the above in mind, the aim of this retrospective study was to investigate postoperative outcomes following PD and to assess the influence of sarcopenia on short-term outcomes. In particular, we focused on the relationship between sarcopenia and infectious postoperative complications in patients following PD.

Methods

Patients
We retrospectively reviewed the medical records of 241 consecutive patients who underwent PD at the Okayama University Hospital between January 2007 and May 2013. This study was approved by the Ethics Committee of the Okayama University Graduate School of Medicine, Dentistry, and Pharmaceutical Sciences and Okayama University Hospital, and was conducted in accordance with the tenets of the Declaration of Helsinki. Due to the retrospective nature of the study, the need for informed consent was waived.

Clinical data
For all enrolled patients, the following demographic and clinical data were evaluated as preoperative factors: sex, age, height, weight, body mass index (BMI), body surface area (BSA), American Society of Anesthesiologists (ASA) physical status, laboratory values (albumin level and total lymphocyte count), liver function according to the Child–Pugh score, comorbidities, etiology of disease, and preoperative biliary drainage. ASA physical status was preoperatively evaluated by an anesthesiologist. Preoperative biliary drainage included endoscopic biliary drainage and percutaneous transhepatic biliary drainage. Data regarding operative time, amount of blood loss, portal vein reconstruction, pancreatic texture (soft or hard) assessed by the surgeon intraoperatively, and main pancreatic duct diameter, were recorded as intraoperative factors.

Surgical procedures and perioperative management
The standard surgical procedure was subtotal stomach-preserving PD. The basic reconstruction of the digestive system was performed by means of a modification of the method described by Child [9]. Pancreatojejunostomy was performed with a duct-to-mucosa anastomosis. Hepatojejunostomy was performed 10 cm distal to the pancreatojejunostomy. Gastrojejunostomy was performed by means of a two-layer anastomosis 50 cm distal to the hepatojejunostomy. A Braun anastomosis was also added.

The details of these surgical techniques have been reported previously [10, 11]. In most cases, three drains were placed around the pancreatic and biliary anastomoses. All patients received prophylactic antibiotics every 3 h intraoperatively and for 3 d postoperatively.

Postoperative care was performed in a specialized surgical unit. Patients did not routinely receive somatostatin analogues and nutritional supplementation during the perioperative period. The drains were removed after postoperative day 5 if the drainage fluid was clear and no bacterial contamination was detected.

Image analysis and definition of sarcopenia
Diagnostic CT images taken within 3 months prior to surgery were chosen and evaluated using a CT image analysis system (Synapse Vincent; Fujifilm Medical, Tokyo, Japan). The total cross-sectional skeletal muscle area (SMA) at the level of the third lumbar vertebra was calculated in the study population using Hounsfield unit thresholds of −29 to +150 for skeletal muscle [12]. The details of the measuring method are as described previously [13, 14]. In this study, the SMA (cm^2) was divided by BSA (m^2) to obtain the SMA/BSA index (SBI; cm^2/m^2), which is our original method of defining sarcopenia [14]. In the present study, patients with values less than the gender-specific lowest quartile of SBI were considered to have radiographic sarcopenia.

Postoperative outcomes
For each patient, data regarding the following parameters were collected: postoperative mortality, morbidity including infectious complications, and postoperative length of hospital stay. Postoperative mortality included all in-hospital deaths before discharge. To analyze morbidity severity, each postoperative event was assessed and graded according to the Clavien–Dindo classification [15]. The major postoperative complications were defined as Clavien grade ≥ 3. POPF and delayed gastric emptying (DGE) were defined according to the International Study Group of Pancreatic Surgery guidelines [16, 17].

Infectious complications
In the present study, we defined infectious complications as all postoperative infectious diseases including wound infections, infected abdominal fluid, intra-abdominal abscess, bacteremia, catheter-related infections, pneumonia, cholangitis, enteritis, and urinary tract infections. The definition of these infectious complications conformed to those of the American College of Surgeons National Surgical Quality Improvement Program criteria (NSQIP) [18]. Infected abdominal fluid was defined as drainage fluid with a positive culture from surgically replaced drains. Intra-abdominal abscess was defined as

intra-abdominal fluid collection with positive cultures identified by ultrasonography or CT with clinical signs. A positive culture was not necessarily required in cases in which the NSQIP criteria were met and clinical signs were consistent with infectious complications.

Risk factors for postoperative infections
Univariate and multivariate analyses were performed to identify the predictors closely related to infectious complications after PD among preoperative and intraoperative factors.

Simple scoring system using perioperative risk factors
A simple scoring system was performed according to the results of multivariate analysis to investigate risk factors for postoperative infections. Patients were divided into three groups according to these risk factors, and the short-term outcomes of each group were then examined.

Statistical analysis
JMP version 11 software (SAS Institute, Cary, NC) was used for all statistical analyses. Data were presented as means, medians, and standard deviations for continuous variables. Categorical data were presented as proportions. Differences between groups were assessed using the Mann-Whitney U-test for continuous variables, and Fisher's exact test or chi-square test for categorical variables. To investigate the impact of prognostic factors associated with postoperative infections, we used a logistic regression model for univariate and multivariate analyses; odds ratios and 95% confidence intervals were calculated. A P–value <0.05 was considered statistically significant.

Results
Study population
Of the 241 patients who underwent PD, 22 were excluded because of the following reasons: unavailable preoperative CT images, 16; emergency surgery, 6. The demographic characteristics of the 219 patients (143 men [65.3%]; mean age, 65.9 years) are shown in Table 1. Pancreatic adenocarcinoma was the most common disease, occurring in 86 patients (39.3%). Preoperative biliary drainage was performed in 101 patients (46.1%). The mean operative time was 448 min (230–733 min) and the mean blood loss was 563 mL (10–3130 mL).

Measurement of body composition
The mean SBI values were 74.7 ± 9.9 cm^2/m^2 for men and 58.3 ± 8.3 cm^2/m^2 for women. The mean SBI was significantly lower for women than for men (P < 0.001). The cut-off values for the lowest quartiles of SBI were 68.5 cm^2/m^2 for men and 52.5 cm^2/m^2 for women. Accordingly, 52 patients were categorized as having sarcopenia.

Table 1 Demographic and clinicopathological factors in patients with and without sarcopenia who underwent pancreaticoduodenectomy

	All patients (n = 219)	Non-sarcopenia (n = 164)	Sarcopenia (n = 55)	P-value
Demographic variables				
Sex (men)	143 (65.3)	107 (65.2)	36 (65.5)	0.98
Age (years)	65.9 (11.7)	65.1 (12.4)	68.2 (9.2)	0.18
BMI (kg/m^2)	21.9 (3.3)	22.0 (3.4)	21.7 (3.0)	0.67
ASA physical status				
1–2/3	203/16	154/10	49/6	0.25
Laboratory value				
Albumin (g/dL)	4.0 (0.5)	4.1 (0.4)	3.9 (0.6)	0.006
Total lymphocyte (/mm^3)	1642 (554)	1665 (561)	1572 (521)	0.30
Child–Pugh score				
A/B	205/14	155/9	50/5	0.36
Comorbidities				
Hypertension	89 (40.6)	68 (41.5)	21 (38.2)	0.67
Diabetes	64 (29.2)	43 (26.2)	21 (38.2)	0.10
Etiology of the disease				
Pancreatic adenocarcinoma	86 (39.3)	61 (37.2)	25 (45.5)	0.31
Bile duct carcinoma	27 (12.3)	20 (12.2)	7 (12.7)	
Ampullary adenocarcinoma	28 (12.8)	18 (11.0)	10 (18.2)	
Duodenal adenocarcinoma	10 (4.6)	9 (5.5)	1 (1.8)	
IPMN	32 (14.6)	26 (15.9)	6 (10.9)	
Others	36 (16.4)	30 (18.3)	6 (10.9)	
Preoperative biliary drainage	101 (46.1)	68 (41.5)	33 (60.0)	0.02
Intraoperative factor				
Operative time (min)	448 (93)	445 (93)	454 (94)	0.64
Blood loss (mL)	563 (486)	543 (443)	624 (596)	0.96
Vascular reconstruction	50 (22.8)	37 (22.6)	13 (23.6)	0.87
Soft pancreatic texture	133 (60.7)	101 (61.6)	32 (58.2)	0.66
Normal pancreatic duct (< 3 mm)	87 (39.7)	69 (42.1)	18 (32.7)	0.22

Data are presented as numbers (percentages) or means (± standard deviation). *BMI* body mass index, *ASA* American Society of Anesthesiologists, *IPMN* intraductal papillary mucinous neoplasm

Postoperative outcomes
The mortality and major complication rates for all 219 patients were 1.4% and 16.4%, respectively (Table 2). All three cases of mortality were caused by severe infectious complications. Of 219 patients, 103 (47.0%) had at least

Table 2 Postoperative outcomes in patients with and without sarcopenia who underwent pancreaticoduodenectomy

	All patients (n = 219)	Non-sarcopenia (n = 164)	Sarcopenia (n = 55)	P-value
Mortality	3 (1.4)	0 (0)	3 (5.5)	0.004
Major complication	36 (16.4)	24 (14.6)	12 (21.8)	0.21
Any infectious complication	103 (47.0)	66 (40.2)	37 (67.3)	<0.001
Wound infection	35 (16.0)	26 (15.9)	9 (16.4)	0.93
Intra-abdominal abscess	12 (5.5)	6 (3.7)	6 (10.9)	0.04
infected abdominal fluid	65 (29.7)	41 (25.0)	24 (43.6)	0.009
Bacteremia	7 (3.2)	2 (1.2)	5 (9.1)	0.004
Catheter-related infection,	9 (4.1)	7 (4.3)	2 (3.6)	0.84
Pneumonia	4 (1.8)	1 (0.6)	3 (5.5)	0.02
Cholangitis	8 (3.7)	4 (2.4)	4 (7.3)	0.10
Enteritis	5 (2.3)	5 (3.1)	0 (0)	0.19
Urinary tract infection	2 (0.9)	1 (0.6)	1 (1.8)	0.42
Pancreatic fistula (Grade B + C)	72 (32.9)	52 (31.7)	20 (36.4)	0.52
Delayed gastric emptying	48 (21.9)	36 (22.0)	12 (21.8)	0.98
Length of stay, median (range)	30 (24–40)	30 (24–38)	30 (25–41)	0.25

Data are presented as numbers (percentages), unless otherwise indicated

one postoperative infection. The most common infectious complications were infected abdominal fluid, 65; wound infections, 35; and intra-abdominal abscess, 12. The incidence rates of clinically relevant POPF (grade B or C) and DGE were 32.9% and 21.9%, respectively. The median length of hospital stay was 30 d (interquartile range, 24–40 d).

The impact of sarcopenia

The clinical demographic characteristics of patients with and without sarcopenia are shown in Table 1. Patients in the sarcopenia group had significantly lower albumin levels and a higher rate of preoperative biliary drainage, but other factors, including intraoperative factors, were not significantly different. Postoperative outcomes associated with the presence or absence of sarcopenia are presented in Table 2. The mortality rate was significantly higher in the sarcopenia group (5.5% vs. 0%, $P = 0.004$). Although the incidences of major complications, POPF, and DGE were not significantly different between the groups, the sarcopenia group had a significantly higher infectious complication rate (67.3% vs. 40.2%, $P < 0.001$). The length of postoperative hospital stay did not significantly differ between the groups.

Comparison between patients with and without postoperative infections

Patient characteristics are shown in Table 3. There were no differences between patients with and without infections with respect to sex, age, BMI, ASA physical status, laboratory values, liver function, comorbidities, etiology of disease, blood loss, vascular reconstruction, and

pancreatic duct diameter. Sarcopenia, preoperative biliary drainage, operative time, and soft pancreatic texture were more common (or longer, in the case of operative time) in patients with infections.

Risk factors for postoperative infections

Table 3 shows the results of univariate and multivariate analyses used to identify the predictors closely related to infectious complications after PD. In univariate analysis, four variables (sarcopenia, preoperative biliary drainage, operative time, and soft pancreatic texture) were found to be significant risk factors. Multivariate analysis showed that sarcopenia (odds ratio = 3.43; $P < 0.001$), preoperative biliary drainage (odds ratio = 2.20; $P = 0.014$), blood loss (odds ratio = 1.92; $P = 0.048$), and soft pancreatic texture (odds ratio = 3.71; $P < 0.001$) were significant risk factors for infectious complications after PD.

Simple scoring system using perioperative risk factors

According to the number of significant risk (R) factors (sarcopenia, preoperative biliary drainage, blood loss, and soft pancreatic texture) in multivariate analysis, patients were divided into three groups: R0/1 group ($n = 91$), R2 group ($n = 89$), and R3/4 group ($n = 39$).

Table 4 shows the short-term outcomes after PD determined using the risk-scoring system. The incidence rates of mortality and major complications were not different between the groups. However, the infectious complication rates after PD were 28.6% for the R0/1 group, 49.4% for the R2 group, and 84.6% for the R3/4 group ($P < 0.001$). In a logistic regression model, all differences

Table 3 Univariate and multivariate analyses of perioperative predictors associated with postoperative infections in patients who underwent pancreaticoduodenectomy

Variable	Non-infection ($n = 116$)	Infection ($n = 103$)	Univariate analysis			Multivariate analysis		
			OR	95% CI	P-value	OR	95% CI	P-value
Sarcopenia	18 (15.5)	37 (35.9)	3.05	1.62–5.91	<0.001	3.43	1.71–7.14	<0.001
Male	77 (66.4)	66 (64.1)	0.90	0.52–1.58	0.72			
Age (≥ 70 years)	45(38.8)	47 (45.6)	1.32	0.77–2.27	0.31			
BMI (≥ 25 kg/m^2)	13 (11.2)	21 (20.4)	2.03	0.97–4.39	0.06	2.01	0.87–4.80	0.10
ASA (≥ grade 3)	6 (5.2)	10 (9.7)	1.97	0.70–5.98	0.20			
Albumin (< 3.6 g/dL)	14 (12.4)	19 (19.4)	1.70	0.81–3.66	0.16			
Child–Pugh score (grade B)	4 (3.4)	10 (9.7)	3.01	0.97–11.3	0.06	1.74	0.48–7.40	0.41
Diabetes	32 (27.6)	32 (31.1)	1.18	0.66–2.12	0.57			
Malignant disease	77 (66.4)	74 (71.8)	1.29	0.73–2.31	0.38			
Preoperative biliary drainage	42 (36.2)	59 (57.3)	2.36	1.38–4.09	0.002	2.20	1.17–4.20	0.014
Operative time (> 425 min)	60 (51.7)	69 (67.0)	1.89	1.10–3.30	0.02	1.57	0.83–2.99	0.17
Blood loss (> 550 mL)	39 (33.6)	46 (44.7)	1.59	0.92–2.76	0.09	1.92	1.00–3.73	0.048
Vascular reconstruction	28 (24.1)	23 (22.3)	0.95	0.50–1.78	0.87			
Soft pancreatic texture	59 (50.9)	74 (71.8)	2.47	1.41–4.37	0.001	3.71	1.96–7.29	<0.001
Normal pancreatic duct (< 3 mm)	42 (36.2)	45 (43.7)	1.37	0.79–2.36	0.26			

Data are presented as numbers (percentages).
OR odds ratio, *CI* confidence interval, *BMI* body mass index, *ASA* American Society of Anaesthesiologists

between the R0/1 group and other groups were significant.

Discussion

This retrospective study demonstrated that sarcopenia is an independent prognostic factor of infectious complications after PD. To the best of our knowledge, this is the first study to identify the prognostic significance of sarcopenia on postoperative infections following PD. Concerning surgical procedures, the standard surgical procedure has changed to subtotal stomach-preserving PD from 2007 at our institution. In addition, the reconstruction of gastrojejunostomy has changed to an antecolic route from 2007 [11]. However, major changes in surgical procedures have not been introduced after 2007, so the results of this study should be valid.

In the entire cohort, the mortality, major complication, and infectious complication rates after PD were 1.4%, 16.4%, and 47.0%, respectively. The results obtained from our institution were better than those reported in previous papers [1, 2, 19]. However, the median length of stay was 30 d in the present study, which was much

longer than the mean value reported from studies performed in Western countries.

Further improvements to surgical procedures and perioperative management are needed in order to improve postoperative outcomes after PD.

Sarcopenia is a syndrome defined by progressive and generalized loss of skeletal muscle mass and strength that occurs with aging or secondary to diseases [20, 21]. In the present study, we used preoperative CT to evaluate sarcopenia. CT is considered to be an objective and precise method for assessing sarcopenia [22–24]. Regarding the definition of sarcopenia, we used SBI to evaluate skeletal muscle mass. We considered that SBI would more precisely evaluate skeletal muscle mass in patients with different physiques, and would be a superior index for evaluating skeletal muscle mass [14]. In the present study, demographic characteristics, including age and body parameters, were not significantly different between the two groups.

The effect of sarcopenia on postoperative complications, especially POPF, has been reported previously [5–8]. In the present study, the incidence rates of major complications

Table 4 Short-term outcomes after pancreaticoduodenectomy based on the results of the risk scoring system

No. of risk factors	Mortality	P-value	Major complication	P-value	Infectious complication	P-value	OR	95% CI	P-value
R0/1 group ($n = 91$)	0 (0)	0.20	11 (12.1)	0.17	26 (28.6)	<0.001	-	-	-
R2 group ($n = 89$)	2 (2.2)		15 (16.9)		44 (49.4)		2.44	1.33–4.57	0.004
R3/4 group ($n = 39$)	1 (2.6)		10 (25.6)		33 (84.6)		13.8	5.47–40.0	<0.001

Data are presented as numbers (percentages).
OR odds ratio, *CI* confidence interval

and POPF were not significantly different between the two groups. This finding differs from the results of previous studies. However, the sarcopenia group had a significantly higher incidence of in-hospital mortality and infectious complications. All cases of mortality were also the result of severe infectious complications. Concerning infectious complications, the incidence rates of intra-abdominal abscess and infected abdominal fluid were significantly higher in the sarcopenia group. Sarcopenia might negatively affect the healing process at the pancreatic anastomosis [6].

Our multivariate analysis revealed that sarcopenia, preoperative biliary drainage, blood loss, and soft pancreatic texture were perioperative risk factors related to postoperative infections after PD. Preoperative biliary drainage has been reported to be a risk factor for postoperative infections following PD. [25] Operative factors and pancreatic factors such as blood loss and soft pancreatic texture have been reported to be associated with POPF after PD, which may also be related to postoperative infections [6]. However, this represents a new finding demonstrating the association between sarcopenia and infections complications after PD.

In this study, we established a simple and comprehensive scoring system that predicted postoperative infections after PD. Thirty-nine patients (17.8%) had three or four risk factors (the R3/4 group), and these patients had 84.6% of all postoperative infectious complications. Assessing and managing these risk factors may improve postoperative outcomes, especially in high-risk patients. Nutritional intervention combined with physical exercise appear to be effective for the management of sarcopenia [26, 27]. Furthermore, perioperative antibiotic strategies to prevent bile contamination could prevent infectious complications after PD. [28] Finally, the development of specialized surgical procedures and techniques might contribute to reducing the rate of infectious complications.

Despite the important findings reported in this study, several limitations should be discussed. First, this was a small, single-center, retrospective study. Because of this, there may be some selection bias with respect to the patients who underwent PD. Second, we did not evaluate functional muscle status in terms of grip strength, walking speed, or exhaustion because of the retrospective nature of the study. The evaluation of both muscle mass and muscle function has been recommended in the diagnosis of sarcopenia [21], and future studies will be required to assess not only muscle mass but also function in sarcopenia. Third, we used the SBI for evaluating sarcopenia, which would be a useful modality for assessing sarcopenia. However, further studies are needed to assess the efficiency of SBI to diagnosis sarcopenia. Fourth, it remains unclear what nutritional interventions and physical exercise regimens would be valid for patients undergoing PD, because few studies have dealt with the effects of such

interventions on sarcopenic patients with PD. Future studies are needed to examine the effects of perioperative interventions focusing on sarcopenia. Finally, there is insufficient evidence in the pathophysiology concerning the interaction between sarcopenia and infections. The depletion of skeletal muscle as a secretory organ of cytokines and peptides, and increasing adipose tissue as a key component of the immune system lead to the synthesis and secretion of several proinflammatory adipocytokines [29]. Thereby, decreased interleukin-15 and increased adipokines levels might be associated with the interaction between sarcopenia and immune depression [30]. Accordingly, We hypothesize that sarcopenia reflects the patients' frailty, including impaired immune function, which ultimately leads to infections [14]. However, further research should investigate the molecular mechanism of sarcopenia's effect on outcomes.

Conclusions

In conclusion, the results of the present study indicate that sarcopenia is an objective and independent preoperative predictor of infectious complications after PD. Furthermore, assessing sarcopenia is easy and practicable. Accordingly, we propose that clinical assessment combined with sarcopenia may help clinicians to understand the risk of postoperative outcomes and determine perioperative management strategies.

Abbreviations
ASA: American Society of Anesthesiologists; BMI: Body mass index; BSA: Body surface area; CT: Computed tomography; DGE: Delayed gastric emptying; NSQIP: National Surgical Quality improvement Program criteria; PD: Pancreaticoduodenectomy; POPF: Postoperative pancreatic fistula; SMA: Skeletal muscle area

Acknowledgements
Not applicable.

Funding
This research has no specific grant from any funding agency in the public, commercial or not-for-profit sectors.

Authors' contributions
Study design: KT, RY, TY. Data collection and analysis: KT, RY, YU, DN, TK. Writing manuscript: KT, RY. Reviewing manuscript: TY, TF. All authors read and approved the final manuscript.

Competing interests
The authors declare that they have no competing interests.

References

1. Yoshioka R, Yasunaga H, Hasegawa K, Horiguchi H, Fushimi K, Aoki T, et al. Impact of hospital volume on hospital mortality, length of stay and total costs after pancreaticoduodenectomy. Br J Surg. 2014;101(5):523–9.
2. Kimura W, Miyata H, Gotoh M, Hirai I, Kenjo A, Kitagawa Y, et al. A pancreaticoduodenectomy risk model derived from 8575 cases from a national single-race population (Japanese) using a web-based data entry system: the 30-day and in-hospital mortality rates for pancreaticoduodenectomy. Ann Surg. 2014;259(4):773–80.
3. Okano K, Hirao T, Unno M, Fujii K, Yoshitomi H, Suzuki S, et al. Postoperative infectious complications after pancreatic resection. Br J Surg. 2015;102(12):1551–60.
4. Levolger S, van Vugt JL, de Bruin RW, IJzermans JN, et al. Systematic review of sarcopenia in patients operated on for gastrointestinal and hepatopancreatobiliary malignancies. Br J Surg. 2015;102(12):1448–58.
5. Sur MD, Namm JP, Hemmerich JA, Buschmann MM, Roggin KK, Dale W. Radiographic Sarcopenia and Self-reported Exhaustion Independently Predict NSQIP Serious Complications After Pancreaticoduodenectomy in Older Adults. Ann Surg Oncol. 2015;22(12):3897–904.
6. Kirihara Y, Takahashi N, Hashimoto Y, Sclabas GM, Khan S, Moriya T, et al. Prediction of pancreatic anastomotic failure after pancreatoduodenectomy: the use of preoperative, quantitative computed tomography to measure remnant pancreatic volume and body composition. Ann Surg. 2013;257(3):512–9.
7. Pecorelli N, Carrara G, De Cobelli F, Cristel G, Damascelli A, Balzano G, et al. Effect of sarcopenia and visceral obesity on mortality and pancreatic fistula following pancreatic cancer surgery. Br J Surg. 2016;103(4):434–42.
8. Nishida Y, Kato Y, Kudo M, Aizawa H, Okubo S, Takahashi D, et al. Preoperative Sarcopenia Strongly Influences the Risk of Postoperative Pancreatic Fistula Formation After Pancreaticoduodenectomy. J Gastrointest Surg. 2016;20(9):1586–94.
9. Child CG. Pancreaticojejunostomy and Other Problems Associated With the Surgical Management of Carcinoma Involving the Head of the Pancreas: Report of Five Additional Cases of Radical Pancreaticoduodenectomy. Ann Surg. 1944;119(6):845–55.
10. Matsuda H, Sadamori H, Umeda Y, Shinoura S, Yoshida R, Satoh D, et al. Preventive effect of omental flap in pancreaticoduodenectomy against postoperative pseudoaneurysm formation. Hepato-Gastroenterology. 2012;59(114):578–83.
11. Takagi K, Yagi T, Yoshida R, Shinoura S, Umeda Y, Nobuoka D, et al. Surgical Outcome of Patients Undergoing Pancreaticoduodenectomy: Analysis of a 17-Year Experience at a Single Center. Acta Med Okayama. 2016;70(3):197–203.
12. Mitsiopoulos N, Baumgartner RN, Heymsfield SB, Lyons W, Gallagher D, Ross R, et al. Cadaver validation of skeletal muscle measurement by magnetic resonance imaging and computerized tomography. J Appl Physiol (1985). 1998;85(1):115–22.
13. Takagi K, Yagi T, Yoshida R, Shinoura S, Umeda Y, Nobuoka D, et al. Sarcopenia and American Society of Anesthesiologists Physical Status in the Assessment of Outcomes of Hepatocellular Carcinoma Patients Undergoing Hepatectomy. Acta Med Okayama. 2016;70(5):363–70.
14. Takagi K, Yagi T, Yoshida R, Umeda Y, Nobuoka N, Kuise T, et al. Sarcopenia predicts postoperative infection in patients undergoing hepato-biliary-pancreatic surgery. Int J Surg Open. 2017;6:12–8.
15. Clavien PA, Barkun J, de Oliveira ML, Vauthey JN, Dindo D, Schulick RD, et al. The Clavien-Dindo classification of surgical complications: five-year experience. Ann Surg. 2009;250(2):187–96.
16. Bassi C, Dervenis C, Butturini G, Fingerhut A, Yeo C, Izbicki J, et al. Postoperative pancreatic fistula: an international study group (ISGPF) definition. Surgery. 2005;138(1):8–13.
17. Wente MN, Bassi C, Dervenis C, Fingerhut A, Gouma DJ, Izbicki JR, et al. Delayed gastric emptying (DGE) after pancreatic surgery: a suggested definition by the International Study Group of Pancreatic Surgery (ISGPS). Surgery. 2007;142(5):761–8.
18. Bilimoria KY, Liu Y, Paruch JL, Zhou L, Kmiecik TE, Ko CY, et al. Development and evaluation of the universal ACS NSQIP surgical risk calculator: a decision aid and informed consent tool for patients and surgeons. J Am Coll Surg. 2013;217(5):833–42.e1-3.
19. Pecorelli N, Balzano G, Capretti G, Zerbi A, Di Carlo V, Braga M. Effect of surgeon volume on outcome following pancreaticoduodenectomy in a high-volume hospital. J Gastrointest Surg. 2012;16(3):518–23.
20. Morley JE, Baumgartner RN, Roubenoff R, Mayer J, Nair KS. Sarcopenia. J Lab Clin Med. 2001;137(4):231–43.
21. Cruz-Jentoft AJ, Baeyens JP, Bauer JM, Boirie Y, Cederholm T, Landi F, et al. Sarcopenia: European consensus on definition and diagnosis: Report of the European Working Group on Sarcopenia in Older People. Age Ageing. 2010;39(4):412–23.
22. Rockwood K, Stadnyk K, MacKnight C, McDowell I, Hébert R, Hogan DB. A brief clinical instrument to classify frailty in elderly people. Lancet. 1999;353(9148):205–6.
23. Fried LP, Tangen CM, Walston J, Newman AB, Hirsch C, Gottdiener J, et al. Frailty in older adults: evidence for a phenotype. J Gerontol A Biol Sci Med Sci. 2001;56(3):M146–56.
24. Rockwood K, Song X, MacKnight C, Bergman H, Hogan DB, McDowell I, et al. A global clinical measure of fitness and frailty in elderly people. CMAJ. 2005;173(5):489–95.
25. Chen Y, Ou G, Lian G, Luo H, Huang K, Huang Y. Effect of Preoperative Biliary Drainage on Complications Following Pancreatoduodenectomy: A Meta-Analysis. Medicine (Baltimore). 2015;94(29):e1199.
26. Calvani R, Miccheli A, Landi F, Bossola M, Cesari M, Leeuwenburgh C, et al. Current nutritional recommendations and novel dietary strategies to manage sarcopenia. J Frailty Aging. 2013;2(1):38–53.
27. Denison HJ, Cooper C, Sayer AA, Robinson SM. Prevention and optimal management of sarcopenia: a review of combined exercise and nutrition interventions to improve muscle outcomes in older people. Clin Interv Aging. 2015;10:859–69.
28. Sudo T, Murakami Y, Uemura K, Hashimoto Y, Kondo N, Nakagawa N, et al. Perioperative antibiotics covering bile contamination prevent abdominal infectious complications after pancreatoduodenectomy in patients with preoperative biliary drainage. World J Surg. 2014;38(11):2952–9.
29. Tilg H, Moschen AR. Adipocytokines: mediators linking adipose tissue, inflammation and immunity. Nat Rev Immunol. 2006;6(10):772–83.
30. Lutz CT, Quinn LS. Sarcopenia, obesity, and natural killer cell immune senescence in aging: altered cytokine levels as a common mechanism. Aging (Albany NY). 2012;4(8):535–46.

22

Major postoperative complications are associated with impaired long-term survival after gastro-esophageal and pancreatic cancer surgery: a complete national cohort study

Eirik Kjus Aahlin[1,2*], Frank Olsen[3], Bård Uleberg[3], Bjarne K. Jacobsen[3,4] and Kristoffer Lassen[1,2]

Abstract

Background: Some studies have reported an association between complications and impaired long-term survival after cancer surgery. We aimed to investigate how major complications are associated with overall survival after gastro-esophageal and pancreatic cancer surgery in a complete national cohort.

Methods: All esophageal-, gastric- and pancreatic resections performed for cancer in Norway between January 1, 2008, and December 1, 2013 were identified in the Norwegian Patient Registry together with data concerning major postoperative complications and survival.

Results: When emergency cases were excluded, there were 1965 esophageal-, gastric- or pancreatic resections performed for cancer in Norway between 1 January 2008, and 1 December 2013. A total of 248 patients (12.6 %) suffered major postoperative complications. Complications were associated both with increased early (90 days) mortality (OR = 4.25, 95 % CI = 2.78–6.50), and reduced overall survival when patients suffering early mortality were excluded (HR = 1.23, 95 % CI = 1.01–1.50).

Conclusions: Major postoperative complications are associated with impaired long-term survival after gastro-esophageal and pancreatic cancer surgery.

Keywords: Postoperative complications, Surgery, Neoplasms

Background

Major complications after surgery have negative effects on health-related quality of life [1], length-of-stay [2] and resource utilization [2]. Major complications may preclude or delay adjuvant cancer treatment [3]. In addition, long-term survival may be negatively affected [4–7].

Khuri and co-workers [5] found that patients experiencing complications from surgery had a markedly reduced long-term survival even when those who died within 30 days after surgery were excluded from analysis. As summarized in a recent meta-analysis, these findings have been corroborated by several reports, but others again have failed to show this connection [6]. It has been suggested that major complications could have long-standing suppressive effects on a patient's immune system and thereby rendering them more susceptible to cancer recurrence [4, 5, 7–9].

Investigating a possible long-standing detrimental effect of postoperative complications on survival after cancer surgery is challenging: Major complications after modern surgery are relatively uncommon and therefore large cohorts are needed for analysis. There is no consensus on the correct cut-off for early mortality and there may be several factors that affect both susceptibility to complications and decreased overall survival - factors that have to

* Correspondence: eirik.kjus.aahlin@unn.no
[1]Department of GI and HPB surgery, University Hospital of Northern Norway, 9038 Breivika, Tromsø, Norway
[2]Department of Clinical Medicine, University of Tromsø - The Arctic University of Norway, Tromsø, Norway
Full list of author information is available at the end of the article

be adequately adjusted for. Naturally, an interventional trial is impossible to conduct.

Patient's level of education is a known indicator of important factors like physical activity and smoking habits [10], factors that are associated with both increased morbidity and impaired survival after surgery [11].

The aim of this study was to investigate whether major complications after gastro-esophageal and pancreatic surgery for cancer are associated with impaired long-term survival or early mortality only. We also aimed to investigate if such an association was influenced by patient's level of education.

Methods

Cohort identification

A database of surgical procedures, major postoperative complications and survival was extracted from the Norwegian Patient Registry (NPR). The Norwegian Patient Registry enables patients to be tracked from one stay to another, thus allowing for identification of an early complication occurring at a local hospital following transfer from a tertiary hospital where index surgery had been performed. All Norwegian hospitals must submit data to the Norwegian Patient Registry for registry and reimbursement purposes. In the present study, we included data from admissions during 2008–2013. Data on educational level were extracted from Statistics Norway, the Norwegian central bureau of statistics.

We identified all resections of the esophagus, stomach and pancreas in the six-year period from January 1, 2008 to December 1, 2013. Complications within 28 days after

surgery (to the end of 2013) are therefore included in the data material. Data on overall survival until June 30, 2014 were retrieved, thus even the last patient subject to surgery included would have seven months follow-up, if not dying. Operations and reoperations were identified from their Nomesco classification of Surgical Procedures (NCSP) code (2014). NCSP is available for download at http://www.nordclass.se/ncsp.htm.

Only cases with an appropriate cancer diagnosis (ICD-10: C15*, C16* and C25* respectively, where * denotes all sub-codes) applied within eight weeks from surgery were included. Emergency cases were excluded to obtain a cohort of patients that were reasonably fit at index surgery.

Overall survival was defined as survival from index surgery. Major complications were defined as equivalent to Accordion score IV or higher, equaling Clavien-Dindo score IIIb or higher [12, 13], i.e. a re-operation in general anesthesia for a complication, and/or single- or multiple organ failure [12]. We did not attempt to identify less severe complications, as these would be difficult to extract from Norwegian Patient Registry data.

All stays in this database (containing an eligible index operation) were coupled with any subsequent stay at any Norwegian hospital with an admission date within 28 days from discharge from the index stay. Hospital stays (single or coupled) containing one or more major complications were identified. This was done by identification of one of the following procedure codes at index or subsequent stay (NCSP): Reoperation for wound dehiscence (JWA00), for deep infection (JWC00/01), for deep hemorrhage (JWE00/01/02), for anastomotic dehiscence (JWF00/01), reoperation for other causes (JWW96/97/98)

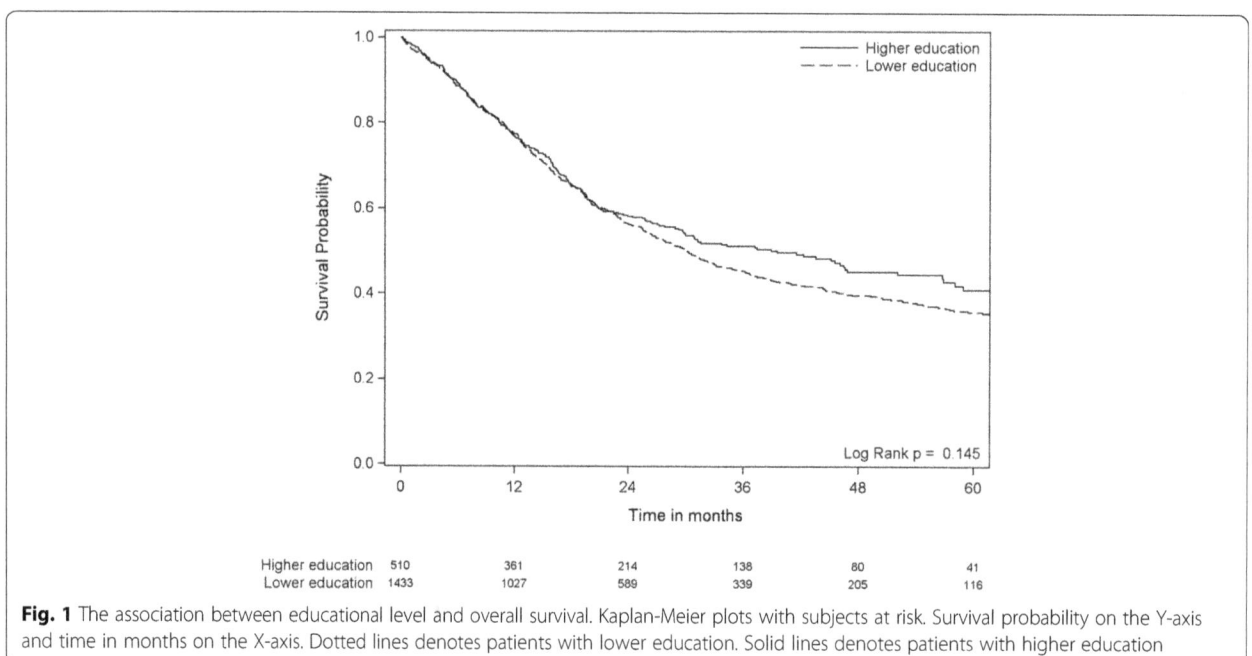

Fig. 1 The association between educational level and overall survival. Kaplan-Meier plots with subjects at risk. Survival probability on the Y-axis and time in months on the X-axis. Dotted lines denotes patients with lower education. Solid lines denotes patients with higher education

or if a tracheostomy was performed (GBB00/03). Also, a major complication was identified from the use of one of the following diagnoses during index or subsequent stays (ICD-10): Bleeding, hematoma or circulatory chock following a procedure (ICD-10: T81.0, T81.1, T81.3).

Validation of algorithm

The algorithms to identify complications were constructed in several wider variations and then validated against hand searched patient files. A tendency to over-score complications (identifying Accordion III or Clavien-Dindo IIIa as "major complications") when using the entire complications section (ICD-10: T81*) was avoided when some sub-codes (ICD-10: T81.2, T81.4, T81.5, T81.6, T81.7, T81.8 and T81.9) were removed from the algorithm. A comparison of the yield from our refined search strings with hand searched patient files in a four-year cohort at our own hospital (150 patients) showed a 100% match in both number of resections and rate of major complications (Accordion IV or higher).

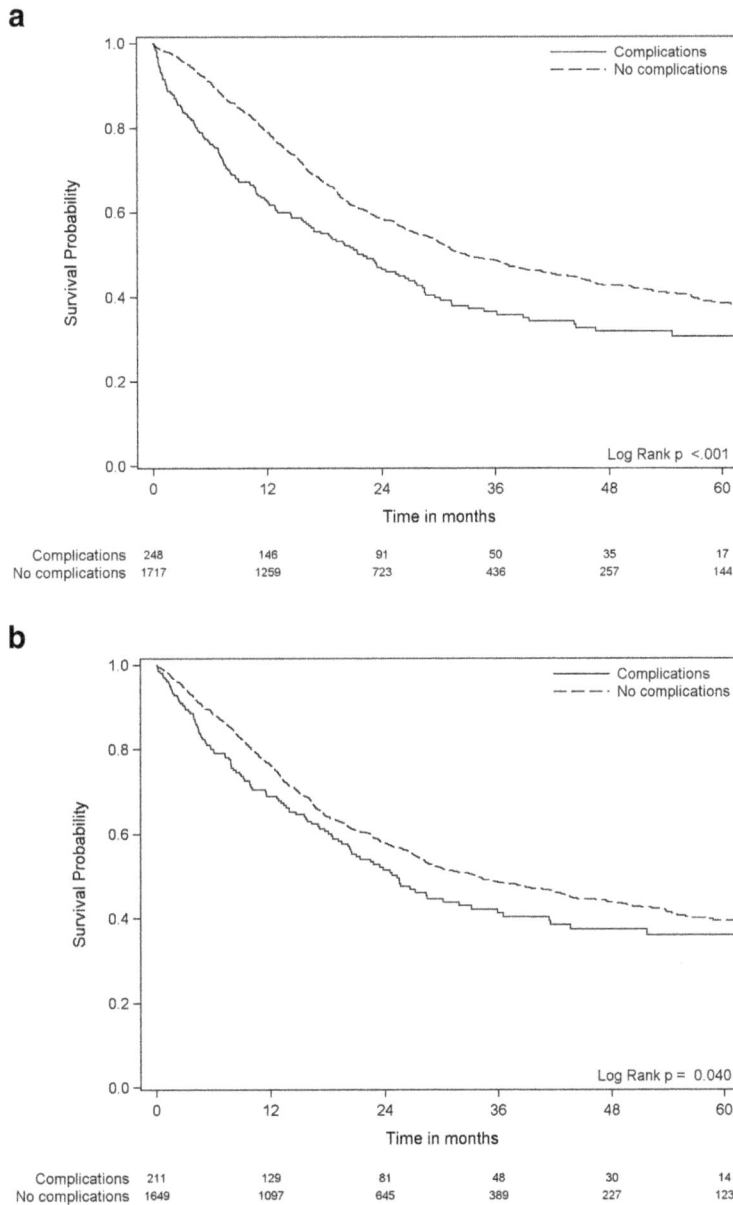

Fig. 2 The association between major postoperative complications and overall survival. Kaplan-Meier plots with subjects at risk. Survival probability on the Y-axis and time in months on the X-axis. Dotted lines denotes patients without any postoperative complications. Solid lines denotes patients who suffered one or more major postoperative complication. **a** All patients included. **b** Patients alive more than 90 days only

Table 1 Cohort characteristics: Number of patients, age, gender, educational level, percentage with complications and estimated median survival according to type of resection

	Esophageal resections	Gastric resections	Pancreatic resections	All patients
Number of patients	331	974	660	1965
Age above 65 years (%)	46.8	67.7	56.4	60.4
Male gender (%)	77.6	62.4	52.7	61.7
Lower educational level (%)	69.5	78.5	68.9	73.7
Complication-rate (%)	17.2	11.1	12.6	12.6
90-day mortality (%)	5.7	6.1	3.9	5.3
Estimated median survival in months	46	36	23	31

Definition of variables

Age at index surgery was analyzed both as a continuous variable and with a cut-off of 65 years. Educational level was divided into higher and lower education. Higher education was defined as education beyond primary and lower secondary school. Surgical resections were stratified into esophageal-, gastric- and pancreatic resections.

Statistics

Statistical analyses were performed with SAS statistics software, SAS Institute, Cary, NC, USA. For comparison of characteristics between different groups and categories, Student t-test for continuous data and Pearson chi-square test for categorical data were used. Logistic regression was used for analyzing associations between age, gender, educational level, type of resection and the risk of a major postoperative complication as well as early (90 days) mortality. Kaplan-Meier survival plots with log-rank test and Cox proportional hazard (PH) regression analysis were used for analysis of overall survival. Both methods were used, as the proportional hazards assumption for Cox regression (constant relative hazards over time) was not met when analyzing the relationships between educational level and survival (Fig. 1) and when analyzing the relationship between complications and survival (Fig. 2). Cox proportional hazard regression analysis using attained age as

the time variable was also used as a supplement, as the proportional hazards assumption was met in this situation. *P*-values according to the log-rank-test are given in the figures (the Kaplan-Meier survival plots) whereas p-value according to the Cox regression analyses (including the analyses adjusted for possible confounders) in Table 3. *P*-values <0.05 were considered statistically significant.

Ethics

Centre of Clinical Documentation and Evaluation has concession from the Norwegian Data Protection Authority and confidentiality exemption from the Regional Committee for Medical and Health Research Ethics (REK –Northern chapter). The concession provides access to unique personal data from Norwegian Patient Registry with information about patients treated at Norwegian hospitals in the period 2008–2013. Encrypted patient serial numbers makes it possible to describe patient pathways involving several hospitals and over several years. The concession also includes permission to pair education data from Statistics Norway.

Results
Patient selection and characteristics

A total of 3080 esophageal-, gastric and pancreatic resections were performed between 1January 2008 and

Table 2 Age, gender, educational level and type of resection, and association with major postoperative complications

Variable	Categories	Percentage[a]	OR (95 % CI)[b]	p-value
Age	Above 65 years	12.2	0.91 (0.70–1.20)	0.515
	65 years or less	13.2	1.0	
Gender	Male	13.7	1.29 (0.98–1.72)	0.071
	Female	10.9	1.0	
Educational level	Lower education	13.5	1.41 (1.02–1.95)	0.039
	Higher education	10.0	1.0	
Type of resection	Esophageal	17.2	1.67 (1.18–2.36)	0.004
	Pancreatic	12.6	1.15 (0.85–1.56)	0.358
	Gastric	11.1	1.0	

[a]Percentage that suffered one or more major postoperative complications
[b]Odds ratio, with 95 % confidence interval, for suffering one or more major postoperative complications

Table 3 The association between postoperative complications and overall survival, with hazard ratio (HR) and 95 % confidence interval (95 % CI)

	Unadjusted			Multivariable adjusted for age, gender and type of resection			Multivariable adjusted for age, gender, resection and educational level		
	HR	95 % CI	p-value	HR	95 % CI	p-value	HR	95 % CI	p-value
All patients	1.48	1.24–1.76	<0.001	1.51	1.27–1.79	<0.001	1.50	1.26–1.79	<0.001
Only patients alive >90 days	1.23	1.01–1.50	0.040	1.26	1.03–1.53	0.023	1.26	1.03–1.54	0.022

1December 2013. Of these, 2792 resections were scheduled. Of the 2792 scheduled resections, 1965 were performed for cancer; 331 esophageal resections (16.8 %), 974 gastric resections (49.6 %) and 660 pancreatic resections (33.6 %). Seventy percent of the gastric resections and almost all of the esophageal (99 %) and pancreatic resections (98 %) were performed at the six university hospitals (only four university hospitals perform esophageal resections). Forty percent of esophageal and half of the pancreatic resections were performed at Norway's largest hospital, Oslo University Hospital (OUS). Only 13% of the gastric resections were performed at OUS.

During the follow-up period, 975 (49.6 %) patients died. Median age at index operation was 68 years. A total of 248 patients (12.6 %) suffered one or more major postoperative complication and 37 (14.9 %) of these patients died within 90 days. Consequently, 1717 patients (87.4 %) did not suffer any major complications within 28 days after surgery and 68 (4.0 %) of these patients died within 90 days. Estimated median survival in the entire cohort was 31 months (Table 1) and the estimated five-year survival rate was 37.3 %.

Major postoperative complications
There were no statistically significant linear changes in the rate of complications from 2008 to 2013 (p = 0.319). The highest (17.2 %) and lowest (11.1 %) complication rate was seen in esophageal resections and gastric resections, respectively (Table 2). Type of resection and lower educational level (OR = 1.41, 95 % CI = 1.02–1.95, p = 0.039) were associated with major postoperative complications. The association with educational level was also present when adjusted for age, gender and type of resection (OR = 1.53, 95 % CI = 1.10–2.13, p = 0.013).

Early mortality
One-hundred-and-five (5.3 %) patients died within 90 days after surgery. Suffering one or more postoperative complications was strongly associated with 90-day mortality (OR = 4.25, 95 % CI = 2.78–6.50, p < 0.001).

Overall survival
There was no association between educational level and overall survival (p = 0.145) (Fig. 1) and this conclusion did not change after multivariable adjustment for age,

gender and type of resection (HR = 1.06, 95 % CI = 0.91–1.23, p = 0.475).

Postoperative complications were negatively associated with overall survival both with all patients included (Fig. 2, panel a) (p < 0.001) and when the first 90 days of the follow-up period (Fig. 2, panel b) (p = 0.040) were excluded. The survival curves (Fig. 2) suggest that the impact of major complications attenuate with time from the index surgery and p-value for interaction with time of follow up was <0.001. The estimated five-year survival rate was 38.2 % in patients who did not suffer any major postoperative complications compared to 30.6 % in patients who did. Major postoperative complications were associated with 23 % higher long term (i.e., excluding early) mortality (HR = 1.23, 95 % CI = 1.01–1.40, p = 0.040) (Table 3). Multivariable adjustment for age, gender, type of resection and educational level did not alter the association between major postoperative complications and overall survival (Table 3). Neither did use of attained age (instead of time in study) as the time variable in the Cox regression analysis. There were no significant interaction between type of resection and complications in the survival analysis, i.e., the association between complications and survival were not statistically significantly different according to type of resection. The association between postoperative complications and survival was similar across all types of resections (Fig. 3). Neither hospital volume (OUS vs. other university hospitals; analyzed for esophageal and pancreatic resections) or hospital teaching status (university hospital vs. non-university hospital; analyzed for gastric resections) did affect the association between complications and survival (data not shown).

Discussion
We present a complete national six-year cohort of gastro-esophageal and pancreatic resections for cancer in Norway with major complications and survival. Suffering one or more major postoperative complications was associated with both considerably increased early mortality and statistically significant decreased long-term survival. Educational level did not affect the relationship between complications and survival.

Several studies have demonstrated an association between postoperative complications and decreased survival [5, 6]. This has led to theories suggesting an immune-

a

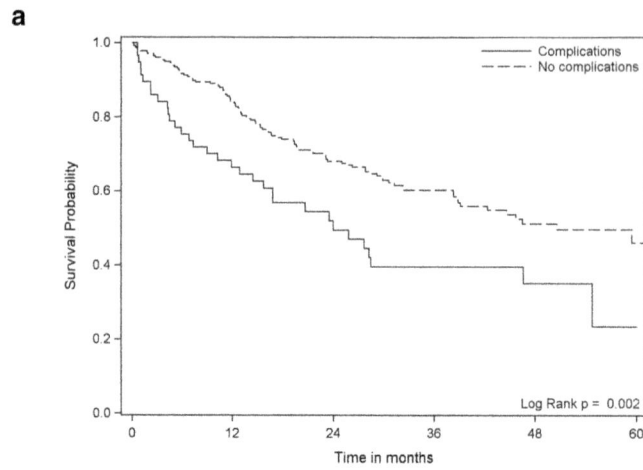

Complications   57   36   20   12   7   1
No complications 274   218   131   75   38   13

b

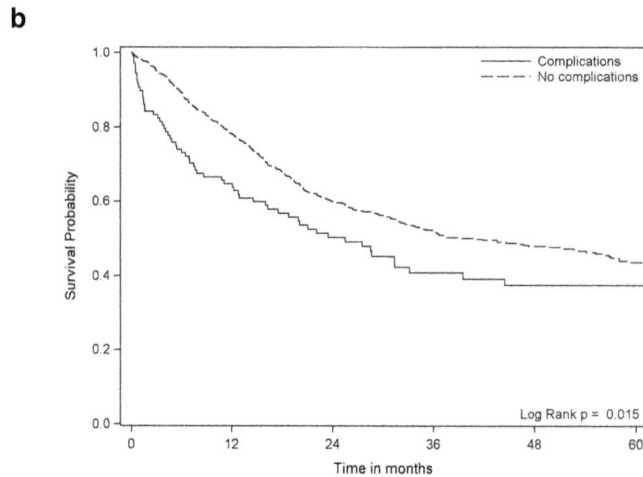

Complications   108   67   45   25   21   13
No complications 866   635   391   258   160   103

c

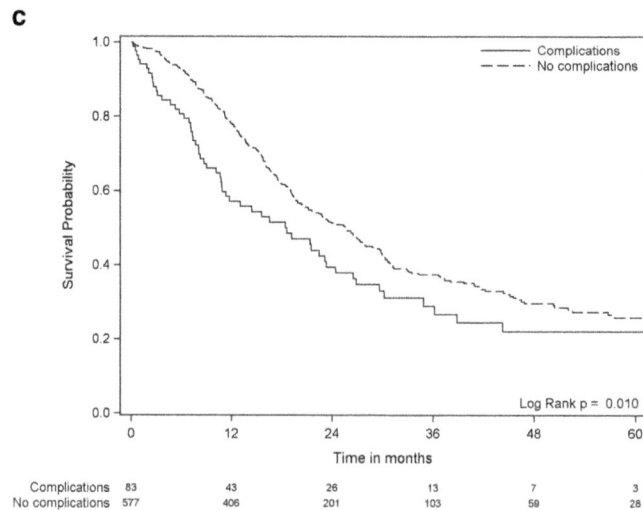

Complications   83   43   26   13   7   3
No complications 577   406   201   103   59   28

Fig. 3 (See legend on next page.)

(See figure on previous page.)

Fig. 3 The association between major postoperative complications and overall survival. Esophageal, gastric and pancreatic resections analyzed separately. Kaplan-Meier plots with subjects at risk. Survival probability on the Y-axis and time in months on the X-axis. Dotted lines denotes patients without any postoperative complications. Solid lines denotes patients who suffered one or more major postoperative complication. **a** Esophageal resections. **b** Gastric resections. **c** Pancreatic resections

suppressive effect of postoperative complications that might lead to cancer recurrence [5, 8, 9]. A recent meta-analysis reported a hazard ratio (HR) of 1.28 for decreased overall survival after any postoperative complication [6], the cut-offs for early mortality were not reported [6]. We found a similar risk of decreased survival associated with major complications if patients suffering early mortality were excluded (HR = 1.23). In this large, nationwide population-based cohort, we found some evidence to support theories concerning long-standing detrimental effects of complications on survival after gastro-esophageal and pancreatic cancer surgery.

Most studies exploring the issue of postoperative complications and long-term survival have either not used a cut-off at all or a 30-days mortality cut-off to exclude patients with fatal complications [5, 6, 8, 9]. Only a few studies report a cut-off for early mortality of 90-days [7]. Therefore, patients who died later than 30 days, but still arguably as a direct result of their complications may still have been included in the analysis, making it more difficult to address a possible long-standing detrimental effect of non-fatal complications.

Reductions in both overall survival and disease-free survival have been observed in colorectal cancer patients who suffered major complications [7, 8, 14]. In a large study of colon cancer patients, complications were associated with precluded or delayed adjuvant chemotherapy [3]. In the same study, complications were not associated with reduced survival if adjuvant chemotherapy were given within appropriate time-limits [3]. While chemotherapy is an important element to achieve increased survival in resectable stage III and IV colon cancer [15, 16], the effect of adjuvant chemotherapy on long-term survival in gastro-esophageal and pancreatic cancer is variable and less certain [17, 18].

The avoidance of postoperative complications is of utmost importance as complications adversely affect health-related quality of life [1] and survival [5, 6]. Complications may preclude or delay adjuvant chemotherapy [3]. Do complications make patients more susceptible to cancer recurrence and therefore cause decreased longevity? Large prospective registries with detailed information on disease-stage, comorbidity, time of recurrence and cause of death are needed to fully investigate this question. The registries used for our study contain complete national data and a large number of patients but lack information on cancer stage and disease-specific survival.

Conclusions

In a national setting, major postoperative complications are associated with both early mortality and decreased long-term survival after gastro-esophageal and pancreatic cancer surgery. Systematic quality improvement to avoid complications may improve the poor prognosis associated these cancers.

Abbreviations
NPR: Norwegian Patient Registry; NCSP: Nomesco Classification of Surgical Procedures; ICD-10: International Classification of Diseases, 10th edition; OUS: Oslo University Hospital.

Competing interests
The authors declare that they have no competing interests.

Authors' contributions
Study conception and design: EKA, BKJ, KL. Data acquisition: FO and BU. Data analysis: FO, BU, BKJ. Data interpretation and manuscript preparation, editing and final approval: All authors.

Acknowledgements
No additional investigators were involved in this research project.

Funding
This investigation and manuscript preparation received no external funding.

Author details
[1]Department of GI and HPB surgery, University Hospital of Northern Norway, 9038 Breivika, Tromsø, Norway. [2]Department of Clinical Medicine, University of Tromsø - The Arctic University of Norway, Tromsø, Norway. [3]Centre of Clinical Documentation and Evaluation, Northern Norway Regional Health Authority, Tromsø, Norway. [4]Department of Community Medicine, University of Tromsø - The Arctic University of Norway, Tromsø, Norway.

References
1. Brown SR, Mathew R, Keding A, et al. The impact of postoperative complications on long-term quality of life after curative colorectal cancer surgery. Ann Surg. 2014;259(5):916–23.
2. Knechtle WS, Perez SD, Medbery RL, et al. The Association Between Hospital Finances and Complications After Complex Abdominal Surgery: Deficiencies in the Current Health Care Reimbursement System and Implications for the Future. Ann Surg. 2015;262(2):273–9.
3. Krarup PM, Nordholm-Carstensen A, Jorgensen LN, et al. Anastomotic Leak Increases Distant Recurrence and Long-Term Mortality After Curative Resection for Colonic Cancer: A Nationwide Cohort Study. Ann Surg. 2014; 259(5):930–8.

4. Tokunaga M, Tanizawa Y, Bando E, et al. Poor survival rate in patients with postoperative intra-abdominal infectious complications following curative gastrectomy for gastric cancer. Ann Surg Oncol. 2013;20(5):1575–83.
5. Khuri SF, Henderson WG, DePalma RG, et al. Determinants of long-term survival after major surgery and the adverse effect of postoperative complications. Ann Surg. 2005;242(3):326–41.
6. Pucher PH, Aggarwal R, Qurashi M, et al. Meta-analysis of the effect of postoperative in-hospital morbidity on long-term patient survival. Br J Surg. 2014;101(12):1499–508.
7. Artinyan A, Orcutt ST, Anaya DA, et al. Infectious postoperative complications decrease long-term survival in patients undergoing curative surgery for colorectal cancer: a study of 12,075 patients. Ann Surg. 2015; 261(3):497–505.
8. Mavros MN, de Jong M, Dogeas E, et al. Impact of complications on long-term survival after resection of colorectal liver metastases. Br J Surg. 2013; 100(5):711–8.
9. Cho JY, Han HS, Yoon YS, et al. Postoperative complications influence prognosis and recurrence patterns in periampullary cancer. World J Surg. 2013;37(9):2234–41.
10. Isaacs SL, Schroeder SA. Class - the ignored determinant of the nation's health. N Engl J Med. 2004;351(11):1137–42.
11. Frederiksen BL, Osler M, Harling H, et al. The impact of socioeconomic factors on 30-day mortality following elective colorectal cancer surgery: a nationwide study. Eur J Cancer. 2009;45(7):1248–56.
12. Porembka MR, Hall BL, Hirbe M, et al. Quantitative weighting of postoperative complications based on the accordion severity grading system: demonstration of potential impact using the american college of surgeons national surgical quality improvement program. J Am Coll Surg. 2010;210(3):286–98.
13. Strasberg SM, Linehan DC, Hawkins WG. The accordion severity grading system of surgical complications. Ann Surg. 2009;250(2):177–86.
14. Mirnezami A, Mirnezami R, Chandrakumaran K, et al. Increased local recurrence and reduced survival from colorectal cancer following anastomotic leak: systematic review and meta-analysis. Ann Surg. 2011; 253(5):890–9.
15. Gill S, Loprinzi CL, Sargent DJ, et al. Pooled analysis of fluorouracil-based adjuvant therapy for stage II and III colon cancer: who benefits and by how much? J Clin Oncol. 2004;22(10):1797–806.
16. Nordlinger B, Sorbye H, Glimelius B, et al. Perioperative chemotherapy with FOLFOX4 and surgery versus surgery alone for resectable liver metastases from colorectal cancer (EORTC Intergroup trial 40983): a randomised controlled trial. Lancet. 2008;371(9617):1007–16.
17. Bringeland EA, Wasmuth HH, Fougner R, et al. Impact of perioperative chemotherapy on oncological outcomes after gastric cancer surgery. Br J Surg. 2014;101(13):1712–20.
18. Rustgi AK, El-Serag HB. Esophageal carcinoma. N Engl J Med. 2014;371(26): 2499–509.

Robotic versus laparoscopic distal pancreatectomy: an up-to-date meta-analysis

Gian Piero Guerrini[1,2]* 🅙, Andrea Lauretta[1], Claudio Belluco[1], Matteo Olivieri[1], Marco Forlin[1], Stefania Basso[1], Bruno Breda[1], Giulio Bertola[1] and Fabrizio Di Benedetto[2]

Abstract

Background: Laparoscopic distal pancreatectomy (LDP) reduces postoperative morbidity, hospital stay and recovery as compared with open distal pancreatectomy. Many authors believe that robotic surgery can overcome the difficulties and technical limits of LDP thanks to improved surgical manipulation and better visualization. Few studies in the literature have compared the two methods in terms of surgical and oncological outcome. The aim of this study was to compare the results of robotic (RDP) and laparoscopic distal pancreatectomy.

Methods: A systematic review and meta-analysis was conducted of control studies published up to December 2016 comparing LDP and RDP. Two Reviewers independently assessed the eligibility and quality of the studies. The meta-analysis was conducted using either the fixed-effect or the random-effect model.

Results: Ten studies describing 813 patients met the inclusion criteria. This meta-analysis shows that the RDP group had a significantly higher rate of spleen preservation [OR 2.89 (95% confidence interval 1.78-4.71, $p < 0.0001$], a lower rate of conversion to open OR 0.33 (95% CI 0.12-0.92), $p = 0.003$] and a shorter hospital stay [MD -0.74; (95% CI -1.34 -0.15), $p = 0.01$] but a higher cost than the LDP group, while other surgical outcomes did not differ between the two groups.

Conclusion: This meta-analysis suggests that the RDP procedure is safe and comparable in terms of surgical results to LDP. However, even if the RDP has a higher cost compared to LDP, it increases the rate of spleen preservation, reduces the risk of conversion to open surgery and is associated to shorter length of hospital stay.

Keywords: Pancreatic cancer, Distal pancreatectomy, Left pancreatectomy, Pancreatic resection, Robotic surgery, Laparoscopic surgery, Review, Meta-analysis

Background

Distal pancreatectomy (DP) is the mainstay surgical procedure for the treatment of body-tail tumors of the pancreas [1]. This type of surgery, generally performed through an open access, a fairly common but potentially demanding procedure, is still burdened with a significant morbidity and mortality up of 5% [2, 3].

Laparoscopic distal pancreatectomy (LDP) is a relatively new procedure as compared with the well-established open distal pancreatectomy [4, 5]. The first

LDP was in fact performed by Cuscheri in 1996 [6]. Since many authors still consider LDP to be a complex operation because of technical problems linked to the vascular control and dissection of the pancreatic gland that is deeply located in the retroperitoneum, this has resulted in a delay in the spread of LDP when compared to other mini-invasive surgical operations. Thanks to the improvement of technology and the experience gained in laparoscopic surgery, it has been shown that LDP has achieved oncological results comparable to open surgery, with an overlapping rate of morbidity, but with the advantage of small surgical incisions, shorter hospital stay and faster recovery [7–10].

The exceptional development of computer technology and its consequent biomedical applications have enabled

* Correspondence: guerrinigp@yahoo.it
[1]Department of Surgical Oncology. Surgical oncology Unit, National Cancer institute-Centro di Riferimento Oncologico IRCCS, Aviano (PN), Italy
[2]Hepato-Pancreato-Biliary Surgery and Liver Transplantation Unit, University of Modena and Reggio Emilia, Modena, Italy

the creation of robotic surgery. Robotic distal pancreatectomy (RDP) is the most recent frontier of minimally invasive surgery applied to the surgical treatment of pancreatic tumors [11, 12]. RDP was first performed by Melvin in 2003 [13].

Robotic surgery has theoretically made it possible to overcome the disadvantages of the laparoscopic approach to the pancreas. In fact, it allows optimal viewing through a three dimensional high definition surgical view, tremor filtration, large range of motion due to an internal articulated endo-wrist, all associated with remarkable ergonomics for the surgeon who performs the procedure [14].

Nevertheless, robotic procedures seem to be longer and have higher costs without a clear advantage in terms of surgical and oncologic outcomes [14, 15]. No randomized controlled trials (RCTs) comparing RDP and LDP have been published on this issue, only retrospective studies [16–26]. Moreover, none of these has reached a uniform conclusion in terms of efficacy and safety [27]. We therefore performed a systematic review and meta-analysis in order to compare the results of laparoscopic vs robotic distal pancreatectomy.

Methods
Literature search strategies and study selection
A systematic literature search was conducted independently by two authors (G.G. and A.L.) using the methods of the Cochrane collaboration. We searched the National library of Medicine (Medline, https://www.ncbi.nlm.nih.gov/pubmed/), the Cochrane central register of controlled trials (Cochrane library www.cochrane.org), and Embase (https://www.embase.com/login) for relevant articles published from January 1980 through December 2016.

The search strategy was set up using the key words or text words combined with a Mesh (Medical subject headings) database search. The terms used were: "Distal pancreatectomy", "Pancreatectomy", "Laparoscopic" and "robotic" with limitation of clinical studies and humans. The search was exploded using the related article term in Pubmed. In addition, the references of searched articles were manually cross-searched for additional publications, and captured citations were filtered for study design in order to identify all control studies. All data extraction was performed in duplicate. We included studies with more than five patients in each arm for comparison of clinical outcomes. Narrative reviews, case series or studies without matched groups were excluded. No unpublished data, or non-English manuscripts or data were used.

The methodological quality of case-control and cohort studies was assessed using the Newcastle-Ottawa scale [28]. Only studies that reached six points or more were considered qualitatively eligible for meta-analysis. To select the titles of relevant studies, abstracts and full text articles were screened.

Quality assessment of the studies and inclusion criteria
We planned to include only randomized controlled trials (RCTs) in this review. However, we found no RCTs on the topic, so we performed a meta-analysis of observational studies. We included studies reported as full text, and studies published as abstract only. All studies with Robotic and Laparoscopic pancreatectomy were considered. Any etiology for distal pancreatectomy was eligible and there were no limitations because of race, gender or age. Two investigators independently reviewed the articles for eligibility and extracted data for the analysis. Any disagreement was resolved through discussion and consensus of the study team. The PRISMA criteria for reporting meta-analyses were used as guidelines in the construction of this analysis [29].

Distal pancreatectomy-related morbidities, such as pancreatic fistula (PF), bleeding rate and all Clavien-Dindo complications grade III or more were used as measures of outcome. Surgical results such as conversion rate, spleen preservation, operative time, length of hospital stay, oncological parameters, cost of operation were principal parameter analyzed in this the meta-analysis.

Data analysis was performed using the software Review Manager (RevMan) [Version 5.1. Copenhagen: The Nordic Cochrane Centre, The Cochrane Collaboration, 2011) and Metanalysis (Tecnopharma 2004 Italy). Results of the meta-analysis are presented as odds ratios (OR) with 95% confidence intervals (CI). The OR was used for dichotomous outcomes as the confirmatory effect size estimate. Continuous variables were analyzed using the weighted mean difference (WMD) with 95% CI. P values of < 0.05 were considered statistically significant. Heterogeneities of treatment effects between the trials were tested using Q statistics and total variation across studies was estimated by I2. A fixed-effect model was adopted if there was no statistically significant heterogeneity in this analysis. If the results of trials had heterogeneity $I^2 > 50\%$, a random-effects model was applied, such as the DerSimonian-Laird method [30]. Potential publication bias was determined by conducting informal visual inspection of the funnel plot, but also using quantitative methods such as the test for asymmetry of the funnel plot.

Definition of complications
Pancreatic fistula (PF) was defined as an amylase-rich fluid from the drain at biochemical evaluation or abnormal communication between the drain and the pancreatic anastomosis seen with fistulography. More recent studies used the definition of pancreatic fistula proposed by the International Study Group on Pancreatic Fistula (ISGPF), where the pancreatic fistula is defined as an output of any measurable volume of fluid

with an amylase content greater than 3 times the upper normal serum value via an operatively (or subsequently) placed drain on or after postoperative day 3 [31]. Postoperative morbidity was defined as any complication in agreement with the Dindo classification [32]. Perioperative mortality was defined as death during the same hospital stay or within 90 days after discharge if the patient was discharged earlier.

Results

Included studies and patient characteristics

The initial search strategy retrieved 844 publications relevant to search words (Fig. 1). After screening all titles and abstracts, a total of 34 full papers were captured, of which 24 were excluded because of missing inclusion criteria. Ten comparative studies were identified for inclusion. The features and quality of the included studies are summarized in Table 1.

Ten studies describing 813 patients were identified for the meta-analysis Table 2. A total of 267 patients underwent robotic distal pancreatectomy and 546 patients laparoscopic distal pancreatectomy. The two groups were similar as regards demographics (age, body mass index (BMI), gender), comorbidities (American Society of Anesthesiologist score) and

pathological characteristics. The number of patients in each study ranged from a minimum of 8 up to 140.

Pancreatic fistula

A fixed-effect model comparing the pancreatic fistula rate after RDP and LDP is shown in Fig. 2. At an Odds Ratio of 1 (central line) there is no difference in the rate of pancreatic fistula between the RDP and LDP groups. Values greater than one represent an increased risk for pancreatic fistula in the Laparoscopic group, while a value less than 1 indicates a reduction in the risk of pancreatic fistula in favor of the Robotic group. A total of 768 patients were included in 9 articles. The rate of pancreatic fistula in the RDP group and LDP group was 30.3% (75/247) and 33.5% (175/521), respectively. The overall pooled results by meta-analysis revealed an OR 0.968 (95% confidence interval 0.66–1.39, $p = 0.84$). The funnel plot showed basic symmetry and the test for the asymmetry applied to the funnel plot was $\alpha = 0.24$, $p = 0.66$ which suggested no publication bias. Specific subgroup analysis was performed in 6 studies that used a standard definition of pancreatic fistula according to the ISGPF classification. The rate of pancreatic fistula was 28.5% in (52/182) in RDP and 28.4% (98/345) in LDP. Meta-analysis showed no differences in the subgroups (OR 0.93 $p = 0.75$).

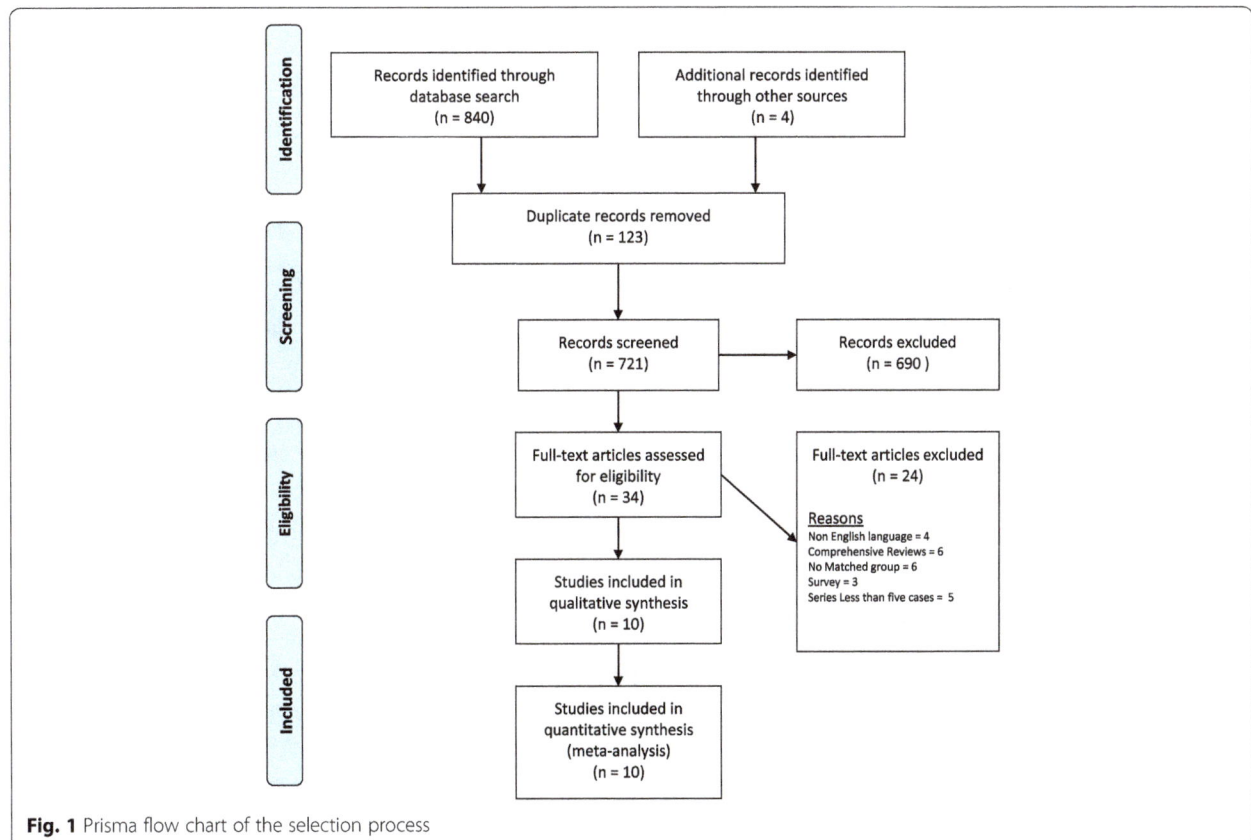

Fig. 1 Prisma flow chart of the selection process

Table 1 Scale assessment of the quality of the studies

Author	Publication Year	Country	Study	Robotic distal pancreatectomy n	Laparoscopic distal pancreatectomy n	Newcastle – Ottawa scale Selection/comparability/ Exposure = total score
Balzano [16]	2014	Italy	Retrospective-Multicenter	31	140	4 / 1 / 2 = 7
Butturini [25]	2015	Italy	Prospective	22	21	4 / 2 / 2 = 8
Chen [17]	2015	China	Prospective	69	50	4 / 2 / 2 = 8
Daouadi [18]	2013	USA	Retrospective	30	94	4 / 2 / 2 = 8
Duran [19]	2014	Spain	Retrospective	16	18	4 / 2 / 2 = 8
Goh [20]	2015	Singapore	Retrospective	8	31	4 / 2 / 2 = 8
Kang [22]	2011	Korea	Retrospective	20	25	4 / 2 / 2 = 8
Lai [23]	2015	China	Retrospective	17	18	4 / 1 / 2 = 7
Lee [24]	2014	USA	Retrospective	37	131	4 / 2 / 2 = 8
Waters [26]	2010	USA	Retrospective	17	18	4 / 2 / 2 = 8

Conversion rate

Eight studies involving 733 patients reported the conversion rate. The conversion Rate in the RDP and LDP groups was 8.2% (19/230) and 21.6% (109/503), respectively. Meta-analysis showed a significant difference in the rate of the conversion between the two groups, with a lower rate in the RDP group (OR 0.33; 95% CI, 0.12–0.92, $p = 0.03$), Fig. 3.

Spleen preservation rate

A total of 479 patients were included in 7 retrospective studies. Spleen conservation rate in the RDP and LDP groups was 48.9% (106/198) and 27% (76/281), respectively. Meta-analysis showed a significant difference in the rate of spleen preservation between the two groups with a higher rate in the RDP group (OR 2.89; 95% CI, 1.78–4.71, $p < 0.0001$), Fig. 4.

Major morbidity (Clavien-Dindo classification ≥ III)

Nine studies involving 637 patients reported morbidity. The morbidity of the RDP and LDP groups was

16% (3/246) and 17% (67/391), respectively. Meta-analysis showed no significant difference in the rate of morbidity between the two groups (OR 1.19, 95% CI 0.73–1.91, $p = 0.52$), whereas 90-day mortality accounted for 1 death in both groups.

Bleeding

The bleeding rate in the RDP and LDP groups was 8.2% (13/157) and 11% (23/5208), respectively. Meta-analysis of five trials showed no significant difference in the rate between the RDP and LDP groups (OR 0.8; 95% CI 0.41–1.79, $p = 0.621$).

Oncologic parameters

Seven of nine studies reported the R0 margin status and six studies reported the number of harvested lymph nodes. All surgical specimens of RDP reported R0 negative margins, while 1% of LDP were diagnosed with positive margins. Five studies reported higher numbers of harvested lymph nodes in the RDP group, while two studies showed a higher number of lymph nodes in the

Table 2 Characteristic of included studies comparing robotic vs laparoscopic distal pancreatectomy, NA not reported

Author	Number of patients RDP vs LDP	Age RDP vs LDP	Female (%) RDP vs LDP	ASA (mean) RDP vs LDP	BMI RDP vs LDP	Malignant (%) RDP vs LDP
Balzano [16]	31 vs 140	Na	NA	NA	Na	18 vs 16
Butturini [25]	22 vs 21	54 vs 55	77 vs 71	1.91 vs 1.76	25.3 vs 24.1	13.6 vs 9.5
Chen [17]	69 vs 50	56.2 vs 56.5	67 vs 64	1.9 vs 1.94	24.6 vs 24.6	23.2 vs 22
Daouadi [18]	30 vs 94	59 vs 59	67 vs 65	2.9 vs 3.2	27.9 vs 29	43 vs 14
Duran [19]	16 vs 18	61 vs 58.3	44 vs 50	2 vs 1.9	Na	56 vs 44
Goh [20]	8 vs 31	57 vs 56	75 vs 62	1.2 vs 1	27.6 vs 23.9	0 vs 12.9
Kang [22]	20 vs 25	44.5 vs 56.5	60 vs 56	NA	24.1 vs 23.4	0 vs 48
Lai [23]	17 vs 18	61.2 vs 63.2	41 vs 78	NA	24.1 vs 25.7	64.7 vs 77.7
Lee [24]	37 vs 131	58 vs 58	73 vs 56	2.5 vs 3	28.7 vs 28.2	10.8 vs 14.5
Waters [26]	17 vs 18	64 vs 55	65 vs 50	2.9 vs 2.8	NA	29 vs 28

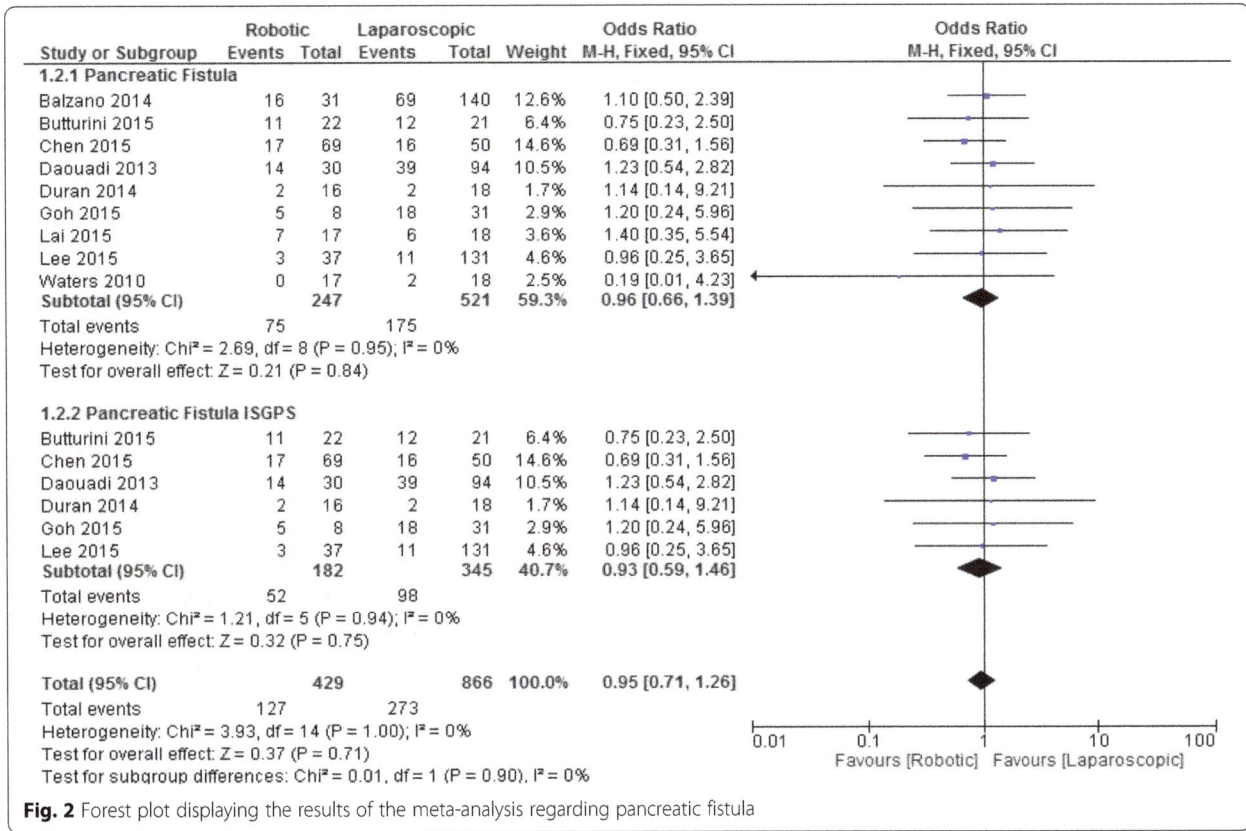

Fig. 2 Forest plot displaying the results of the meta-analysis regarding pancreatic fistula

LDP group (Table 3). Meta-analysis of the oncological variable could not be performed because of the impossibility to retrieve the standard deviation from the studies.

Length of hospital stay
Eight studies reported the length of hospital stay. The mean hospital stay was 7.18 days in the RDP group and 9.08 in the LDP group. Meta-analysis showed that the hospital stay was slightly shorter in the RDP group than

in the LDP group with statistic significant difference (mean difference = -0.7495% CI -1.34 -0.15; $p = 0.01$), Fig. 5.

Cost of the operation
Three studies reported cost analysis. Meta-analysis showed that the cost of the operation was higher in RDP group (Standard mean difference 5.24, 95% CI 3.52 -6.95, $p < 0.00001$), Fig. 6.

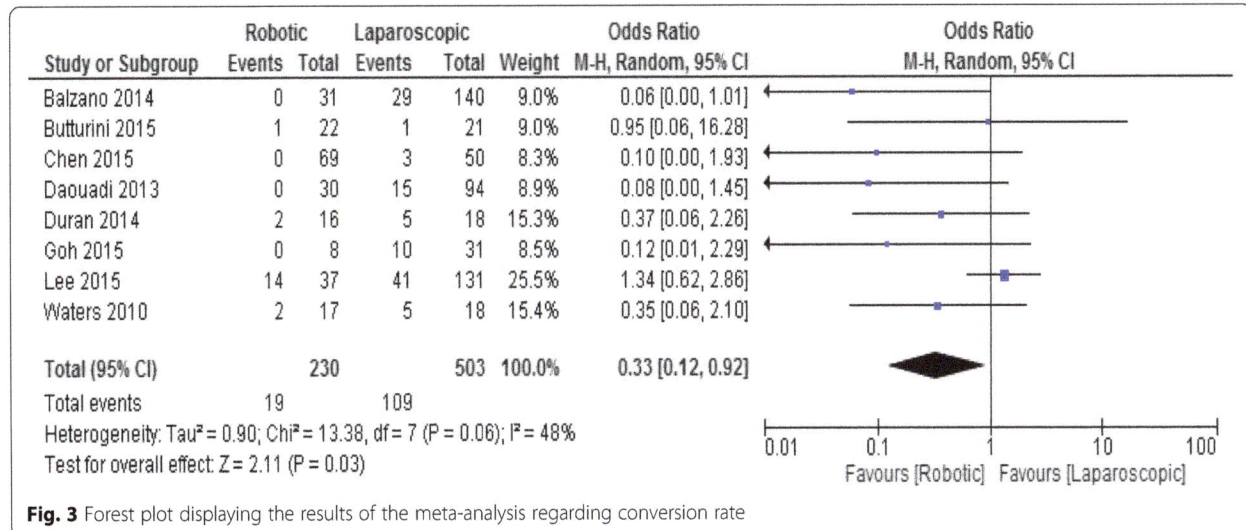

Fig. 3 Forest plot displaying the results of the meta-analysis regarding conversion rate

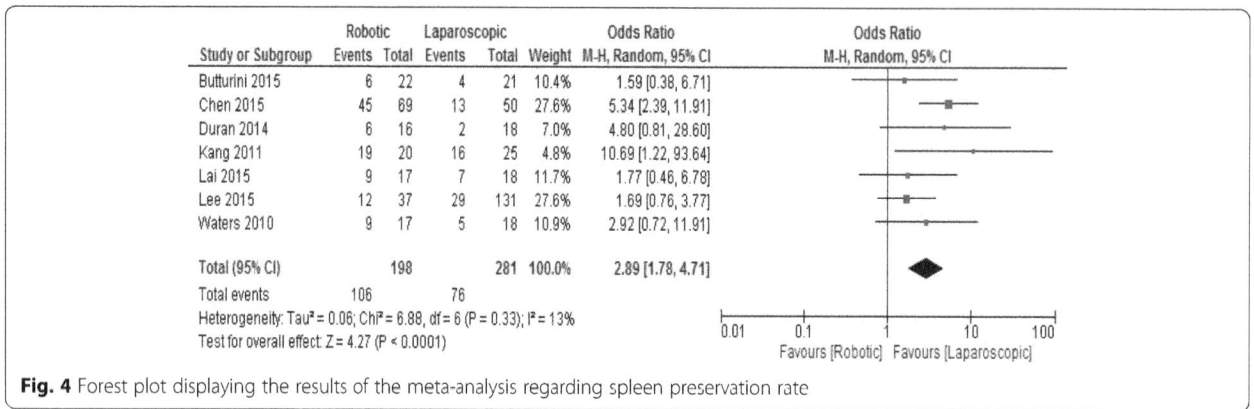

Study or Subgroup	Robotic Events	Total	Laparoscopic Events	Total	Weight	Odds Ratio M-H, Random, 95% CI
Butturini 2015	6	22	4	21	10.4%	1.59 [0.38, 6.71]
Chen 2015	45	69	13	50	27.6%	5.34 [2.39, 11.91]
Duran 2014	6	16	2	18	7.0%	4.80 [0.81, 28.60]
Kang 2011	19	20	16	25	4.8%	10.69 [1.22, 93.64]
Lai 2015	9	17	7	18	11.7%	1.77 [0.46, 6.78]
Lee 2015	12	37	29	131	27.6%	1.69 [0.76, 3.77]
Waters 2010	9	17	5	18	10.9%	2.92 [0.72, 11.91]
Total (95% CI)		198		281	100.0%	2.89 [1.78, 4.71]
Total events	106		76			
Heterogeneity: Tau² = 0.06; Chi² = 6.88, df = 6 (P = 0.33); I² = 13%						
Test for overall effect: Z = 4.27 (P < 0.0001)						

Fig. 4 Forest plot displaying the results of the meta-analysis regarding spleen preservation rate

Operative time

Eight studies reported the operative time which was respectively 262.8 min in the RDP group and 233.2 in the LDP group. The difference between the two groups was not statistic significant (mean difference = 26.91 95% CI -11.8 + 65.6; $p = 0.17$), Fig. 7.

Discussion

This meta-analysis demonstrates the safety and feasibility of the robotic approach to distal pancreatectomy. Specifically, the results of our study reveal that RDP does not increase the rate of post-operative complications, is associated to higher rate of spleen preservation, reduces hospital stay and decreases conversion rate.

Many studies of minimally invasive distal pancreatectomy have been published in the literature, highlighting the increasing surgical community interest in this new technique [33, 34].

Several studies have compared open versus laparoscopic distal pancreatectomy, demonstrating the superiority of the latter in terms of less blood loss, faster recovery and less hospital stay [10, 35–37].

Robotic surgery is the latest development of mini-invasive surgery of the pancreas. This technology maintains the advantages of laparoscopic technique in terms of smaller surgical scars and faster functional recovery, but adds the specific advantages of robotic surgery; in fact, thanks to the stability of articulated instruments and magnification of the 3D high definition view, the robot allows more complex surgical operations to be performed. This added value of RDP could increase the chance to increase the rate of spleen preservation [38, 39].

This meta-analysis shows that the RDP increases the rate of splenic preservation; in fact, 7 studies indicated a better spleen preservation rate through robotic surgery. The preservation of the spleen has been shown to be important in preventing postoperative complications and particularly the overwhelming post-splenectomy infection syndrome. The preservation of the spleen, however, depends not only on technical factors but primarily on the indication for pancreatectomy. In fact, malignant tumors are not an indication for the conservation of the spleen, which is instead generally taken into account for benign or neuroendocrine tumors [40]. Two spleen-

Table 3 Oncological characteristic of study population

Author	Lymph nodes Harvested Number LDP vs RDP	Rate of R1 resection Number of patients (% percentage) LDP vs RDP	Tumor size Centimeter (cm) LDP vs RDP
Balzano [16]	NA	NA	NA
Butturini [25]	15 (1–47 range) vs 11.5 (0–37)	0 vs 0	3.45 (1.5–1.7) vs 2.5 (0.5–9)
Chen [17]	9 vs 15	0 vs 0	3.5 (2.5–4 IQ) vs 3.5(2.1–3.5 IQ)
Daouadi [18]	9 (7–11 IQ) vs 19 (17–24 IQ)	5 (36) vs 0	3.4 ± 1.6 vs 3.1 ± 1.7
Duran [19]	5 ± 2 vs 12.5 ± 7.2	0 vs 0	4.1 ± 2.3 vs 2.9 ± 1.6
Goh [20]	NA	1(3.2) vs 1(12.5)	2.5 (0.8–7) vs 3 (1–6.9)
Kang [22]	NA	NA	3.0 ± 1.4 vs 3.5 ± 1.3
Lai [23]	NA	NA	NA
Lee [24]	10 ± 8 vs 12 ± 7	0 vs 0	NA
Waters [26]	11 vs 5	0 vs 0	3 ± 1 vs 2 ± 1

NA not reported

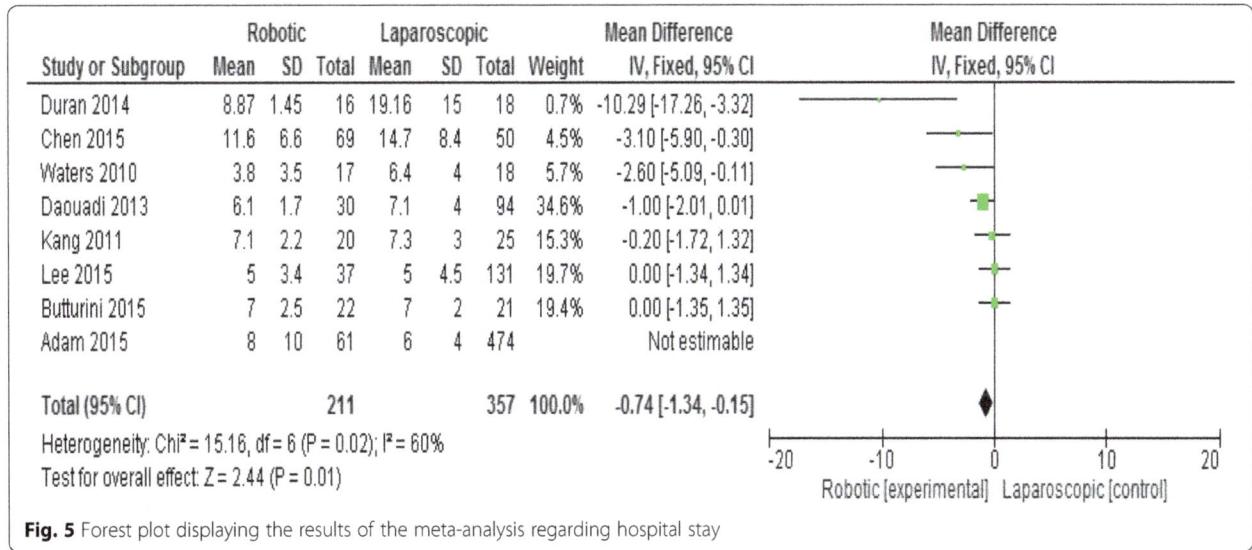

Study or Subgroup	Robotic Mean	SD	Total	Laparoscopic Mean	SD	Total	Weight	Mean Difference IV, Fixed, 95% CI
Duran 2014	8.87	1.45	16	19.16	15	18	0.7%	-10.29 [-17.26, -3.32]
Chen 2015	11.6	6.6	69	14.7	8.4	50	4.5%	-3.10 [-5.90, -0.30]
Waters 2010	3.8	3.5	17	6.4	4	18	5.7%	-2.60 [-5.09, -0.11]
Daouadi 2013	6.1	1.7	30	7.1	4	94	34.6%	-1.00 [-2.01, 0.01]
Kang 2011	7.1	2.2	20	7.3	3	25	15.3%	-0.20 [-1.72, 1.32]
Lee 2015	5	3.4	37	5	4.5	131	19.7%	0.00 [-1.34, 1.34]
Butturini 2015	7	2.5	22	7	2	21	19.4%	0.00 [-1.35, 1.35]
Adam 2015	8	10	61	6	4	474		Not estimable
Total (95% CI)			211			357	100.0%	-0.74 [-1.34, -0.15]

Heterogeneity: Chi² = 15.16, df = 6 (P = 0.02); I² = 60%
Test for overall effect: Z = 2.44 (P = 0.01)

Fig. 5 Forest plot displaying the results of the meta-analysis regarding hospital stay

preservation surgical techniques have been described: the Kimura [41] and the Warshaw method [42]. In the Kimura's technique the artery and splenic vein are skeletonized and preserved in order to maintain the vascular flow to the spleen. The Warshaw method consists in the section of splenic vessels while preserving short gastric vessels and left gastroepiplonic artery, which provide adequate vascular flow to the spleen. This second technique seems to increase the risk of spleen infarction. The studies considered in our review do not provide the details of the surgical technique used to preserve the spleen and therefore a comparison between the two methods has not been performed [43].

With regard to overall postoperative complications, these were similar between two groups. The most frequently reported complication was intra-abdominal fluid collection. However, severe complications, defined as Dindo-Clavien ≥ 3, were similar in the two groups, as was the reported mortality.

The pancreatic fistula is still the Achilles heel of pancreatic surgery [44–46]. This complication remains a very serious problem because it increases morbidity and lengthens hospital stay. Regardless of the technique used to cut and close the pancreatic stump, the incidence of postoperative pancreatic fistula varies from 0 to 47% [47]. A recent meta-analysis compared different methods of treating pancreatic parenchyma after distal pancreatectomy, but none of the techniques used was superior to the others in reducing the incidence of pancreatic fistula [48]. In this meta-analysis, nine studies compared the rate of pancreatic fistula between RDP and LDP failing to show any significant differences. In particular, the rate of severe pancreatic fistulas grade B / C was not statistically different between the two groups.

Blood transfusion during surgery for malignant disease is associated with an increased risk of long-term relapse [49]. In the meta-analysis we did not observe statistically significant differences in the rate of blood transfusions between the two groups.

In relation to oncological parameters, we did not observe significant differences in the considered studies. It was interesting to note that the surgical margins were

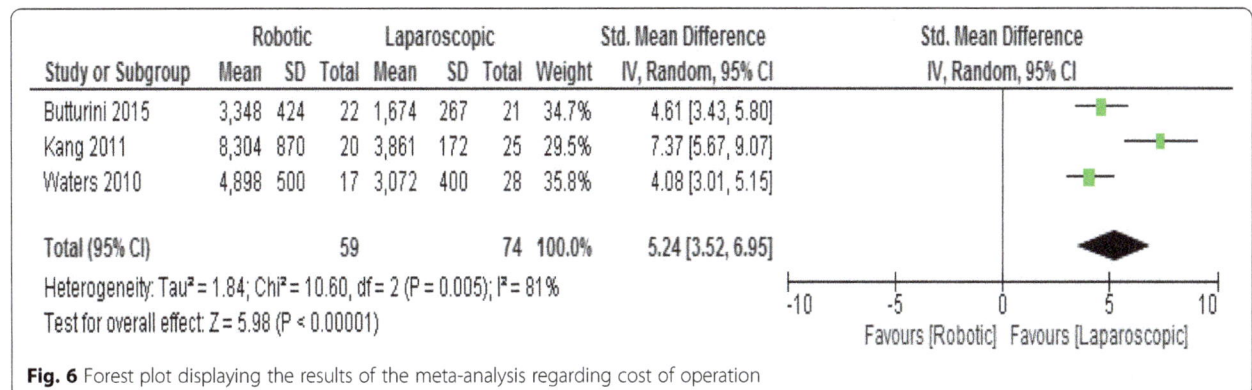

Study or Subgroup	Robotic Mean	SD	Total	Laparoscopic Mean	SD	Total	Weight	Std. Mean Difference IV, Random, 95% CI
Butturini 2015	3,348	424	22	1,674	267	21	34.7%	4.61 [3.43, 5.80]
Kang 2011	8,304	870	20	3,861	172	25	29.5%	7.37 [5.67, 9.07]
Waters 2010	4,898	500	17	3,072	400	28	35.8%	4.08 [3.01, 5.15]
Total (95% CI)			59			74	100.0%	5.24 [3.52, 6.95]

Heterogeneity: Tau² = 1.84; Chi² = 10.60, df = 2 (P = 0.005); I² = 81%
Test for overall effect: Z = 5.98 (P < 0.00001)

Fig. 6 Forest plot displaying the results of the meta-analysis regarding cost of operation

Study or Subgroup	Robotic			Laparoscopic			Weight	Mean Difference IV, Random, 95% CI	Mean Difference IV, Random, 95% CI
	Mean	SD	Total	Mean	SD	Total			
Butturini 2015	265	70	22	195	60	21	12.9%	70.00 [31.09, 108.91]	
Chen 2015	150	80	69	200	90	50	13.5%	-50.00 [-81.28, -18.72]	
Daouadi 2013	293	93	30	372	141	94	12.5%	-79.00 [-122.82, -35.18]	
Duran 2014	315	62	16	250	45	18	13.1%	65.00 [28.19, 101.81]	
Kang 2011	348	121.8	20	258	118.6	25	9.9%	90.00 [19.21, 160.79]	
Lai 2015	221	73.2	17	173.6	45.6	18	12.8%	47.40 [6.72, 88.08]	
Lee 2015	213	55.7	37	193	45.3	131	14.3%	20.00 [0.45, 39.55]	
Waters 2010	298	98.5	17	224	79	18	11.0%	74.00 [14.63, 133.37]	
Total (95% CI)			228			375	100.0%	26.91 [-11.83, 65.65]	

Heterogeneity: Tau² = 2631.91; Chi² = 59.54, df = 7 (P < 0.00001); I² = 88%
Test for overall effect: Z = 1.36 (P = 0.17)

-100   -50   0   50   100
Favours [Robotic] Favours [Laparoscopic]

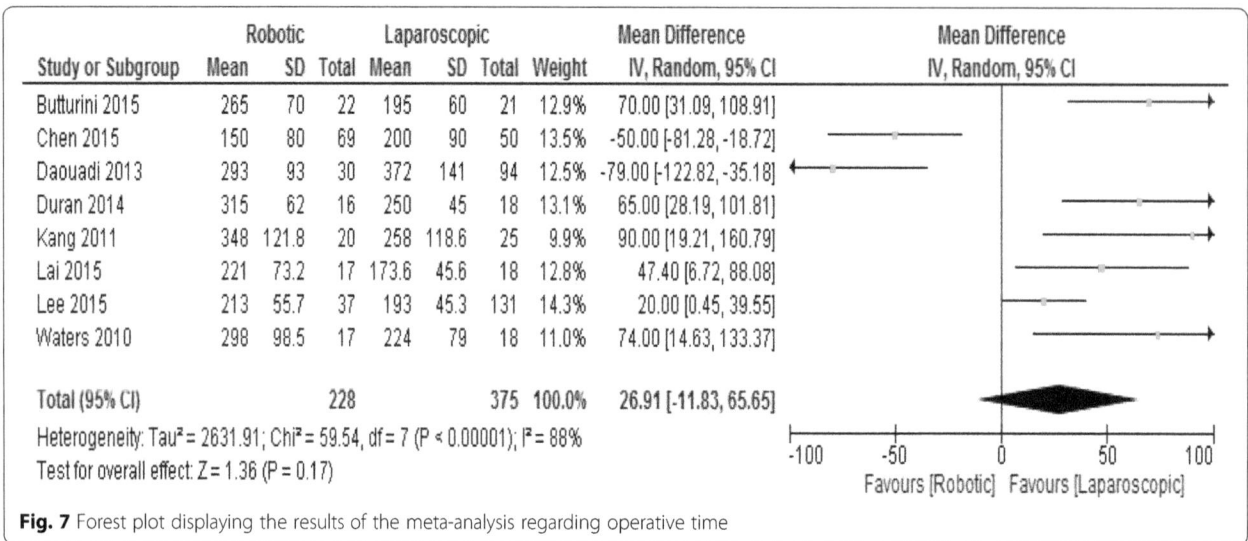

Fig. 7 Forest plot displaying the results of the meta-analysis regarding operative time

negative (R0) with a near 100% rate in the two groups and good lymphadenectomy was performed in both groups. However, no indication was provided by the authors regarding chemo-radiotherapy treatments with adjuvant or neoadjuvant purposes. No specific data were also available regarding disease free survival and tumor recurrence. Therefore it is not possible to draw final conclusion on the oncological adequacy of the robotic approach in this type of surgery.

Since minimally invasive surgery is typically associated with a faster recovery, the length of hospital stay is a very important index in the evaluation of this type of surgical approach [38, 50].

A shorter hospital stay was observed in the RDP group in our study. This result could be an argument in favor of robotic surgery in reducing the overall impact of the cost, which is still considered very high by several authors. Each robotic procedure generally costs from 1000 to 3000 dollars more than a laparoscopic procedure. Our meta-analysis shows that the robotic procedure is more expensive than the laparoscopic one. However, in calculating the cost of the operation Waters et al. [26] took into account the associated cost of the hospital stay. In this case, robotic surgery showed a greater economic advantage over laparoscopic surgery with an estimated cost of 10,588 and 12,986 dollars respectively for the RDP and the LDP group. It should be noted also that prices often vary considerably among the different surgical centers, even in the same country, so the this comparison may be misleading and at risk of bias.

Our systematic review summarizes most of the available evidence in this context. However, it has some limitations. Although most of the included studies showed a high methodological quality according to the Newcastle-Ottawa scale, the studies were retrospective and not randomized. The absence of randomization and the retrospective nature involves some structural bias that could lead to inaccurate or incorrect conclusions. Further prospective randomized studies are therefore needed to understand which of the two methods is superior to the other in terms of cancer, complications and long-term results.

Conclusions

This meta-analysis suggests that the RDP procedure is safe and comparable in terms of surgical results to LDP. However even if the RDP has a higher cost than the LDP, it increases the rate of preservation of the spleen, reduces the risk of conversion to open surgery and is associated to shorter length of hospital stay. Nevertheless, due to the high risk of bias of these retrospective studies, the benefits of RDP proven in our meta-analysis should be confirmed through further RCTs.

Abbreviations

C.I.: Confidence interval; DP: Distal pancreatectomy; LDP: Laparoscopic distal pancreatectomy; MD: Mean difference; OR: Odds ratio; PF: Pancreatic fistula; RDP: Robotic distal pancreatectomy

Acknowledgements

Not applicable.

Funding

The authors have no grant or financial support to report.

Authors' contributions

Protocol/project development: GG, AL. Data acquisition and interpretation of data: SB, CB, MO, MF. Statistics analysis of data: GG. Manuscript drafting: GG. Manuscript Revision and accountable for all aspects of the work: FB, GB, BB, GG. All authors read and approved the final manuscript.

Competing interests
The authors declare that they have no competing interests.

References
1. Fujino Y. Perioperative management of distal pancreatectomy. World J Gastroenterol. 2015;21(11):3166–9.
2. Zhang YH, Zhang CW, ZM H, Hong DF. Pancreatic cancer: open or minimally invasive surgery? World J Gastroenterol. 2016;22(32):7301–10.
3. Wellner UF, Lapshyn H, Bartsch DK, Mintziras I, Hopt UT, Wittel U, Kramling HJ, Preissinger-Heinzel H, Anthuber M, Geissler B, et al. Laparoscopic versus open distal pancreatectomy-a propensity score-matched analysis from the German StuDoQ|pancreas registry. Int J Color Dis. 2017;32(2):273–80.
4. Borja-Cacho D, Al-Refaie WB, Vickers SM, Tuttle TM, Jensen EH. Laparoscopic distal pancreatectomy. J Am Coll Surg. 2009;209(6):758–65. quiz 800
5. Sulpice L, Farges O, Goutte N, Bendersky N, Dokmak S, Sauvanet A, Delpero JR and ACHBT French Pancreatectomy Study Group. Laparoscopic distal Pancreatectomy for pancreatic Ductal Adenocarcinoma: time for a randomized controlled trial? Results of an all-inclusive National Observational Study. Ann Surg. 2015;262(5):868-73.
6. Cuschieri A, Jakimowicz JJ, van Spreeuwel J. Laparoscopic distal 70% pancreatectomy and splenectomy for chronic pancreatitis. Ann Surg. 1996; 223(3):280–5.
7. Jin T, Altaf K, Xiong JJ, Huang W, Javed MA, Mai G, Liu XB, WM H, Xia Q. A systematic review and meta-analysis of studies comparing laparoscopic and open distal pancreatectomy. HPB (Oxford). 2012;14(11):711–24.
8. Jusoh AC, Ammori BJ. Laparoscopic versus open distal pancreatectomy: a systematic review of comparative studies. Surg Endosc. 2012;26(4):904–13.
9. Riviere D, Gurusamy KS, Kooby DA, Vollmer CM, Besselink MG, Davidson BR, van Laarhoven CJ. Laparoscopic versus open distal pancreatectomy for pancreatic cancer. Cochrane Database Syst Rev. 2016, Apr 4;4:CD011391.
10. Venkat R, Edil BH, Schulick RD, Lidor AO, Makary MA, Wolfgang CL. Laparoscopic distal pancreatectomy is associated with significantly less overall morbidity compared to the open technique: a systematic review and meta-analysis. Ann Surg. 2012;255(6):1048–59.
11. Cirocchi R, Partelli S, Coratti A, Desiderio J, Parisi A, Falconi M. Current status of robotic distal pancreatectomy: a systematic review. Surg Oncol. 2013; 22(3):201–7.
12. Strijker M, van Santvoort HC, Besselink MG, van Hillegersberg R, Borel Rinkes IH, Vriens MR, Molenaar IQ. Robot-assisted pancreatic surgery: a systematic review of the literature. HPB (Oxford). 2013;15(1):1–10.
13. Melvin WS, Needleman BJ, Krause KR, Ellison EC. Robotic resection of pancreatic neuroendocrine tumor. J Laparoendosc Adv Surg Tech A. 2003; 13(1):33–6.
14. Jung MK, Buchs NC, Azagury DE, Hagen ME, Morel P. Robotic distal pancreatectomy: a valid option? Minerva Chir. 2013;68(5):489–97.
15. Magge D, Zureikat A, Hogg M, Zeh HJ 3rd. Minimally invasive approaches to pancreatic surgery. Surg Oncol Clin N Am. 2016;25(2):273–86.
16. Balzano G, Bissolati M, Boggi U, Bassi C, Zerbi A, Falconi M. A multicenter survey on distal pancreatectomy in Italy: results of minimally invasive technique and variability of perioperative pathways. Updat Surg. 2014;66(4): 253–63.
17. Chen S, Zhan Q, Chen JZ, Jin JB, Deng XX, Chen H, Shen BY, Peng CH, Li HW. Robotic approach improves spleen-preserving rate and shortens postoperative hospital stay of laparoscopic distal pancreatectomy: a matched cohort study. Surg Endosc. 2015;29(12):3507–18.
18. Daouadi M, Zureikat AH, Zenati MS, Choudry H, Tsung A, Bartlett DL, Hughes SJ, Lee KK, Moser AJ, Zeh HJ. Robot-assisted minimally invasive distal pancreatectomy is superior to the laparoscopic technique. Ann Surg. 2013;257(1):128–32.
19. Duran H, Ielpo B, Caruso R, Ferri V, Quijano Y, Diaz E, Fabra I, Oliva C, Olivares S, Vicente E. Does robotic distal pancreatectomy surgery offer similar results as laparoscopic and open approach? A comparative study from a single medical center. Int J Med Robot. 2014;10(3):280–5.
20. Goh BK, Chan CY, Soh HL, Lee SY, Cheow PC, Chow PK, Ooi LL, Chung AY. A comparison between robotic-assisted laparoscopic distal pancreatectomy versus laparoscopic distal pancreatectomy. Int J Med Robot. 2017;13(1) epub.
21. Ito M, Asano Y, Shimizu T, Uyama I, Horiguchi A. Comparison of standard laparoscopic distal pancreatectomy with minimally invasive distal pancreatectomy using the da Vinci S system. Hepato-Gastroenterology. 2014;61(130):493–6.

22. Kang CM, Kim DH, Lee WJ, Chi HS. Conventional laparoscopic and robot-assisted spleen-preserving pancreatectomy: does da Vinci have clinical advantages? Surg Endosc. 2011;25(6):2004–9.
23. Lai EC, Tang CN. Robotic distal pancreatectomy versus conventional laparoscopic distal pancreatectomy: a comparative study for short-term outcomes. Front Med. 2015;9(3):356–60.
24. Lee SY, Allen PJ, Sadot E, D'Angelica MI, DeMatteo RP, Fong Y, Jarnagin WR, Kingham TP. Distal pancreatectomy: a single institution's experience in open, laparoscopic, and robotic approaches. J Am Coll Surg. 2015;220(1):18–27.
25. Butturini G, Damoli I, Crepaz L, Malleo G, Marchegiani G, Daskalaki D, Esposito A, Cingarlini S, Salvia R, Bassi C. A prospective non-randomised single-center study comparing laparoscopic and robotic distal pancreatectomy. Surg Endosc. 2015;29(11):3163–70.
26. Waters JA, Canal DF, Wiebke EA, Dumas RP, Beane JD, Aguilar-Saavedra JR, Ball CG, House MG, Zyromski NJ, Nakeeb A, et al. Robotic distal pancreatectomy: cost effective? Surgery. 2010;148(4):814–23.
27. Zhou JY, Xin C, Mou YP, XW X, Zhang MZ, Zhou YC, Lu C, Chen RG. Robotic versus laparoscopic distal Pancreatectomy: a meta-analysis of short-term outcomes. PLoS One. 2016;11(3):e0151189.
28. Stang A. Critical evaluation of the Newcastle-Ottawa scale for the assessment of the quality of nonrandomized studies in meta-analyses. Eur J Epidemiol. 2010;25(9):603–5.
29. Liberati A, Altman DG, Tetzlaff J, Mulrow C, Gotzsche PC, Ioannidis JP, Clarke M, Devereaux PJ, Kleijnen J, Moher D. The PRISMA statement for reporting systematic reviews and meta-analyses of studies that evaluate healthcare interventions: explanation and elaboration. BMJ. 2009;339:b2700.
30. Higgins JP, Thompson SG. Quantifying heterogeneity in a meta-analysis. Stat Med. 2002;21(11):1539–58.
31. Bassi C, Dervenis C, Butturini G, Fingerhut A, Yeo C, Izbicki J, Neoptolemos J, Sarr M, Traverso W, Buchler M. Postoperative pancreatic fistula: an international study group (ISGPF) definition. Surgery. 2005;138(1):8–13.
32. Vonlanthen R, Slankamenac K, Breitenstein S, Puhan MA, Muller MK, Hahnloser D, Hauri D, Graf R, Clavien PA. The impact of complications on costs of major surgical procedures: a cost analysis of 1200 patients. Ann Surg. 2011;254(6):907–13.
33. Al-Taan OS, Stephenson JA, Briggs C, Pollard C, Metcalfe MS, Dennison AR. Laparoscopic pancreatic surgery: a review of present results and future prospects. HPB (Oxford). 2010;12(4):239–43.
34. Mesleh MG, Stauffer JA, Asbun HJ. Minimally invasive surgical techniques for pancreatic cancer: ready for prime time? J Hepatobiliary Pancreat Sci. 2013; 20(6):578–82.
35. Edwin B, Sahakyan MA, Hilal MA, Besselink MG, Braga M, Fabre JM, Fernandez-Cruz L, Gayet B, Kim SC, Khatkov IE. Laparoscopic surgery for pancreatic neoplasms: the European association for endoscopic surgery clinical consensus conference. Surg Endosc. 2017;31(5):2023–41.
36. de Rooij T, Klompmaker S, Abu Hilal M, Kendrick ML, Busch OR, Besselink MG. Laparoscopic pancreatic surgery for benign and malignant disease. Nat Rev Gastroenterol Hepatol. 2016;13(4):227–38.
37. Kang CM, Lee SH, Lee WJ. Minimally invasive radical pancreatectomy for left-sided pancreatic cancer: current status and future perspectives. World J Gastroenterol. 2014;20(9):2343–51.
38. Kendrick ML. Laparoscopic and robotic resection for pancreatic cancer. Cancer J. 2012;18(6):571–6.
39. Eckhardt S, Schicker C, Maurer E, Fendrich V, Bartsch DK. Robotic-assisted approach improves vessel preservation in spleen-preserving distal Pancreatectomy. Dig Surg. 2016;33(5):406–13.
40. Doi R. Determinants of surgical resection for pancreatic neuroendocrine tumors. J Hepatobiliary Pancreat Sci. 2015;22(8):610–7.
41. Kimura W, Inoue T, Futakawa N, Shinkai H, Han I, Muto T. Spleen-preserving distal pancreatectomy with conservation of the splenic artery and vein. Surgery. 1996;120(5):885–90.
42. Warshaw AL. Conservation of the spleen with distal pancreatectomy. Arch Surg. 1988;123(5):550–3.
43. Baker MS, Bentrem DJ, Ujiki MB, Stocker S, Talamonti MS. A prospective single institution comparison of peri-operative outcomes for laparoscopic and open distal pancreatectomy. Surgery. 2009;146(4):635–43. discussion 643-635
44. Adam U, Makowiec F, Riediger H, Trzeczak S, Benz S, Hopt UT. Distal pancreatic resection–indications, techniques and complications. Zentralbl Chir. 2001;126(11):908–12.

45. Wilson C, Robinson S, French J, White S. Strategies to reduce pancreatic stump complications after open or laparoscopic distal pancreatectomy. Surg Laparosc Endosc Percutan Tech. 2014;24(2):109–17.

46. Mahvi D. Defining, controlling, and treating a pancreatic fistula. J Gastrointest Surg. 2009;13(7):1187–8.

47. Miyasaka Y, Mori Y, Nakata K, Ohtsuka T, Nakamura M. Attempts to prevent postoperative pancreatic fistula after distal pancreatectomy. Surg Today. 2017;47(4):416–24.

48. Zhou W, Lv R, Wang X, Mou Y, Cai X, Herr I. Stapler vs suture closure of pancreatic remnant after distal pancreatectomy: a meta-analysis. Am J Surg. 2010;200(4):529–36.

49. Partelli S, Cirocchi R, Randolph J, Parisi A, Coratti A, Falconi M. A systematic review and meta-analysis of spleen-preserving distal pancreatectomy with preservation or ligation of the splenic artery and vein. Surgeon. 2016;14(2):109–18.

50. Nakamura M, Nakashima H. Laparoscopic distal pancreatectomy and pancreatoduodenectomy: is it worthwhile? A meta-analysis of laparoscopic pancreatectomy. J Hepatobiliary Pancreat Sci. 2013;20(4):421–8.

Radical antegrade modular pancreatosplenectomy versus standard procedure in the treatment of left-sided pancreatic cancer: A systemic review and meta-analysis

Feng Cao[†], Jia Li[†], Ang Li and Fei Li[*]

Abstract

Background: Radical antegrade modular pancreatosplenectomy (RAMPS), first reported by Strasberg in 2003, has attracted increasing attention in the treatment of left-sided pancreatic cancer. The limited number of cases eligible for RAMPS makes it difficult to perform any prospective randomized trial of RAMPS versus the standard procedure. Therefore, we performed this systemic review and meta-analysis of the current data to clarify the role of the RAMPS procedure.

Methods: A literature search was performed in electronic databases, including PubMed, Medline, Embase, CNKI and the Cochrane Library. Studies comparing RAMPS with the standard procedure were included in this meta-analysis. R0 resection rate, recurrence rate at the end of the follow-up, overall survival (OS) and disease-free survival (DFS) were measured as primary outcomes. Revman 5.3 was used to perform the analysis.

Results: Six retrospective cohort studies with a total number of 378 patients were included in our analysis. Meta-analysis revealed that RAMPS was correlated with higher R0 resection rates [Odds Ratio (OR) 95% confidence interval (CI), 2.19 (1.16 ~ 4.13); $P = 0.02$] and successful harvest of more lymph nodes [weighted mean difference (WMD) 95% CI, 7.06 (4.52 ~ 9.60); $P < 0.01$] compared with the standard procedure. However, no statistically significant difference was found between the procedures with respect to recurrence rates [OR 95% CI, 0.66 (0.40 ~ 1.09); $P = 0.10$], OS [Hazard ratio (HR) 95% CI, 0.65 (0.42 ~ 1.00); $P = 0.05$] or DFS [HR 95% CI, 1.02 (0.62 ~ 1.68); $P = 0.93$].

Conclusions: RAMPS is safe and oncologically superior to the standard procedure for the treatment of left-sided pancreatic cancer. However, high-grade evidence will be necessary to confirm the potential survival benefits of RAMPS.

Keywords: Pancreatic body/tail cancer, Surgery, R0, Overall survival, Disease-free survival

Background

Distal pancreatectomy is the standard surgical approach for left-sided pancreatic cancer. However, the long-term survival of these patients remains unsatisfactory, with a median survival time of 10–28 months and a 5-year overall survival of 6–30% [1–5]. In recent years, new surgical approaches for resectable or borderline resectable pancreatic cancer, including the artery-first approach [6–9], superior mesenteric vein/portal vein resection and reconstruction [10–13], intraoperative radiotherapy [14, 15] and preoperative chemo-radiotherapy [16–18], have been increasingly applied to pancreaticoduodenectomy to achieve R0 resection for carcinomas of the head of the pancreas. Despite the highly aggressive nature of the disease and early regional lymph node metastasis, adenocarcinomas of the body and tail of the pancreas have attracted significantly less clinical attention. However, in 2003, Strasberg described a new distal pancreatectomy

* Correspondence: feili36@ccmu.edu.cn
[†]Equal contributors
Department of General Surgery, Xuanwu Hospital, Capital Medical University, Beijing 100053, People's Republic of China

technique, termed radical antegrade modular pancreatosplenectomy (RAMPS), to achieve negative posterior resection margins and to completely remove the N1 lymph nodes [19]. In the past decade, the RAMPS procedure has been increasingly applied, particularly in Japan and Korea [20–24]. However, the number of patients eligible for RAMPS is too small to consider any prospective randomized trial of RAMPS versus the standard procedure. Therefore, systemic review and meta-analysis of the current retrospective data comparing RAMPS and the standard procedure are necessary and useful to clarify the role the RAMPS in the treatment of left-sided pancreatic cancer.

Methods
Search strategy and selection of trials
A computerized search was performed in July 2016 using the following terms: "radical antegrade modular pancreatosplenectomy" or "RAMPS". The following electronic databases were included: PubMed, Medline, Embase, CNKI and the Cochrane Library. The reference list of selected articles was also reviewed.

Randomized controlled trials (RCTs) and retrospective cohort studies (RCSs) comparing RAMPS and the standard procedure for the treatment of left-sided pancreatic cancer were included in this systemic review and meta-analysis. There were no limitations with respect to language or date. Case reports, review articles and letters were not included, and studies without any major postoperative outcomes were excluded from the search results.

Data extraction and quality assessment
Two reviewers (FC and JL) independently considered the eligibility of potential titles and extracted the data. Discrepancies were resolved by mutual discussion. Inclusion and exclusion criteria, country and year of publication, study type, number of patients operated on with each technique and the general characteristics of patients (age, gender, perioperative outcome and postoperative results) were extracted. The risk of bias for the trials enrolled in the meta-analysis was evaluated according to the Cochrane Handbook for Systematic Reviews of Interventions, and the quality of the non-randomized studies was assessed using the criteria suggested by the Newcastle-Ottawa quality assessment (NOS) tool [25]. This scale rates studies on a scale of one to nine, with nine representing the highest methodological quality, a NOS score of 7 or above considered high quality, and a NOS score of 3 or below considered low quality.

Outcome measurements
The primary outcomes of this study were R0 resection rate, overall survival (OS) and disease-free survival (DFS); secondary outcomes included recurrence rate at the end of the follow-up, postoperative complication rate, intraoperative blood loss, operative time, the number of lymph nodes harvested, combined resection rate and duration of hospital stay.

Statistical analysis
Meta-analysis was performed according to recommendations from the Cochrane Collaboration. Hazard ratios (HRs) and 95% confidence intervals (CIs), derived from values reported explicitly in the published studies or calculated from the Kaplan-Meier survival curve using the methods reported by Tierney and colleagues [26], were combined to measure the survival rates. Odds ratios (ORs) and weighted mean differences (WMDs) were used to measure dichotomous and continuous data, respectively. A combined $HR/OR > 1$ and $WMD > 0$ indicated poor outcomes for patients in the RAMPS group (except R0 resection and the number of lymph node harvested). Heterogeneity was evaluated using the Chi-square test, and a P value less than 0.1 was considered statistically significant. The fixed effect model was used throughout the analysis unless significant heterogeneity was detected. Funnel plot and Egger's test were used to investigate the publication bias. Analysis was performed using the Review Manager version 5.3 (Cochrane Collaboration, Software Update, Oxford, UK) and STATA/SE software version 12.0 (STATA Corporation, College Station, TX, USA).

Results
Characteristics of the trials
Six retrospective trials that met the inclusion criteria were included in the meta-analysis for a total of 378 patients, including 152 patients undergoing RAMPS and 226 patients undergoing the standard procedure [20, 24, 27–30]. Figure 1 summarized the study flow. The patient characteristics and surgical outcomes of the included trials are summarized in Tables 1 and 2. No RCTs had been published at the time of our search. The risk of bias was evaluated by the Newcastle-Ottawa scale. Three studies earned a score of 7 or more and were considered high quality [20, 24, 30] (Additional file 1: Table S1). Outcomes may have been influenced by allocation bias in all studies for patients who underwent RAMPS or the standard procedure. Furthermore, the follow-up method was unclear in all of the studies.

Meta-analysis results
Primary outcome

R0 resection rate All of the included studies reported R0 resection rates [20, 24, 27–30]. The R0 resection rate was 89.5% (136/152) in the RAMPS group and 83.6% (189/226) in the standard surgery group. The overall

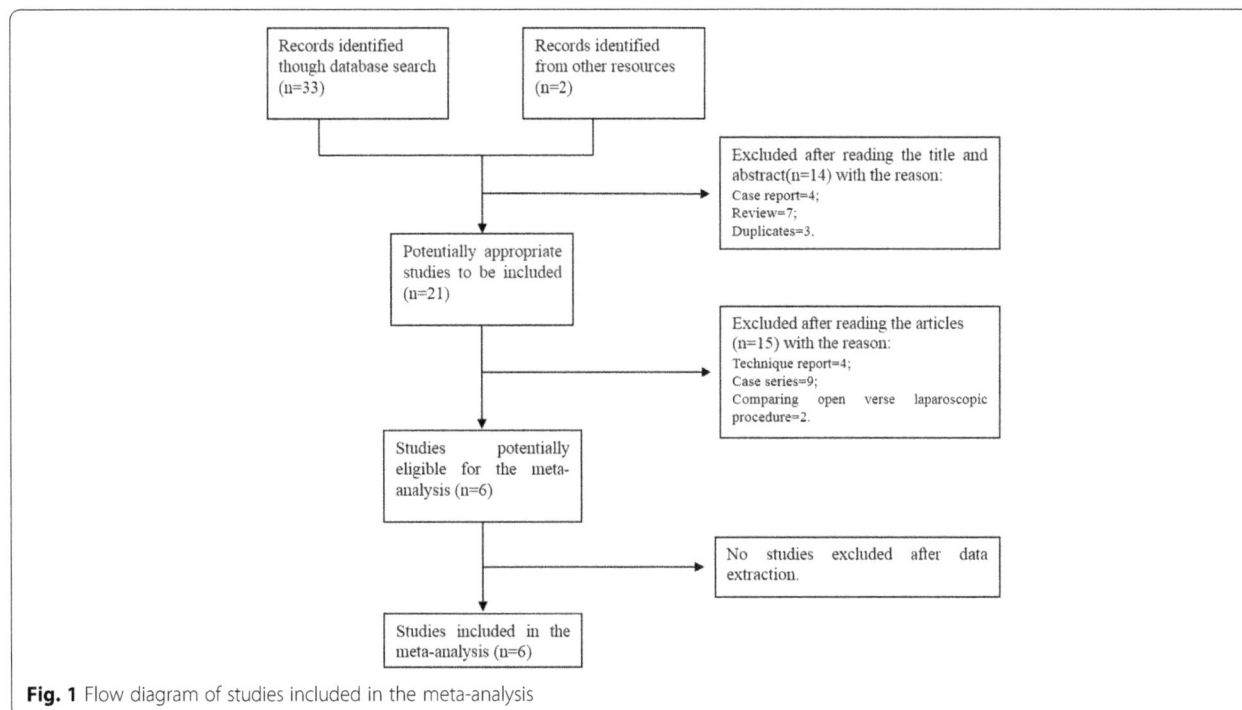

Fig. 1 Flow diagram of studies included in the meta-analysis

analysis revealed that the R0 resection rate was significantly higher in the RAMPS group than in the standard surgery group [OR 95% CI, 2.19 (1.16 ~ 4.13); $P = 0.02$] (Fig. 2a). Heterogeneity was not detected ($P = 0.57$, $I^2 = 0\%$), and the fixed-effects model was used.

Recurrence rate at the end of the follow-up The four large studies reported recurrence rates at the end of the follow-up [20, 24, 29, 30]: 52.6% and 58.1% in the RAMPS and standard groups, respectively. Overall analysis revealed that there was no statistically significant difference between the groups with respect to the recurrence rate [OR 95% CI, 0.66 (0.40 ~ 1.09); $P = 0.10$] (Fig. 2b).

Overall survival Four of the included studies reported the overall survival rate [20, 24, 28, 30]. Heterogeneity was not detected among these studies ($P = 0.56$, $I^2 = 0\%$), and the fixed-effected model was used. Overall analysis revealed no significant difference between the RAMPS and standard surgery groups [HR 95% CI, 0.65 (0.42 ~ 1.00); $P = 0.05$] (Fig. 2c).

Disease-free survival Three studies reported disease-free survival rates [20, 28, 30]. No significant difference was found when comparing RAMPS with the standard procedure [HR 95% CI, 1.02 (0.62 ~ 1.68); $P = 0.93$] using a fixed-effect model ($P = 0.87$, $I^2 = 0\%$) (Fig. 2d).

Secondary outcomes
Meta-analysis results for secondary outcomes, including postoperative complication rate, intraoperative blood loss, operative time, number of lymph nodes harvested, combined resection rate and duration of hospital stay, are summarized in Table 3. The number of lymph nodes harvested in the RAMPS group was significantly greater than that in the standard operation group [WMD 95% CI, 7.06 (4.52 ~ 9.60); $P < 0.01$] without increased intraoperative blood loss [−85.11 (−278.08 ~ 107.85); $P = 0.39$]. Despite the tendency toward higher combined resection rates [OR 95% CI, 3.30 (1.00 ~ 10.93); $P = 0.05$], the incidence of complications in the RAMPS group did not increase [OR 95% CI, 0.94 (0.56 ~ 1.59); $P = 0.83$]. There were no statistically significant differences between the groups with respect to operative time or duration of hospital stay (Additional file 2: Figure S1, Additional file 3: Figure S2, Additional file 4: Figure S3, Additional file 5: Figure S4, Additional file 6: Figure S5, Additional file 7: Figure S6).

Sensitivity analyses
To test the stability of the overall meta-analysis results, sensitivity analyses were conducted by excluding low quality studies [27–29]. The results of these analyses revealed no significant differences when compared with the former estimates (Additional file 8: Table S2).

Publication bias
Funnel plots for primary results were drawn to assess potential publication bias (Additional file 9: Figure S7). All of

Table 1 Characteristics of patients of included studies

References	Country	Published Year	Group	No. of patients	Age(year)	M/F	Tumor size (cm)	CA19-9 level (U/ml)	T3 + T4	N+	Well differentiation	Quality of study[a]
Latorre [28]	Italy	2013	RAMPS	8	61	5/3	5.1 ± 1.9	NA	NA	NA	3	6
			Standard	17	60	11/6		NA	NA	NA		
Park [24]	Korea	2014	RAMPS	38	62.17 (40–75)	23/15	3.1 (2–8.0)	18.2 (3.0–82.1)	37	22	4	7
			Standard	54	61.25 (37–79)	35/19	3.8 (1–11)	15.7 (4.4–148.5)	51	22	3	
Trottman [27]	USA	2014	RAMPS	6	NA	NA	NA	NA	NA	NA	NA	3
			Standard	20	NA	NA	NA	NA	NA	NA	NA	
Abe [20]	Japan	2016	RAMPS	53	68.6 ± 10.7	1.40:1	NA	136.4 ± 291.0	38	28	3	7
			Standard	40	65.2 ± 8.6	2.63:1	NA	390.4 ± 1157.1	34	26	7	
Xu [29]	China	2016	RAMPS	21	62 ± 11	11/10	5(4.3–6.6)	70.2(20.7–594.2)	21	11	NA	6
			Standard	78	63 ± 9	41/37	3.8(3.0–5.0)	158.7(35.6–692.2)	63	26	NA	
Kim [30]	Korea	2016	RAMPS	30	63.7 ± 8.2	13/17	4.6 ± 1.6	NA	25	14	3	8
			Standard	19	62.1 ± 8.5	7/12	4.5 ± 1.5	NA	13	6	2	

M/F male/female, NA not available. [a]according to Newcastle-Ottawa quality assessment scale

Table 2 Surgical outcomes of patients of included studies

References	Group	Intraoperative blood loss(ml)	Operative time (min)	Lymph node harvested	Complication	R0 resection	Combined resection	Hospital stay (days)	Recurrence	HR(95% CI) for DFS	HR(95% CI) for OS
Latorre [28]	RAMPS	342	315	20.7 ± 8.9	2	7(87.5%)	4	12.1	NA	1.32 (0.45–3.92)	1.26 (0.45–3.57)
	Standard	369	265	16.2 ± 4.2	5	15(88.2%)		9.9	NA		
Park [24]	RAMPS	325 (50–3400)	210 (125–480)	14(5–52)	7	34(89.5%)	15	11.5(7–32)	25(65.6%)	NA	0.56 (0.32–0.98)
	Standard	400 (50–3300)	185 (80–390)	9(1–36)	12	46(85.2%)	11	10.7(6–42)	35(64.8%)		
Trottman [27]	RAMPS	500.0 ± 260.8	300.0 ± 87.0	11.2 ± 6.0	3	6(100%)	NA	7.7 ± 3.0	NA	NA	NA
	Standard	581.3 ± 559.2	295.3 ± 83.8	4.3 ± 5.4	12	19(95%)	NA	6.9 ± 1.4	NA		
Abe [20]	RAMPS	485.4 ± 63.3	267.3 ± 11.5	28.4 ± 11.6	19	48(90.6%)	8	35.7 ± 19.6	32(60.4%)	0.96 (0.54–1.71)	0.66 (0.21–2.11)
	Standard	682.3 ± 72.8	339.4 ± 13.2	20.7 ± 10.1	14	27(67.5%)	5	26.7 ± 25.5	30(75.0%)		
Xu[a] [29]	RAMPS	400(350–650)	235(180–278)	NA	16	19(90.5%)	13	15(13–23)	6(33.3%)	NA	NA
	Standard	225(200–400)	180(130–210)	NA	48	71(91.0%)	10	12(10–16)	31(45.6%)		
Kim[b] [30]	RAMPS	300 ± 220	277.8 ± 55.6	21.5 ± 8.3	14	22(84.6%)	NA	6.4 ± 4.3	8(30.8%)	0.90 (0.08–9.92)	0.48 (0.13–1.83)
	Standard	260 ± 180	253.3 ± 41.0	13.7 ± 7.4	8	11(64.%7)	NA	8.2 ± 3.3	8(47.1%)		

NA not available. [a]Three and 10 patients in RAMPS and standard group were loss of follow-up (median 18 months, range 5–37 months) in the study period. [b]Two patients who had neuroendocrine carcinoma and two who had metastatic renal cell carcinoma in RAMPS group and two patients who had neuroendocrine carcinoma in standard group were excluded from the analyses of R0 and recurrence rate

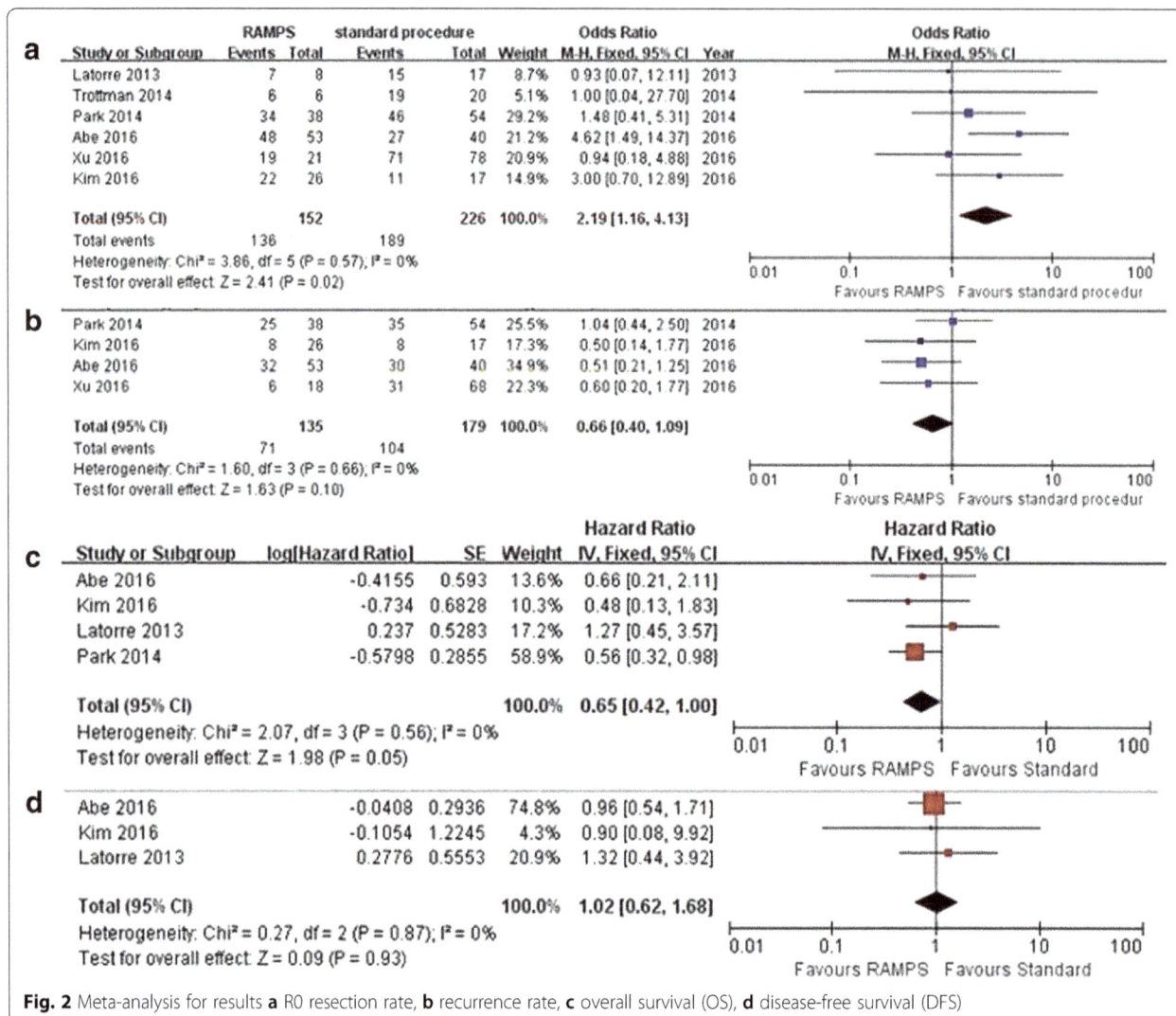

Fig. 2 Meta-analysis for results **a** R0 resection rate, **b** recurrence rate, **c** overall survival (OS), **d** disease-free survival (DFS)

the plots were symmetrical, suggesting no reporting bias among the studies. Egger's test for OS ($t = 0.51$, $P = 0.659$) and DFS ($t = 0.33$, $P = 0.795$) revealed no publication bias.

Discussion

The RAMPS procedure, first reported in 2003, was designed to establish an operation with oncologic safety both with respect to the dissection planes used to achieve negative margins as well as the extent of lymph node dissection, thereby improving patient outcomes. According to the original paper by Strasberg, if the tumour did not penetrate the posterior capsule of the pancreas on preoperative CT scans, the resection plane lay just behind the anterior renal fascia, and anterior RAMPS was performed; otherwise,

Table 3 Secondly results of meta-analysis for RAMPS verse standard procedure in treatment of left-sided pancreatic cancer

Outcome	Ref. included	No. of patients with RAMPS vs no standard	Heterogeneity Chi-square test	Model used	OR or Mean difference	95% CI	P value
Intraoperative blood loss(ml)	[20, 27, 30]	89 vs 79	$P < 0.01$; $I^2 = 88\%$	Random effect	−85.11	−278.08-107.85	0.39
Operating time (min)	[20, 27, 30]	89 vs 79	$P < 0.01$; $I^2 = 96\%$	Random effect	−16.81	−95.19-61.57	0.67
Lymph node harvested	[20, 27, 28]	93 vs 94	$P = 0.86$; $I^2 = 0\%$	Fixed effect	7.06	4.52-9.60	<0.01
Complication	[20, 24, 27–29]	135 vs 150	$P = 0.97$; $I^2 = 0\%$	Fixed effect	0.94	0.56-1.59	0.83
Combined resection	[20, 24, 29]	112 vs 172	$P = 0.02$; $I^2 = 73\%$	Random effect	3.30	1.00-10.93	0.05
Hospital stay (days)	[20, 27, 30]	89 vs 79	$P = 0.04$; $I^2 = 68\%$	Random effect	0.49	−2.97-3.94	0.78

OR odds ratio, CI confidence intervals

posterior RAMPS was applied, and the left adrenal gland and Gerota fascia were removed [19]. Deep resection is performed because tumours can spread microscopically beyond their radiographically visible or palpable margins. The systemic review of descriptive studies concerning the RAMPS procedure for the treatment of left-sided pancreatic cancer is summarized in Table 4. R0 resection was achieved in 77–100% of patients after RAMPS, and an R0 rate > 85% was observed in most case series. In this meta-analysis, we found that the R0 resection rate was significantly higher in the RAMPS group than in the standard surgery group [89.5% vs 83.6%, OR 95% CI, 2.19 (1.16 ~ 4.13); P = 0.02]. However, the combined resection rates were comparable between the RAMPS and standard groups [OR 95% CI, 3.30 (1.00 ~ 10.93); P = 0.05], which might be attributable to the low rate of posterior RAMPS procedures in present practices [24, 31, 32].

Lymph node metastasis has been reported to be an independent prognostic risk factor for resected left-sided pancreatic cancer [33, 34]. The extent of lymph node dissection is one of the key points of pancreatosplenectomy. However, guidelines from Eastern and Western countries differ significantly. In the RAMPS procedure, the lymph nodes along the superior and inferior borders of the left-sided pancreas (No. 10, 11, and 18 according to Japanese classification), the celiac lymph nodes (No. 9) and the nodes along the front and left side of the superior mesenteric artery (No. 14p, 14d) are considered N1 lymph nodes and are completely removed; in the standard operation, only lymph nodes No. 10, 11, and 18 are resected [35]. Therefore, in this meta-analysis, we found that the number of lymph nodes harvested in the RAMPS procedure was significantly greater than in the standard operation [WMD 95% CI, 7.06 (4.52–9.60); P < 0.01]. Compared with the standard operation, the RAMPS procedure is reported to require greater technical skill for extensive resection as well as longer operating times [24, 28]. However, these differences were not detected in our meta-analysis [WMD 95% CI, –16.81 (–95.19–61.57); P = 0.67]. Additionally, RAMPS procedures were not correlated with longer hospital stays [WMD 95% CI, 0.49 (–2.97–3.94); P = 0.78]. These findings may be influenced by a recent study with a large volume of patients and more experienced surgeons.

Improving the survival of patients with resectable or borderline resectable tumours is the major aim of the RAMPS procedure. The 5-year survival rate after RAMPS ranged from 25.1% to 55.6% (Table 4). In a recent study, when comparing RAMPS and the standard procedure, RAMPS exhibited a greater tendency towards improvement of median survival times relative to the standard procedure (47 vs 34 months, P = 0.192), but no significant differences in the recurrence rates were detected (66.6 vs 75.0%;

P = 0.1386) [20]. In the study by Park, the 5-year overall survival rate was 40.1% in RAMPS patients and 12.0% in the standard group (p = 0.014). However, by multivariate analysis, adjuvant chemoradiotherapy but not RAMPS reached statistical significance with respect to overall survival [24]. In the present study, no favourable overall survival outcomes were detected when comparing RAMPS with the standard procedure. The recurrence rate after RAMPS did not decrease (65.7% vs 64.8%, P = 0.482), which was consistent with our meta-analysis [OR 95% CI, 0.66 (0.40 ~ 1.09); P = 0.10] and led to similar DFS rates in the two groups [OR 95% CI, 1.02 (0.62 ~ 1.68); P = 0.93]. With respect to recurrence, we believed that it is important to differentiate local recurrence from systemic recurrence. RAMPS increased the R0 resection rate and theoretically may decrease local recurrence. Unfortunately, few studies reported the local recurrence rate. In these studies, systemic recurrence alone, such as liver, lung and peritoneum, was reported most often, and the local recurrence rate did not decrease significantly after RAMPS [20, 31].

Recently, a modified RAMPS procedure including a superior mesenteric artery (SMA)-first approach has been attempted [22, 36–38]. The artery-first approach, initially designed for the early determination of cancer resectability during pancreatoduodenectomy, is now applied in the RAMPS procedure. As described by Strasberg, dissection of the SMA is performed after transection of the pancreas or wide detachment of the distal pancreas and spleen, which may reach the point of no return. However, carcinoma of the pancreatic body and tail exhibits high aggressive potential, and the celiac axis (CA) and SMA are often involved. Although left-sided pancreatic cancer with CA invasion can be treated by distal pancreatectomy combined with celiac axis resection (DP-CAR), SMA encroachment usually indicates that the tumour is a late-stage lesion and may be completely unresectable. SMA-first RAMPS provides an opportunity to determine resectability before pancreas transection. Dissection further along the aorta and exposure of the left renal vein and the left adrenal gland can help prepare the correct RAMPS dissection plane in advance. When the renal vein is reached, the surgeon can accurately assess the extent of tumour penetration to help decide whether anterior or posterior RAMPS is optimal. Data from Japan has demonstrated the safety and reliability of this procedure even in borderline resectable tumours [22, 36, 37].

Laparoscopic or robotic RAMPS operations have also been performed with satisfactory oncological results and survival outcomes [39–41]. However, this procedure is limited to highly selective cases. According to the Yonsei criteria developed by Lee, only patients meeting the following characteristics can be treated with minimally invasive RAMPS: (1) tumour confined to the pancreas, (2) intact fascial layer between the distal pancreas and

Table 4 Systemic review of descriptive studies about RAMPS procedure in treatment of left-sided pancreatic cancer

Reference	Year	No. of patients	A/P RAMPS	Tumor size (cm)	N+(%)	R0(%)	Lymph Node harvested	Median follow-up time(months)	Recurrence rate (%)	Median survival time (months)	5-year overall survival (%)
Strasberg [19]	2003	10	6/4	4(2–15)	NA	90	1–28	NA	3(30.0%)	NA	NA
Strasberg [32]	2007	23	15/8	5.1 ± 2.6	48	87	14.3 ± 7.8	17 for alive	11(47.3%)	NA	NA
Kang[a] [41]	2010	5	5/0	2.4 ± 0.7	20	100	8.2 ± 5.9	13(4–21)	1(20%)	NA	NA
Ikegami [42]	2011	6	3/3	3.0 ± 0.9	NA	100	NA	NA	NA	NA	NA
Mitchem [43]	2012	47	32/15	4.4 ± 2.1	55	80.1	18.0 ± 11.7	26.4 for alive	27(57.4%)	25.9	35.5
Chang [44]	2012	24	19/5	4.09 ± 2.15	70.8	91.7	20.92 ± 11.24	20.06	21(87.5%)	18.2	NA
Kim [45]	2013	12	12/0	2(0.8–4.0)	50	NA	17(5–29)	NA	NA	NA	NA
Rosso [46]	2013	10	1/9	4.65(1.0–8.0)	70	90	17(13–95)	19.1 ± 10.1	NA	20.5%	NA
Lee[b] [39]	2014	12	12/0	2.75 ± 1.32	25	100	10.5 ± 7.14	39	5(41.7%)	60.0	55.6
Kitagawa[c] [38]	2014	24	19/5	3.5 ± 1.4	54.2	88	28 ± 12	52 for alive	10(41.7%)	NA	53
Kawabata[d] [37]	2015	11	NA	3.35(1.9–5.5)	91	77	26(9–80)	12.4(3.5–16.4)	1(9.1%)	NA	NA
Murakawa [12]	2015	49	NA	0.5–8.3	55	83.7	15	41.4	30(61.2%)	22.6	27
Grossman [31]	2016	78	56/22	4.71	47	85	20 ± 12.2	20.6 (0.3–145.3)	49(62.8%)	24.6	25.1

A/P anterior/posterior, NA not available. [a]laparoscopic or robot-assisted anterior RAMPS; [b]laparoscopic modified anterior RAMPS; [c]modified RAMPS; [d]RAMPS in well-selected patients with Yonsei criteria; [c]modified RAMPS; [d]RAMPS with artery-first approach the left adrenal gland and kidney, and (3) tumour located more than 1–2 cm from the celiac axis [39].

An important limitation of this review is the small number of included studies and cases. In addition, the nature of the included retrospective studies may lead to allocation and publication biases and could distort the conclusions of this review. However, this study represents the initial attempt to perform a systemic review and meta-analysis of RAMPS versus the standard procedure in the treatment of left-sided pancreatic cancer. Our systematic review and meta-analysis presents evidence to suggest that RAMPS is the optimal procedure to increase R0 resection rates but has no increased benefit with respect to tumour recurrence or patient survival.

Conclusion
The RAMPS procedure for the treatment of left-sided pancreatic cancer can achieve higher rates of R0 resection without increasing complication rates compared with the standard procedure. However, high-grade evidence is required before any conclusions may be made concerning the survival benefit of RAMPS.

Additional files

Additional file 1: Table S1. Risk of bias in the included retrospective cohort studies (by the Newcastle–Ottawa quality assessment tool). (DOCX 12 kb)

Additional file 2: Figure S1. Meta-analysis for lymph node harvested showed significantly greater in RAMPS group. (PNG 9 kb)

Additional file 3: Figure S2. Meta-analysis revealed compared result for intraoperative blood loss. (PNG 10 kb)

Additional file 4: Figure S3. Meta-analysis for combined resection rate. RAMPS procedure did not combined resection rate. (PNG 9 kb)

Additional file 5: Figure S4. Meta-analysis revealed that RAMPS did not increase the complication. (PNG 10 kb)

Additional file 6: Figure S5. Meta-analysis for operation time showed compared result between RAMPS and standard procedure. (PNG 10 kb)

Additional file 7: Figure S6. Meta-analysis revealed similar hospital stay in RAMPS and standard procedure. (PNG 9 kb)

Additional file 8: Table S2. Results of sensitivity analyses which revealed no significant differences when compared with main analyses. (DOCX 13 kb)

Additional file 9: Figure S7. Funnel plots for (a) R0 resection, (b) recurrence, (c) OS and (d) DFS revealed no publication bias. (PNG 182 kb)

Acknowledgements
None.

Funding
This work is partly supported by Beijing Municipal Administration of Hospitals' Youth Programme, code: QML20160806.

Authors' contributions
FC and FL designed this study. FC, AL and JL collected and analyzed the data. FC wrote the first draft of the manuscript. All authors contributed to review the manuscript. All authors read and approved the final manuscript.

Competing interests
The authors declare that they have no competing interest.

References
1. Wu X, Tao R, Lei R, Han B, Cheng D, Shen B, Peng C. Distal pancreatectomy combined with celiac axis resection in treatment of carcinoma of the body/tail of the pancreas: a single-center experience. Ann Surg Oncol. 2010;17(5):1359–66.
2. Yamamoto J, Saiura A, Koga R, Seki M, Katori M, Kato Y, Sakamoto Y, Kokudo N, Yamaguchi T. Improved survival of left-sided pancreas cancer after surgery. Jpn J Clin Oncol. 2010;40(6):530–6.
3. Reddy SK, Tyler DS, Pappas TN, Clary BM. Extended resection for pancreatic adenocarcinoma. Oncologist. 2007;12(6):654–63.
4. van Gulik TM, Nakao A, Obertop H. Extended resection for pancreatic adenocarcinoma. HPB (Oxford). 2002;4(3):101–3.
5. Dalton RR, Sarr MG, van Heerden JA, Colby TV. Carcinoma of the body and tail of the pancreas: is curative resection justified? Surgery. 1992;111(5):489–94.
6. Pandanaboyana S, Bell R, Windsor J. Artery first approach to pancreatoduodenectomy: current status. ANZ J Surg. 2016;86(3):127–32.
7. Inoue Y, Saiura A, Yoshioka R, Ono Y, Takahashi M, Arita J, Takahashi Y, Koga R. Pancreatoduodenectomy with systematic Mesopancreas dissection using a Supracolic anterior artery-first approach. Ann Surg. 2015;262(6):1092–101.
8. Nagakawa Y, Hosokawa Y, Sahara Y, Takishita C, Nakajima T, Hijikata Y, Tago T, Kasuya K, Tsuchida A. A novel "artery first" approach allowing safe resection in laparoscopic Pancreaticoduodenectomy: the Uncinate process first approach. Hepato-Gastroenterology. 2015;62(140):1037–40.
9. Pittau G, Sanchez-Cabus S, Laurenzi A, Gelli M, Cunha AS. Laparoscopic Pancreaticoduodenectomy: right posterior superior mesenteric artery "first" approach. Ann Surg Oncol. 2015;22(Suppl 3):S345–8.
10. Xing-Mao Z, Hua F, Jian-Tao K, Xin-Xue Z, Ping L, Yang D, Qiang H. Resection of portal and/or superior mesenteric vein and reconstruction by using allogeneic vein for pT3 pancreatic cancer. J Gastroenterol Hepatol. 2016;31(8):1498–503.
11. Ramacciato G, Nigri G, Petrucciani N, Pinna AD, Ravaioli M, Jovine E, Minni F, Grazi GL, Chirletti P, Tisone G, et al. Pancreatectomy with mesenteric and portal vein resection for borderline Resectable pancreatic cancer: multicenter study of 406 patients. Ann Surg Oncol. 2016;23(6):2028–37.
12. Murakami Y, Satoi S, Motoi F, Sho M, Kawai M, Matsumoto I, Honda G. Portal or superior mesenteric vein resection in pancreatoduodenectomy for pancreatic head carcinoma. Br J Surg. 2015;102(7):837–46.
13. Wang WL, Ye S, Yan S, Shen Y, Zhang M, Wu J, Zheng SS. Pancreaticoduodenectomy with portal vein/superior mesenteric vein resection for patients with pancreatic cancer with venous invasion. Hepatobiliary Pancreat Dis Int. 2015;14(4):429–35.
14. Jingu K, Tanabe T, Nemoto K, Ariga H, Umezawa R, Ogawa Y, Takeda K, Koto M, Sugawara T, Kubozono M, et al. Intraoperative radiotherapy for pancreatic cancer: 30-year experience in a single institution in Japan. Int J Radiat Oncol Biol Phys. 2012;83(4):e507–11.
15. Ogawa K, Karasawa K, Ito Y, Ogawa Y, Jingu K, Onishi H, Aoki S, Wada H, Kokubo M, Etoh H, et al. Intraoperative radiotherapy for resected pancreatic cancer: a multi-institutional retrospective analysis of 210 patients. Int J Radiat Oncol Biol Phys. 2010;77(3):734–42.
16. Hirata T, Teshima T, Nishiyama K, Ogawa K, Otani K, Kawaguchi Y, Konishi K, Tomita Y, Takahashi H, Ohigashi H, et al. Histopathological effects of preoperative chemoradiotherapy for pancreatic cancer: an analysis for the impact of radiation and gemcitabine doses. Radiother Oncol. 2015;114(1):122–7.
17. Eguchi H, Nagano H, Tanemura M, Takeda Y, Marubashi S, Kobayashi S, Kawamoto K, Wada H, Hama N, Akita H, et al. Preoperative chemoradiotherapy, surgery and adjuvant therapy for resectable pancreatic cancer. Hepato-Gastroenterology. 2013;60(124):904–11.
18. Vento P, Mustonen H, Joensuu T, Karkkainen P, Kivilaakso E, Kiviluoto T. Impact of preoperative chemoradiotherapy on survival in patients with resectable pancreatic cancer. World J Gastroenterol. 2007;13(21):2945–51.
19. Strasberg SM, Drebin JA, Linehan D. Radical antegrade modular pancreatosplenectomy. Surgery. 2003;133(5):521–7.

20. Abe T, Ohuchida K, Miyasaka Y, Ohtsuka T, Oda Y, Nakamura M. Comparison of surgical outcomes between radical Antegrade modular Pancreatosplenectomy (RAMPS) and standard retrograde Pancreatosplenectomy (SPRS) for left-sided pancreatic cancer. World J Surg. 2016;40(9):2267–75.

21. Murakawa M, Aoyama T, Asari M, Katayama Y, Yamaoku K, Kanazawa A, Higuchi A, Shiozawa M, Kobayashi S, Ueno M, et al. The short- and long-term outcomes of radical antegrade modular pancreatosplenectomy for adenocarcinoma of the body and tail of the pancreas. BMC Surg. 2015;15:120.

22. Ome Y, Hashida K, Yokota M, Nagahisa Y, Michio O, Kawamoto K. Laparoscopic radical antegrade modular pancreatosplenectomy for left-sided pancreatic cancer using the ligament of Treitz approach. Surg Endosc. 2017. doi:10.1007/s00464-017-5561-6. [Epub ahead of print].

23. Han DH, Kang CM, Lee WJ, Chi HS. A five-year survivor without recurrence following robotic anterior radical antegrade modular pancreatosplenectomy for a well-selected left-sided pancreatic cancer. Yonsei Med J. 2014;55(1):276–9.

24. Park HJ, You DD, Choi DW, Heo JS, Choi SH. Role of radical antegrade modular pancreatosplenectomy for adenocarcinoma of the body and tail of the pancreas. World J Surg. 2014;38(1):186–93.

25. Stang A. Critical evaluation of the Newcastle-Ottawa scale for the assessment of the quality of nonrandomized studies in meta-analyses. Eur J Epidemiol. 2010;25(9):603–5.

26. Tierney JF, Stewart LA, Ghersi D, Burdett S, Sydes MR. Practical methods for incorporating summary time-to-event data into meta-analysis. Trials. 2007;8:16.

27. Trottman P, Swett K, Shen P, Sirintrapun J. Comparison of standard distal pancreatectomy and splenectomy with radical antegrade modular pancreatosplenectomy. Am Surg. 2014;80(3):295–300.

28. Latorre M, Ziparo V, Nigri G, Balducci G, Cavallini M, Ramacciato G. Standard retrograde pancreatosplenectomy versus radical antegrade modular pancreatosplenectomy for body and tail pancreatic adenocarcinoma. Am Surg. 2013;79(11):1154–8.

29. Xu D, Jiang KR, Lu ZP, Guo F, Chen JM, Wei JS, Yin J, Zhang K, Wu PF, Cai BB, Lv N, Miao Y. Clinical effect of radical antegrade modular pancreatosplenectomy for carcinoma of pancreatic body and tail. Zhong Hua Xiao Hua Wai Ke Za Zhi. 2016;15(6):567–73.

30. Kim EY, You YK, Kim DG, Hong TH. Initial experience with radical antegrade modular pancreatosplenectomy in a single institution. Ann Surg Treat Res. 2016;91(1):29–36.

31. Grossman JG, Fields RC, Hawkins WG, Strasberg SM. Single institution results of radical antegrade modular pancreatosplenectomy for adenocarcinoma of the body and tail of pancreas in 78 patients. J Hepatobiliary Pancreat Sci. 2016;23(7):432–41.

32. Strasberg SM, Linehan DC, Hawkins WG. Radical antegrade modular pancreatosplenectomy procedure for adenocarcinoma of the body and tail of the pancreas: ability to obtain negative tangential margins. J Am Coll Surg. 2007;204(2):244–9.

33. Fujita T, Nakagohri T, Gotohda N, Takahashi S, Konishi M, Kojima M, Kinoshita T. Evaluation of the prognostic factors and significance of lymph node status in invasive ductal carcinoma of the body or tail of the pancreas. Pancreas. 2010;39(1):e48–54.

34. Shimada K, Sakamoto Y, Sano T, Kosuge T. Prognostic factors after distal pancreatectomy with extended lymphadenectomy for invasive pancreatic adenocarcinoma of the body and tail. Surgery. 2006;139(3):288–95.

35. Tol JA, Gouma DJ, Bassi C, Dervenis C, Montorsi M, Adham M, Andren-Sandberg A, Asbun HJ, Bockhorn M, Buchler MW, et al. Definition of a standard lymphadenectomy in surgery for pancreatic ductal adenocarcinoma: a consensus statement by the international study group on pancreatic surgery (ISGPS). Surgery. 2014;156(3):591–600.

36. Aosasa S, Nishikawa M, Hoshikawa M, Noro T, Yamamoto J. Inframesocolic superior mesenteric artery first approach as an introductory procedure of radical Antegrade modular Pancreatosplenectomy for carcinoma of the pancreatic body and tail. J Gastrointest Surg. 2016;20(2):450–4.

37. Kawabata Y, Hayashi H, Takai K, Kidani A, Tajima Y. Superior mesenteric artery-first approach in radical antegrade modular pancreatosplenectomy for borderline resectable pancreatic cancer: a technique to obtain negative tangential margins. J Am Coll Surg. 2015;220(5):e49–54.

38. Kitagawa H, Tajima H, Nakagawara H, Makino I, Miyashita T, Terakawa H, Nakanuma S, Hayashi H, Takamura H, Ohta T. A modification of radical antegrade modular pancreatosplenectomy for adenocarcinoma of the left pancreas: significance of en bloc resection including the anterior renal fascia. World J Surg. 2014;38(9):2448–54.

39. Lee SH, Kang CM, Hwang HK, Choi SH, Lee WJ, Chi HS. Minimally invasive RAMPS in well-selected left-sided pancreatic cancer within Yonsei criteria: long-term (>median 3 years) oncologic outcomes. Surg Endosc. 2014;28(10):2848–55.

40. Poves I, Burdio F, Membrilla E, Alonso S, Grande L. Laparoscopic radical antegrade modular pancreatosplenectomy. Cir Esp. 2010;88(1):51–3.

41. Kang CM, Kim DH, Lee WJ. Ten years of experience with resection of left-sided pancreatic ductal adenocarcinoma: evolution and initial experience to a laparoscopic approach. Surg Endosc. 2010;24(7):1533–41.

42. Ikegami T, Maeda T, Oki E, Kayashima H, Ohgaki K, Sakaguchi Y, Shirabe K, Maehara Y. Antegrade en bloc distal pancreatectomy with plexus hanging maneuver. J Gastrointest Surg. 2011;15(4):690–3.

43. Mitchem JB, Hamilton N, Gao F, Hawkins WG, Linehan DC, Strasberg SM. Long-term results of resection of adenocarcinoma of the body and tail of the pancreas using radical antegrade modular pancreatosplenectomy procedure. J Am Coll Surg. 2012;214(1):46–52.

44. Chang YR, Han SS, Park SJ, Lee SD, Yoo TS, Kim YK, Kim TH, Woo SM, Lee WJ, Hong EK. Surgical outcome of pancreatic cancer using radical antegrade modular pancreatosplenectomy procedure. World J Gastroenterol. 2012;18(39):5595–600.

45. Kim SH, Kang CM, Satoi S, Sho M, Nakamura Y, Lee WJ. Proposal for splenectomy-omitting radical distal pancreatectomy in well-selected left-sided pancreatic cancer: multicenter survey study. J Hepatobiliary Pancreat Sci. 2013;20(3):375–81.

46. Rosso E, Langella S, Addeo P, Nobili C, Oussoultzoglou E, Jaeck D, Bachellier P. A safe technique for radical antegrade modular pancreatosplenectomy with venous resection for pancreatic cancer. J Am Coll Surg. 2013;217(5):e35–9.

25

Prognostic role of nodal ratio, LODDS, pN in patients with pancreatic cancer with venous involvement

Giovanni Ramacciato[1], Giuseppe Nigri[1*] (iD), Niccolo' Petrucciani[1], Antonio Daniele Pinna[2], Matteo Ravaioli[2], Elio Jovine[3], Francesco Minni[4], Gian Luca Grazi[5], Piero Chirletti[6], Giuseppe Tisone[7], Fabio Ferla[8], Niccolo' Napoli[9] and Ugo Boggi[9]

Abstract

Background: The UICC/AJCC TNM staging system classifies lymph nodes as N0 and N1 in pancreatic cancer. Aim of the study is to determine whether the number of examine nodes, the nodal ratio (NR) and the logarithm odds of positive lymph nodes (LODDS) may better stratify the prognosis of patients undergoing pancreatectomy combined with venous resection for pancreatic cancer with venous involvement.

Methods: A multicenter database of 303 patients undergoing pancreatectomy in 9 Italian referral centers was analyzed. The prognostic impact of number of retrieved and examined nodes, NR, LODDS was analyzed and compared with ROC curves analysis, Pearson test, univariate and multivariate analysis.

Results: The number of metastatic nodes, pN, the NR and LODDS was significantly correlated with survival at multivariate analyses. The corresponding AUC for the number of metastatic nodes, pN, the NR and LODDS were 0.66, 0.69, 0.63 and 0.65, respectively. The Pearson test showed a significant correlation between the number of retrieved lymph nodes and number of metastatic nodes, pN and the NR. LODDS had the lower coefficient correlation. Concerning N1 patients, the NR, the LODDS and the number of metastatic nodes were able to significantly further stratify survival ($p = 0.040$; $p = 0.046$; $p = 0.038$, respectively).

Conclusions: The number of examined lymph nodes, the NR and LODDS are useful for further prognostic stratification of N1 patients in the setting of pancreatectomy combined with PV/SMV resection. No superiority of one over the others methods was detected.

Keywords: Pancreatic cancer, Tnm, Nodal ratio, Lodds, Prognosis, Nodal staging, Venous invasion, Portal vein, Superior mesenteric vein, Pancreatectomy

Background

Pancreatic cancer represents the fourth-leading cause of cancer-related mortality in the United States with an estimated 53,670 new cases in 2017 and 43,090 deaths [1]. In Europe, an estimated 103,773 new cases were reported in 2012 [2]. Lymph nodal status is an important prognostic factor in these patients, as a determinant for the appropriate prognostic stratification and therapeutic

decision-making [3]. Patients with pancreatic carcinoma with portal vein (PV) and/or superior mesenteric vein (SMV) invasion represent a particular challenge regarding prognostic analysis and treatment. The seventh edition of the International Union against Cancer (UICC) and the American Joint Committee on Cancer (AJCC) Tumor Node Metastasis (TNM) staging system classify regional lymph nodes as N0 and N1, according to the presence of none or one or more nodal metastases [4]. The number of lymph nodes should be reported because it represents a prognostic factor, and N0 patients have a better prognosis with an increasing number of examined lymph nodes [5–8]. For optimal staging, the analysis of

* Correspondence: giuseppe.nigri@uniroma1.it; http://w3.uniroma1.it/nigri
[1]Department of Medical and Surgical Sciences and Translational Medicine, Faculty of Medicine and Psychology, St Andrea Hospital, Sapienza University, General Surgery Unit, Via di Grottarossa 1037, 00189 Rome, Italy
Full list of author information is available at the end of the article

11–17 lymph nodes is recommended [5–9]. However, extended lymphadenectomy does not provide a survival advantage, according to randomized trials and meta-analyses [10–13]. In light of these data, the International Study Group of Pancreatic Surgery (ISGPS) agreed on a definition of standard lymphadenectomy [14]. Inaccurate surgical dissection, pathological evaluation or both may cause understaging for the suboptimal number of analyzed nodes, and subsequent inappropriate prognostic evaluation and error in clinical decisions [15].

To optimize nodal staging in patients with pancreatic cancer, different systems have been proposed and studied. The nodal ratio (NR) (ratio between metastatic and retrieved nodes) permits a subclassification of N1 patients, but it does not provide more information than TNM for N0 patients. Several authors have shown that the NR is a significant prognostic factor for overall survival [16, 17]. LODDS (log odds of positive lymph nodes), defined as the logarithm of the ratio between the number of positive nodes and number of negative nodes, has thus been proposed as more effective than the NR in N0 patients [15].

Until now, few studies have compared all nodal staging systems in patients with pancreatic carcinoma and no data have been published on patients with PV/SMV venous invasion. Therefore, our aim is to analyze and compare different nodal staging systems in a subgroup of patients who underwent pancreatectomy with combined venous resection in nine Italian referral centers in order to identify the more advantageous nodal classification in this subset of patients.

Methods

The study included 303 patients who underwent pancreatectomy combined with PV or SMV resection for pancreatic carcinoma. The procedures were performed at nine Italian referral institutions. Some data retrieved from this multicenter database have already been published [18]. Written informed consent for participation in the study was obtained from participants.

Preoperative work-up and surgical treatment

The diagnosis of pancreatic adenocarcinoma was confirmed by pathological examination in all cases. Regarding neoadjuvant treatment, the multidisciplinary board of each unit established the indication and protocol, after imaging discussion among radiologists and clinicians.

Pancreaticoduodenectomy, left spleno-pancreatectomy or total pancreatectomy were performed according to the site of the lesion. Lymphadenectomy was performed as previously described in a standard fashion [14].

Definition of clinical outcomes and pathological examination

Postoperative mortality was defined as death during hospitalization or during the the first 30 days after pancreatectomy. For postoperative complications, ISGPS definitions were used [19, 20]. The presence of tumor cells within 1 mm from the margin was defined as R1 resection. Evidence of macroscopic residual tumor was defined as R2. ISGPS recommendations were followed [21].

Lymph nodal staging systems

N status was defined according to the AJCC staging system. The nodal ratio (NR) was defined as the ratio between the number of positive nodes and total harvested nodes. The classification system validated by Malleo et al. was chose for NR, after a careful review of the literature. Interval values were as follows: 0, 0.01–0.2, 0.21–0.4 and more than 0.4 [3]. LODDS were calculated by $\log (\text{pnod} + 0.5)/(\text{tnod-pnod} + 0.5)$, where pnod was the number of positive lymph nodes and tnod was the total number of examined nodes; 0.5 was added to both the numerator and the denominator to avoid an infinite number [15]. Patients were divided into two groups, dichotomizing the LODDS values around the median value. Each subgroup was further divided into two, dichotomizing again around the median LODDS value, resulting in four LODDS groups. The classification reported by Strobel et al. was chosen for the number of positive nodes, [8].

Adjuvant therapies and follow-up

The multidisciplinary tumor board of each institution validated the indication for adjuvant chemotherapy or radiochemotherapy. Decision was based on patients' performance status and pathological results. During follow-up, physical examination and CA 19–9 determination were scheduled every 3 months in the first 2 years and than every 6 months, and thoraco-abdominal CT scan every 6 months in the first 2 years.

Statistical analysis

The multicenter database was prospectively collected by each center and retrospectively analyzed. T-test for continuous variables and the chi-square test for categorical variables were used to calculate differences in distribution. Overall survival rates were calculated according to the Kaplan–Meier method, and we used the log-rank test to assess the statistical differences between different groups. Univariate and multivariate analyses were used to identify the most significant. Correlation between nodal staging systems and prognosis was assessed with univariate and multivariate analyses. Variables significant in the univariate analysis were used for the multivariate

Prognostic role of nodal ratio, LODDS, pN in patients with pancreatic cancer with venous...

173

model, analyzing separately each nodal staging system. Overall survival rates were calculated according to different pN, NR, LODDS, number of metastatic nodes and number of retrieved nodes. ROC curves analysis was used to evaluate the accuracy of the different nodal staging systems, using nodal classifications as variables and 5-year survival as classification variables. The method of Delong et al. [22] was used. Pearson correlation coefficient was used to calculate the correlations between number of retrieved nodes, number of metastatic nodes, NR and LODDS. $p < 0.05$ was considered as statistically significant. Statistical analyses were performed by using MedCalc for Windows, version 10.2.0.0 (MedCalc Software, Belgium).

Results
Patients' characteristics, preoperative work-up and treatment and surgery
The study population was composed of 165 men (54.5%) and 138 women (45.5%). The majority of patients were classed as N1 (70.6%). Patients' characteristics according to nodal status are listed in Table 1. One hundred and eighty-seven patients (61.7%) had one or more comorbidity. Cardiovascular comorbidities were detected in 49.5% of patients, respiratory comorbidities in 12.2% and metabolic comorbidities in 29.0%.

Mean tumor diameter according to the CT scan was 32.9 ± 15.4 mm. Preoperative biliary drainage was performed in 28.6% of cases, and neoadjuvant chemotherapy was administered to 6.4% of patients.

The majority of patients underwent pancreaticoduodenectomy (PD) (76.9%), 60 (19.8%) underwent left

pancreatectomy (LP) and 10 (3.3%) total pancreatectomy (TP) (Table 1). All patients underwent portal or superior mesenteric vein resection. Mean operative time was 462.6 ± 134.2 min and blood loss 475.2 ± 401.6 ml.

Postoperative outcomes, pathological and lymph nodal analysis and survival
Complications occurred in 49.8% of patients and mortality in 6.6% (Table 2). Postoperative pancreatic fistula occurred in 11.9% and delayed gastric emptying in 23.1%. Mean intensive care unit stay was 3.2 ± 4.6 days. Mean hospital stay was 20.4 ± 11.6 days. Histological venous invasion was found in 53.8% of venous specimens. Mean tumor diameter was 35.0 ± 20.7 mm. The mean number of retrieved lymph nodes was 33.5 ± 22.6 and ranged from 2 to 131. The mean number of metastatic nodes was 3.4 ± 4.5, ranging from 0 to 25. Patients undergoing LP had a significantly higher number of retrieved lymph nodes than patients undergoing PD (47.9 ± 25 versus 29.6 ± 20.2; $p < 0.0001$). The mean number of metastatic nodes was not different in patients submitted to PD (3.1 ± 4), LP (4.4 ± 5.8) and TP (3.7 ± 4.9). The resection margin was tumor-free in 73.3% of cases. Adjuvant therapy was administered to 72.1% of patients. Mean follow-up duration was 37.9 months. Median overall survival was 25 months and five-year survival rate was 25.2%.

Analysis of prognostic factors
Table 3 shows survival according to patient and tumor characteristics. Factors that significantly correlated with overall survival were the number of metastatic nodes, pN, the NR and LODDS, whereas no correlation was

Table 1 Patients' characteristics and procedures. Data are presented for the entire cohort and according to nodal status. Continuous variables are presented as mean ± SD

Variable	N0 (89)	N1 (214)	Total (303)	p
Age	65.7 ± 10.7	67.4 ± 10.5	66.9 ± 10.6	0.223
Sex, Females	40.7%	47.5%	45.5%	0.348
ASA score	2.3 ± 0.7	2.5 ± 0.7	2.4 ± 0.7	0.379
BMI	23.8 ± 2.9	24.1 ± 3.2	24.0 ± 3.1	0.651
Comorbidities	57.0%	63.5%	61.7%	0.381
CEA (UI/ml)	15.7 ± 33.7	10.7 ± 19.1	12.0 ± 23.6	0.452
CA 19.9 (UI/ml)	592 ± 1276	644 ± 1375	637.0 ± 1345	0.831
Albumin (g/dl)	3.8 ± 0.6	3.7 ± 0.6	3.7 ± 0.6	0.258
Bilirubin (mg/dl)	6.7 ± 15.7	6.2 ± 6.3	6.3 ± 9.7	0.745
Tumor diameter at CT, mm	36.3 ± 22.6	31.6 ± 11.7	32.9 ± 15.4	0.103
Surgery				0.747
PD, number	68	165	233	
LP, number	18	42	60	
TP, number	3	7	10	

SD standard deviation, ASA American Society of Anesthesiology, BMI Body Mass Index, CEA carcinoembryonic antigen, CA 19.9 Carbohydrate Antigen 19.9, CT computed tomography, PD pancreaticoduodenectomy, LP left pancreatectomy, TP total pancreatectomy

Table 2 Postoperative complications and mortality in 303 patients submitted to pancreatectomy with portal vein and/or superior mesenteric vein resection

Variable	N.	%
Overall complications	151	49.8%
Mortality	20	6.6%
Pancreatic fistula	36	11.9%
Grade A	16	
Grade B	14	
Grade C	6	
DGE	70	23.1%
Grade A	32	
Grade B	25	
Grade C	13	
Non pancreatic leak	9	3.0%
Postoperative bleeding	18	5.9%
Re-laparotomy	21	6.9%
PV-SMV thrombosis	5	1.7%
Abdominal collection	33	10.9%
Need of postoperative abdominal drain	36	11.9%
Wound infection	16	5.3%
Urinary tract infection	3	1.0%
Cardiovascular complications	6	2.0%
DVT/PE	5	1.6%
Acute renal failure	3	1.0%
Pneumonia	4	1.3%

N number, *DGE* delayed gastric emptying, *PV-SMV* portal vein-superior mesenteric vein, *DVT/PE* deep venous thrombosis/pulmonary embolism

found for age, sex, comorbidities, tumor size, number of retrieved nodes, T stage and resection margin. Figs. 1, 2, 3 and 4 show the survival curves according to the number of metastatic nodes, pN, the NR and LODDS, respectively. According to the multivariate analyses, the number of metastatic nodes, pN, the NR and LODDS were significantly correlated with survival (Table 4).

Comparison between pN staging, the NR and LODDS methods

The corresponding AUC for the number of metastatic nodes, pN, the NR and LODDS were 0.66 (95% CI 0.58 to 0.73), 0.69 (95% CI 0.62 to 0.76), 0.63 (95% CI 0.55 to 0.70) and 0.65 (95% CI 0.57 to 0.72), respectively, with no significant differences (Fig. 5). The scatter plot of the relationship between LODDS and the NR is reported in Fig. 6. The LODDS value increased with the ratio of metastatic lymph nodes, showing correlation between LODDS and the NR. Values of LODDS were still heterogeneous, even in cases with NR = 0. A significant

Table 3 Clinicopathological data and univariate survival analysis results of 303 patients submitted to pancreatectomy with portal vein and/or superior mesenteric vein resection

Variable	Patients (%)	Median survival (months)	p (univariate analysis)
Age			0.531
< 70	53.2	28.3	
≥ 70	46.8	24	
Sex			0.094
Males	54.5	25	
Females	45.5	26	
Comorbidities			0.058
No	38.3	26	
Yes	61.7	24	
Tumor size			0.193
<30 mm	37.3	28	
≥30 mm	62.7	24	
Resection margin			0.850
R0	73.3	27	
R1	26.7	23	
T stage			0.506
1	0.7	na	
2	6.6	28	
3	86.1	24	
4	6.6	22	
Number of retrieved lymph nodes			0.797
< 17	24.1	26	
≥ 17	75.9	24	
Number of metastatic lymph nodes			0.0005
0–2	56.1	35	
≥ 3	43.9	22	
N stage		0.0002	
N0	29.4	46	
N1	70.6	23	
NR		0.0005	
0	29.4	43	
0.01–0.2	48.2	24	
0.21–0.4	16.2	17	
> 0.4	6.3	22	
LODDS			0.0013
Lodds <−0.005	23.4	72	
−0.005 ≤ Lodds <0.012	24.8	32	
0.012 ≤ Lodds <0.026	26.1	22	
Lodds ≥0.026	25.7	22	

NR nodal ratio, *LODDS* log odds of positive lymph nodes

correlation between the number of retrieved lymph nodes and number of metastatic nodes was found at Pearson test (Table 5). The correlation values were lower for pN and the NR, and LODDS had the lower

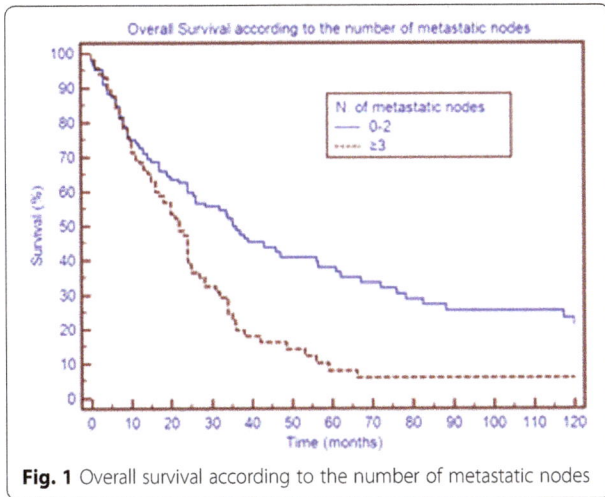

Fig. 1 Overall survival according to the number of metastatic nodes

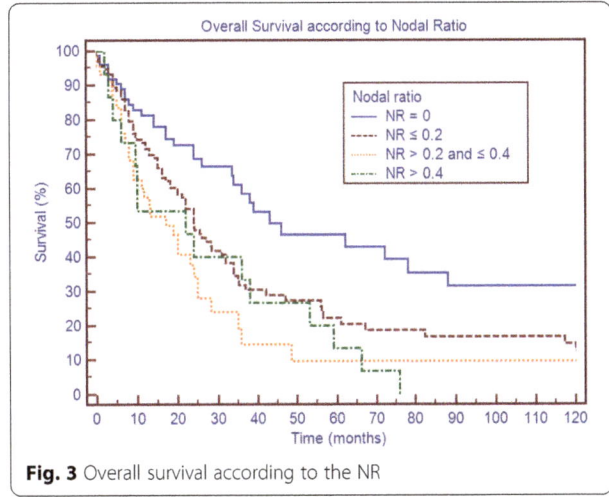

Fig. 3 Overall survival according to the NR

coefficient correlation (0.079) with the number of retrieved nodes ($p = 0.154$).

Further stratification of N1 and N0 patients

Concerning N1 patients, the NR was able to further stratify survival, with patients with NR < 0.2 having better prognosis (median survival of 24 versus 19 months, $p = 0.040$). Further, LODDS stratified N1 patients into two groups with different prognoses, with patients of LODDS >0.03 having significantly worse survival (20 versus 24 months, $p = 0.046$). In addition, the number of metastatic nodes was able to stratify N1 patients in this series, according to the classification reported by Strobel et al. ($p = 0.038$). In the group of patients with <17 retrieved lymph nodes, pN, the NR and LODDS were all able to stratify patient survival ($p = 0.01$, $p = 0.023$ and $p = 0.05$, respectively). The LODDS classification was used to stratify the 89 N0 patients; LODDS1 patients had a median survival of 72 months, whereas

LODDS2 patients had a median survival of 36 months (not statistically significant; $p = 0.229$).

Discussion

Lymph nodal status is considered to be one of the most important prognostic factors after pancreatectomy for adenocarcinoma. The most used nodal staging system is the N status of the AJCC classification, which identifies N0 and N1 patients, according to the presence or absence of nodal metastases. Previous studies have analyzed the prognostic role of the number of examined lymph nodes, number of pathologic lymph nodes, the NR and LODDS in patients with pancreatic cancer, with different results [5, 6, 8, 23, 24]. The number of positive nodes has been suggested to stratify N1 patients, adding prognostic information [8, 25]. Strobel and colleagues reported a median survival of 31.1, 26.1, 21.9 and 18.3 months in patients with 1, 2–3, 4–7 and >7 positive nodes, respectively [8]. The role of the number of positive nodes was also shown in patients submitted to

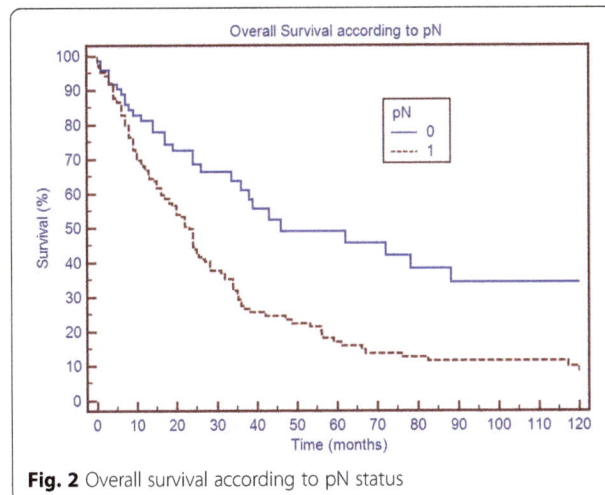

Fig. 2 Overall survival according to pN status

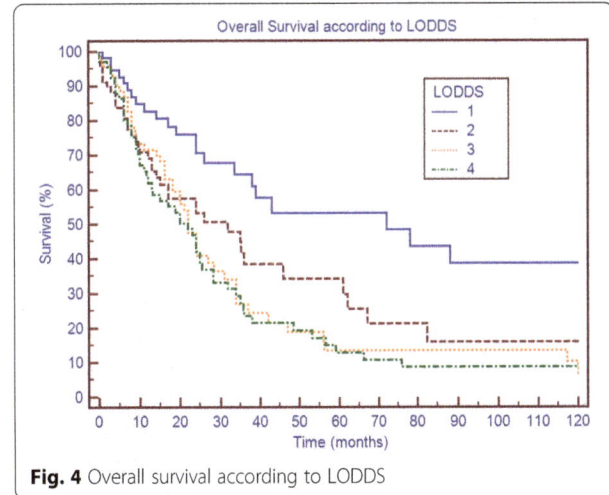

Fig. 4 Overall survival according to LODDS

Table 4 Multivariate analyses using the Cox proportional hazard method. Evaluation of prognostic impact of number of metastatic nodes, pN, nodal ratio and LODDS

Variable	b	SE	P	Exp (b)	95% CI
Age	−0.100	0.184	0.585	0.905	0.633 to 1.294
Sex	−0.244	0.188	0.196	0.784	0.543 to 1.132
Tumor size	0.176	0.197	0.372	1.192	0.813 to 1.749
R status	−0.089	0.221	0.686	0.915	0.594 to 1.407
T stage	−0.059	0.193	0.759	0.942	0.646 to 1.374
N. met. Nodes	0.427	0.186	0.022	1.533	1.066 to 2.23
Age	−0.013	0.183	0.945	0.987	0.691 to 1.411
Sex	−0.247	0.189	0.192	0.781	0.540 to 1.130
Tumor size	0.190	0.197	0.336	1.209	0.823 to 1.775
R status	−0.085	0.218	0.698	0.919	0.600 to 1.407
T stage	−0.115	0.195	0.555	0.892	0.610 to 1.303
N stage	0.603	0.239	0.011	1.828	1.148 to 2.911
Age	−0.0812	0.183	0.655	0.922	0.646 to 1.316
Sex	−0.195	0.190	0.305	0.823	0.568 to 1.192
Tumor size	0.206	0.196	0.293	1.229	0.838 to 1.803
R status	−0.170	0.221	0.441	0.843	0.548 to 1.298
T stage	−0.019	0.188	0.920	0.981	0.680 to 1.416
Nodal ratio	0.384	0.108	0.001	1.468	1.189 to 1.811
Age	−0.010	0.183	0.955	0.989	0.692 to 1.415
Sex	−0.229	0.188	0.221	0.795	0.551 to 1.146
Tumor size	0.184	0.197	0.349	1.202	0.819 to 1.764
R status	−0.189	0.222	0.395	0.828	0.537 to 1.277
T stage	−0.114	0.197	0.563	0.892	0.608 to 1.310
LODDS	0.273	0.089	0.002	1.313	1.105 to 1.562

N. met. Nodes number of metastatic nodes, *NR* nodal ratio, *LODDS* log odds of positive lymph nodes

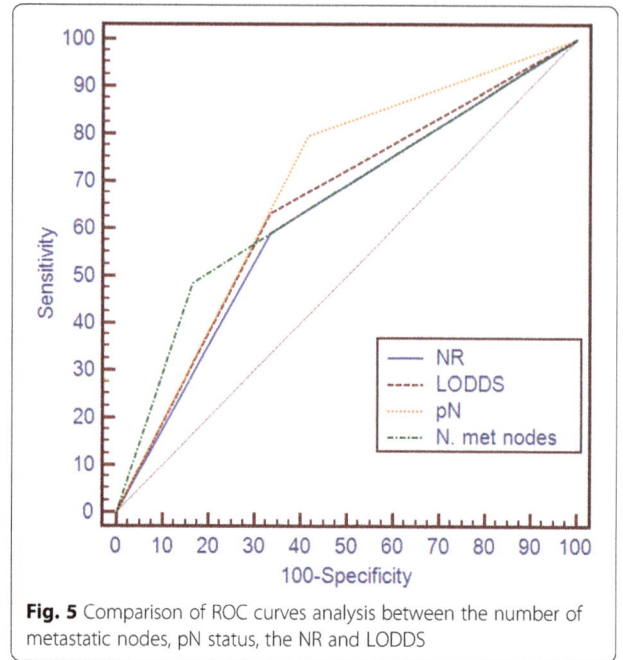

Fig. 5 Comparison of ROC curves analysis between the number of metastatic nodes, pN status, the NR and LODDS

pancreatic surgery after neoadjuvant therapy [25]. Concerning the NR, a number of authors have demonstrated its ability to further stratify node-positive patients [26, 27].

LODDS are new prognostic parameters, which aim to better stratify patients regarding their nodal metastases status. In the setting of gastric, colorectal, breast and other neoplasms, promising data have been reported [28–30]. Comparing to NR, which is a function of the number of retrieved nodes, LODDS is a function of the number of negative lymph nodes. In the setting of pancreatic cancer, only one study has analyzed this parameter, suggesting the advantage of LODDS over the NR in node-negative patients [15]. Patients with pancreatic cancer and portal vein/superior mesenteric vein axes involvement represent a peculiar and challenging subset of patients. Several questions are still open in this setting regarding better perioperative treatment, surgical strategies and prognostic stratification. No study has thus far

analyzed the nodal staging system in this subset of patients to our knowledge, and for these reasons we reviewed a multicenter database to report our data about nodal prognostic factors in patients with venous invasion.

Our study analyzed a population of 303 patients undergoing pancreatectomy combined with venous resection. Patients were treated in referral centers for pancreatic pathology, and standard lymphadenectomy, as recommended by the ISGPS, was performed. The mean number of retrieved lymph nodes was high (33.5), and the majority of patients (70.6%) had at least one metastatic node. Patients submitted to LP had a higher number of retrieved nodes, whereas the number of metastatic nodes was not different in patients

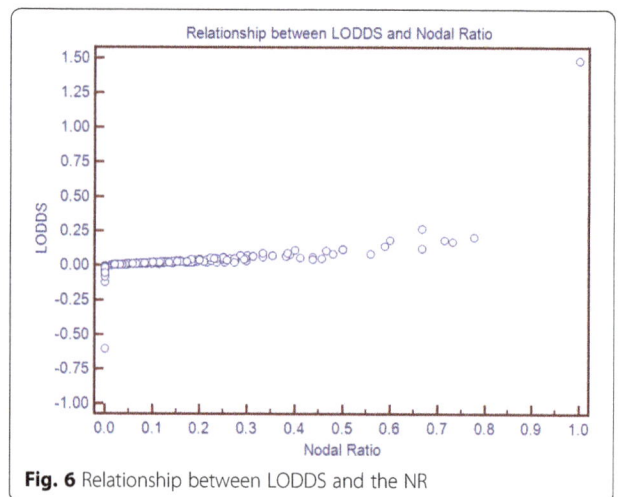

Fig. 6 Relationship between LODDS and the NR

Table 5 Pearson correlation test between number of retrieved lymph nodes and number of metastatic nodes, N status, NR, LODDS

Correlation between of retrieved lymph nodes and number or metastatic nodes	
Sample size	303
Correlation coefficient r	0.298
Significance level	$p < 0.0001$
95% coefficient interval for r	0.192 to 0.398
Correlation between of retrieved lymph nodes and N status	
Sample size	303
Correlation coefficient r	0.1276
Significance level	$p = 0.026$
95% coefficient interval for r	0.015 to 0.237
Correlation between of retrieved lymph nodes and N ratio	
Sample size	303
Correlation coefficient r	−0.193
Significance level	$p = 0.001$
95% coefficient interval for r	−0.299 to −0.082
Correlation between of retrieved lymph nodes and LODDS	
Sample size	303
Correlation coefficient r	−0.082
Significance level	$p = 0.154$
95% coefficient interval for r	−0.193 to 0.031

NR nodal ratio, LODDS log odds of positive lymph nodes

undergoing PD, LP or TP. Univariate and multivariate analyses of prognostic factors were performed. Nodal staging indexes were significant predictors of survival, and the multivariate analysis confirmed the significant prognostic value of the number of metastatic nodes, pN, the NR, and LODDS. A comparison of the different systems was attempted to demonstrate the superiority of one of them. The ROC curves' comparison did not show any significant differences. LODDS had a lower and non-significant correlation with the number of retrieved nodes according to the Pearson test, which may be advantageous in the case of inadequate lymphadenectomy (in this series, only 12.5% of patients has fewer than 11 retrieved nodes). A scatter plot was presented to show that LODDS has the power to discriminate patients with the same NR (0 or 1) but a different prognosis. However, in the entire cohort, all nodal staging systems seemed to be efficacious with a strong prognostic significance.

We further studied the group of patients having at least one nodal metastasis. Clearly, pN classification is limited in this setting, because all patients are classified as N1. The comparison of survival curves via the log-rank test demonstrated that the NR, the number of positive nodes and LODDS might all provide further

stratification for these patients. This result is concordant with those of previous studies, and confirms that pN staging may also be integrated by further information. The number of positive nodes is easy to retrieve and does not require calculation. However, patients with different prognosis may have the same values. For example, the number of positive nodes is the same for patients having 4 metastatic nodes out of 4 retrieved (100% of metastatic nodes) or 4 out of 40 (10%), for example. The NR is simple to calculate. NR carries information that are related to both the number of metastatic and retrieved nodes. However, for values approaching 1 its accuracy seems to diminish (no difference between a patient with 1/1 metastasis and one with 40/40). Furthermore, further stratification of N0 patients is not possible using NR and number of positive nodes. LODDS represent a nodal prognostic index, which is more complex to understand. Furthermore, calculation is less simple, which explain why is rarely used in clinical practice. Theoretically, LODDS have several advantages, including the possibility to further stratify N0 patients. In our series, we failed to demonstrate a statistically significant difference in the 89 N0 patients using LODDS, but these results were limited by the sample size of N0 patients in our study population.

The novelty of this study is that it is the first one evaluating different nodal staging systems in the setting of patients undergoing pancreatectomy with synchronous venous resection. Patients with portal vein or superior mesenteric vein invasion represent a challenging subset of patients, and optimal prognostic stratification is needed in their clinical management. We demonstrated that N1 patients might be further classified using the number of examined lymph nodes, the NR and LODDS. Furthermore, our study adds useful information on the role of LODDS and pancreatic cancer, which is still controversial. Only a few studies have been published about LODDS in pancreatic cancer staging, with some authors suggesting its utility [15] and others recommending avoiding its use [31].

We point out some limitations of this study. Data regarding disease-free survival were not analyzed, because not all included centres reported the information. Furthermore, the study is retrospective. However, use of ISGPS definition and the numbers of included patients represent some remarkable aspects of this series. In this study, neoadjuvant therapy was administered only to a minority of patients. We can explain this data analyzing NCCN guidelines until 2014. Up-front surgery was indicated in fit patients with venous invasion at CT scan suitable to resection and reconstruction with complete tumor clearance. Furthermore, neoadjuvant therapy is a factor that may modify nodal status; hence, the low rate of neoadjuvant therapy in this study represents an advantage regarding the analysis of nodal prognostic factors.

Conclusions

In conclusion, in patients undergoing pancreatectomy with combined PV/SMV resection for pancreatic cancer, the number of examined lymph nodes, the NR and LODDS are useful for the further prognostic stratification of N1 patients. All these staging systems permit the better stratification of patients with nodal metastases and are useful in clinical practice. No superiority of one over the others was detected in patients undergoing pancreatectomy with venous resection.

Acknowledgements
Not applicable

Funding
No founding was received.

Authors' contributions
GR, GN, NP, have made substantial contributions to conception and design, acquisition of data, analysis and interpretation of data; 2) have been involved in drafting the manuscript and revising it critically for important intellectual content; 3) have given final approval of the version to be published; and 4) agree to be accountable for all aspects of the work in ensuring that questions related to the accuracy or integrity of any part of the work are appropriately investigated and resolved. ADP, MR, EJ, FM, GLG, PC, GT, FF, NN, UB have made substantial contributions to acquisition of data, analysis and interpretation of data; 2) have been involved in revising the manuscript critically for important intellectual content; 3) have given final approval of the version to be published; and 4) agree to be accountable for all aspects of the work in ensuring that questions related to the accuracy or integrity of any part of the work are appropriately investigated and resolved.

Competing interests
The authors declare that they have no competing interests. Prof. Giuseppe Nigri is a member of the board (Associate Editor) of BMC Series journal.

Author details
[1]Department of Medical and Surgical Sciences and Translational Medicine, Faculty of Medicine and Psychology, St Andrea Hospital, Sapienza University, General Surgery Unit, Via di Grottarossa 1037, 00189 Rome, Italy. [2]Department of Medical and Surgical Sciences-DIMEC, S. Orsola-Malpighi Hospital, Alma Mater Studiorum, University of Bologna, General Surgery and Transplantation Unit, Bologna, Italy. [3]General Surgery Unit, 'Maggiore' Hospital, Bologna, Italy. [4]Department of Medical and Surgical Sciences (DIMEC), Alma Mater Studiorum, S. Orsola-Malpighi Hospital, University of Bologna, General Surgery Unit, Bologna, Italy. [5]Regina Elena National Cancer Institute IFO, Hepato-pancreato-biliary Surgery Unit, Rome, Italy. [6]Department of Surgical Sciences, Sapienza University of Rome, Policlinico Umberto I Hospital, General Surgery Unit, Rome, Italy. [7]Department of Experimental Medicine and Surgery, Liver Unit, Tor Vergata University of Rome, Rome, Italy. [8]Division of General Surgery and Transplantation Surgery, Niguarda Hospital, Milan, Italy. [9]Division of General Surgery and Transplantation Surgery, Pisa University Hospital, Pisa, Italy.

References
1. Siegel RL, Miller KD, Jemal A. Cancer statistics, 2017. CA Cancer J Clin. 2017; 67:7–30.
2. New European Cancer Observatory – IARC; Cancer factsheets. Available at: http://eco.iarc.fr/eucan/Cancer.aspx?Cancer=15. Accessed 13 Jul 2015.
3. Malleo G, Maggino L, Capelli P, et al. Reappraisal of nodal staging and study of lymph node station involvement in pancreaticoduodenectomy with the standard international study group of pancreatic surgery definition of lymphadenectomy for cancer. J Am Coll Surg. 2015;221:367–79.
4. Pancreas Cancer Staging, American Joint Committee on Cancer, 7th Edition. Available at: https://cancerstaging.org/references-tools/quickreferences/ Documents/PancreasSmall.pdf. Accessed 1 Apr 2016.
5. Valsangkar NP, Bush DM, Michaelson JS, et al. N0/N1, PNL, or LNR? The effect of lymph node number on accurate survival prediction in pancreatic ductal adenocarcinoma. J Gastrointest Surg. 2013;17:257–66.
6. Huebner M, Kendrick M, Reid-Lombardo KM, et al. Number of lymph nodes evaluated: prognostic value in pancreatic adenocarcinoma. J Gastrointest Surg. 2012;16:920–6.
7. Opfermann KJ, Wahlquist AE, Garrett-Mayer E, Shridhar R, Cannick L, Marshall DT. Adjuvant radiotherapy and lymph node status for pancreatic cancer: results of a study from the surveillance, epidemiology, and end results (SEER) registry data. Am J Clin Oncol. 2014;37:112–6.
8. Strobel O, Hinz U, Gluth A, et al. Pancreatic adenocarcinoma: number of positive nodes allows to distinguish several N categories. Ann Surg. 2015;261:961–9.
9. Ashfaq A, Pockaj BA, Gray RJ, Halfdanarson TR, Wasif N. Nodal counts and lymph node ratio impact survival after distal pancreatectomy for pancreatic adenocarcinoma. J Gastrointest Surg. 2014;18:1929–35.
10. Michalski CW, Kleeff J, Wente MN, Diener MK, Büchler MW, Friess H. Systematic review and meta-analysis of standard and extended lymphadenectomy in pancreaticoduodenectomy for pancreatic cancer. Br J Surg. 2007;94:265–73.
11. Sun J, Yang Y, Wang X, et al. Meta-analysis of the efficacies of extended and standard pancreatoduodenectomy for ductal adenocarcinoma of the head of the pancreas. World J Surg. 2014;38:2708–15.
12. Jang JY, Kang MJ, Heo JS, et al. A prospective randomized controlled study comparing outcomes of standard resection and extended resection, including dissection of the nerve plexus and various lymph nodes, in patients with pancreatic head cancer. Ann Surg. 2014;259: 656–64.
13. Dasari BV, Pasquali S, Vohra RS, et al. Extended versus standard lymphadenectomy for pancreatic head cancer: meta-analysis of randomized controlled trials. J Gastrointest Surg. 2015;19:1725–32.
14. Tol JA, Gouma DJ, Bassi C, et al. Definition of a standard lymphadenectomy in surgery for pancreatic ductal adenocarcinoma: a consensus statement by the international study group on pancreatic surgery (ISGPS). Surgery. 2014;156:591–600.
15. La Torre M, Nigri G, Petrucciani N, et al. Prognostic assessment of different lymph node staging methods for pancreatic cancer with R0 resection: pN staging, lymph node ratio, log odds of positive lymph nodes. Pancreatology. 2014;14:289–94.
16. Liu ZQ, Xiao ZW, Luo GP, et al. Effect of the number of positive lymph nodes and lymph node ratio on prognosis of patients after resection of pancreatic adenocarcinoma. Hepatobiliary Pancreat Dis Int. 2014;13:634–41.
17. Slidell MB, Chang DC, Cameron JL, et al. Impact of total lymph node count and lymph node ratio on staging and survival after pancreatectomy for pancreatic adenocarcinoma: a large, population-based analysis. Ann Surg Oncol. 2008;15:165–74.
18. Ramacciato G, Nigri G, Petrucciani N, et al. Pancreatectomy with mesenteric and portal vein resection for borderline resectable pancreatic cancer: multicenter study of 406 patients. Ann Surg Oncol. 2016; [Epub ahead of print]
19. Bassi C, Dervenis C, Butturini G, et al. Postoperative pancreatic fistula: an international study group (ISGPF) definition. Surgery. 2005;138:8–13.
20. Wente MN, Bassi C, Dervenis C, et al. Delayed gastric emptying (DGE) after pancreatic surgery: a suggested definition by the international study Group of Pancreatic Surgery (ISGPS). Surgery. 2007;142:761–8.
21. Bockhorn M, Uzunoglu FG, Adham M, et al. Borderline resectable pancreatic cancer: a consensus statement by the international study Group of Pancreatic Surgery (ISGPS). Surgery. 2014;155:977–88.

Prognostic role of nodal ratio, LODDS, pN in patients with pancreatic cancer with venous...

179

22. DeLong ER, DeLong DM, Clarke-Pearson DL. Comparing the areas under two or more correlated receiver operating characteristic curves: a nonparametric approach. Biometrics. 1988;44:837–45.

23. Kang MJ, Jang JY, Chang YR, Kwon W, Jung W, Kim SW. Revisiting the concept of lymph node metastases of pancreatic head cancer: number of metastatic lymph nodes and lymph node ratio according to N stage. Ann Surg Oncol. 2014;21:1545–51.

24. Riediger H, Keck T, Wellner U, et al. The lymph node ratio is the strongest prognostic factor after resection of pancreatic cancer. J Gastrointest Surg. 2009;13:1337–44.

25. Fischer LK, Katz MH, Lee SM, et al. The number and ratio of positive lymph nodes affect pancreatic cancer patient survival after neoadjuvant therapy and pancreaticoduodenectomy. Histopathology. 2016;68:210–20.

26. Yamada S, Fujii T, Hirakawa A, Kanda M, Sugimoto H, Kodera Y. Lymph node ratio as parameter of regional lymph node involvement in pancreatic cancer. Langenbeck's Arch Surg. 2016; [Epub ahead of print]

27. Robinson SM, Rahman A, Haugk B, et al. Metastatic lymph node ratio as an important prognostic factor in pancreatic ductal adenocarcinoma. Eur J Surg Oncol. 2012;38:333–9.

28. Wen J, Ye F, He X, et al. Development and validation of a prognostic nomogram based on the log odds of positive lymph nodes (LODDS) for breast cancer. Oncotarget. 2016;

29. Song YX, Gao P, Wang ZN, et al. Which is the most suitable classification for colorectal cancer, log odds, the number or the ratio of positive lymph nodes? PLoS One. 2011;6:e28937.

30. Aurello P, Petrucciani N, Nigri GR, et al. Log odds of positive lymph nodes (LODDS): what are their role in the prognostic assessment of gastric adenocarcinoma? J Gastrointest Surg. 2014;18:1254–60.

31. Riediger H, Kulemann B, Wittel U, et al. Prognostic role of log odds of lymph nodes after resection of pancreatic head cancer. J Gastrointest Surg. 2016;20:1707–15.

26

Delayed gastric emptying following pancreatoduodenectomy with alimentary reconstruction according to Roux-en-Y or Billroth-II

Tim R. Glowka[1*], Markus Webler[2], Hanno Matthaei[1], Nico Schäfer[1], Volker Schmitz[3], Jörg C. Kalff[1], Jens Standop[4] and Steffen Manekeller[1]

Abstract

Background: Delayed gastric emptying (DGE) remains the most frequent complication following pancreatoduodenectomy (PD) with published incidences as high as 61%. The present study investigates the impact of bowel reconstruction techniques on DGE following classic PD (Whipple-Kausch procedure) with pancreatogastrostomy (PG).

Methods: We included 168 consecutive patients who underwent PD with PG with either Billroth II type (BII, $n = 78$) or Roux-en-Y type reconstruction (ReY, $n = 90$) between 2004 and 2015. Excluded were patients with conventional single loop reconstruction after pylorus preserving procedures. DGE was classified according to the 2007 International Study Group of Pancreatic Surgery definition. Patients were analyzed regarding severity of DGE, morbidity and mortality, length of hospital stay and demographic factors.

Results: No difference was observed between BII and ReY regarding frequency of DGE. Overall rate for clinically relevant DGE was 30% (ReY) and 26% (BII). BII and ReY did not differ in terms of demographics, morbidity or mortality. DGE significantly prolongs ICU (four vs. two days) and hospital stay (20.5 vs. 14.5 days). Risk factors for DGE development are advanced age, retrocolic reconstruction, postoperative hemorrhage and major complications.

Conclusions: The occurrence of DGE can not be influenced by the type of alimentary reconstruction (ReY vs. BII) following classic PD with PG. Old age and major complications could be identified as important risk factors in multivariate analysis.

Keywords: Delayed gastric emptying, DGE, Pancreatoduodenectomy, Billroth II, Whipple, Roux-en-Y

Background

Pancreatoduodenectomy (PD) is the standard surgical procedure for malignant pancreatic head and periampullary tumors [1]. In specialized centers, the surgery can be performed with a relatively low mortality rate of 0–6% [2–4]. Nevertheless, the morbidity rate remains high, ranging from 30% to above 50% [5]. Apart from pancreatic fistula as the most frequent *major* complication following PD [6], delayed gastric emptying (DGE) is even more common with up to 61% reported rates [5, 7]. The type of reconstruction technique after PD is considered to influence the frequency of DGE. While antecolic position of the gastro-/duodenojejunal loop has been considered superior in terms of DGE [8, 9], recent studies demonstrated comparable benefits of retrocolic reconstruction [7, 10, 11]. In terms of DGE frequency, this could also be shown for pylorus-preserving PD compared to classic PD with antrectomy (Kausch-Whipple procedure) [12]. However, in recent years, pylorus resection without antrectomy has been increasingly advocated [13–15]. Furthermore,

* Correspondence: tim.glowka@ukb.uni-bonn.de
[1]Department of Surgery, University of Bonn, Sigmund-Freud-Str. 25, 53105 Bonn, Germany
Full list of author information is available at the end of the article

regarding DGE, single loop ("conventional reconstruction") and Roux-en-Y (dual loop) reconstruction show no difference [16].

Classic PD with pyloric resection and reconstruction according to Billroth II (BII) and Roux-en-Y (ReY) as standard procedures are performed with decreasing frequency since single loop reconstruction methods and pyloric preservation have proven comparable in terms of fistula formation and DGE with reduced surgery duration and blood loss [8, 17]. However, antral resection with BII or ReY reconstructions are still performed in case of local tumor infiltration to the distal stomach. Apart from the above mentionend perioperative options, Whipple-Kausch procedure as well as pylorus-preserving single-loop PD are equally effective in the treatment of periampullary malignancies [18]. Outside tertiary referral centers, BII and ReY remain in use, but only limited data are available on the incidence of DGE when comparing BII and ReY following PD. To our knowledge, only one study compared BII and ReY reconstructions after pancreatojejunal anastomosis for their impact on DGE [19]. To date, these two reconstruction methods have not been compared after pancreatogastrostomy (PG).

Methods

Between 2004 and 2015, 390 patients underwent anatomical pancreatic resection at our department. Of these, 168 patients underwent a classic pancreatoduodenectomy with antral resection and reconstruction according to BII or ReY. Excluded were patients with pylorus preserving procedures and conventional reconstruction with a single jejunal loop, and patients who had previous gastrectomy (Fig. 1). All pancreatic resections were prospectively recorded in a pancreatic resection database with the approval of the institutional ethics committee (Ethik-Kommission der Medizinischen Fakultät der Rheinischen Friedrich-Wilhelms-Universität, 347/13) and with obtaining written informed consent from the participants. Morbidity and mortality were consistently documented according to the Dindo-Clavien- classification [20].

Perioperative management was conducted according to an institutional recovery programm: sip feeds were provided in case of preoperative malnutrition; parenteral nutrition was only administered when the oral route was inaccesible. No endoscopic biliary drainage was performed if serum bilirubin was below 250 μmol/l and surgery was scheduled within the next ten days. No oral bowel preparation was used and oral fasting was limited to 2 h for liquids and 6 h for solids. A mid-thoracic epidural catheter was placed by default, while in case of contraindications, missing placement options or catheter disfunction, patient-controlled analgesia was considered as alternative. Anesthesia was carried out according to guidelines (postoperative nausea and vomiting prophylaxis if required, near zero fluid balance, tranfusion according to patient blood mangement guidelines and close glycemic control).

PD was performed via a bilateral subcostal incision. After complete abdominal exploration and exclusion of arterial infiltation, PD was carried out with antrectomy, standard lymphadenectomy by default and PG as previously described [21]. Infiltration to the portal or superior mesenteric vene was resected en-bloc with the pancreas.

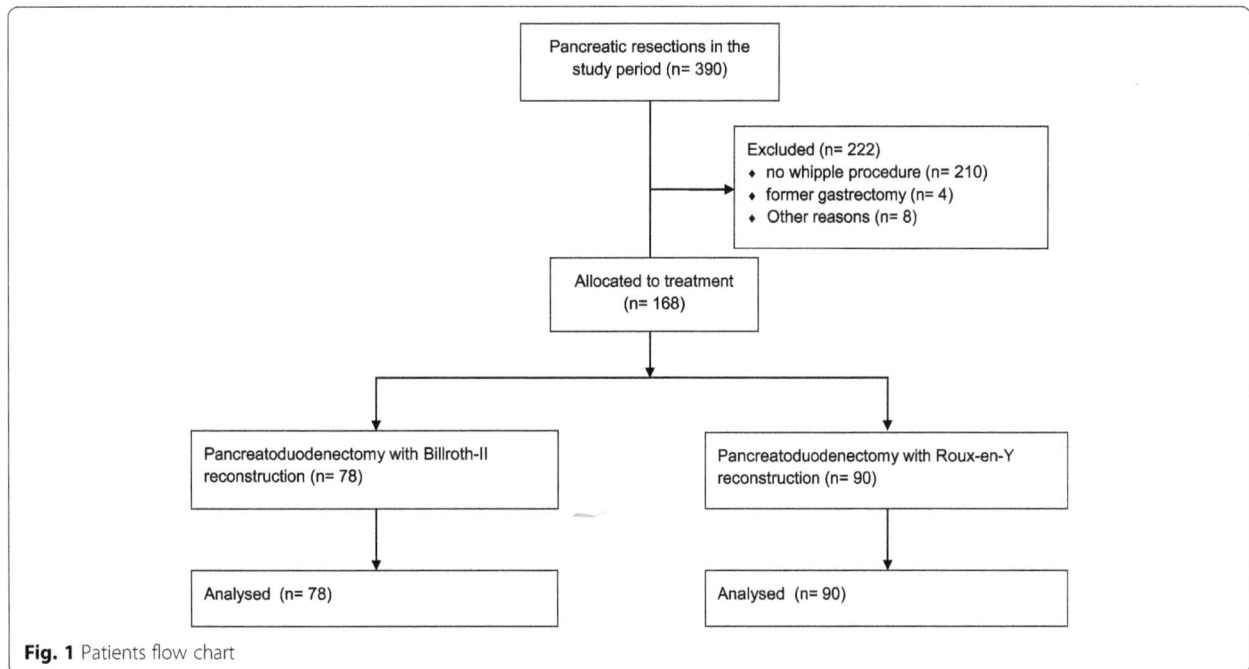

Fig. 1 Patients flow chart

If simple suture led to narrowing of the vein, resection and end-to-end anastomosis was performed. Choledochojejunostomy was carried out to the oral jejunal loop with a retrocolic single-layer end-to-side running suture (4/0 absorbable). Reconstruction method was chosen in a pragmatic manner according to the surgeon's preference [22]. In BII reconstruction, a double layer end-to-side running suture gastrojejunostomy (4/0 absorbable) was performed 40 cm aboral to the biliary anstomosis, while 15 cm below, reconstruction was completed by a (stapled) Braun enteroenterostomy (Fig. 2a). ReY reconstruction was performed with the same gastrojejunal anstomosis with an isolated jejunal loop and enteroenterostomy 30 cm aborally (Fig. 2b). Two soft drains were placed at the sites of PG and choledochojejunostomy before closure of the abdomen. These drains were removed between postoperative days (POD) 3–5 if no elevated amylase content (compared to serum amylase) could be detected in measurements. By default, all patients spent at least one night in the intensive care unit. A 14 French nasogastric tube (NGT) was placed and subsequently removed on POD 3 when output fell below 500 ml/day. Patients were allowed to drink water on the day of surgery, liquid diet was introduced from POD 2, and solid food from POD 3 and increased according to a standard protocol (POD 3 fat reduced/easily digestible, POD 4 fiber reduced/easily digestible, POD 5 basic diet (no pulses/no brassica), POD 6 normal diet). If no bowel movement had occurred by POD 3, oral laxative (magnesium sulfate) was administered. Transition to a normal diet was discontinued in case of vomiting. All patients received perioperative antibiotic prophylaxis (aminopenicillin plus β-lactamase inhibitor) and weight-adapted thrombosis prophylaxis (continued for four weeks after surgery plus support stockings) but no secretion inhibitor (octreotide) on a regular basis. DGE was recorded as stipulated by the 2007 International Study Group of Pancreatic Surgery (ISGPS) definition [5]. Based on duration of NGT, need for reinsertion, the day, when solid food was first tolerated, occurrence of

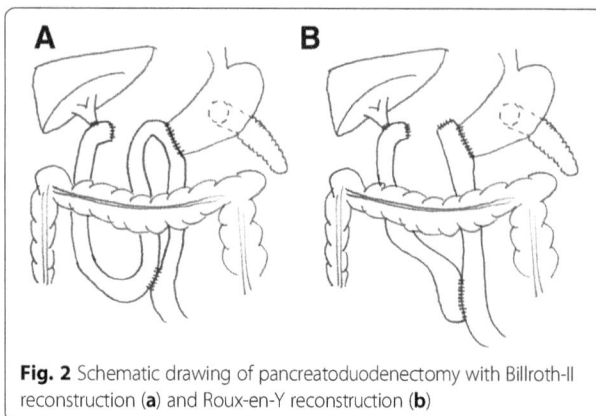

Fig. 2 Schematic drawing of pancreatoduodenectomy with Billroth-II reconstruction (**a**) and Roux-en-Y reconstruction (**b**)

vomiting and use of prokinetics, DGE was classified according to three grades. Since the ISGPS definition tends to overestimate DGE at °A [23], some authors report the clinically relevant °B and °C when specific treatment is indicated. Prior to 2007, patients were retrospectively graded according to the ISGPS definition based on their medical records.

Data were recorded and analyzed with Excel 2013 (Microsoft Corporation, Redmond, Washington, USA) and SPSS 23 (IBM Corporation, Armonk, New York, USA). Continuously and normally distributed variables were expressed as medians ± standard deviation and analyzed using Student's t test, while non-normally distributed data was expressed as medians and interquartile range and analyzed using the Mann–Whitney U test. Categorical data was expressed as proportions and compared with the Pearson χ^2 or the Fisher's exact test as appropriate. Factors with P <0.1 in the univariate analysis were included in multivariate stepwise logistic regression analysis. The relative risk was described by the estimated odds ratio with 95% confidence intervals. A P-value <0.05 was considered statistically significant.

Results

ReY and BII groups were comparable in age, gender, diagnosis and preoperative characteristics. Intra- and perioperative data were equal. There was no difference between morbidity factors or mortality. Clinically significant DGE occurred in 30% ($n = 27$, ReY) and 26% ($n = 20$, BII), respectively (Table 1). Patients suffering from DGE were significantly older (68 vs. 62 years), while no significant difference in other demographic factors, such as diagnosis or preoperative risk factors, could be shown (Table 2). Surgery duration and blood loss did not differ in patients with and without DGE (Table 3). In the DGE group, more patients were reconstructed with a retrocolic gastrojejunostomy (89/98 (91%) vs. 66/80 (80%), $P = 0.047$) and ICU stay (four vs. two days, $P < 0.001$) as well as hospital stay (20.5 vs. 14.5 days, $P < 0.001$) were significantly longer. Major complications (Dindo-Clavien °3-5) were associated with DGE (42% vs. 23%, $P = 0.01$), while pancreatic fistula was only slightly more common in the DGE group compared with patients not suffering from DGE (30% vs. 38%, $P = 0.297$). Secondary DGE (following other intraabdominal complications) was more common than primary DGE (56 vs. 42, $P = 0.068$) and DGE was more severe in secondary DGE (°A 25 vs. 26, $P = 0.971$; °B 9 vs. 11, $P = 0.717$; °C 8 vs. 19, $P = 0.030$). Significantly more patients with DGE suffered from post pancreatectomy hemorrhages (PPH; 28% vs. 14%, $P = 0.041$), which was also a risk factor for the severity of DGE (°C 12/37 vs. 15/131 (PPH yes/no), $P = 0.002$). If no DGE developed, solid food was tolerated on average on POD

Table 1 Preoperative and perioperative characteristics

		ReY		BII		P
		n = 90		n = 78		
Age, years		65 (55–74)		67 (54–70)		0.948
Gender						0.092
female		29	(32%)	35	(45%)	
male		61	(68%)	43	(55%)	
BMI		25,2 ± 3,5		23,4 ± 4,3		0.066
Diagnosis						
Malignant		71	(79%)	59	(76%)	0.616
Ductal adenocarcinoma		39	(43%)	32	(41%)	
Ampullary carcinoma		13	(14%)	16	(21%)	
Distal bile duct carcinoma		8	(9%)	8	(10%)	
Benign		19	(21%)	19	(24%)	
Pancreatitis		11	(12%)	17	(22%)	
DM	pre	14	(16%)	17	(22%)	0.298
	post	14	(16%)	21	(27%)	0.076
Alcohol		23	(26%)	15	(19%)	0.328
Smoker		43	(48%)	26	(33%)	0.058
Weight loss		39	(43%)	25	(32%)	0.133
Preoperative biliary drainage		56	(62%)	45	(58%)	0.618
Cholangitis		21	(23%)	16	(21%)	0.66
Time of operation	min	434 ± 104		410 ± 77		0.104
Red blood cell transfusion	units	2 (0–4)		2 (1,5–4)		0.518
Blood loss		1000 (500–1600)		800 (400–1300)		0.262
Clavien classification						0.145
minor		55	(61%)	56	(72%)	
major		35	(39%)	22	(28%)	
Mortality		1	(1%)	1	(1%)	1.0
Pancreatic fistula		36	(40%)	22	(28%)	0.109
Post pancretectomy hemorrhage		20	(22%)	17	(22%)	0.947
DGE		49	(54%)	49	(63%)	0.272
	B/C	27	(30%)	20	(26%)	0.53

Data are expressed as mean ± SD, *number (%), or* median (interquartile range)

6 and NGT was then removed on POD 2 (Table 4). If DGE developed, solid food was tolerated on POD 11 ($P < 0.001$), NGT removal occurred on POD 4 ($P < 0.001$) and NGT reinsertion was required in 39% of the patients ($P < 0.001$). Vomiting and use of prokinetics were significantly more common in the DGE group. DGE was graded as °A in 52%, °B in 20% and °C in 28% of the patients. In univariate analysis, the following factors qualified for multivariate analysis: patient age (dichotomized for multivariate analysis), weight loss, cholangitis, antecolic reconstruction, extended lymphadenectomy, PPH and major complications (Table 5). Age above 70 years ($P = 0.009$) and major complications ($P = 0.003$) proved to be significant risk factors in multivariate analysis.

Discussion

Delayed gastric emptying is the most common complication following pancreatoduodenectomy (PD), occuring in 19–61% of patients [5, 7]. Since the first description of DGE following PD by Warshaw in 1985 [24], many attempts have been made to further understand the mechanisms leading to DGE. Proposed factors are a decrease of plasma motlin levels due to resection of the duodenum, ischemia and denervation of the stomach due to mobilisation and lymphadenectomy, or DGE caused by postoperative intra-abdominal complications [25]. Only limited data exist on the effect of dual loop reconstruction on DGE formation, with DGE occurrence ranging from 9.5 to 72% [26–29]. At our department, as

Table 2 Preoperative Characteristics

		No DGE		DGE		P
		n = 70		n = 98		
Age, years		62 (51–69)		68 (60–74)		*0.003*
Gender						0.39
female		24	(34%)	40	(41%)	
male		46	(66%)	58	(59%)	
BMI		24,6 ± 3,8		24,4 ± 4		0.888
Diagnosis						
Malignant		54	(77%)	76	(78%)	0.95
Ductal adenocarcinoma		31	(44%)	40	(41%)	
Ampullary carcinoma		10	(14%)	19	(19%)	
Distal bile duct carcinoma		7	(10%)	9	(9%)	
Benign		16	(23%)	22	(22%)	
Pancreatitis		13	(19%)	15	(15%)	
DM	pre	12	(17%)	19	(19%)	0.712
	post	15	(21%)	20	(20%)	0.835
Alcohol		19	(27%)	19	(19%)	0.236
Smoker		31	(44%)	38	(39%)	0.474
Weight loss		32	(46%)	32	(33%)	0.086
Preoperative biliary drainage		43	(61%)	58	(59%)	0.831
Cholangitis		20	(29%)	17	(17%)	0.083

Data are expressed as mean ± SD, *number (%), or* median (interquartile range). Statistical significance indicated by italics

in most centers for pancreatic surgery, pylorus-preserving PD with single loop reconstruction is the established standard procedure due to reduced surgery duration and blood loss and equal complication rates [8, 17]. Nevertheless, in case of tumor infiltration to the distal stomach, or after previous gastrectomy, classic PD with dual loop reconstruction is required. Very little is known about the effect of BII and ReY reconstruction on DGE. In 2015, a meta-analysis comparing ReY and BII reconstruction after PD found that DGE frequency can be lowered when using BII reconstruction [30]. A limitation of this study was the different understanding of the surgical reconstruction methods. Two studies compared conventional single loop reconstruction with ReY reconstruction [29, 31], while only one study intentionally compared ReY and BII, again favoring BII reconstruction [19]. However, differences regarding the local setting (e.g. overall length of hospital stay) make their and our findings difficult to compare. Moreover, the authors based their findings on pancreatojejunostomy (PJ) as pancreato-enteric anastomosis. The existing studies did not find a difference in DGE frequency between PJ and PG [4, 32]. However, in these studies, reconstruction was neither specified or performed as conventional single loop reconstruction. Thus, especially after PG, knowledge about DGE after dual loop reconstruction is very limited. In our study, we identified PPH

rather than pancreatic fistula as a significant factor contributing to DGE. Most studies comparing PG and PJ found no difference in PPH frequency [33–35], whereas the biggest randomized study, involving 440 patients, found PPH more common after PG [4]. In fact, it was found to be more than twice as common (PJ 11% vs. PG 21%), which is exactly the PPH frequency we observed. Most bleedings (PPH °A 3/0, °B 18/8 and °C 6/2 [DGE yes/no]) were °A/B, which in most cases, could be treated conservatively or endoscopically. The option of easy endoscopic access is one of the advantages of PG reconstruction compared to PJ, making intraluminal PPH easily treatable with interventional gastroscopy [36]. Endoscopic access in PPH after PD with dual loop reconstruction using PJ is more difficult. Other advantages claimed for PG over PJ after PD is a reduced rate of pancreatic and bile leakage [32]. However, the afore mentioned German multicenter trial (RECOPANC) could not confirm this finding [4]. Apart from the treatment of acute postoperative bleeding, long term endoscopic access is still under debate: successful endoscopic retrograde cholangiography is more likely to be achieved after BII than after ReY reconstruction [37]. However, following distal gastrectomy, ReY was found superior to BII in terms of related symptoms, weight gain, as well as regarding endoscopic findings and bile reflux [38]. For PD, no long-term endoscopic examinations exist. Therefore, BII and ReY reconstruction have certain advantages and disadvantages. Both procedures have the same DGE frequency following PD. In our department, BII reconstruction with a Braun enterostomy is performed by default. A recent assessment of Braun enterostomy after PD found it to be beneficial in lowering DGE frequency [39, 40]. In our opinion, Braun enterostomy is obligatory after antrectomy (or subtotal gastrectomy) to prevent biliary reflux, ulceration and long-term impairments associated with subtotal gastrectomy (especially gastric stump carcinoma). In our cohort, patient age was identified as a uni- and multivariate risk factor for DGE. The impact of age on morbidity and mortality after PD varies [41]. Two nationwide surveys from the US and the Netherlands found more complications and a higher morbidity in the elderly [42, 43]. When DGE occurs, ICU stay as well as general hospital stay as markers for health care costs are signifcantly prolonged, while complications after pancreatic surgery generally lead to a cost increase [44]. In today's age of diagnosis-related groups with case-related reimbursement, prophylaxis of DGE is also of important economic interest. In Germany, PD can only be performed cost-neutrally when the complication rate is low [45]. Therefore, prevention of DGE after PD is not only of major medical, but also economical interest. As DGE is more severe following other intraabdominal complications, thus requiring a longer hospital stay, intraabdominal complications should be avoided as a

Table 3 Perioperative characteristics and morbidity

		No DGE		DGE		P
		n = 70		n = 98		
Time of operation	min	427 ± 90		421 ± 97		0.721
Red blood cell transfusion	units	2 (0–4)		2 (0–4)		0.091
Blood loss	ml	750 (500–1500)		1000 (400–1800)		0.324
Antecolic reconstruction		14	(20%)	9	(9%)	*0.047*
Extended lymphadenectomy		31	(44%)	31	(32%)	0.094
Venous resection		4	(6%)	13	(13%)	0.11
Roux-en-Y reconstruction		41	(59%)	49	(50%)	0.272
ICU stay	days	2 (2–4)		4 (3–7)		*<0.001*
Primary DGE				42		0.068
Secondary DGE				56		
Clavien classification						
minor		54	(77%)	57	(58%)	
major		16	(23%)	41	(42%)	*0.010*
Mortality		0	(0%)	2	(2%)	0.511
Redo operation		10	(14%)	24	(24%)	0.105
Pancreatic fistula		21	(30%)	37	(38%)	0.297
A		13	(19%)	24	(25%)	0.361
B		3	(4%)	5	(5%)	1.0
C		5	(7%)	8	(8%)	0.807
Post pancreatectomy hemorrhage		10	(14%)	27	(28%)	*0.041*
Wound infection		9	(13%)	17	(14%)	0.428
Intraabdominal abscess formation		6	(9%)	9	(9%)	0.891
Hospital stay	days	14,5 (13–21,5)		20,5 (16–30)		*<0,001*

Data are expressed as mean ± SD, *number (%), or median (inter*quartile range). Statistical significance indicated by italics

matter of priority. In particular, secure hemostasis at the pancreatic surface, safe closure of resected vessels (gastroduodenal artery) by non-resorbable sutures and standardized pancreatic anastomosis technique are the cornerstones following pancreatic resections [46]. In the

Table 4 DGE and DGE-related parameters

	No DGE		DGE		P
	n = 70		n = 98		
Tolerate solid diet (days)	6 (5–6,25)		11 (8–15)		*<0.001*
Nasogastric tube (NGT)					
NGT duration (days)	2 (1–3)		4 (2,75-5,25)		*<0.001*
NGT reinsertion	5	(7%)	38	(39%)	*<0.001*
Vomiting	14	(20%)	49	(50%)	*<0.001*
Use of prokinetics	16	(23%)	61	(62%)	*<0.001*
DGE °A			51	(52%)	
DGE °B			20	(20%)	
DGE °C			27	(28%)	

Data are expressed as mean ± SD, number (%), or median (interquartile range). Statistical significance indicated by italic

therapy of DGE, it is important to distinguish DGE from postoperative ileus and to rule out mechanical obstruction as previosly described [47]. When DGE is diagnosed, first therapy steps include NGT and prokinetics (erythromycin) [25]. When secondary DGE occurs, the treatment of the underlying cause must be top prioritiy. If DGE persists after the complication was properly treated or in case of longer lasting primary DGE, we recommend endoscopic insertion of a jejunal feeding tube, followed by low-dose (20 mL/h) enteral feeding. In our experience, DGE will then resolve within a few days. This is especially beneficial if nutritional support commences within ten postoperative days [48]. Routine placement of a jejunal tube during surgery can not be recommended at present [49].

Conclusions
When antrectomy and subsequent dual loop reconstruction is necessary, DGE frequency is equal to pylorus-preserving procedures. DGE occurrence can not be influenced by either BII or ReY reconstruction. Since patient age can not be modified, the primary focus should

Table 5 Risk factors for DGE

	Odds ratio	95% CI	P
univariate			
Age >70 years	2.323	1.136 – 4.749	*0.019*
Weight loss	0.576	0.306 – 1.083	0.086
Cholangitis	0.525	0.251 – 1.096	0.083
Antecolic reconstruction	0.409	0.166 – 1.008	*0.047*
Extended lymphadenectomy	0.582	0.308 – 1.099	0.094
Post pancreatectomy hemorrhage	2.282	1.022 – 5.092	*0.041*
Major complications (Dindo-Clavien °3-5)	2.428	1.221 – 4.827	*0.01*
multivariate			
Age >70 years	2.745	1.29 – 5.841	*0.009*
Major complications (Dindo-Clavien °3-5)	3.03	1.458 – 6.297	*0.003*

CI confidence interval. Statistical significance indicated by italic

be to lower postoperative complications. In particular, PPH should be prevented through extensive hemostasis at the pancreatic remnant and the sourrounding vessels. Anteoclic gastrojejunostomy, if technically possible, was helpful in our cohort to further reduce DGE.

Abbreviations
BII: Billroth-II; DGE: Delayed gastric emptying; ISGPS: International Study Group of Pancreatic Surgery; NGT: Nasogastric tube; PD: Pancreatoduodenectomy; PG: Pancreatogastrostomy; PJ: Pancreatojejunostomy; POD: Psotoperative day; PPH: Post pancreatectomy hemorrhage; ReY: Roux-en-Y

Acknowledgements
Not applicable.

Funding
No funding.

Authors' contributions
TRG, JS and SM are responsible for study conception and design. NS, JCK, JS and SM performed the operations. VS performed the endoscopies. TRG and MW collected the data. TRG, MW, HM, NS, VS, JCK, JS, SM analyzed and interpreted the data. TRG drafted the manuscript. TRG, MW, HM, NS, VS, JCK, JS, SM revised the manuscript and gave their final approval.

Competing interests
The authors declare that they have no competing interests.

Author details
[1]Department of Surgery, University of Bonn, Sigmund-Freud-Str. 25, 53105 Bonn, Germany. [2]Department of Orthopedic and Trauma Surgery, University of Bonn, Sigmund-Freud-Str. 25, 53105 Bonn, Germany. [3]Department of Gastroenterology, St. Marienwörth Hospital, Mühlenstr. 39, 55543 Bad Kreuznach, Germany. [4]Department of Surgery, Maria Stern Hospital, Am Anger 1, 53424 Remagen, Germany.

References
1. Gouma DJ, Nieveen van Dijkum EJ, Obertop H. The standard diagnostic work-up and surgical treatment of pancreatic head tumours. Eur J Surg Oncol. 1999;25:113–23.
2. Gordon TA, Bowman HM, Tielsch JM, Bass EB, Burleyson GP, Cameron JL. Statewide regionalization of pancreaticoduodenectomy and its effect on in-hospital mortality. Ann Surg. 1998;228:71–8.
3. van Heek NT, Kuhlmann KF, Scholten RJ, de Castro SM, Busch OR, van Gulik TM, et al. Hospital volume and mortality after pancreatic resection: a systematic review and an evaluation of intervention in the Netherlands. Ann Surg. 2005;242:781–8. discussion.
4. Keck T, Wellner UF, Bahra M, Klein F, Sick O, Niedergethmann M, et al. Pancreatogastrostomy versus pancreatojejunostomy for RECOnstruction after PANCreatoduodenectomy (RECOPANC, DRKS 00000767): perioperative and long-term results of a multicenter randomized controlled trial. Ann Surg. 2016;263:440–9.
5. Wente MN, Bassi C, Dervenis C, Fingerhut A, Gouma DJ, Izbicki JR, et al. Delayed gastric emptying (DGE) after pancreatic surgery: a suggested definition by the International Study Group of Pancreatic Surgery (ISGPS). Surgery. 2007;142:761–8.
6. Bassi C, Dervenis C, Butturini G, Fingerhut A, Yeo C, Izbicki J, et al. Postoperative pancreatic fistula: an international study group (ISGPF) definition. Surgery. 2005;138:8–13.
7. Eshuis WJ, van Eijck CHJ, Gerhards MF, Coene PP, de Hingh IHJT, Karsten TM, et al. Antecolic versus retrocolic route of the gastroenteric anastomosis after pancreatoduodenectomy: a randomized controlled trial. Ann Surg. 2014;259:45–51.
8. Tani M, Terasawa H, Kawai M, Ina S, Hirono S, Uchiyama K, et al. Improvement of delayed gastric emptying in pylorus-preserving pancreaticoduodenectomy: results of a prospective, randomized, controlled trial. Ann Surg. 2006;243:316–20.
9. Kurahara H, Shinchi H, Maemura K, Mataki Y, Iino S, Sakoda M, et al. Delayed gastric emptying after pancreatoduodenectomy. J Surg Res. 2011;171:e187–92.
10. Imamura M, Kimura Y, Ito T, Kyuno T, Nobuoka T, Mizuguchi T, et al. Effects of antecolic versus retrocolic reconstruction for gastro/duodenojejunostomy on delayed gastric emptying after pancreatoduodenectomy: a systematic review and meta-analysis. J Surg Res. 2016;200:147–57.
11. Joliat G-R, Labgaa I, Demartines N, Schäfer M, Allemann P. Effect of antecolic versus retrocolic gastroenteric reconstruction after pancreaticoduodenectomy on delayed gastric emptying: a meta-analysis of six randomized controlled trials. Dig Surg. 2016;33:15–25.
12. Diener MK, Knaebel H-P, Heukaufer C, Antes G, Büchler MW, Seiler CM. A systematic review and meta-analysis of pylorus-preserving versus classical pancreaticoduodenectomy for surgical treatment of periampullary and pancreatic carcinoma. Ann Surg. 2007;245:187–200.
13. Kurahara H, Takao S, Shinchi H, Mataki Y, Maemura K, Sakoda M, et al. Subtotal stomach-preserving pancreaticoduodenectomy (SSPPD) prevents postoperative delayed gastric emptying. J Surg Oncol. 2010;102:615–9.
14. Kawai M, Tani M, Hirono S, Miyazawa M, Shimizu A, Uchiyama K, et al. Pylorus ring resection reduces delayed gastric emptying in patients undergoing pancreatoduodenectomy: a prospective, randomized, controlled trial of pylorus-resecting versus pylorus-preserving pancreatoduodenectomy. Ann Surg. 2011;253:495–501.
15. Hackert T, Hinz U, Hartwig W, Strobel O, Fritz S, Schneider L, et al. Pylorus resection in partial pancreaticoduodenectomy: impact on delayed gastric emptying. Am J Surg. 2013;206:296–9.
16. Klaiber U, Probst P, Knebel P, Contin P, Diener MK, Büchler MW, et al. Meta-analysis of complication rates for single-loop versus dual-loop (Roux-en-Y) with isolated pancreaticojejunostomy reconstruction after pancreaticoduodenectomy. Br J Surg. 2015;102:331–40.
17. Hüttner FJ, Fitzmaurice C, Schwarzer G, Seiler CM, Antes G, Büchler MW, et al. Pylorus-preserving pancreaticoduodenectomy (pp Whipple) versus pancreaticoduodenectomy (classic Whipple) for surgical treatment of periampullary and pancreatic carcinoma. Cochrane Database Syst Rev. 2016;2:CD006053.
18. Seiler CA, Wagner M, Bachmann T, Redaelli CA, Schmied B, Uhl W, et al. Randomized clinical trial of pylorus-preserving duodenopancreatectomy versus classical Whipple resection-long term results. Br J Surg. 2005;92:547–56.

19. Shimoda M, Kubota K, Katoh M, Kita J. Effect of billroth II or Roux-en-Y reconstruction for the gastrojejunostomy on delayed gastric emptying after pancreaticoduodenectomy: a randomized controlled study. Ann Surg. 2013;257:938–42.

20. Dindo D, Demartines N, Clavien PA. Classification of surgical complications: a new proposal with evaluation in a cohort of 6336 patients and results of a survey. Ann Surg. 2004;240:205–13.

21. Standop J, Overhaus M, Schaefer N, Decker D, Wolff M, Hirner A, et al. Pancreatogastrostomy after pancreatoduodenectomy: a safe, feasible reconstruction method? World J Surg. 2005;29:505–12.

22. Murray GD. Statistical aspects of research methodology. Br J Surg. 1991;78: 777–81.

23. Kunstman JW, Fonseca AL, Ciarleglio MM, Cong X, Hochberg A, Salem RR. Comprehensive analysis of variables affecting delayed gastric emptying following pancreaticoduodenectomy. J Gastrointest Surg. 2012;16:1354–61.

24. Warshaw AL, Torchiana DL. Delayed gastric emptying after pylorus-preserving pancreaticoduodenectomy. Surg Gynecol Obstet. 1985;160:1–4.

25. Lytras D, Paraskevas KI, Avgerinos C, Manes C, Touloumis Z, Paraskeva KD, et al. Therapeutic strategies for the management of delayed gastric emptying after pancreatic resection. Langenbecks Arch Surg. 2007;392:1–12.

26. Sugiyama M, Abe N, Ueki H, Masaki T, Mori T, Atomi Y. A new reconstruction method for preventing delayed gastric emptying after pylorus-preserving pancreatoduodenectomy. Am J Surg. 2004;187:743–6.

27. Grobmyer SR, Hollenbeck ST, Jaques DP, Jarnagin WR, Dematteo R, Coit DG, et al. Roux-en-Y reconstruction after pancreaticoduodenectomy. Arch Surg. 2008;143:1184–8.

28. Ballas K, Symeonidis N, Rafailidis S, Pavlidis T, Marakis G, Mavroudis N, et al. Use of isolated Roux loop for pancreaticojejunostomy reconstruction after pancreaticoduodenectomy. World J Gastroenterol. 2010;16:3178–82.

29. Ke S, Ding XM, Gao J, Zhao AM, Deng GY, Ma RL, et al. A prospective, randomized trial of Roux-en-Y reconstruction with isolated pancreatic drainage versus conventional loop reconstruction after pancreaticoduodenectomy. Surgery. 2013;153:743–52.

30. Yang J, Wang C, Huang Q. Effect of Billroth II or Roux-en-Y reconstruction for the gastrojejunostomy after pancreaticoduodenectomy: meta-analysis of randomized controlled trials. J Gastrointest Surg. 2015;19:955–63.

31. Tani M, Kawai M, Hirono S, Okada KI, Miyazawa M, Shimizu A, et al. Randomized clinical trial of isolated Roux-en-Y versus conventional reconstruction after pancreaticoduodenectomy. Br J Surg. 2014;101:1084–91.

32. Menahem B, Guittet L, Mulliri A, Alves A, Lubrano J. Pancreaticogastrostomy is superior to pancreaticojejunostomy for prevention of pancreatic fistula after pancreaticoduodenectomy: an updated meta-analysis of randomized controlled trials. Ann Surg. 2015;261:882–7.

33. Bassi C, Falconi M, Molinari E, Salvia R, Butturini G, Sartori N, et al. Reconstruction by pancreaticojejunostomy versus pancreaticogastrostomy following pancreatectomy: results of a comparative study. Ann Surg. 2005; 242:767–71.

34. Figueras J, Sabater L, Planellas P, Muñoz-Forner E, Lopez-Ben S, Falgueras L, et al. Randomized clinical trial of pancreaticogastrostomy versus pancreaticojejunostomy on the rate and severity of pancreatic fistula after pancreaticoduodenectomy. Br J Surg. 2013;100:1597–605.

35. Topal B, Fieuws S, Aerts R, Weerts J, Feryn T, Roeyen G, et al. Pancreaticojejunostomy versus pancreaticogastrostomy reconstruction after pancreaticoduodenectomy for pancreatic or periampullary tumours: a multicentre randomised trial. Lancet Oncol. 2013;14:655–62.

36. Standop J, Schafer N, Overhaus M, Schmitz V, Ladwein L, Hirner A, et al. Endoscopic management of anastomotic hemorrhage from pancreatogastrostomy. Surg Endosc. 2008;23:2005–10.

37. Shimatani M, Matsushita M, Takaoka M, Koyabu M, Ikeura T, Kato K, et al. Effective "short" double-balloon enteroscope for diagnostic and therapeutic ERCP in patients with altered gastrointestinal anatomy: a large case series. Endoscopy. 2009;41:849–54.

38. Zong L, Chen P. Billroth I vs. Billroth II vs. Roux-en-Y following distal gastrectomy: a meta-analysis based on 15 studies. Hepatogastroenterology. 2011;58:1413–24.

39. Xu B, Meng H, Qian M, Gu H, Zhou B, Song Z. Braun enteroenterostomy during pancreaticoduodenectomy decreases postoperative delayed gastric emptying. Am J Surg. 2015;209:1036–42.

40. Huang M, Li M, Mao J, Tian B. Braun enteroenterostomy reduces delayed gastric emptying: a systematic review and meta-analysis. Int J Surg. 2015;23:75–81.

41. Miyazaki Y, Kokudo T, Amikura K, Kageyama Y, Takahashi A, Ohkohchi N, et al. Age does not affect complications and overall survival rate after pancreaticoduodenectomy: single-center experience and systematic review of literature. Biosci Trends. 2016;10:300–6.

42. Langan RC, Zheng C, Harris K, Verstraete R, Al-Refaie WB, Johnson LB. Hospital-level resource use by the oldest-old for pancreaticoduodenectomy at high-volume hospitals. Surgery. 2015;158:366–72.

43. van der Geest LGM, Besselink MGH, Busch ORC, de Hingh IHJT, van Eijck CHJ, Dejong CHC, et al. Elderly patients strongly benefit from centralization of pancreatic cancer surgery: a population-based study. Ann Surg Oncol. 2016;23:2002–9.

44. Enestvedt CK, Diggs BS, Cassera MA, Hammill C, Hansen PD, Wolf RF. Complications nearly double the cost of care after pancreaticoduodenectomy. Am J Surg. 2012;204:332–8.

45. Tittelbach-Helmrich D, Abegg L, Wellner U, Makowiec F, Hopt UT, Keck T. Insurance costs in pancreatic surgery : does the pecuniary aspect indicate formation of centers? Chirurg. 2011;82:154–9.

46. Standop J, Overhaus M, Schafer N, Turler A, Hirner A, Kalff JC. [Technique of pancreatogastrostomy after pancreaticoduodenectomy]. Zentralbl Chir. 2009;134:113–9.

47. Glowka TR, von Websky M, Pantelis D, Manekeller S, Standop J, Kalff JC, et al. Risk factors for delayed gastric emptying following distal pancreatectomy. Langenbecks Arch Surg. 2016;401:161–7.

48. Beane JD, House MG, Miller A, Nakeeb A, Schmidt CM, Zyromski NJ, et al. Optimal management of delayed gastric emptying after pancreatectomy: an analysis of 1,089 patients. Surgery. 2014;156:939–46.

49. Waliye HE, Wright GP, McCarthy C, Johnson J, Scales A, Wolf A, et al. Utility of feeding jejunostomy tubes in pancreaticoduodenectomy. Am J Surg. 2016;213(3):530–3.

27

Rapid progressive long esophageal stricture caused by gastroesophageal reflux disease after pylorus-preserving pancreatoduodenectomy

Masahide Fukaya[*], Tetsuya Abe and Masato Nagino

Abstract

Background: Delayed gastric emptying (DGE) is a major postoperative complication after pylorus-preserving pancreatoduodenectomy (PpPD) and sometimes causes reflux esophagitis. In most cases, this morbidity is controllable by proton-pump inhibitor (PPI) and very rarely results in esophageal stricture. Balloon dilation is usually performed for benign esophageal stricture, and esophagectomy was rarely elected. In the present case, there were two important problems of surgical procedure; how to perform esophageal reconstruction after PpPD and whether to preserve the stomach or not.

Case presentation: A 63-year-old man underwent PpPD and Child reconstruction with Braun anastomosis for lower bile duct carcinoma. Two weeks after surgery DGE occurred, and a 10 cm long stricture from middle esophagus to cardia developed one and a half month after surgery in spite of the administration of antacids. Balloon dilation was performed, but perforation occurred. It was recovered with conservative treatment. Even the administration of a proton pump inhibitor (PPI) for approximately five mouths did not improve esophageal stricture. Simultaneous 24-h pH and bilirubin monitoring confirmed that this patient was resistant to PPI. We performed middle-lower esophagectomy with total gastrectomy to prevent gastric acid from injuring reconstructed organ and remnant esophagus through a right thoracoabdominal incision, and we also performed reconstruction with transverse colon, adding Roux-Y anastomosis, to prevent bile reflux to the remnant esophagus. Minor leakage developed during the postoperative course but was soon cured by conservative treatment. The patient started oral intake on the 25th postoperative day (POD) and was discharged on the 34th POD in good condition.

Conclusion: Long esophageal stricture after PpPD was successfully treated by middle-lower esophagectomy and total gastrectomy with transverse colon reconstruction through a right thoracoabdominal incision. Conventional PD or SSPPD with Roux-en Y reconstruction rather than PpPD should be selected to reduce the risk of DGE and prevent bile reflux, in performing PD for patients with hiatal hernia or rapid metabolizer CYP2C19 genotype; otherwise, fundoplication such as Nissen and Toupet should be added.

Keywords: Esophageal stricture, Esophagectomy, Pancreatoduodenectomy, Delayed gastric emptying

* Correspondence: mafukaya@med.nagoya-u.ac.jp
Division of Surgical Oncology, Department of Surgery, Nagoya University
Graduate School of Medicine, 65 Tsurumai-cho Showa-ku, Nagoya 466-8550,
Japan

Rapid progressive long esophageal stricture caused by gastroesophageal reflux disease...

189

Background

Delayed gastric emptying (DGE) is a major postoperative complication after pylorus-preserving pancreatoduodenectomy (PpPD) and sometimes causes reflux esophagitis [1, 2]. In most cases, this morbidity is controllable by proton-pump inhibitor (PPI) and very rarely results in esophageal stricture. Conservative therapy, such as balloon dilation and the temporary placement of a self-expanding plastic stent, is usually performed for benign esophageal stricture, and surgical treatment was rarely elected [3]. Moreover, there have so far been few such reports on esophageal reconstruction after pancreatoduodenectomy. We report a patient with rapid progressive long esophageal stricture caused by gastroesophageal reflux disease (GERD) after PpPD in whom balloon dilation failed and subsequent esophagectomy with colon reconstruction was required.

Case presentation

A 63-year-old man underwent PpPD and Child reconstruction with Braun anastomosis for lower bile duct carcinoma at another hospital. Two weeks after surgery, he vomited several times due to DGE, and a nasogastric tube was inserted into the stomach. On the 32nd POD, however, DGE improved and the nasogastric tube was removed, as dysphagia persisted. On the 41st POD, gastrointestinal endoscopy was performed, revealing stricture of the middle esophagus. PPI did not improve esophageal stricture; the patient then underwent balloon dilation on the 70th POD, but the esophagus was perforated. The esophagus recovered with fasting, antibiotics, and PPI without surgical treatment. As the stricture still remained, he was referred to our hospital for further treatment on the 148th POD.

The upper gastrointestinal series revealed a long stricture extending from the middle esophagus to just above the cardia portion, the length of which was approximately 10 cm, and the sliding esophageal hiatal hernia (Fig. 1). Gastrointestinal endoscopy showed circumferential stricture of the middle esophagus with longitudinal esophageal ulcer scars (Fig. 2a). The narrow lesion was biopsied, and the result showed no malignancy. Preoperative gastrointestinal endoscopy before PpPD revealed a sliding esophageal hiatal hernia and mild esophagitis (Fig. 2b). We speculated that postoperative DGE, hiatal hernia, and gastric hyperacidity exacerbated the patient's reflex esophagitis. The patient was treated with an H2 blocker for 2 weeks just after the surgery and with PPI from the 14th POD until the 140th POD. PPI was replaced to the H2 blocker due to the decreased numbers of white blood cells to less than 2000/µl from the 141th POD. The number of white blood cells recovered to normal level soon. Severe extensive stricture remained observed. We suspected that this patient had

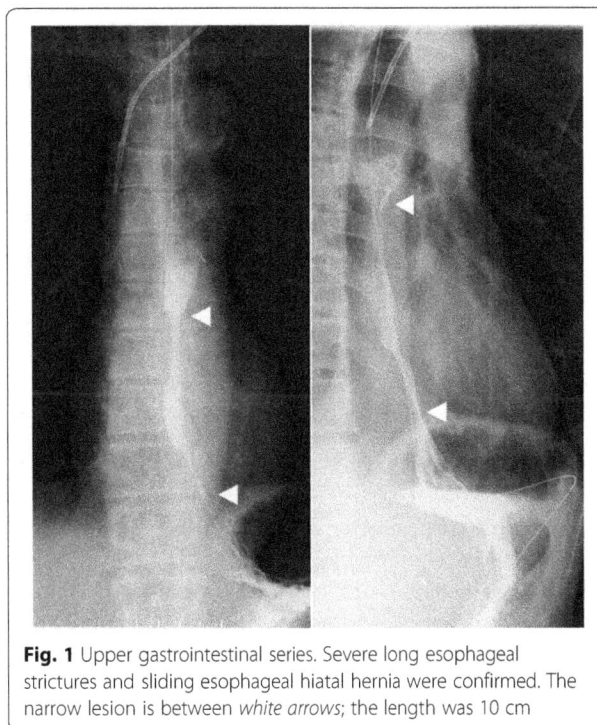

Fig. 1 Upper gastrointestinal series. Severe long esophageal strictures and sliding esophageal hiatal hernia were confirmed. The narrow lesion is between *white arrows*; the length was 10 cm

resistance to PPI; thus, we performed simultaneous 24-h pH and bilirubin monitoring to estimate the extent to which gastric acid secretion was inhibited by omeprazole (20 mg/drip/twice a day). Proximal and distal pH sensors were positioned in the narrow lesion and in the stomach, respectively, and a bilirubin sensor was positioned just beyond the narrow lesion. In the stomach, a $pH < 4$ was observed 89.3 % of the time (Fig. 3). Usually, in patients with GERD or intermediate and poor metabolizer CYP2C19 genotype, the proportion of time for which the stomach is characterized by $pH < 4$ decreases to approximately 50 % with PPI [4, 5]. In this study, after treatment with omeprazole for 6 days, the white blood cell count decreased from 4000 to 1700/µl; this level increased to normal levels soon after the course of medication had been completed. We recognized that this patient was resistant to PPI. Neither an H2 blocker nor PPI could prevent the exacerbation of reflux esophagitis. We therefore concluded that medication therapy could not suppress gastric acid and considered performing total gastrectomy to prevent gastric acid from injuring reconstructed organs and the remnant esophagus.

On the 158th POD, we performed resection of the middle-lower esophagus and total gastrectomy through a right thoracoabdominal approach. The middle-lower esophagus was hard; we therefore cut the esophagus just beyond the azygos arch. The length of the jejunum was not sufficient to pull up to the cut end of the esophagus due to Child reconstruction after PpPD, and we performed reconstruction using the transverse colon (Fig. 4).

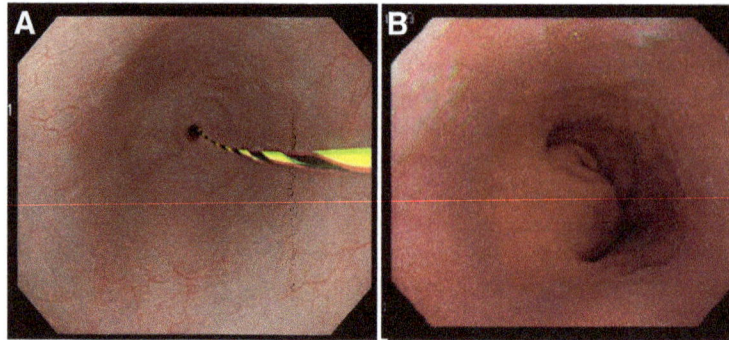

Fig. 2 a. Endoscopic findings on the 150th POD after PpPD showed severe stricture of the middle thoracic esophagus and longitudinal esophageal ulcer scars on the oral side. **b** Endoscopic findings before PpPD showed sliding esophageal hiatal hernia and mild esophagitis, which was classified as Grade A according to the Los Angeles classification

The resected specimen showed wall thickening of the middle-lower esophagus, an ulcer scar on the 8-cm oral side of the cardia, an ulcer at the esophagogastric junction, and a petechial hemorrhage in the stomach. Pathological examination revealed no malignancy.

Minor leakage of the esophagocolonostomy developed postoperatively; the patient recovered rapidly under conservative treatment. He started oral intake on the 23rd POD and was discharged on the 34th POD in good condition. The CYP2C19 genotyping test performed after the second operation showed that the patient had a rapid metabolizer genotype. Two and a half years after the second surgery, gastroendoscopy and simultaneous 24-h pH and bilirubin monitoring were performed. There was no sign of either esophagitis or Barrett's esophagus. Simultaneous 24-h pH and bilirubin

monitoring revealed that the rate of fraction time bilirubin absorbance >0.14 was 0.7 % in the remnant esophagus; there was little bile reflux to the remnant esophagus. Nine years after surgery, the patient has good oral intake with good nutrition, without reflux esophagitis, symptom, or any evidence of recurrence. However, he has undergone gastrointestinal endoscopy once a year to detect early stage colon cancer which can be treated by endoscopic submucosal dissection in preventing surgical resection of reconstructed colon.

Discussion

DGE is one of the major postoperative complications after PpPD, and the incidence has been reported to be 22–45 % [6]. The main pathogenesis of DGE after PpPD has been thought to be preservation of the pylorus ring

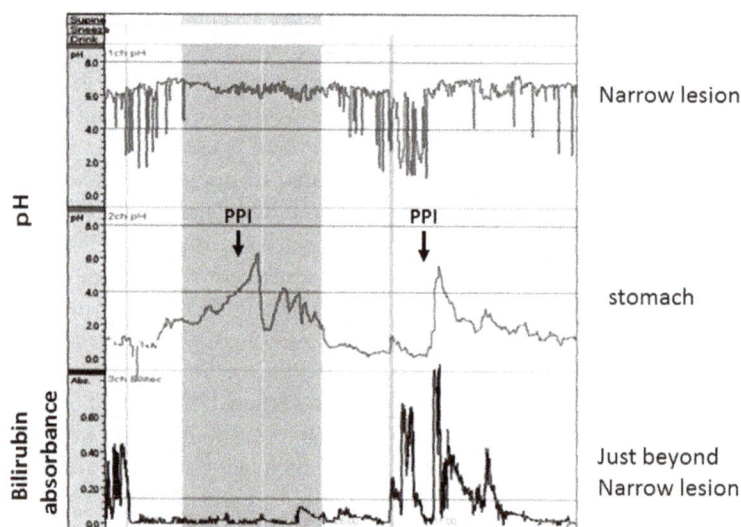

Fig. 3 Simultaneous 24-h pH and bilirubin monitoring. In the narrow lesion, the proportion of time at pH < 4 was 3.0 %. With a drip of omeprazole of 20 mg, pH in the stomach rapidly increased to approximately 6 and but then rapidly decreased to less than 4. (Omeprazole treatment was started 3 days before the test.) The fraction of time with pH < 4 was 89.3 %. Just beyond the narrow lesion, the proportion of time at bilirubin absorbance >0.14 was 20.4 %

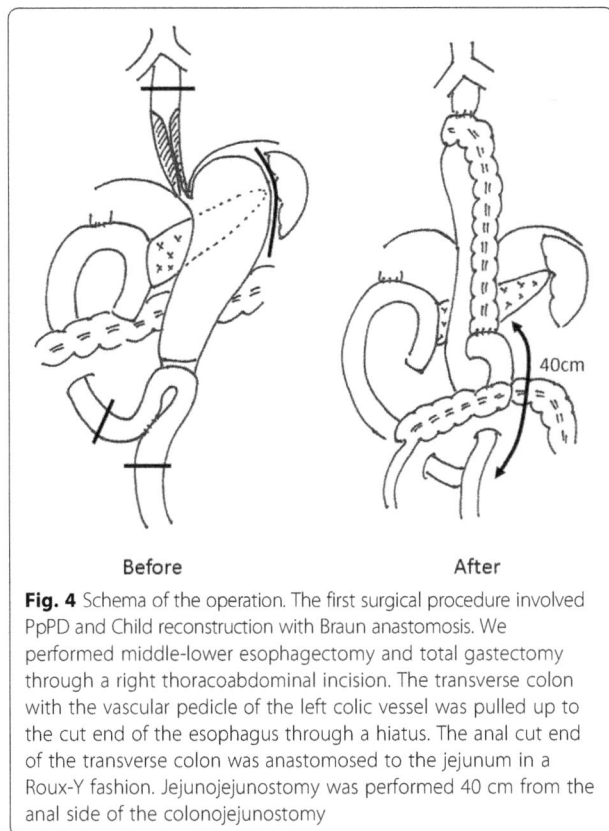

Before   After

Fig. 4 Schema of the operation. The first surgical procedure involved PpPD and Child reconstruction with Braun anastomosis. We performed middle-lower esophagectomy and total gastectomy through a right thoracoabdominal incision. The transverse colon with the vascular pedicle of the left colic vessel was pulled up to the cut end of the esophagus through a hiatus. The anal cut end of the transverse colon was anastomosed to the jejunum in a Roux-Y fashion. Jejunojejunostomy was performed 40 cm from the anal side of the colonojejunostomy

without innervation. Conventional PD and subtotal stomach-preserving pancreatoduodenectomy (SSPPD), in which the pylorus and duodenum are removed and more than 90 % of the stomach is preserved, has recently been reported to reduce the incidence of DGE compared with PpPD [7–10]. In this patient, a sliding hernia was detected by preoperative gastroendoscopy. If DGE happened after surgery, substantial gastric acid reflux to the esophagus was expected to lead to severe esophagitis. Simultaneous 24-h pH and bilirubin monitoring revealed the reflux of not only gastric acid but also bile, resulting in severe esophagitis (Fig. 3). Conventional PD may reduce the risk of acid reflux because an antrectomy induces the reduction of the gastric acid secretion. Therefore, conventional PD or SSPPD with Roux-en Y anastomosis should have been selected to reduce the gastric acid secretion or the risk of DGE, and prevent bile reflux; otherwise, fundoplication such as Nissen and Toupet should have been added.

In this case, 24-h pH monitoring revealed that omeprazole could not sufficiently suppress gastric acid. The CYP2C19 genotyping test performed after the second operation showed that the patient had a rapid metabolizer genotype. Several studies have reported on the effects of CYP2C19 genotypic differences on PPI-mediated cure of GERD [11]. We suggest that the rapid metabolizer CYP2C19 genotype was one reason why

extensive esophageal stricture happened so rapidly. In this patient, the decrease of white blood cell occurred due to the administration of PPI after the initial surgery and on the 24-h pH and bilirubin monitoring. We considered that PPI could not be administered after the second surgery due to the decrease in the white blood cell count caused by PPI. The results of simultaneous 24-h pH and bilirubin monitoring and the decrease of the white blood cell due to PPI could allow us to decide to perform total gastrectomy to protect the reconstructed organ and remnant esophagus from gastric acid. Simultaneous 24-h pH and bilirubin monitoring were very valuable in evaluating the pathogenesis of this case and choosing the operative procedure most likely to preserve the stomach.

Esophageal stricture of GERD is generally treated by endoscopic balloon dilation and continuous PPI administration; surgical resection is rarely performed due to the associated high morbidity and mortality [12]. Herein, we considered less invasive procedure such as balloon dilation or temporary stent replacement; however, because these treatments were expected to cause perforation again and because this patient had medication-resistant GERD, we decided to perform esophagectomy. There were some problems regarding surgical procedures, including the approach, the reconstructed organ, and the reconstructive route. We thought that mediastinitis due to perforation during balloon dilation might scar the tissue surrounding the esophagus and noted that it was difficult to separate the esophagus form adjacent tissue. As the transhiatal approach requires a blind separation maneuver, the right transthoracic approach was chosen. Esophageal stricture extended the middle esophagus, and the esophagus was cut just beyond the bifurcation of the trachea. Alimentary tract reconstruction was performed using the transverse colon (not the jejunum) because of the shortage of useful jejunum due to Child reconstruction after PpPD. With respect to the route of reconstruction, we elected to perform intrathoracic anastomosis because the patient refused the percutaneous route due to the poor cosmetic consequences. Roux-Y anastomosis was also added to prevent bile reflux to remnant esophagus. In fact, postoperative simultaneous 24-h pH and bilirubin monitoring revealed little bile reflux to the remnant esophagus.

Conclusion

Long esophageal stricture after PpPD was successfully treated by middle-lower esophagectomy and total gastrectomy with transverse colon reconstruction through a right thoracoabdominal incision. Conventional PD or SSPPD with Roux-en Y reconstruction rather than PpPD should be selected to reduce the risk of DGE and prevent postoperative bile reflux, in performing PD for patients with hiatal hernia or rapid metabolizer CYP2C19 genotype; otherwise, fundoplication such as Nissen and Toupet should be added.

Abbreviations

DGE: delayed gastric emptying; GERD: gastroesophageal reflux disease; POD: postoperative day; PPI: proton-pump inhibitor; PpPD: pylorus-preserving pancreatoduodenectomy; SSPPD: subtotal stomach-preserving pancreatoduodenectomy.

Competing interests

Masahide Fukaya and other co-authors have no conflict of interest.

Authors' contributions

AT and MF performed the surgery. MF took charge of postoperative care and prepared the manuscript. MN assisted in drafting the manuscript and reviewed the article. All authors read and approved the final manuscript.

Acknowledgements

The authors acknowledge all the medical and surgical staffs that took care of the patient. All authors report no source of funding for conducting this manuscript.

References

1. Nakai T, Kawabe T, Shiraishi O, Okuno K, Shiozaki H. Pylorotomy in pylorus-preserving pancreaticoduodenectomy. Hepato-Gastroenterology. 2006; 53(72):947–9.
2. Wu JM, Tsai MK, Hu RH, Chang KJ, Lee PH, Tien YW. Reflux esophagitis and marginal ulcer after pancreaticoduodenectomy. J Gastrointest Surg. 2011; 15(5):824–8.
3. Ferguson DD. Evaluation and management of benign esophageal strictures. Dis Esophagus. 2005;18(6):359–64.
4. Johnson DA, Stacy T, Ryan M, Wootton T, Willis J, Hornbuckle K, et al. A comparison of esomeprazole and lansoprazole for control of intragastric pH in patients with symptoms of gastro-oesophageal reflux disease. Aliment Pharmacol Ther. 2005;22(2):129–34.
5. Sugimoto M, Shirai N, Nishino M, Kodaira C, Uotani T, Sahara S, et al. Comparison of acid inhibition with standard dosages of proton pump inhibitors in relation to CYP2C19 genotype in Japanese. Eur J Clin Pharmacol. 2014;70(9):1073–8.
6. Kawai M, Yamaue H. Pancreaticoduodenectomy versus pylorus-preserving pancreaticoduodenectomy: the clinical impact of a new surgical procedure; pylorus-resecting pancreaticoduodenectomy. J Hepatobiliary Pancreat Sci. 2011;18(6):755–61.
7. Lin PW, Shan YS, Lin YJ, Hung CJ. Pancreaticoduodenectomy for pancreatic head cancer: PPPD versus Whipple procedure. Hepato-Gastroenterology. 2005;52(65):1601–4.
8. Kawai M, Tani M, Hirono S, Miyazawa M, Shimizu A, Uchiyama K, et al. Pylorus ring resection reduces delayed gastric emptying in patients undergoing pancreatoduodenectomy: a prospective, randomized, controlled trial of pylorus-resecting versus pylorus-preserving pancreatoduodenectomy. Ann Surg. 2011;253(3):495–501.
9. Hanna MM, Gadde R, Tamariz L, Allen CJ, Meizoso JP, Sleeman D, et al. Delayed gastric emptying after pancreaticoduodenectomy: is subtotal stomach preserving better or pylorus preserving? J Gastrointest Surg. 2015; 19(8):1542–52.
10. Zhou Y, Lin L, Wu L, Xu D, Li B. A case-matched comparison and meta-analysis comparing pylorus-resecting pancreaticoduodenectomy with pylorus-preserving pancreaticoduodenectomy for the incidence of postoperative delayed gastric emptying. HPB. 2015;17(4):337–43.
11. Kawamura M, Ohara S, Koike T, Iijima K, Suzuki H, Kayaba S, et al. Cytochrome P450 2C19 polymorphism influences the preventive effect of lansoprazole on the recurrence of erosive reflux esophagitis. J Gastroenterol Hepatol. 2007;22(2):222–6.
12. Young MM, Deschamps C, Allen MS, Miller DL, Trastek VF, Schleck CD, et al. Esophageal reconstruction for benign disease: self-assessment of functional outcome and quality of life. Ann Thorac Surg. 2000;70(6):1799–802.

28

One visceral artery may be enough; successful pancreatectomy in a patient with total occlusion of the celiac and superior mesenteric arteries

Evangelos Tagkalos[1], Florian Jungmann[2], Hauke Lang[1] and Stefan Heinrich[1*]

Abstract

Background: The anatomic variations of the visceral arteries are not uncommon. The liver arterial blood supply shows 50% variability between humans, with the most common anatomy being one hepatic artery arising from the celiac trunk and one pancreatico-duodenal arcade between the celiac trunk and the superior mesenteric artery. Occlusion of one artery are mostly asymptomatic but may become clinically relevant when surgery of the liver, bile duct or the pancreas is required. If these pathologies are not reversible, an oncologic pancreatic head resection cannot be performed.

Case presentation: We report the case of a 64-year-old Caucasian female patient with a locally advanced, resectable adenocarcinoma of the pancreas with complete atherosclerotic occlusion of the celiac trunk and the superior mesenteric artery. This vascular anomaly was missed on the preoperative imaging and became known postoperatively. A collateral circulation from a hypertrophic inferior mesenteric artery to the celiac trunk and the superior mesenteric artery compensated the blood supply to the visceral organs. The postoperative course was complicated by an elevation of the transaminases AST/ALT, which normalized under conservative treatment with alprostadil (prostavasin™) and anticoagulation, since angiographic recanalization failed. The patient recovered fully and was discharged at the 14th postoperative day. Two years later, she required endovascular repair of an aortic rupture during which the inferior mesenteric artery was preserved.

Conclusion: This case underlines the natural potential of the human body to adapt to chronic arterial malperfusion by creating a collateral circulation and supports the need for adequate preoperative imaging, including a proper arterial phase before upper abdominal surgery.

Keywords: Pancreaticoduodenectomy, Mesenteric arteries, Occlusion, Celiac trunk

Background

The blood supply of the liver is variable and only 50% of humans present with a standard vascular anatomy of one hepatic artery arising from the celiac trunk and a pancreatico-duodenal arcade between the hepatic and the superior mesenteric arteries (SMA) [1]. Chronic occlusion of one artery exists in approximately 10–20% of patients, but can often be compensated and therefore usually remains asymptomatic due to the dual blood supply [2–5]. The most frequent compensation is the hypertrophy of the pancreatico-duodenal arcade [6].

Asymptomatic occlusion may become clinically relevant when surgery of the liver, bile duct or the pancreas is required; the oncologic resection of the pancreatic head (e.g. Whipple procedure) requires the ligation of the gastroduodenal (GDA), and the pancreatico-duodenal arteries (PDA). Gastrointestinal and biliary anastomoses require adequate arterial flow. Therefore, a celiac trunk stenosis is critical and a complete occlusion is considered a contraindication for many of these procedures.

* Correspondence: stefan.heinrich@unimedizin-mainz.de
[1]Department of General, Visceral and Transplantation Surgery, Johannes Gutenberg University Hospital, Langenbeckstrasse 1, 55131 Mainz, Germany
Full list of author information is available at the end of the article

We report the case of a patient with a locally advanced, resectable adenocarcinoma of the pancreas with complete atherosclerotic occlusion of the celiac trunk and the SMA.

Case presentation

A 64-year-old female patient suspicious of cancer of the pancreatic head with a recent history of acute pancreatitis and cholangitis was admitted to our department for further treatment in April 2012. The patient had had coronary artery bypass surgery, diabetes and arterial hypertension. Laboratory findings revealed cholestasis, and endoscopic retrograde cholangiopancreatography (ERCP) showed a stenosis in the distal bile duct which was highly suspicious of a pancreatic malignancy. Computed tomography (CT) scan and magnetic resonance imaging (MRI) images, 2 months and 3 weeks prior to surgery, were demonstrated by a radiologist in the preoperative conference: a double duct sign, but no signs of metastases were found, and the tumor had contact to the superior mesenteric artery without suspect of a vascular invasion (Fig. 1).

The patient underwent a classic Whipple procedure (partial duodenopancreatectomy) with regional lymphadenectomy in May 2012. Intraoperatively, the arterial pulse in the liver hilum appeared weak, but flow increased after test clamping of the GDA. Therefore, resection was completed. The dissection of the mesopancreas was performed on the SMA. The pancreatico-jejunostomy was performed according to Warren & Kartell using 4–0 PDS and 6–0 PDS sutures for the duct-to-duct anastomosis. About 15 cm distal to this anastomosis, the hepatico-jejunostomy was done with 5–0 PDS interrupted sutures. The intestinal passage was reconstructed by a gastroenterostomy (3–0 PDS) and a Braun anastomosis using 4–0 PDS.

Postoperative course

Postoperative transaminases were elevated and peaked on postoperative day (POD) 3 (AST 713 U/L, ALT 1222 U/L). Therefore, abdominal CT with intravenous contrast was performed and revealed a chronic occlusion of both the celiac trunk and the SMA. A large-caliber inferior mesenteric artery (IMA) had strong collaterals to the SMA and celiac trunk (Fig. 2). Emergency angiography confirmed chronic occlusion of the SMA and celiac trunk without any possibility for interventional therapy. In the absence of treatment alternatives, continuous alprostadil (prostavasin™) infusion and anticoagulation with unfractionated heparin were initiated and continued over 7 days. During this treatment, transaminases decreased continuously and remained normal thereafter (Fig. 3).

Histopathological findings

The final histology revealed a 3.2 cm poorly differentiated adenocarcinoma of the pancreatic head with infiltration of the distal bile duct and the peripancreatic tissue. Moreover, the tumor had spread to 4/18 lymph nodes, and perineural and vascular infiltration were detected (pT3, pN1 (4/18), M0, G3, V1, Pn1, R0).

Outcome

No further complications occurred in the postoperative course. In particular, no signs of intestinal hypoperfusion or anastomotic leak occurred. The patient was discharged 2 weeks after the operation in a very good condition.

Follow-up

The patient received 6-months of adjuvant gemcitabine chemotherapy and presented in excellent general condition for a follow-up 12 months after surgery. Two years after surgery, the patient required emergency endovascular treatment (EVAR) of an aortic rupture. The aortic rupture extended from the aortic bifurcation to the renal arteries. At that time, also tumor recurrence was found (Fig. 4). The IMA was spared during stent placement in

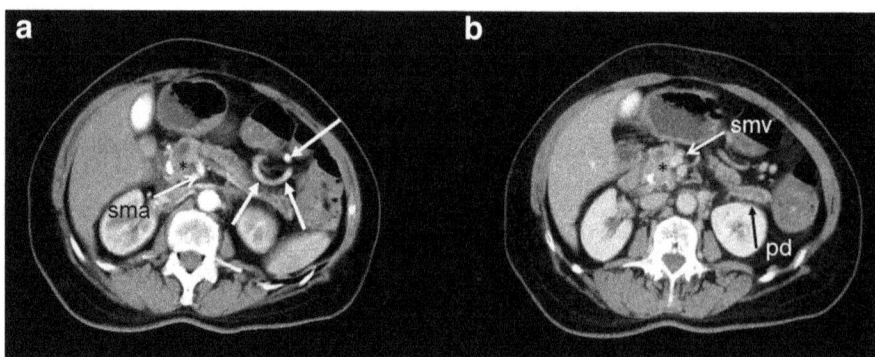

Fig. 1 Transverse CT images preoperatively with arterial (a) and venous (b) phases: the pancreatic duct (pd) is dilated, a stent had been implanted into the bile duct due to biliary obstruction of the tumor in the pancreatic head (*). The arterial collaterals are visible in the left upper abdomen (arrows) (sma): superior mesenteric artery, smv: superior mesenteric vein)

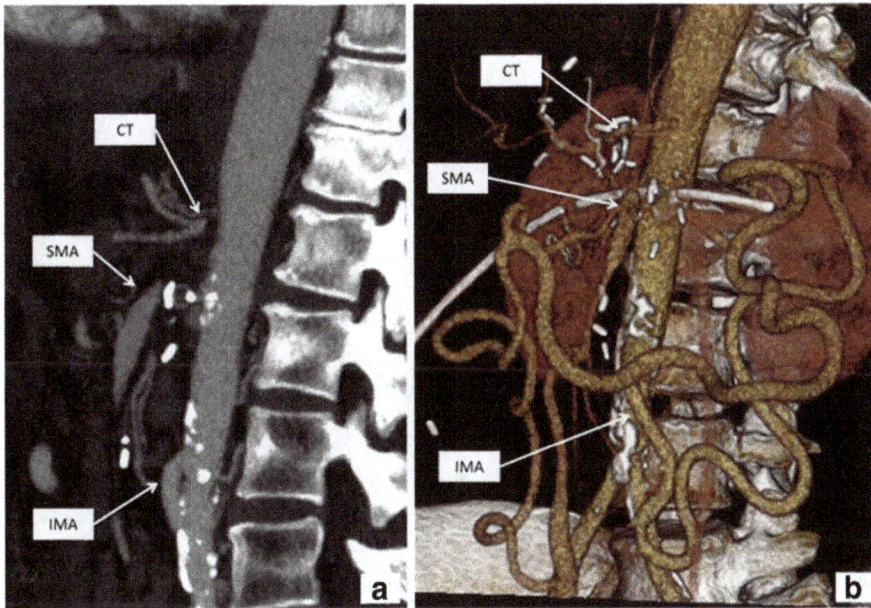

Fig. 2 Sagittal reconstruction of a computed tomography scan (**a**) demonstrates proximal occlusion of celiac trunk (CT) and SMA with poststenotic dilatation of the SMA. Note the hypertrophic IM. Volume rendering (**b**) shows collateral arteries from IMA to SMA (hypertrophic anastomosis of Riolan)

order to preserve intestinal perfusion. After this intervention, the patient received 5 cycles of palliative gemcitabine chemotherapy and later changed to FOLFOX4 in December 2014 due to tumor progression. The patient died 34 months after the pancreas resection.

Discussion and conclusions

Splanchnic vascular stenosis or occlusion can be caused by a variety of diseases. One of the most frequent causes of a stenosis of the celiac trunk is a hypertrophic arcuate ligament resulting in an extrinsic obstruction of the artery [3, 7, 8], which can usually be solved intraoperatively by

dissecting the ligament [9]. Angiographic studies revealed asymptomatic severe stenosis of celiac or superior mesenteric arteries in up to 50% of patients with atherosclerosis, and synchronous severe stenosis of both arteries are present in up to 5% of these patients [7, 10]. A percutaneous transluminal stent placement or even a vascular bypass surgery may be performed to improve the perfusion of the celiac trunk. If these interventions are not feasible, a Whipple procedure is considered impossible. In contrast, the hypertrophic pancreaticogastroduodenal arcade may be preserved during distal pancreas resection [11, 12].

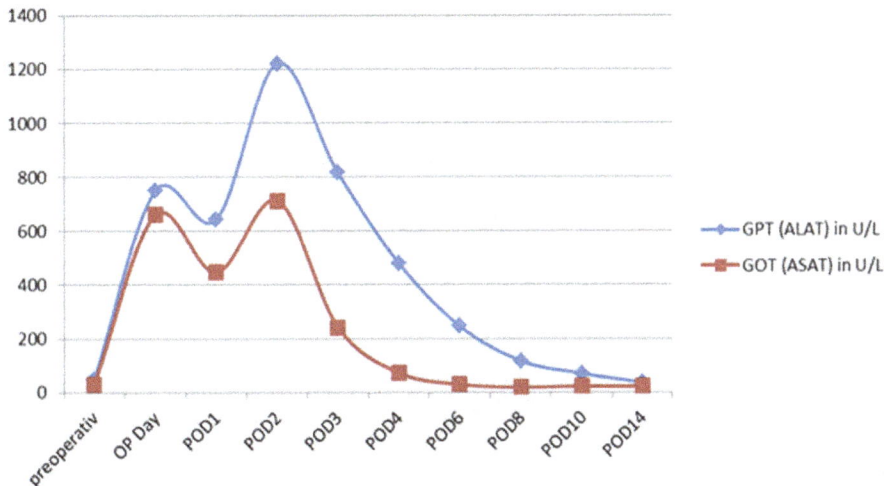

Fig. 3 Postoperative course of transaminases AST/ALT

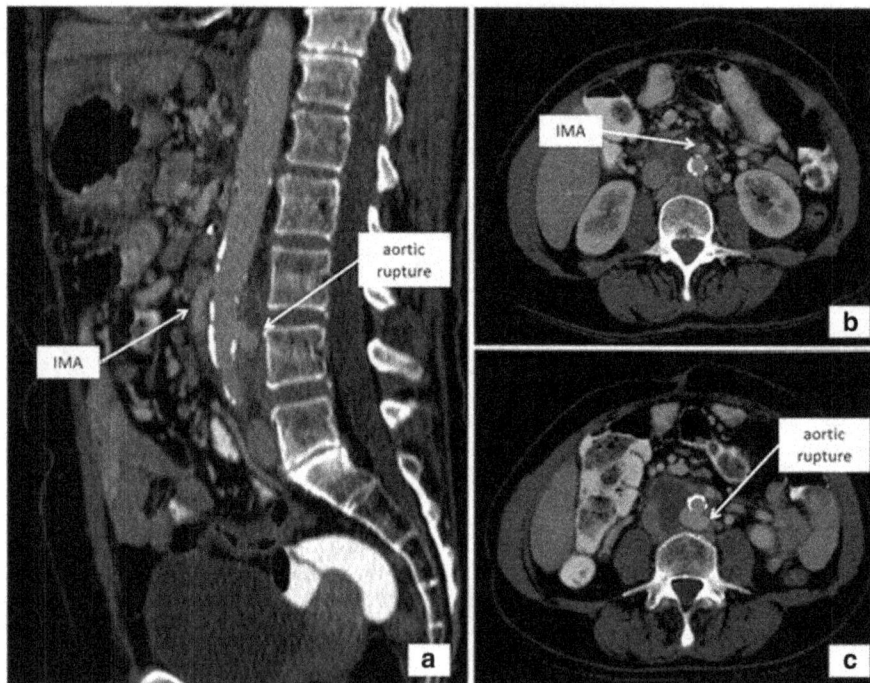

Fig. 4 Sagittal reconstruction of computed tomography scan (**a**) and axial images (**b**, **c**) revealed abdominal aortic pseudoaneurysm at the dorsal circumference of the aorta below the ostium of the IMA due to tumor relapse

In this case, the arterial collaterals as consequence of the arterial occlusion were misdiagnosed as venous collaterals during the preoperative conference. Upon postoperative CT scan, the late arterial phase clearly demonstrated the occlusion of both vessels. Due to the chronicity of the arterial occlusion, hypertrophic collaterals, e.g. through the anastomosis of Riolan, had been formed and prevented severe complications. In contrast, the resection of the celiac trunk or the SMA without development of collaterals may have fatal consequences.

In summary, the synchronous chronic occlusion of the celiac trunk and the SMA, as reported in this case, is extremely rare, while cases of occlusion of one of both is well known in the literature. If this arterial situation would have been detected preoperatively, a bypass procedure would have been performed during pancreas resection in order to prevent serious complications, or surgery would have been denied. Although our patient tolerated major pancreas surgery well, procedures impairing the IMA (i.e. left hemicolectomy) could have been lethal for her. Since this arterial situation was well documented, the IMA was preserved during the emergency treatment of an aortic rupture 24 months postoperatively.

Although chronic arterial occlusion can be compensated through collateralization, cases as the above emphasize the importance of proper arterial imaging prior to operations of the upper abdomen. Moreover, careful assessment of the available imaging by trained radiologists is mandatory.

Abbreviations
CT: Computed tomography; ERCP: Endoscopic retrograde cholangiopancreatography; EVAR: Endovascular aneurysm repair; GDA: Gastroduodenal artery; IMA: Inferior mesenteric artery; MRI: Magnetic resonance imaging; PDA: Pancreatico-duodenal artery; POD: Postoperative day; SMA: Superior mesenteric artery; SMV: Superior mesenteric vein

Acknowledgements
None.

Funding
No funding was received.

Authors' contributions
ET conception and writing of the manuscript as well as assessment of the data. FJ carried out the reconstruction of radiological images and contributed to the radiological findings of the case. HL conception and critical discussion of this case report. SH conception and coordination of this case report. All authors read and approved the final manuscript.

Competing interests
The authors declare that they have no competing interests.

Author details
[1]Department of General, Visceral and Transplantation Surgery, Johannes Gutenberg University Hospital, Langenbeckstrasse 1, 55131 Mainz, Germany. [2]Department of Diagnostic and Interventional Radiology, Johannes Gutenberg University Hospital, Mainz, Germany.

References

1. Catalano OA, Singh AH, Uppot RN, Hahn PF, Ferrone CR, Sahani DV. Vascular and biliary variants in the liver: implications for liver surgery. Radiographics. 2008;28(2):359–78.
2. Park CM, Chung JW, Kim HB, Shin SJ, Park JH. Celiac axis stenosis: incidence and etiologies in asymptomatic individuals. Korean J Radiol. 2001;2(1):8–13.
3. Lindner HH, Kemprud E. A clinicoanatomical study of the arcuate ligament of the diaphragm. Arch Surg. 1971;103(5):600–5.
4. Sakorafas GH, Sarr MG, Peros G. Celiac artery stenosis: an underappreciated and unpleasant surprise in patients undergoing pancreaticoduodenectomy. J Am Coll Surg. 2008;206(2):349–56.
5. Zeller T, Rastan A, Sixt S. Chronic atherosclerotic mesenteric ischemia (CMI). Vasc Med. 2010;15(4):333–8.
6. Song SY, Chung JW, Kwon JW, Joh JH, Shin SJ, Kim HB, et al. Collateral pathways in patients with celiac axis stenosis: angiographic-spiral CT correlation. Radiographics. 2002;22(4):881–93.
7. Thomas JH, Blake K, Pierce GE, Hermreck AS, Seigel E. The clinical course of asymptomatic mesenteric arterial stenosis. J Vasc Surg. 1998;27(5):840–4.
8. Levin DC, Baltaxe HA. High incidence of celiac axis narrowing in asymptomatic individuals. Am J Roentgenol Radium Therapy, Nucl Med. 1972;116(2):426–9.
9. Gaujoux S, Sauvanet A, Vullierme MP, Cortes A, Dokmak S, Sibert A, et al. Ischemic complications after pancreaticoduodenectomy: incidence, prevention, and management. Ann Surg. 2009;249(1):111–7.
10. Valentine RJ, Martin JD, Myers SI, Rossi MB, Clagett GP. Asymptomatic celiac and superior mesenteric artery stenoses are more prevalent among patients with unsuspected renal artery stenoses. J Vasc Surg. 1991;14(2):195–9.
11. Kurosaki I, Hatakeyama K, Nihei KE, Oyamatsu M. Celiac axis stenosis in pancreaticoduodenectomy. J Hepato-Biliary-Pancreat Surg. 2004;11(2):119–24.
12. Pelloni A, Gertsch P. Cephalic duodenopancreatectomy with preservation of pancreaticoduodenal arcades in coeliac trunk occlusion. Ann Chir. 2000;125(7):660–4.

29

Clinical impact of duodenal pancreatic heterotopia – Is there a need for surgical treatment?

Alexander Betzler[1], Soeren T. Mees[1], Josefine Pump[1], Sebastian Schölch[1], Carolin Zimmermann[1], Daniela E. Aust[2], Jürgen Weitz[1], Thilo Welsch[1] and Marius Distler[1*] (ID)

Abstract

Background: Pancreatic heterotopia (PH) is defined as ectopic pancreatic tissue outside the normal pancreas and its vasculature and duct system. Most frequently, PH is detected incidentally by histopathological examination. The aim of the present study was to analyze a large single-center series of duodenal PH with respect to the clinical presentation.

Methods: A prospective pancreatic database was retrospectively analyzed for cases of PH of the duodenum. All pancreatic and duodenal resections performed between January 2000 and October 2015 were included and screened for histopathologically proven duodenal PH. PH was classified according to Heinrich's classification (Type I acini, ducts, and islet cells; Type II acini and ducts; Type III only ducts).

Results: A total of 1274 pancreatic and duodenal resections were performed within the study period, and 67 cases of PH (5.3%) were identified. The respective patients were predominantly male (72%) and either underwent pancreatoduodenectomy ($n = 60$); a limited pancreas resection with partial duodenal resection ($n = 4$); distal pancreatectomy with partial duodenal resection ($n = 1$); total pancreatectomy ($n = 1$); or enucleation ($n = 1$). Whereas 65 patients (83.5%) were asymptomatic, 11 patients (18.4%) presented with symptoms related to PH (most frequently with abdominal pain [72%] and duodenal obstruction [55%]). Of those, seven patients (63.6%) had chronic pancreatitis in the heterotopic pancreas. The risk of malignant transformation into adenocarcinoma was 2.9%.

Conclusions: PH is found in approximately 5% of pancreatic or duodenal resections and is generally asymptomatic. Chronic pancreatitis is not uncommon in heterotopic pancreatic tissue, and even there is a risk of malignant transformation. PH should be considered for the differential diagnosis of duodenal lesions and surgery should be considered, especially in symptomatic cases.

Keywords: Pancreatic heterotopia, Pancreatic resection, Heinrich's classification, Pancreatic cancer, Chronic pancreatitis

Background

Pancreatic heterotopia (PH) was first reported by Jean-Schultz in 1729 and is defined as pancreatic tissue without anatomical or vascular connection to the pancreas [1, 2].

The ectopic pancreatic tissue possesses its own duct system and vascular supply [3, 4]. It is mostly found in the upper gastrointestinal tract (GIT), but may occur anywhere in the GIT [5, 6]. Frequent locations are the duodenum (93.6%), stomach (24–38%), jejunum (0.5–27%), and Meckel's diverticulum (2–6.5%) [7]. The most widespread explanation of the origin of PH is that the ectopic tissue separates itself from the pancreas during embryonic rotation and fusion of the dorsal and ventral pancreatic buds (misplacement theory) [3, 8]. For a clinical understanding of PH it is important to know that all diseases arising in the genuine pancreas can also develop in heterotopic tissue [3, 6, 9, 10].

* Correspondence: Marius.Distler@uniklinikum-dresden.de
[1]Department of General, Thoracic and Vascular Surgery, University Hospital Carl Gustav Carus, TU Dresden, Fetscher Str. 74, 01037 Dresden, Germany
Full list of author information is available at the end of the article

Among all abdominal surgeries the incidence of PH ranges from 0.25–1.2%, and specific symptoms have not been described until now [11]. Most patients with PH are asymptomatic, and PH is detected incidentally by histological examination of the specimen. Although malignant transformation originating from PH is extremely rare, it has been reported in several cases in the literature [12, 13]. Because of the scarcity of symptomatic PH cases in the literature [6, 14–16], we investigated our series of duodenal PH with a special focus on its clinical relevance and impact.

Methods

We retrospectively analyzed our prospective pancreatic database for cases with PH of the duodenum. All pancreatic and duodenal resections performed at the Department of Visceral, Thoracic and Vascular Surgery, University Hospital, TU Dresden between January 2000 and October 2015 were included. Partial results have been published elsewhere [17]. Clinical symptoms, surgical procedures and pathological findings were documented for each case. At histological examination, the specimens were stained with hematoxylin and eosin, and a senior GI pathologist (DEA) reviewed each sample regarding the components of pancreatic tissue (including acini, ducts, and islets of Langerhans). PH was classified according to Heinrich's classification (Fig. 1) [18]. Briefly,

PH Type I includes acini, ducts and endocrine islet cells, Type II contains acini and ducts, but no islet cells, and Type III contains only pancreatic ducts.

PH was classified as "symptomatic" if the surgery was directly indicated for PH-associated pathologies, whereas incidental PH diagnosed on postoperative histopathological examination was classified as "asymptomatic". We compared these two groups regarding type of PH, associated disease and treatment.

In accordance with the guidelines for human subject research, approval was obtained from the ethics committee at the Carl Gustav Carus University Hospital (decision number EK 435102015).

Results

Patient cohort

In total, 1274 pancreatic and duodenal resections were performed in our department during the study period. Some 67 cases (5.3%) with histologically proven duodenal PH were identified (19 women and 49 men). The mean age of the whole cohort was 54 years (range 24–76 years). The postoperative histology showed chronic pancreatitis (CP) (n = 25; 37.3%), pancreatic ductal adenocarcinomas (PDAC) (n = 11; 16.4%), and cystic neoplasms (n = 11; 16.4%). Nine operated patients (13.4%) had papillary carcinomas (AP) and six (9%) presented with neuroendocrine tumors (NET). More rare

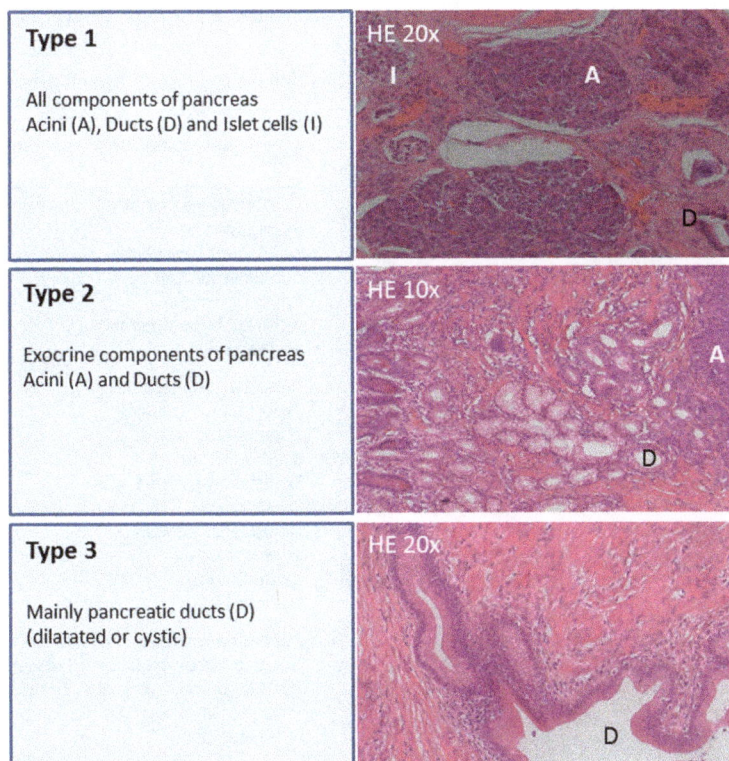

Type 1	
All components of pancreas Acini (A), Ducts (D) and Islet cells (I)	HE 20x
Type 2	
Exocrine components of pancreas Acini (A) and Ducts (D)	HE 10x
Type 3	
Mainly pancreatic ducts (D) (dilatated or cystic)	HE 20x

Fig. 1 Heinrich's classification of pancreatic heterotopia

indications for operation included duodenal polyps (two cases; 2.9%), one cholangiocarcinoma, one pancreas divisum, and one duodenal carcinoma (Tables 1 and 2). Pancreatic head resections including pylorus-preserving pancreatoduodenectomies (PPPD) and Whipple procedures represented the vast majority of the operations (n = 60; 89.5%). In four cases (5.9%) a segmental pancreatic resection with partial duodenal resection was performed. Furthermore, one patient each underwent a distal pancreatectomy with partial duodenal resection, a total pancreatectomy and an enucleation of the pancreas and the duodenum (1.4%). According to Heinrich's classification, Type I PH was found in 32 patients (47.9%), Type II in 28 patients (41.7%), and Type III in 7 patients (10.4%) (Tables 1 and 2).

"Asymptomatic" subgroup

Fifty-six of the 67 patients (83.5%) were classified as asymptomatic. Performed operations, and postoperative histology are shown on Table 1. In this subgroup the following types of heterotopia were diagnosed: Type I, n = 26; Type II, n = 24; and Type III, n = 6. The patients in the "asymptomatic" cohort presented with the following complaints of the underlying non-PH associated disease (e.g., pancreatic malignancy or chronic pancreatitis): obstructive jaundice, upper abdominal pain, vomiting/nausea, weight loss or duodenal obstruction (Table 1).

"Symptomatic" subgroup

In 11 cases (16.4%) duodenal PH was responsible for the clinical symptoms (symptomatic subgroup) (Table 2). In this subgroup Heinrich's Type I and II were predominantly found (Type I n = 6; Type II n = 4 and Type III n = 1). Interestingly, the most frequent PH-related symptom was upper abdominal pain (n = 8, 72%), and duodenal obstruction (n = 6, 55%). The postoperative histological examination of the symptomatic patients revealed chronic pancreatitis in 7 patients (64%), PDAC in two patients (18%), and duodenal tumors in two cases (18%) originating from the existing duodenal PH. There was no difference in age, sex and type of surgery between the two groups, and there was no significant difference regarding related disease or Heinrich type (p > 0.05) between the symptomatic and asymptomatic cases (Table 3).

Discussion

PH is described as a rare pathological entity, and a preoperative clinical diagnosis is difficult because characteristic clinical symptoms are frequently camouflaged by the multitude of underlying diseases [3, 6, 19]. Clinical series are rare and most data in the literature stem from case reports.

The present study focused on duodenal PH. Approximately 5% of the patients undergoing pancreatic and/or duodenal resections in our cohort were diagnosed with PH, and thus PH was not a particularly

Table 1 Characteristics of "asymptomatic patients" with duodenal PH (n = 56) (Indication for operation due to clinical presentation and symptoms)

Type of duodenal PH (according to Heinrich)	Age (mean) Sex (m/f)	Operation	Clinical presentation and symptoms[a]	Histology
Type 1 n = 26	57.4 years (16/10)	1xpancreatectomie; 3xWhipple; 19× PPPD; 2× partial duodenal resection; 1× enucleation of the pancreas and the duodenum	11xobstructive jaundice 9xepigastric pain 6xrecurrent pancreatitis duodenal stenosis 5xloss of weight recurrent hypoglycemia acid reflux	SCN 5xPDAC 5xIPMN 6xCP 5xAP 4xNET
Type 2 n = 24	55.9 years (18/6)	19xPPPD 4xWhipple Pancreas left resection	9xrecurrent pancreatitis 7xobstructive jaundice 10xepigastric pain diarrhoe 3xdilatation pancreas duct 2xpseudocyst 2xduodenal stenosis 5xweight loss gastric stenosis 2xcholestasis	4xIPMN Carcinoma of the bile duct 3xAP 9xCP 2xNET 4xPDAC SCN
Type 3 n = 6	57.2 years (4/2)	5xPPPD 1xWhipple	2xrecurrent pancreatitis; 3xobstructive jaundice; 3xepigastric pain; 1xpseudocyst; 1xcystic tumor; 1xampullary tumor; 1xduodenal stenosis; 1× dilatation pancreatic duct	1xPDAC; 3xCP; 1xAP; 1xpancreas divisum

[a]multiple answers possible;
PDAC pancreatic ductal adenocarcinoma, *CP*chronic pancreatitis, *AP*ampullary carcinoma, *SCN* serous cystic neoplasia, *IPMN* intraductal papillary mucinous neoplasia, *NET* Neuroendocrine tumor

Table 2 Characteristics of "symptomatic patients" with lesions originating from duodenal PH or symptoms due to duodenal PH (*n* = 11)

Type of duodenal PH (according to Heinrich)	Age (mean) Sex (m/f)	Operation	Clinical presentation and symptoms[a]	Histology
Type 1 *n* = 6	58.6 years (5/1)	3xWhipple; 3xPPPD	3xduodenal stenosis; 4xepigastric pain; 1xnausea/vomiting; 1xobstructive jaundice; 1xweigth loss; 1xpseudocysts	3xCP in PH; 2xPDAC in PH; 1× PH in duodenal wall
Type 2 *n* = 4	47.8 years (4/0)	2xpartial duodenal resection; 1xWhipple; 1xPPPD	3xduodenal stenosis; 3xepigastric pain; 1xNausea/vomiting; 1xobstructive jaundice; 1xpseudocysts	1× PH in duodenal wall; 3xCP in PH
Type 3 *n* = 1	47.0 years male	PPPD	recurrent epigastric pain	CP in PH

[a]multiple answers possible
PDAC pancreatic ductal adenocarcinoma, *CP* chronic pancreatitis, *PH* pancreatic heterotopia

rare finding. Our study confirms that most of the patients with PH were asymptomatic, and therefore PH was discovered incidentally. However, depending on its location and diameter, heterotopic pancreatic tissue can lead to nonspecific symptoms [20–22]. According to the literature, lesions are more likely to be symptomatic if they are >2 cm in diameter [23]. This seems to be especially true for tumors that are located in the duodenum due to the anatomic character of this region of the digestive tract. Nevertheless, due to a lack of data concerning the diameter of the duodenal PH-lesions we could not make a clear statement to this point. But abdominal pain is the most common –but nonspecific– symptom of pancreatic heterotopia, [4] as found in the present study (73%). Consequently, the nonspecific set of symptoms makes the clinical diagnosis of PH challenging; none of the patients in the present analysis was diagnosed with PH preoperatively.

Table 3 Comparison of the asymptomatic and symptomatic subgroups

	Asymptomatic Subgroup *n* = 56	Symptomatic Subgroup *n* = 11	*p*-value
Mean age y (±SD)	56,7 (12.5)	53,6 (12.3)	*p* = 0.45
Sex (m/f)	38/18	10/1	*p* = 0.12 (X^2 = 2.405)
Type of surgery (n=)			
PPPD	*n* = 43	*n* = 5	*p* = 0.10 (X^2 = 4.515)
Whipple	*n* = 8	*n* = 4	
Other	*n* = 5	*n* = 2	
Associated disease (n=)			
PDAC	*n* = 10	*n* = 2	*p* = 0.05 (X^2 = 10.47)
CP	*n* = 18	*n* = 7	
Cystic neoplasia	*n* = 11	*n* = 0	
NET	*n* = 6	*n* = 0	
AP	*n* = 9	*n* = 0	
Other	*n* = 2	*n* = 2	
Heinrich Type			
I	26	6	*p* = 0.88 (X^2 = 0.2428)
II	24	4	
III	6	1	

PDAC pancreatic ductal adenocarcinoma, *CP* chronic pancreatitis, *NET* neuroendocrine tumor

Differential diagnosis of duodenal heterotopia

In general, PH lesions in the GIT are detectable by endoscopy. PH often presents as a submucosal swelling covered by normal mucosa and can easily be mistaken as gastrointestinal stroma tumor (GIST) or leiomyoma using endoscopy, ultrasonography or CT scanning [24]. In addition the risk of false negative biopsy results is high because ectopic tissue is most commonly located in the submucosal layer (76%), and sporadically appears in the muscular layer (15%), or in the subserosa (9%) [25]. Therefore, most biopsies are inconclusive, because of inadequate tissue samples [22]. In this context, endoscopic ultrasound-guided fine-needle aspiration (EUS-FNA) has been found to be valuable in the diagnosis of upper GIT lesions [26, 27].

In the present study, endoscopic ultrasound was not one of the standard preoperative investigations but the lesions were differentiated by preoperative CT and/or MRI scans (Fig. 2). If one looks on the presented CT-scan of a duodenal PH, it was especially difficult to distinguish the tumor from the original pancreas because of the close proximity of the two organs (Fig. 2). Based on current data on the value of EUS in the diagnosis of upper GIT lesions, EUS should be performed if a submucosal lesion is suspected. From the clinical point of view it is often impossible to distinguish GIST, lymphomas, peptic ulcer disease, or malignancies from heterotopic pancreatic tissue [16, 20, 22]. To diagnose PH, histopathological examination is therefore essential.

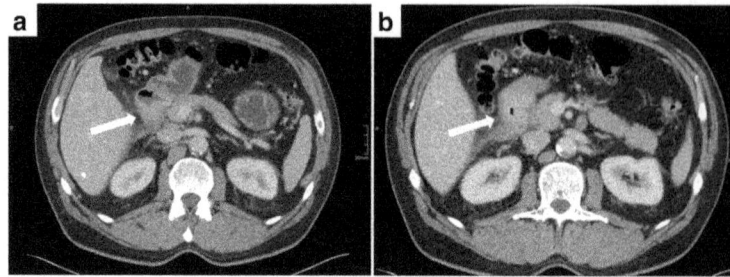

Fig. 2 Computed tomography (CT) scans (**a/b**) of a duodenal pancreatic heterotopia (arrows) with a duodenal stenosis

Malignant transformation of pancreatic heterotopia

Several studies have demonstrated that any disease of the ordinary pancreas can also arise in the heterotopic tissue, such as acute and chronic pancreatitis, the occurrence of pseudocystic changes, or even a malignant transformation to adenocarcinoma or acinar cell carcinoma [3, 6, 10, 16, 28–30]. The present results are in line with these findings, as two out of 67 patients with PH developed adenocarcinoma by malignant transformation of the heterotopic pancreatic tissue (2.9%). Guillou et al. stated that the incidence of malignancy due to heterotopic pancreatic tissue is 0.7% and therefore is extremely rare [13]. They studied the frequency of malignant transformations among 146 cases of PH between 1975 and 1991, including surgical and autopsy specimens. In a study by Makhlouf et al. two out of 109 patients (1.8%) with PH of the gastrointestinal tract were diagnosed with adenocarcinoma between 1970 and 1997 [12]. Malignancy is therefore a differential diagnosis and should be excluded. Furthermore, histopathological examination of the resected specimen of the 11 symptomatic patients in the present study showed chronic pancreatitis in seven cases (63.6%) and a duodenal tumor (adenoma) with no signs of chronic pancreatitis or malignancy in two cases (18%). Interestingly cystic lesions or NET arising from a duodenal PH were not found in our symptomatic subgroup. Furthermore, no specific Heinrich's type was associated with symptoms or malignancy.

Management of PH

For patients with symptomatic PH, local resection of the lesion seems to be the most appropriate therapy [16]. Patients underwent partial duodenal resections in two cases due to a symptomatic PH with suspicion of a duodenal tumor after intraoperative exclusion of malignancy by frozen section. Although endoscopic therapy is currently being evaluated for removal of ectopic pancreatic tissue, surgery remains the standard therapy [31, 32]. If histologically proven PH is asymptomatic and malignancy is definitely excluded, it can be treated conservatively. Nevertheless, if PH is found incidentally during a surgical procedure, excision should be considered due to its potential for becoming symptomatic and malignant. If malignancy is suspected extended oncological surgical resection (e.g., PPPD) is justified. The prognosis of patients with adenocarcinoma arising from PH seems to be better compared to patients with tumors arising from the pancreas itself, probably due to earlier presentation [16, 33].

Conclusion

In summary, PH of the duodenum represents a rare diagnosis and most patients are asymptomatic. Duodenal PH is mostly diagnosed by histological evaluation of surgical specimens resected for different pathologies. Nevertheless, the present results indicate that nearly all diseases of the genuine pancreas can occur in heterotopic pancreatic tissue. Therefore, depending on the current disease, different symptoms can appear and lead to another diagnosis. Ectopic duodenal pancreatic tissue should be considered in the differential diagnosis when a duodenal lesion is detected. Surgical resection is indicated if the lesion is symptomatic or malignancy cannot be excluded.

Abbreviations
PDAC: Pancreatic ductal adenocarcinoma; NET: Neuroendocrine tumors; GIT: Gastrointestinal tract; PH: Pancreatic heterotopia; PPPD: Pylorus-preserving pancreatoduodenectomy; EUS-FNA: Endoscopic ultrasound-guided fine-needle aspiration

Acknowledgements
We acknowledge the service of "PRS -Proof Reading Service" (Herfordshire, UK) for English language editing of the paper.

Funding
There is no supporting fund.

Authors' contributions
AB and MD wrote the manuscript, collected the data, interpreted the results and analyzed the data, STM and CZ interpreted the results and critically revised the manuscript, JP collected the data and wrote parts of the manuscript, SS analyzed the data statistically and corrected the manuscript,

DEA performed histological examinations, JW and TW gave important manuscript corrections. All authors read and approved the final manuscript.

Competing interests
The authors declare that they have no competing interests.

Author details
[1]Department of General, Thoracic and Vascular Surgery, University Hospital Carl Gustav Carus, TU Dresden, Fetscher Str. 74, 01037 Dresden, Germany.
[2]Institute for Pathology, University Hospital Carl Gustav Carus, TU Dresden, Fetscher Str. 74, 01307 Dresden, Germany.

References
1. Cano DA, Hebrok M, Zenker M. Pancreatic development and diseases. Gastroenterology. 2007;132:745–62.
2. Jiang LX, Xu J, Wang XW, et al. Gastric outlet obstruction caused by heterotopic pancreas: a case report and a quick review. World J Gastroenterol. 2008;14:6757–9.
3. Barbosa JC, Dockerty M, Waugh JM. Pancreatic heterotopia. Review of the literature and report of 41 authenticated surgical cases of which 25 were clinically significant. Surg Gynecol Obstet. 1946;82:527–42.
4. Dolan RV, ReMine WH, Dockerty MB. The fate of heterotopic pancreatic tissue. A study of 212 cases. Arch Surg. 1974 Dec;109(6):762–5.
5. Shetty A, Paramesh AS, Dwivedi AJ, et al. Symptomatic ectopic pancreas. Clinical Review. 2002;58:203–7.
6. Pang LC. Pancreatic heterotopia: a reappraisal and clinicopathologic analysis of 32 cases. South Med J. 1988 Oct;81(10):1264–75.
7. Thoeni RF, Gedgaudas RK. Ectopic pancreas: usual and unusual features. Gastrointestinal Radiol. 1980;5:37–42.
8. Cattell RB, Warren KW. Surgery of the pancreas. Philadelphia: WB Saunders Co; 1953. p. 26–37.
9. Hennings J, Garske U, Botling J, et al. Malignant insulinoma in ectopic pancreatic tissue. Dig Surg. 2005;22(5):377–9.
10. Jeong HY, Yang HW, Seo SW, et al. Adenocarcinoma arising from an ectopic pancreas in the stomach. Endoscopy. 2002 Dec;34(12):1014–7.
11. Tanaka K, Tsunoda T, Eto T, et al. Diagnosis and management of heterotopic pancreas. Int Surg. 1993 Jan–Mar;78(1):32–5.
12. Makhlouf HR, Almeida JL, Sobin LH. Carcinoma in jejunal pancreatic heterotopia. Arch Pathol Lab Med. 1999;123:707–11.
13. Guillou L, Nordback P, Gerber C, et al. Ductal adenocarcinoma arising in a heterotopic pancreas situated in a hiatal hernia. Arch Pathol Lab Med. 1994;118:568–71.
14. Yuan Z, Chen J, Zheng Q, et al. Heterotopic pancreas in the gastrointestinal tract. World J Gastroenterol. 2009;15829:3701–3.
15. Chandan VS, Wang W. Pancreatic heterotopia in the gastric antrum. Arch Pathol Lab Med. 2004;128(1):111–2.
16. Eisenberger CF, Gocht A, Knoefel WT, et al. Heterotopic pancreas—clinical presentation and pathology with review of the literature. Hepato-Gastroenterology. 2004 May–Jun;51(57):854–8. Review
17. Distler M, Rückert F, Aust D, et al. Pancreatic heterotopia of the duodenum: anatomic anomaly or clinical challenge ? J Gastrointest Surg. 2011;15:631–6.
18. Von Heinrich H. Ein Beitrag zur Histologie des sogenannten akzessorischen Pankreas. Virchows Arch A Pathol Anat Histopathol. 1909;198:392–440.
19. Elfving G, Hästbacka J. Pancreatic heterotopia and its clinical importance. Acta Chir Scand. 1965 Dec;130(6):593–602.
20. Armstrong CP, King PM, Dixon JM, et al. The clinical significance of heterotopic pancreas in the gastrointestinal tract. Br J Surg. 1981 Jun;68(6):384–7.
21. Christodoulidis G, Zacharoulis D, Barbanis S, et al. Heterotopic pancreas in the stomach: a case report and literature review. World J Gastroenterol. 2007 Dec 7;13(45):6098–100.
22. Hsia CY, Wu CW, Lui WY. Heterotopic pancreas: a difficult diagnosis. J Clin Gastroenterol. 1999 Mar;28(2):144–7.
23. Trifan A, Tarcoveanu E, Danciu M, et al. Gastric heterotopic pancreas: an unusual case and review of the literature. J Gastrointestin Liver Dis. 2012;21:209–12.
24. Kim JY, Lee JM, Kim KW, et al. Ectopic pancreas: CT findings with emphasis on differentiation from small gastrointestinal stromal tumor and leiomyoma. Radiology. 2009;252(1):92–100.
25. Martinez NS, Morlock CG, Dockerty MB, et al. Heterotopic pancreatic tissue involving the stomach. Ann Surg. 1958 Jan;147(1):1–12.
26. Chak A, Canto MI, Rösch T, et al. Endosonographic differentiation of benign and malignant stromal cell tumors. Gastrointest Endosc. 1997 Jun;45(6):468–73.
27. Philipper M, Hollerbach S, Gabbert HE, et al. Prospective comparison of endoscopic ultrasound-guided fine-needle aspiration and surgical histology in upper gastrointestinal submucosal tumors. Endoscopy. 2010;42:300–5.
28. Burke GW, Binder SC, Barron AM, et al. Heterotopic pancreas: gastric outlet obstruction secondary to pancreatitis and pancreatic pseudocyst. Am J Gastroenterol. 1989 Jan;84(1):52–5.
29. Green PH, Barratt PJ, Percy JP, et al. Acute pancreatitis occurring in gastric aberrant pancreatic tissue. Am J Dig Dis. 1977 Aug;22(8):734–40.
30. Emerson L, Layfield LJ, Rohr LR, et al. Adenocarcinoma arising in association with gastric heterotopic pancreas: a case report and review of the literature. J Surg Oncol. 2004 Jul 15;87(1):53–7.
31. Vitello JM. Gastric intramural pseudocyst with associated gastric outlet obstruction: recognition and management. South Med J. 1996;89:534–7.
32. Holman GA, Parasher G. Extra-pancreatic pancreatitis: a rare cause of abdominal pain. Dig Dis Sci. 2014;59:1714–6.
33. Okamoto H, Kawaoi A, Ogawara T, et al. Invasive ductal carcinoma arising from an ectopic pancreas in the gastric wall: a long-term survival case. Case Rep Oncol. 2012;5:69–73.

30

Negative pressure irrigation and endoscopic necrosectomy through man-made sinus tract in infected necrotizing pancreatitis: a technical report

Zhihui Tong[1†], Lu Ke[1†], Baiqiang Li[1], Gang Li[1], Jing Zhou[1], Xiao Shen[1], Weiqin Li[1,3*], Ning Li[2] and Jieshou Li[2]

Abstract

Background: In recent years, a step-up approach based on minimally invasive techniques was recommended by latest guidelines as initial invasive treatment for infected pancreatic necrosis (IPN). In this study, we aimed to describe a novel step-up approach for treating IPN consisting of four steps including negative pressure irrigation (NPI) and endoscopic necrosectomy (ED) as a bridge between percutaneous catheter drainage (PCD) and open necrosectomy

Methods: A retrospective review of a prospectively collected internal database of patients with a diagnosis of IPN between Jan, 2012 to Dec, 2012 at a single institution was performed. All patients underwent the same drainage strategy including four steps: PCD, NPI, ED and open necrosectomy. The demographic characteristics and clinical outcomes of study patients were analyzed.

Results: A total of 71 consecutive patients (48 males and 23 females) were included in the analysis. No significant procedure-related complication was observed and the overall mortality was +21.1 % (15 of 71 patients). Seven different strategies like PCD+ NPI, PCD+NPI+ED, PCD+open necrosectomy, etcetera, were applied in study patients and a half of them received PCD alone. In general, each patient underwent a median of 2 drainage procedures and the median total drainage duration was 11 days (interquartile range, 6–21days).

Conclusions: This four-step approach is effective in treating IPN and adds no extra risk to patients when compared with other latest step-up strategies. The two novel techniques (NPI and ED) could offer distinct clinical benefits without posing unanticipated risks inherent to the procedures.

Keywords: Infected pancreatic necrosis, Negative pressure irrigation, Endoscopic necrosectomy, Percutaneous catheter drainage

Background

Secondary infection of pancreatic necrosis (IPN), either pancreatic or peripancreatic, has been proved to be one of the most important determinants of severity in patients with acute necrotizing pancreatitis [1]. When compared with patients with sterile necrosis, patients with IPN suffered substantial increase in mortality ranging from 14 to 69 % due to sepsis and multiple organ failure, despite advances in critical care and antibiotics [2]. Traditionally, primary open necrosectomy has long been center of treatment in IPN patients [3], but in recent years, a step-up approach based on minimally invasive techniques was recommended by latest guidelines as initial invasive treatment [4]. In previous studies, percutaneous catheter drainage (PCD) is the cornerstone of step-up approaches and open necrosectomy always the last choice for those who did not respond to minimally invasive treatment [3]. However, techniques using

* Correspondence: njzy_pancrea@163.com
†Equal contributors
[1]SICU, Department of General Surgery, Jinling Hospital, Nanjing University School of Medicine, Nanjing 210002, People's Republic of China
[3]Department of SICU, Research Institute of General Surgery, Jinling Hospital, 305 East Zhongshan Road, Nanjing 210002, Jiangsu Province, China
Full list of author information is available at the end of the article

either endoscope or laparoscope applied between PCD and open necrosectomy vary in different studies [5–8] and the optimal choice remains unknown.

In the present study, we aimed to describe both the technical and clinical aspects of a new step-up approach for treating IPN consisting of four steps including negative pressure irrigation (NPI) and endoscopic necrosectomy (ED) as a bridge between PCD and open necrosectomy. By evaluating its feasibility and safety, we aimed to establish a framework for further studies comparing clinical effectiveness of currently available minimally invasive strategies.

Methods

Using an prospectively collected internal database, a retrospective review on all patients with a diagnosis of IPN between Jan, 2012 and Dec, 2012 at the Jinling Hospital, Nanjing University was performed. Study procedures were approved by the Jinling Hospital Institutional Review Board. The inclusion criteria included: 1) diagnosed with AP based on the Atlanta Criteria [9]; 2) age between 18 and 70 years old; 3) confirmation of IPN when one or more of the following was present: gas bubbles within pancreatic necrosis seen on Computed Tomography (CT); a positive culture obtained by fine-needle aspiration or during the first drainage and/or operative necrosectomy [1]. Patients were excluded if 1) they were pregnant; 2) they had received operative necrosectomy in other hospitals during the current episode of AP; 3) they had received abdominal surgery before IPN was present due to abdominal compartment syndrome (ACS), perforation of a visceral organ, bleeding, etc.; 4) treatment strategy was not completed due to non-medical reasons. All the patients initially received standard medical treatment according to the guidelines when IPN was not clinically diagnosed [10, 11]. Organ failure was managed with organ-specific treatment if needed, including mechanical ventilation, continuous renal replacement therapy (CRRT), vasoactive agents, invasive hemodynamic monitor (Picco2), etc.

Definitions

The criteria for organ dysfunction were described for 3 organ systems based on recently published international consensus [1, 12]: cardiovascular (need for inotropic agent), renal (creatinine ≥171 μmol/L), and respiratory ($PaO2/FiO2 \leq 300$ mmHg). Persistent organ failure was defined as organ failure in the same organ system for 48 h or more. Sepsis and septic shock was diagnosed according to SSC 2012 [13]. Gastrointestinal fistula was diagnosed when either small- or large-bowel contents were discharged from a drain or from the surgical wound. New-onset complication was defined as a complication not present at any time during the 24 h before first intervention. The severities of patients were classified at discharge or hospital death by the criteria of both the Revised Atlanta Classification (RAC) and the Determinant-based Classification (DBC) [1, 12].

The minimally invasive approach

The drainage strategy includes four procedures (Fig. 1): PCD, NPI, ED trough man-made sinus tract and operative necrosectomy (ON). Image-guided PCD was well described in previous studies and was also considered as the first choice in this study, the route could be through the retroperitoneum or the peritoneum depending on the location of IPN and adjacent organs [7, 14]. When the following criteria was met: 1) clinical improvement (improved organ dysfunction including circulatory, respiratory and renal, at least 10 % drop of APACHE [Acute Physiology and Chronic Health Evaluation] II score) could not be achieved through PCD alone in 3 days after procedure and CT results showed the drain was adequate, 2) mean CT density of necrotic tissue ≥30Hu or 3) suspicious or diagnosed gastrointestinal fistula, NPI would be applied as the first intervention or in addition to the drain catheters already existed and followed by ED when necessary (through the sinus tract created by NPI) before consideration of ON. NPI was implemented using "double catheterization cannula" (Fig. 2) which enables continuous irrigation of the cavity.

During the minimally invasive treatment, if patients presented one or more of 1) ACS developed and non-operative measure failed; 2) abdominal bleeding can not be controlled by conservative treatment; 3) diagnosed gastrointestinal fistula can not be well drained (judged by the treating physician); 4) progression of septic shock; 5) clinical improvement could not be achieved after 3 times of repeated ED. open necrosecotomy would be arranged to avoid life-threatening complications and facilitate the drainage process. Moreover, at whatever stage, return to one or more of the previous steps was allowed (e.g. patients already received ON was allowed to receive postoperative PCD as additional drainage).

The "double catheterization cannula" was made of a 24–30F tube for continuous negative pressure drainage and a 12F urethral catheter for continuous infusion (see the operating mechanism of this tube in the Additional file 1, similar instrument was also described in previous literature [15]). The diameter of the hole around the tube is 5 mm and the number of the hole is 14–30 depending on the length of the tube. This cannula could be placed mini-invasively under the guidance of CT or during the operation and the route could be either peritoneal or retroperitoneal. Briefly, after the access to the necrotic cavity was obtained with a 18G hollow needle (150 mm long), a guide wire was placed into the cavity and CT scan was repeated to confirm the puncture route. Then the tract was

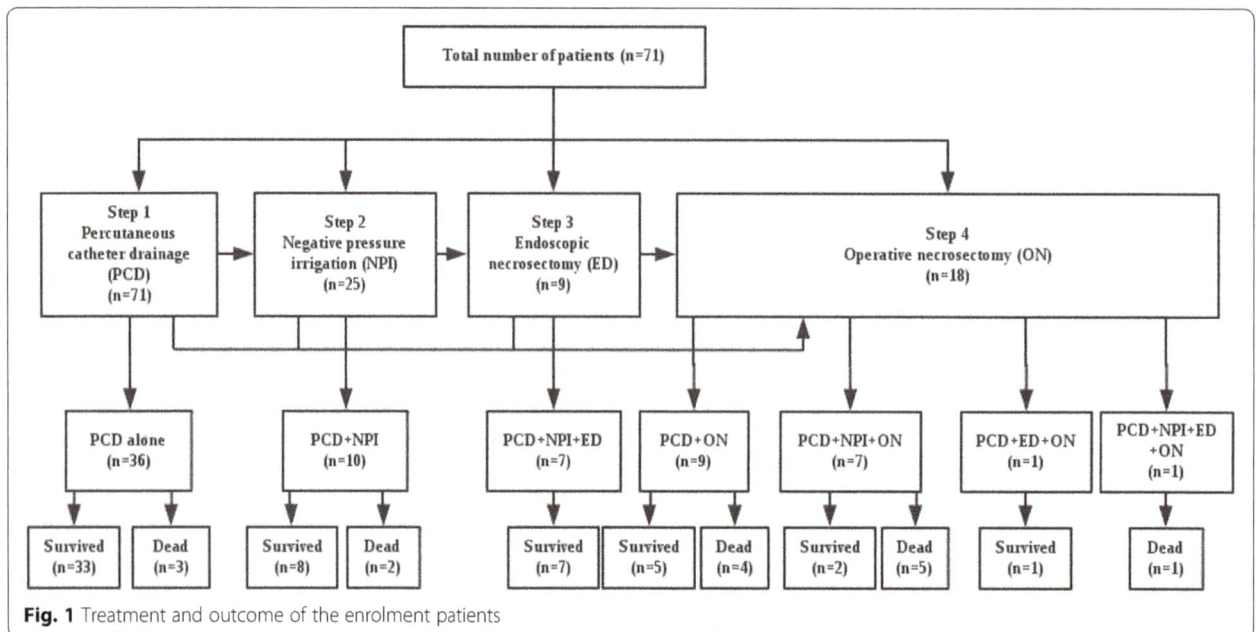

Fig. 1 Treatment and outcome of the enrolment patients

dilated to 28F using serial renal dilators over the guide wire and the catheter was then inserted. The catheters were routinely changed every week to maximize the effect of continuous drainage. In patients received NPI, PCD would usually be additionally applied and the route would be delicately designed to construct a "drainage system" (Fig. 3) in the cavity which could potentially facilitate the drainage process.

ED was performed using electronic gastroscope (30F) through the sinus tract created by the "double catheterization cannulas" and a snare was used to drag out massive bulk of necrotic tissue (see the videos in Additional files 2 and 3) that could hardly be drained by NPI and PCD. ED can be repeated whenever deemed to be necessary, and NPI would be continuously applied in the same port during the intervals between EDs. The ON was similar to previous reports, briefly, a laparotomy through a bilateral subcostal incision was performed and

several "double catheterization cannulas" or drains were inserted for postoperative lavage. All interventions were performed by the same team who were experienced in pancreatic surgery and also PCD and NPI therapy. EN procedures were performed by two experienced endoscopists who were well trained for this intervention.

Data collection

Demographic data including age, sex, etiology, APACHE II score, Sequential Organ Failure Assessment (SOFA) score, interval between symptom onset and admission of all study patients were recorded on admission. Outcome assessment included a composite of clinical metric to evaluate the feasibility and safety of the four-step approach such as mortality and morbidity, length of hospital and intensive care unit (ICU) stay, total treatment duration, treatment strategy for each patient, economical cost, etc. Contrast enhanced CT (CECT) was performed

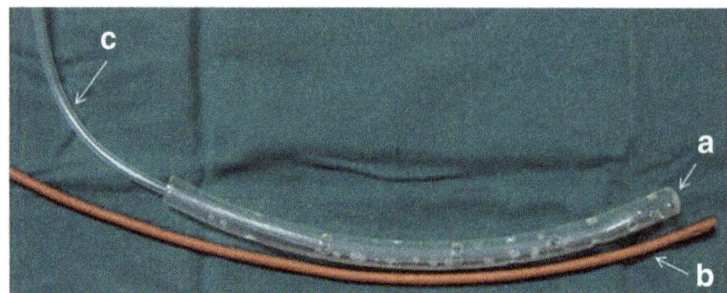

Fig. 2 Sketch map for double catheterization cannula, which is made of 3 parts. Part a is a plastic dead-end tube with a diameter between 24F and 30F. There are 14–30 side apertures along the tube according to the length of the tube and the diameter of each side aperture is 5 mm. Part b is a 12F urinary catheter for continuous infusion of irrigation fluid. Part c is a plastic drainage tube inside part and it is used for continuous negative pressure drainage. The diameter of Part c is about half of Part a

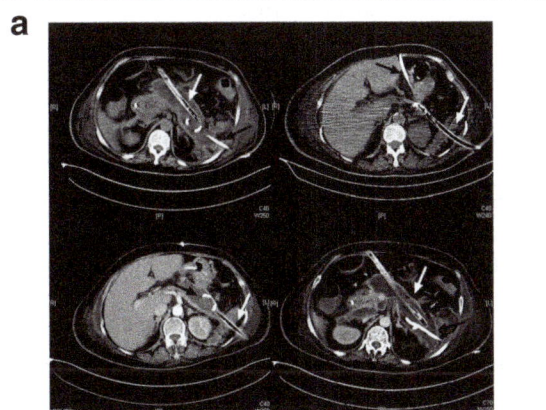

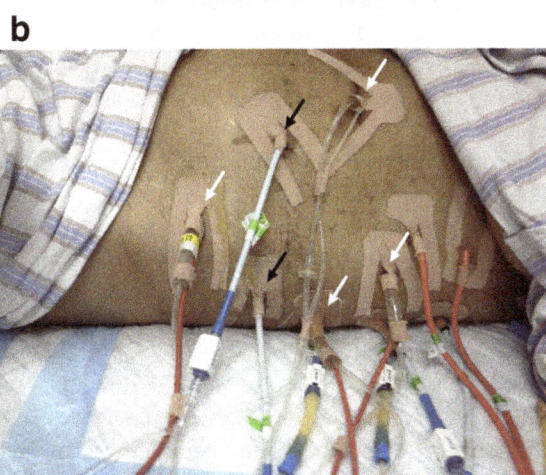

Fig. 3 a Samples of "drainage system" (pig-tail catheter and double catheterization cannula within the same necrosis cavity for continuous irrigation); **b** A patient with multiple drainage catheters and double catheterization cannulas, namely, multiple "drainage systems". The *black arrows* indicate pig-tail catheters and the *white arrows* indicate double catheterization cannulas

after admission, before discharge and on demand of the treating physician, and the CT severity index was assessed according to Balthazar's CT score [16]. All patients were followed up for at least 3 months after discharge. The clinical characteristics of patients admitted from Jan to Jun and from Jul to Dec were compared.

Statistically analysis

Continuous variables were expressed as medians (interquartile ranges) due to the limited sample size and the variability of the study patients. Categoric variables were described in absolute numbers and in percentages.

Results

During the study period, a total of 71 patients underwent the minimally invasive procedure were included in the analysis. No significant treatment-related complication was observed and the overall mortality was 21.1 %

(15 of 71 patients). Most patients (11 of 15) died of uncontrolled pancreatic infection with associated organ dysfunction, 3 patients died of recurrent major abdominal bleeding and another elderly patient (76 years old) died of respiratory dysfunction due to respiratory tract infection and co-existing chronic obstructive pulmonary disease (COPD). It is notable that the mortality in patients received operation (10 of 18 patients, 56 %) was significantly higher than the other patients.

Demographics

The demographic characteristics of all 71 patients were shown in Table 1. Most patients in this study suffered the most severe type of AP (critical AP in DBC and severe AP in RAC) and the CT severity index (CTSI) score was also extremely high. Moreover, as 90 % of the study patients were transferred from other hospitals, the median time from onset of AP to admission were 23 days (interquartile range, 6–53 days). Although our patients did not show very high APACHE II score and SOFA score (Table 1), organ dysfunction at admission was very common in study population and respiratory dysfunction could be seen in more than half of the patients (71.8 %). In addition, more than a fourth of patients were admitted with existing sepsis (19 of 71, 26.7 %).

Table 1 Demographic data and clinical characteristics

Demographic and clinical variables ($n = 71$)	
Age (years)	45 (35 to 53)
Gender	48 males/23 females
Etiology	34 Biliary origin
	9 Alcohol abuse
	24 Hyperlipidemia
	4 Idiopathic
APACHE II score at admission	10 (7 to 15)
SOFA score at admission	3 (1 to 6)
CT severity index	10 (8–10)
Revised Atlanta Classification	Moderate AP 23 (32.4 %)
	Severe AP 48 (67.6 %)
Determinant-based Classification	Severe AP 23 (32.4 %)
	Critical AP 48 (67.6 %)
Onset of symptom to admission (days)	23 (6 to 53)
Tertiary referral	64 (90.1 %)
Organ dysfunction at admission	Respiratory 51 (71.8 %)
	Renal 21 (29.6 %)
	Cardiovascular 12 (16.9 %)
Sepsis at admission	19 (26.7 %)

Feasibility metrics

As shown in Table 2, a total of 7 different strategies were applied in our patients and a half of the study patients received PCD only. Other commonly used strategies include PCD + NPI, PCD+ ON, PCD + NPI + ED and PCD+ NPI +ON and only one patients underwent all four steps. In general, a median of 2 drainage procedures were applied for each patient and the median total drainage duration was 11 days (interquartile range, 6–21days). About one fourth of all patients received operative necrosectomy and the mortality in these patients was noticeably high (10 of 18 patients, 56 %). The indications for the first operation included: 1) dissatisfactory drainage by minimally invasive measures and no clinical improvement (6 patients) 2) major abdominal bleeding (3 patients) 3) progress of septic complications like multiple organ dysfunction (6 patients); 4) operational enterostomy and drainage for intestinal or colonic fistulas that can not be well drainage with minimally invasive interventions (3 patients). Reoperation was rare (3 patients) and abdominal bleeding was the only reason for all cases.

For PCD, all patients received PCD either as the initial step of drainage or as a supplement and the median times and numbers of catheters placed were shown in Table 2. Similar to PCD, repeated NPI tube placement was quite common, and most patients received more than one "double catheterization cannula" for continuous irrigation. Moreover, ED was also usually applied in a repeated manner with a median of 2 times (interquartile range, 2–4 times)

Clinical outcome and safety metrics

As shown in Table 3, the median hospital duration of our cohort was significantly long with a median of 41 day (interquartile range, 23–61 days), as well as the ICU duration. During the drainage process, new-onset organ dysfunction was seldom seen and new-onset cardiovascular dysfunction was the one with highest incidence (6 of 71 patients). In contrast, gastrointestinal fistula (colonic and duodenal for the most), pancreatic fistula and intra-abdominal bleeding were the three most commonly seen complications (Table 3). Most patients with gastrointestinal fistula were managed non-operatively (laparotomic neostomy was done in only 5 patients) and topical irrigation around the fistula site was the major intervention. According to our 6-month follow-up data, pancreatic fistula was the most common long-term complication in this cohort, incision hernia also developed in one patient.

Regarding other complications, none of the study patients suffered internal bleeding during the procedure of NPI. Two patients (8.0 %) developed severe abdominal bleeding during the period of NPI drainage and required interventional embolization. According to the DSA results, the bleeding events were more likely to be caused by continuous corrosion due to infected pancreatic necrosis rather than the NPI instrument, as the bleeding site is far away from the NPI tube. All bleeding events were retroperitoneal and operation was applied in

Table 2 Metrics for feasibility

Metrics for feasibility (n = 71)	
Treatment approach	PCD alone 36 (50.1 %)
	PCD+NPI 10 (14.1 %)
	PCD+ON 9 (12.7 %)
	PCD + NPI + ED 7 (9.9 %)
	PCD+ NPI +ON 7 (9.9 %)
	PCD+ ED +ON 1 (1.4 %)
	PCD+NPI+ED+ON 1 (1.4 %)
Times of PCD in patients received PCD (n = 71)	2 (1 to 3)
No. of drainage catherters in patients received PCD (n = 71)	3 (2–4)
Times of NPI in patients received NPI (n = 25)	2 (1 to 3)
No. of NPI in patients received NPI (n = 25)	2 (1 to 3)
Times of ED in patients received ED (n = 9)	2 (2 to 4)
Patients needing operative intervention (%)	18 (25.4 %)
Patients needing reoperation (%)	3 (4.2 %)
Patients needing readmission (%)	5 (7.0 %)
Total no. of drainage procedures per patient	2 (2 to 4)
Total drainage duration (day)	11 (6–21)

Table 3 Metrics for safety and clinical outcome

Clinical outcome measures	
Mortality (%)	15 (21.1 %)
New-onset organ dysfunction	Cardiovascular 6 (8.4 %)
	Respiratory 1 (1.4 %)
	Renal 5 (7.0 %)
New-onset Sepsis	10 (14.1 %)
Gastrointestinal fistula	17 (23.9 %)
	Colonic alone 7 (9.9 %)
	Duodenal alone 5 (7.0 %)
	Jejunal or gastric alone 1 (1.4 %)
	Multiple 4 (5.6)
Pancreatic fistula	14 (19.7 %)
Chylous fistula	3 (4.2 %)
Intra-abdominal bleeding	11 (15.5 %)
Portal venous system thrombosis	3 (4.2 %)
Positive culture result for fungi	12 (16.9 %)
Gastric outlet obstruction	2 (2.8 %)
Hospital duration (day)	41 (23–61)
ICU duration (day)	17 (7–43)
Total cost (10,000 rmb)	18.2 (8.6–32.4)

8 case in which bleeding could not be stopped by interventional embolization. Moreover, 10 patients developed new-onset sepsis or septic shock during treatment and only 3 of them were reversed. Other less common complications include chylous fistula, portal venous system thrombosis and gastric outlet obstruction and all of which showed an incidence rate less than 5 %.

Discussion

As minimally invasive approach became the mainstream for treating IPN in recent years, we developed a new drainage protocol combining three minimally invasive techniques and operation together. With this novel four-step approach, the overall mortality in our series was 21.1 %, which is comparable to that reported in previous series [7, 17], despite that most of our patients were deemed as the most severe type of AP according to latest classifications [12, 13]. The incidence of major complications such as intra-abdominal bleeding, enterocutaneous fistula, etc. also did not dramatically differ from the largest series of step-up approach [7, 17]. Moreover, the total number of drainage procedures including all the steps was lower than that in previous major studies [7, 14]. These results suggest that this novel four-step approach, when applied by an experienced team, does not place subjects at greater risk of mortality and morbidity and it has the potential to improve the cost-effectiveness of currently available treatment.

With the dint of PCD, NPI and ED, about three fourth of study patients avoid open surgery and most of them successfully survived (48 of 53 patients, 91 %). No procedure-related complication was observed during the study period. It is noteworthy that patients who received open necrosectomy suffered a mortality as high as 56 %, which is significantly higher than those without operation. Our rigorous indication for surgical intervention might be responsible for that. Moreover, most patients in this series received multiple minimally invasive sessions for removal of necrosis, which is in accordance to the previous reports [7, 8].

The use of NPI had been long in our center, but the tube was routinely placed during open surgery for continuous "active" drainage in the past. In the recent years, we managed to place the "double catheterization cannula" minimal-invasively under CT guidance and therefore the use of NPI could be much more extensive. As the "double catheterization cannula" can access the necrosis either peritoneally or retroperitoneally, the drainage route can be as variable as PCD and offer not only a route for continuous lavage, but also much bigger sinus tract for draining bulk of necrosis. Moreover, NPI catheter together with other pig-tail catheters could form a "drainage system" to extend the range of continuous active drainage. Briefly, lavage fluid can be infused through one or multiple pig-tails catheter and drained out by a NPI tube as shown in Fig. 3. Although the NPI catheter is very similar to the instrument described by Raraty et al. [15], our "drainage system" combining different catheters can make full use of continuous irrigation.

Different from the well-known videoscopic assisted retroperitoneal debridement (VARD), endoscopic transgastric necrosectomy (ETN) and percutaneous endoscopic necrosectomy (PEN) [5, 6, 8] techniques, we can access the target site both peritoneally or retroperitoneally through the sinus tract constructed by the "double catheterization cannula" and perform ED. Therefore no surgical incision was needed to enter the necrosis before ED and the whole procedure could be performed under conscious condition with only topical anesthesia. As it is easy to operate with very limited impairment, ED could even be repeated on a daily basis if necessary. In contrast, the previously reported techniques including VARD, ETN or PEN, need basal anesthesia to obtain a temporary access (either incision or dilation) to the necrosis before debridement and the route were relatively rigid [5, 6]. However, similar to other minimally invasive necrosectomy, our ED also face great difficulty in removing bulk of necrosis due to the limited size of access tract. An alternative temporary trocar may offer better outlet for removing necrosis and we have started to work with that.

Conclusion

In conclusion, our four-step approach is effective in treating IPN and add no extra risk to patients when compared with other latest step-up strategies. The two novel techniques (NPI and ED) could offer distinct clinical benefits without posing unanticipated risks inherent to the procedures and work well together to debride IPN.

Additional files

Additional file 1: The mechanism of the "double catheterization cannula". The "double catheterization cannula" was made of a 24–30F tube for continuous negative pressure drainage and a 12F urethral catheter for continuous infusion. (GIF 483 kb)

Additional file 2: Movie S1. Video one of endoscopic necrosectomy. Endoscopic necrosectomy was performed using electronic gastroscope (30F) through the sinus tract created by the "double catheterization cannulas" and a snare was used to drag out massive bulk of necrotic tissue.

Additional file 3: Movie S2. Video two of endoscopic necrosectomy. Endoscopic necrosectomy was performed using electronic gastroscope (30F) through the sinus tract created by the "double catheterization cannulas" and a snare was used to drag out massive bulk of necrotic tissue.

Abbreviations

ACS: Abdominal compartment syndrome; APACHE: Acute Physiology and Chronic Health Evaluation; CECT: Contrast enhanced Computed Tomography; COPD: Chronic obstructive pulmonary disease; CRRT: Continuous renal replacement therapy; CT: Computed Tomography; CTSI: CT severity index; DBC: Determinant-based Classification; ED: Endoscopic necrosectomy;

ETN: Endoscopic transgastric necrosectomy; ICU: Intensive care unit; IPN: Infected pancreatic necrosis; NPI: Negative pressure irrigation; ON: Operative necrosectomy; PCD: Percutaneous catheter drainage; PEN: Percutaneous endoscopic necrosectomy; RAC: Revised Atlanta classification; SOFA: Sequential Organ Failure Assessment; VARD: Videoscopic assisted retroperitoneal debridement

Acknowledgements
We would like to thank Yuhui Chen and Wei Jiang for their contributions in data acquisition.

Funding
This study was supported by the National Science Foundation of China (81170438 and 81200334).

Authors' contributions
ZT and LK contributed to design, data acquisition, statistical analysis and drafted the manuscript. BL and GL contributed to data acquisition, data analysis and presentation. JZ contributed to data acquisition and data analysis. XS participated in data acquisition and statistical analysis. WL, NL and JL contributed to study control, study design and manuscript drafting. WL contributed to manuscript drafting and revision. ZT and LK contribute equally to the paper. All authors have read and approved the final manuscript.

Authors' information
WL is pancreatic disease specialists. ZT, LK, BL, GL, JZ and XS are also intensivists at the Research Institute of General Surgery, Jinling Hospital, Medical School of Nanjing University. NL is the associate director of the Research Institute of General Surgery, Jinling Hospital, Medical School of Nanjing University. JL is the director of the Research Institute of General Surgery, Jinling Hospital, Medical School of Nanjing University.

Competing interests
The authors declare that they have no competing interest.

Author details
[1]SICU, Department of General Surgery, Jinling Hospital, Nanjing University School of Medicine, Nanjing 210002, People's Republic of China. [2]Department of General Surgery, Jinling Hospital, Nanjing University School of Medicine, Nanjing 210002, People's Republic of China. [3]Department of SICU, Research Institute of General Surgery, Jinling Hospital, 305 East Zhongshan Road, Nanjing 210002, Jiangsu Province, China.

References
1. Dellinger EP, Forsmark CE, Layer P, Levy P, Maravi-Poma E, Petrov MS, Shimosegawa T, Siriwardena AK, Uomo G, Whitcomb DC, Windsor JA, Pancreatitis Across Nations Clinical R, Education A. Determinant-based classification of acute pancreatitis severity: an international multidisciplinary consultation. Ann Surg. 2012;256:875–80.
2. Tenner S, Baillie J, Dewitt J, Vege SS. American College of Gastroenterology Guidelines: management of acute pancreatitis. Am J Gastroenterol. 2013; 108:1400-15. 1416.
3. Hollemans RA, Bollen TL, van Brunschot S, Bakker OJ, Ahmed Ali U, van Goor H, Boermeester MA, Gooszen HG, Besselink MG, van Santvoort HC, Dutch Pancreatitis Study G. Predicting Success of Catheter Drainage in Infected Necrotizing Pancreatitis. Ann Surg. 2015;263:787–92.
4. Working Group IAPAPAAPG. IAP/APA evidence-based guidelines for the management of acute pancreatitis. Pancreatology. 2013;13:e1–e15.
5. Dhingra R, Srivastava S, Behra S, Vadiraj PK, Venuthurimilli A, Shalimar, Dash NR, Madhusudhan KS, Gamanagatti SR, Garg PK. Single or multiport percutaneous endoscopic necrosectomy performed with the patient under conscious sedation is a safe and effective treatment for infected pancreatic necrosis (with video). Gastrointest Endosc. 2015;81:351–9.
6. van Santvoort HC, Besselink MG, Horvath KD, Sinanan MN, Bollen TL, van Ramshorst B, Gooszen HG, Dutch Acute Pancreatis Study G. Videoscopic assisted retroperitoneal debridement in infected necrotizing pancreatitis. HPB (Oxford). 2007;9:156–9.
7. van Santvoort HC, Besselink MG, Bakker OJ, Hofker HS, Boermeester MA, Dejong CH, van Goor H, Schaapherder AF, van Eijck CH, Bollen TL, van Ramshorst B, Nieuwenhuijs VB, Timmer R, Lameris JS, Kruyt PM, Manusama ER, van der Harst E, van der Schelling GP, Karsten T, Hesselink EJ, van Laarhoven CJ, Rosman C, Bosscha K, de Wit RJ, Houdijk AP, van Leeuwen MS, Buskens E, Gooszen HG. A step-up approach or open necrosectomy for necrotizing pancreatitis. N Engl J Med. 2010;362:1491–502.
8. Bakker OJ, van Santvoort HC, van Brunschot S, Geskus RB, Besselink MG, Bollen TL, van Eijck CH, Fockens P, Hazebroek EJ, Nijmeijer RM, Poley JW, van Ramshorst B, Vleggaar FP, Boermeester MA, Gooszen HG, Weusten BL, Timmer R, Dutch Pancreatitis Study G. Endoscopic transgastric vs surgical necrosectomy for infected necrotizing pancreatitis: a randomized trial. JAMA. 2012;307:1053–61.
9. Bradley 3rd EL. A clinically based classification system for acute pancreatitis. Summary of the International Symposium on Acute Pancreatitis, Atlanta, Ga, September 11 through 13, 1992. Arch Surg. 1993;128:586–90.
10. Banks PA, Freeman ML. Practice guidelines in acute pancreatitis. Am J Gastroenterol. 2006;101:2379–400.
11. Muddana V, Whitcomb DC, Papachristou GI. Current management and novel insights in acute pancreatitis. Expert Rev Gastroenterol Hepatol. 2009;3:435–44.
12. Banks PA, Bollen TL, Dervenis C, Gooszen HG, Johnson CD, Sarr MG, Tsiotos GG, Vege SS, Acute Pancreatitis Classification Working G. Classification of acute pancreatitis–2012: revision of the Atlanta classification and definitions by international consensus. Gut. 2013;62:102–11.
13. Dellinger RP, Levy MM, Rhodes A, Annane D, Gerlach H, Opal SM, Sevransky JE, Sprung CL, Douglas IS, Jaeschke R, Osborn TM, Nunnally ME, Townsend SR, Reinhart K, Kleinpell RM, Angus DC, Deutschman CS, Machado FR, Rubenfeld GD, Webb S, Beale RJ, Vincent JL, Moreno R. Surviving sepsis campaign: international guidelines for management of severe sepsis and septic shock, 2012. Intensive Care Med. 2013;39:165–228.
14. Babu BI, Genovese T, Mazzon E, Riccardi L, Paterniti I, Galuppo M, Crisafulli C, Siriwardena AK, Cuzzocrea S. Recombinant human activated protein C (Xigris) attenuates murine cerulein-induced acute pancreatitis via regulation of nuclear factor kappaB and apoptotic pathways. Pancreas. 2012;41:619–28.
15. Raraty MG, Halloran CM, Dodd S, Ghaneh P, Connor S, Evans J, Sutton R, Neoptolemos JP. Minimal access retroperitoneal pancreatic necrosectomy: improvement in morbidity and mortality with a less invasive approach. Ann Surg. 2010;251:787–93.
16. Balthazar EJ. Acute pancreatitis: assessment of severity with clinical and CT evaluation. Radiology. 2002;223:603–13.
17. Babu RY, Gupta R, Kang M, Bhasin DK, Rana SS, Singh R. Predictors of surgery in patients with severe acute pancreatitis managed by the step-up approach. Ann Surg. 2013;257:737–50.

31

Primary pancreatic-type acinar cell carcinoma of the jejunum with tumor thrombus extending into the mesenteric venous system: a case report and literature review

Kosei Takagi[1]* [ID], Takahito Yagi[1], Takehiro Tanaka[2], Yuzo Umeda[1], Ryuichi Yoshida[1], Daisuke Nobuoka[1], Takashi Kuise[1] and Toshiyoshi Fujiwara[1]

Abstract

Background: Although ectopic pancreatic tissue is common in the upper gastrointestinal tract, the incidence of ectopic pancreatic tissue in the jejunum is low, and malignant transformation in ectopic pancreatic tissue is rare. Furthermore, pancreatic-type acinar cell carcinoma (ACC) developing in the jejunum and ACC accompanied by tumor thrombus are extremely rare.

Case presentation: A 78-year-old-woman presented with melena. Abdominal computed tomography images and endoscopic examination revealed a submucosal jejunal mass with tumor thrombus extending into a jejunal vein. The patient underwent a curative resection combined with a partial jejunectomy and partial pancreatectomy. Histopathological examination of the resected tissue showed tumor cells with a homogeneous acinar architecture identical to pancreatic-type ACC and tumor thrombus. Postoperatively, she was followed for 10 months and had no recurrence.

Conclusion: We present an extremely rare case of pancreatic-type ACC in the jejunum with extensive tumor thrombus invading into the mesenteric venous system. This type of cancer has not been reported previously but should be considered in the differential diagnosis of a jejunal mass.

Keywords: Acinar cell carcinoma, Jejunum, Ectopic pancreas, Tumor thrombus

Background

Ectopic pancreatic tissue is most frequently found in the upper gastrointestinal tract, and malignant transformation of ectopic pancreatic tissue is rare. In the English literature, approximately 30 cases of adenocarcinoma arising from ectopic pancreatic tissue have been reported, and most occurred in the upper gastrointestinal tract [1, 2]. Only seven cases of adenocarcinoma arising from ectopic pancreatic tissue in the jejunum have been reported [3].

Acinar cell carcinoma (ACC) is a rare malignant tumor that accounts for 1–2% of all exocrine pancreatic neoplasms and usually arises in the pancreatic parenchyma [4]. ACC derived from ectopic pancreatic tissue is very rare, with only 12 previous reports [1, 2, 5–14]. Among these reports, only one described ACC in jejunal pancreatic heterotopia [14]. Furthermore, ACC accompanied by tumor thrombus is very rare. In the English literature, there have been only two reports of ACC with portal vein tumor thrombus [15, 16].

We herein report an extremely rare case of pancreatic-type ACC presenting as a submucosal jejunal tumor accompanied by tumor thrombus and review the previously reported cases of heterotopic ACC.

* Correspondence: kotakagi15@gmail.com
[1]Department of Gastroenterological Surgery, Okayama University Graduate School of Medicine, Dentistry and Pharmaceutical Sciences, 2-5-1 Shikata-cho, Kita-ku, Okayama 700-8558, Japan
Full list of author information is available at the end of the article

Case presentation

A 78-year-old woman was admitted to another hospital complaining of melena and transferred to our facility for further examination. Her physical examination was unremarkable. The laboratory values were as follows: white blood count, 4220 cells/μL; hemoglobin level, 12.4 g/dL;

platelet count, 16.4×10^4 cells/μL; aspartate transaminase, 25 IU/L; alanine aminotransferase, 16 IU/L; total bilirubin, 0.8 mg/dL; albumin, 3.6 g/dL; and creatinine, 0.48 mg/dL. Tumor markers (carcinoembryonic antigen, carbohydrate antigen 19–9, s-pancreas-1 antigen, and Duke pancreatic monoclonal antigen type 2) were within normal limits.

Abdominal computed tomography scans revealed an 8.5×4.0 cm exophytic submucosal tumor in the jejunum (Fig. 1a). The tumor extended to the uncinate process of the pancreas and compressed the posterior aspect of the superior mesenteric vein. The first jejunal vein was thrombosed, and we suspected a tumor thrombus. Tumor thrombus was not identified in the superior mesenteric vein (Fig. 1b). We also observed significant thickening of the jejunal mesentery, but no distant metastasis was found (Fig. 1c).

Double-balloon enteroscopy showed an approximately 3 cm submucosal tumor with central ulceration in the jejunum (Fig. 2a). Endoscopic biopsy revealed a poorly

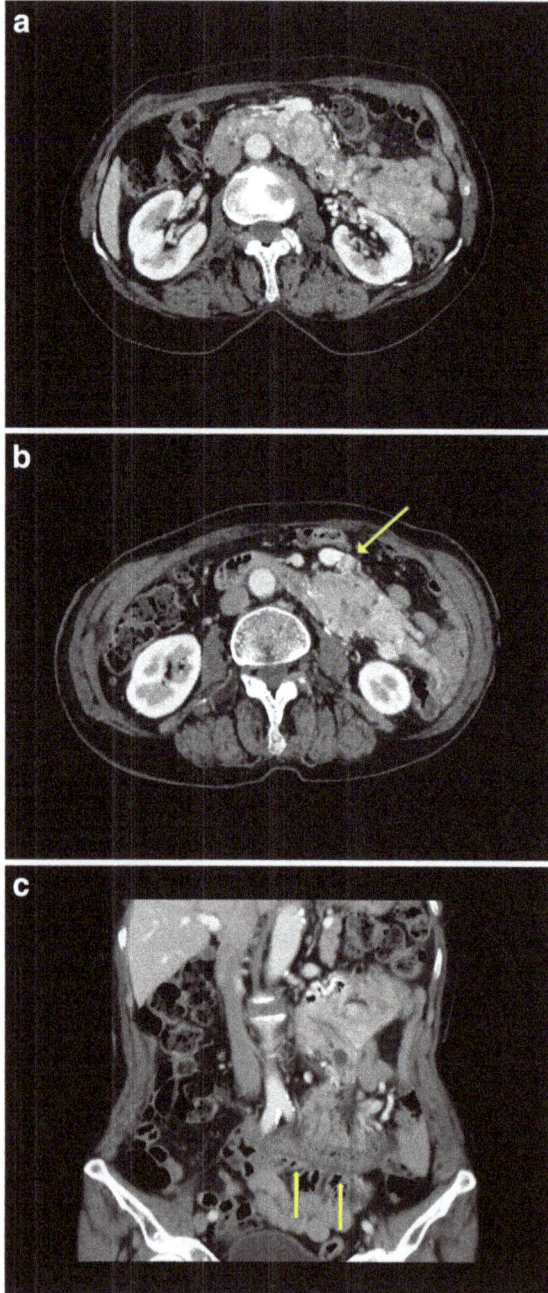

Fig. 1 Preoperative computed tomography scans: **a**. An 8.5 × 4.0 cm exophytic submucosal tumor located in the jejunum. The posterior aspect of the superior mesenteric vein is compressed by the tumor, and the tumor extends to the uncinate process of the pancreas; **b**. The tumor thrombus invades the first jejunal vein (*arrow*); **c**. The jejunal mesentery shows significant thickening (*arrow*)

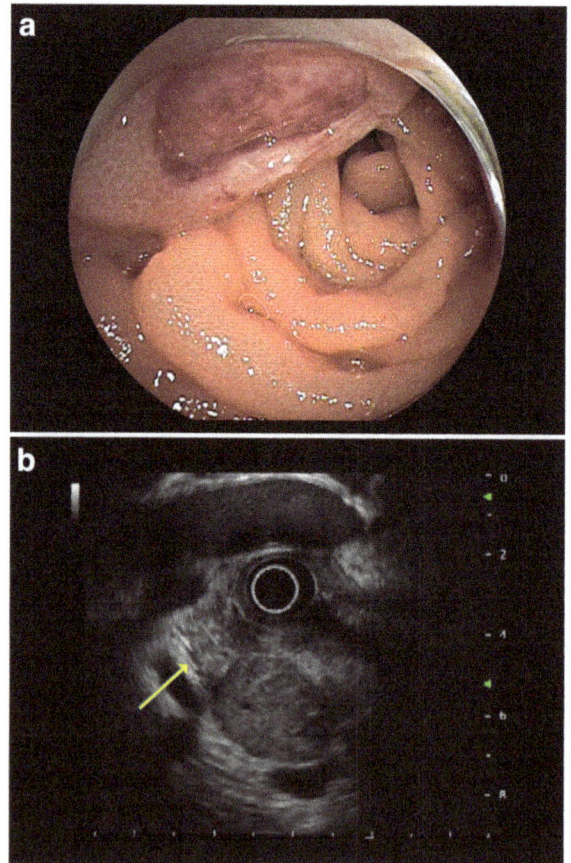

Fig. 2 Endoscopic examination: **a**. Double-balloon enteroscopy reveals a centrally ulcerated submucosal jejunal lesion measuring approximately 3 cm; **b**. Endoscopic ultrasonography shows a submucosal tumor touching the uncinate process of the pancreas, suggesting the possibility of pancreatic infiltration (*arrow*, pancreas)

differentiated adenocarcinoma. Endoscopic ultrasonography showed a submucosal jejunal tumor which touched the uncinate process of the pancreas and suggested possible pancreatic infiltration (Fig. 2b).

Our preoperative diagnosis was a jejunal adenocarcinoma. Although there was tumor thrombus in the mesenteric venous system and the possibility of pancreatic invasion, we considered the tumor resectable.

At surgery, there was neither peritoneal dissemination nor liver metastasis. The tumor was located mainly in the mesentery of the upper jejunum. No invasion of the superior mesenteric artery or vein was found. We did not observe invasion of the pancreatic uncinate process grossly, but we resected it. Accordingly, the patient underwent a curative resection combined with a partial jejunectomy (approximately 50 cm of the jejunum) and a partial pancreatectomy (uncinate process).

The gross examination revealed an 8.5 cm, soft, circumscribed, yellowish-white, submucosal mass in the jejunum (Fig. 3a). Histologically, the tumor showed an acinar and solid growth pattern (Fig. 3b). Marked vascular invasion was observed, and the tumor thrombus extended into the first jejunal vein (Fig. 3c). The tumor was confined to the jejunal wall without pancreatic parenchymal invasion (Fig. 3d). Immunohistochemically, the tumor cells were positive for trypsin and negative for chromogranin A, synaptophysin, and CD56 (Figs. 3e, f, g, and h). The resected margins were free of tumor cells. Although residual ectopic pancreas was not identified, the tumor was diagnosed as pancreatic-type ACC of the jejunum based on the architectural patterns of ACC and immunohistochemical findings.

The postoperative course was uneventful. The patient received adjuvant chemotherapy with S-1 (TS-1; Taiho Pharmaceutical, Tokyo, Japan) after the curative resection. She was alive and without recurrence at her last follow-up visit 10 months postoperatively.

Discussion and conclusions

To the best of our knowledge, this is the first report of pancreatic-type ACC in the jejunum accompanied by tumor thrombus in the mesenteric venous system. This report highlights the clinicopathological findings of an extremely rare case and reviews the features of previously reported cases of heterotopic ACC.

There have been only 13 cases, including our case, reporting heterotopic ACC in a digestive organ (Table 1). The cases included seven women and six men with a mean age of 61.8 years. Heterotopic ACC was most frequently found in the upper gastrointestinal tract. The average tumor size was relatively large (4.5 cm). Interestingly, no case was preoperatively diagnosed as ACC. Indeed, five cases were diagnosed as poorly differentiated adenocarcinoma by biopsy, and other tumor types were suspected in four cases. ACCs usually develop submucosally, so preoperative diagnosis by histological examination might be difficult. Furthermore, the histological examination of the resected specimen revealed ectopic pancreatic tissue in only two cases.

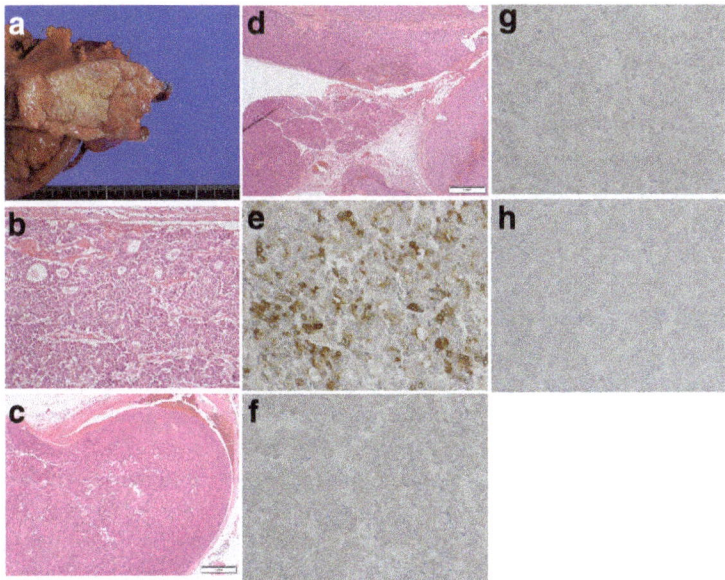

Fig. 3 Pathological examination of the jejunal tumor: **a**. Gross examination shows an 8.5 cm, soft, circumscribed, yellowish-white, submucosal mass in the jejunum; **b**. Microscopic examination reveals acinar and solid architectural patterns; **c**. Marked vascular invasion, including tumor thrombus, extends into the first jejunal vein; **d**. No invasion to the pancreatic parenchyma is identified; Immunohistochemically, the tumor cells are positive for trypsin (**e**) and negative for chromogranin A (**f**), synaptophysin (**g**), and CD56 (**h**)

Table 1 Demographic and clinicopathological features in reported cases of acinar cell carcinoma arising from heterotopic pancreas

Reports	Age[a]/Sex	Site	Size (cm)	Preoperative diagnosis	Metastasis	Tumor characteristics	Treatment	Adjuvant chemo	EPT	Outcome
Sun et al. 2004 [5]	86/F	Stomach	5.0	PDA	None	Exophytic, ulcerated	Partial gastrectomy	NM	A	NM
Mizuno et al. 2007 [6]	73/M	Stomach	7.6	GIST/L	LN	Submucosal	PD	NM	A	11 months alive, liver metastasis at 7 months
Ambrosini-Spaltro et al. 2009 [7]	52/M	Stomach	4.0	PDA	None	Ulcerated	Subtotal gastrectomy	NM	P	NM
Coyne et al. 2012 [8]	77/F	Stomach	4.5	PDA	None	Ulcerated, submucosal	Partial gastrectomy	NM	A	NM
Yonenaga et al 2016 [2]	63/M	Stomach	6.5	PDA	Liver	Borrmann type-2 lesion	Chemo	None	A	5 month died, sepsis
Kim et al. 2017 [9]	54/M	Stomach	2.7	GIST/L	None	Submucosal	Wedge resection	None	A	33 months alive, NR
Bookman 1932 [10]	28/F	Duodenum	NM	Benign[b]	None	NM	Partial resection	NM	A	NM
Jahromi et al. 2013 [1]	58/M	Duodenum	2.7	NM	None	Submucosal	Partial resection	Cap + Oxal	A	18 months alive, NR
Kawakami et al. 2007 [11]	65/F	AoV	1.2	NM	None	Exophytic	PD	NM	A	19 months alive, NR
Hervieu et al. 2008 [12]	35/F	Liver	4.0	HCC	None	Well-limited	Hepatectomy	None	A	6 years alive, NR
Chiaravalli et al. 2009 [13]	65/F	Colon	4.0	NM	LN	Ulcerated	Partial resection	NM	A	24 months died, bone metastasis at 18 months
Makhlouf et al. 1999 [14]	71/M	Jejunum	3.5	NM	None	Ulcerated	Partial resection	NM	P	1 year alive, liver metastasis at 1 year
Our case	76/F	Jejunum	8.5	PDA	None	Exophytic, ulcerated, submucosal, mass with tumor thrombus	Partial resection with partial pancreatectomy	S-1	A	10 months alive, NR

F female, M male, P present, A absent, PDA poorly differentiated adenocarcinoma, NM not mentioned, GIST/L gastrointestinal stromal tumor or lymphoma, HCC hepatocellular carcinoma, AoV ampulla of Vater, Cap + Oxal Capecitabine + Oxaliplatin, PD pancreaticoduodenectomy, Chemo chemotherapy, EPT ectopic pancreatic tissue, NR no recurrence, LN lymph node
[a]Reported in years; [b]Benign tumor such as a polyp

Ectopic pancreatic tissue is found in 0.5–13.7% of laparotomy and autopsy cases and is usually located in the upper gastrointestinal tract [3]. The pathological classification of ectopic pancreas was diagnosed by the Heinrich classification [17]. Malignant transformation of ectopic pancreas tissue most frequently occurs in the upper digestive organs, and the reported incidence ranges from 0.7–1.8% [3]. The following three criteria have been proposed for ectopic pancreas carcinoma: the tumor must be found within or near the ectopic pancreas, a transition between pancreatic structures and carcinoma must be observed, and the non-neoplastic pancreatic tissue must comprise fully developed acini and ductal structures [18]. However, similar to most previous cases, in our case, no ectopic pancreas tissue was identified (Table 1). It has been proposed that a carcinoma arising from ectopic pancreas destroys the primary benign lesion [14].

ACC is typically relatively circumscribed and large with extensive hemorrhage and necrosis [19]. The characteristic microscopic architectural patterns are the acinar pattern, with neoplastic cells arranged in small acinar units, and solid pattern, with solid nests of neoplastic cells lacking luminal formations [20]. In the histopathologic diagnosis of ACC, an immunohistochemical evaluation of pancreatic exocrine enzymes is helpful; both trypsin and chymotrypsin are positive in more than 95% cases [20]. Furthermore, neuroendocrine markers such as chromogranin A, synaptophysin, and CD56 should be assessed when ACC is in the differential diagnosis [9]. In our case, the tumor showed both acinar and solid growth patterns, trypsin-positivity, and neuroendocrine marker-negativity. Therefore, we diagnosed a pure pancreatic-type ACC of the jejunum.

Although ACC has been considered to have a poor prognosis, the surgical resection and 5-year survival rates after resection have been reported as 76.5 and 43.9%, respectively, in a nationwide survey performed in Japan [21]. Furthermore, patients with ACC had a significantly better prognosis than those with pancreatic ductal adenocarcinoma [22]. Aggressive surgical resection with negative margins is also associated with longer survival [23]. However, the prognosis of heterotopic ACC remains unclear because of the limited number of reported cases.

Pancreatic cancers frequently invade the portal venous system leading to extrinsic portal vein obstruction. However, intrinsic venous obstruction by tumor thrombus, while a common occurrence in hepatocellular carcinoma, rarely occurs in pancreatic cancer [16]. Indeed, there have been only a few cases of pancreatic cancer with portal vein tumor thrombus, including two cases of ACC accompanied by tumor thrombus [15, 16]. Furthermore, distinguishing tumor thrombus from a blood clot is very important, because it is well recognized that a tumor thrombus involving the mesenteric venous system is associated with liver metastases. The treatment strategy will also be affected by the preoperative evaluation. In our case, although tumor thrombus was present in the first jejunal vein accompanied by significant mesenteric thickening, we considered the tumor resectable because there were no distant metastases.

The efficacy of neoadjuvant or adjuvant chemotherapy for ACC arising in ectopic pancreatic tissue is still unknown. In patients with unresectable ACC, fluorouracil-based chemotherapy should be considered a neoadjuvant or palliative treatment [24]. However, in the previous 12 reports of heterotopic ACC, only one patient received adjuvant treatment with capecitabine and oxaliplatin after curative resection (Table 1).

In our case, the patient had a high risk of recurrence because of extensive tumor thrombus. Therefore, administered S-1 as adjuvant chemotherapy according to the treatment for pancreatic cancer after curative resection [25]. The patient continued chemotherapy without severe adverse effects or recurrence postoperatively. Future studies are required to assess heterotopic ACC's sensitivity to chemotherapy and long-term treatment outcomes.

In conclusion, we have presented an extremely rare case of pancreatic-type ACC arising in the jejunum with extensive tumor thrombus into the mesenteric venous system. Although it is difficult to diagnose heterotopic ACC because of its rarity, such lesions may develop in the gastrointestinal tracts as submucosal tumors, sometimes accompanied by tumor thrombus. Curative resection in these cases could be associated with increased survival.

Abbreviation
ACC: Acinar cell carcinoma

Acknowledgements
We would like to thank Editage (www.editage.jp) for English language editing.

Funding
The authors declare that they received no funding for this case report.

Authors' contributions
KT and TT wrote the draft. KT, TY, YU, RY, DN, and TK performed the surgery and perioperative care. TT contributed to the pathological diagnosis. TY and TF revised and finalized the draft. All authors read and approved the final manuscript.

Author's information
Not applicable.

Competing interests
The authors declare that they have no competing interests.

Author details
[1]Department of Gastroenterological Surgery, Okayama University Graduate School of Medicine, Dentistry and Pharmaceutical Sciences, 2-5-1 Shikata-cho, Kita-ku, Okayama 700-8558, Japan. [2]Department of Diagnostic Pathology, Okayama University Hospital, 2-5-1 Shikata-cho, Kita-ku, Okayama 700-8558, Japan.

References
1. Hamidian Jahromi A, Shokouh-Amiri H, Wellman G, Hobley J, Veluvolu A, Zibari GB. Acinar cell carcinoma presenting as a duodenal mass: review of the literature and a case report. J La State Med Soc. 2013;165:20–3. 25
2. Yonenaga Y, Kurosawa M, Mise M, Yamagishi M, Higashide S. Pancreatic-type Acinar cell carcinoma of the stomach included in multiple primary carcinomas. Anticancer Res. 2016;36:2855–64.
3. Yamaoka Y, Yamaguchi T, Kinugasa Y, Shiomi A, Kagawa H, Yamakawa Y, et al. Adenocarcinoma arising from jejunal ectopic pancreas mimicking peritoneal metastasis from colon cancer: a case report and literature review. Surg Case Rep. 2015;1:114.
4. Ordóñez NG. Pancreatic acinar cell carcinoma. Adv Anat Pathol. 2001;8:144–59.
5. Sun Y, Wasserman PG. Acinar cell carcinoma arising in the stomach: a case report with literature review. Hum Pathol. 2004;35:263–5.
6. Mizuno Y, Sumi Y, Nachi S, Ito Y, Marui T, Saji S, et al. Acinar cell carcinoma arising from an ectopic pancreas. Surg Today. 2007;37:704–7.
7. Ambrosini-Spaltro A, Potì O, De Palma M, Filotico M. Pancreatic-type acinar cell carcinoma of the stomach beneath a focus of pancreatic metaplasia of the gastric mucosa. Hum Pathol. 2009;40:746–9.
8. Coyne JD. Pure pancreatic-type acinar cell carcinoma of the stomach: a case report. Int J Surg Pathol. 2012;20:71–3.
9. Kim KM, Kim CY, Hong SM, Jang KY. A primary pure pancreatic-type acinar cell carcinoma of the stomach: a case report. Diagn Pathol. 2017;12:10.
10. Bookman MR. Carcinoma in the Duodenum: originating from aberrant pancreatic cells. Ann Surg. 1932;95:464–7.
11. Kawakami H, Kuwatani M, Onodera M, Hirano S, Kondo S, Nakanishi Y, et al. Primary acinar cell carcinoma of the ampulla of Vater. J Gastroenterol. 2007;42:694–7.
12. Hervieu V, Lombard-Bohas C, Dumortier J, Boillot O, Scoazec JY. Primary acinar cell carcinoma of the liver. Virchows Arch. 2008;452:337–41.
13. Chiaravalli AM, Finzi G, Bertolini V, La Rosa S, Capella C. Colonic carcinoma with a pancreatic acinar cell differentiation. A case report. Virchows Arch. 2009;455:527–31.
14. Makhlouf HR, Almeida JL, Sobin LH. Carcinoma in jejunal pancreatic heterotopia. Arch Pathol Lab Med. 1999;123:707–11.

15. Ueda T, Ku Y, Kanamaru T, Hasegawa Y, Kuroda Y, Saitoh Y. Resected acinar cell carcinoma of the pancreas with tumor thrombus extending into the main portal vein: report of a case. Surg Today. 1996;26:357–60.
16. Igarashi H, Shinozaki S, Mukada T. A case of acinar cell carcinoma of the pancreas that formed extensive tumor thrombus of the portal vein. Clin J Gastroenterol. 2009;2:96–102.
17. Saad RS, Essig DL, Silverman JF, Liu Y. Diagnostic utility of CDX-2 expression in separating metastatic gastrointestinal adenocarcinoma from other metastatic adenocarcinoma in fine-needle aspiration cytology using cell blocks. Cancer. 2004;102:168–73.
18. Guillou L, Nordback P, Gerber C, Schneider RP. Ductal adenocarcinoma arising in a heterotopic pancreas situated in a hiatal hernia. Arch Pathol Lab Med. 1994;118:568–71.
19. Klimstra DS, Heffess CS, Oertel JE, Rosai J. Acinar cell carcinoma of the pancreas. A clinicopathologic study of 28 cases. Am J Surg Pathol. 1992;16:815–37.
20. Bosman FT, Carneiro F, Hruban RH, Theise ND. WHO classification of tumours of the digestive system. In: Klimstra DS, Hruban RH, Kloppel G, Morohoshi T, Ohike N, editors. Acinar cell neoplasms of the pancreas. Lyon: IARC Press; 2010. p. 314–8.
21. Kitagami H, Kondo S, Hirano S, Kawakami H, Egawa S, Tanaka M. Acinar cell carcinoma of the pancreas: clinical analysis of 115 patients from pancreatic cancer registry of Japan pancreas society. Pancreas. 2007;35:42–6.
22. Wisnoski NC, Townsend CM Jr, Nealon WH, Freeman JL, Riall TS. 672 patients with acinar cell carcinoma of the pancreas: a population-based comparison to pancreatic adenocarcinoma. Surgery. 2008;144:141–8.
23. Schmidt CM, Matos JM, Bentrem DJ, Talamonti MS, Lillemoe KD, Bilimoria KY. Acinar cell carcinoma of the pancreas in the United States: prognostic factors and comparison to ductal adenocarcinoma. J Gastrointest Surg. 2008;12:2078–86.
24. Distler M, Rückert F, Dittert DD, Stroszczynski C, Dobrowolski F, Kersting S, et al. Curative resection of a primarily unresectable acinar cell carcinoma of the pancreas after chemotherapy. World J Surg Oncol. 2009;7:22.
25. Sudo K, Nakamura K, Yamaguchi T. S-1 in the treatment of pancreatic cancer. World J Gastroenterol. 2014;20:15110–8.

32

Initial experience with laparoscopic radical antegrade modular pancreatosplenectomy for left-sided pancreatic cancer in a single institution: technical aspects and oncological outcomes

Eun Young Kim and Tae Ho Hong[*]

Abstract

Background: Laparoscopic surgery has been performed less frequently in the era of pancreatic cancer due to technical difficulties and concerns about oncological safety. Radical antegrade modular pancreatosplenectomy (RAMPS) is expected to be helpful to obtain a negative margin during radical lymph node dissection. We hypothesized that it would also be favorable as a laparoscopic application due to unique features.

Methods: Fifteen laparoscopic RAMPS for well-selected patients with left-sided pancreatic cancer were performed from July 2011 to April 2016. Five trocars were usually used, and the operative procedures and range of dissection were similar to or the same as those of open RAMPS described by *Strasberg*. All medical records and follow-up data were reviewed and analyzed.

Results: All patients had pancreatic ductal adenocarcinoma. Mean operative time was 219.3 ± 53.8 min, and estimated blood loss was 250 ± 70 ml. The length of postoperative hospital stay was 6.1 ± 1.2 days, and postoperative morbidities developed in two patients (13.3%) with urinary retention. The median number of retrieved lymph nodes was 18.1 ± 6.2 and all had negative margins. Median follow-up time was 46.0 months, and the 3-year disease free survival and overall survival rates were 56.3% and 74.1%, respectively.

Conclusion: Our early experience with laparoscopic RAMPS achieved feasible perioperative results accompanied by acceptable survival outcomes. Laparoscopic RAMPS could be a safe and oncologically feasible procedure in well-selected patients with left-sided pancreatic cancer.

Keywords: Distal pancreatectomy, Laparoscopy, Left-sided pancreas cancer

Background

While the oncologic feasibility of laparoscopic surgery has been accepted for colon, stomach, and liver malignancies [1–5], only a few surgeons have performed laparoscopic surgery in the era of pancreatic cancer due to its fastidiousness for adequate dissection and the safety margin [6]. However, several studies have reported that a laparoscopic approach for pancreatic malignancies can result in favorable outcomes [1–5, 7, 8], and the need for discussion has emerged.

In 2003, Strasberg described an approach to resect left-sided pancreatic cancer called radical antegrade modular pancreatosplenectomy (RAMPS), which is a novel procedure that includes a horizontal dissection plane from right-to-left and radical resection of regional lymph nodes based on anatomic drainage of the pancreas. RAMPS has been performed more frequently with the expectation that it could be helpful to obtain negative tangential margins and a favorable survival rate [9–11]. RAMPS has some unique features that are favorable for

* Correspondence: gshth@catholic.ac.kr
Department of Hepato-biliary and Pancreas Surgery, Seoul St. Mary's Hospital, College of Medicine, The Catholic University of Korea, 222, Banpo-daero, Seocho-gu, Seoul 06591, Republic of Korea

application to laparoscopic surgery. The direction of dissection (from right-to-left) in RAMPS is familiar to operators with conventional laparoscopic distal pancreatectomy experience for benign or borderline malignant tumors, and this RAMPS feature helps the operator feel more comfortable during laparoscopic RAMPS.

The aim of this study was to describe the technical aspects of our laparoscopic RAMPS experience and present survival outcomes of laparoscopic RAMPS in selected patients with left-sided pancreatic cancer.

Methods

Fifteen laparoscopic RAMPS for well-selected patients with left-sided pancreatic cancer were performed from July 2011 to April 2016 at the Department of Surgery, Seoul St. Mary's Hospital. All patients were evaluated preoperatively using abdominal computed tomography (CT) scans and magnetic resonance cholangiopancreatography to accurately identify the location of the cancer. A positron emission tomography scan was used to detect the distant metastasis. Laparoscopic RAMPS was selectively applied to cases diagnosed as left-sided pancreatic cancer that was less than stage T3 without distant metastasis or peritoneal seeding on the preoperative imaging study. Cases in which we were unable to secure a safety margin from a major vessel, such as the superior mesenteric artery (SMA) or vein or celiac axis, were excluded from the laparoscopic approach. Cases exceeding the T4 stage or in which adjacent organs, such as the stomach, colon, or kidney, had been invaded, except the left adrenal gland, were also treated using an open method. The study was approved by the ethics committee of the Seoul St. Mary's Hospital (IRB No. KC15RISI0939). Patients provided written informed consent from each participant, and the procedures were in compliance with Helsinki Declaration.

Operative technique

The patient was placed with legs apart in the supine position and tilted to the right side in the reverse Trendelenburg position. The operator was positioned to the right side of the patient, and the first assistant and scrub nurse stood on the opposite side. The second assistant held the laparoscope and was positioned between the patient's legs. We created a pneumoperitoneum through the umbilicus using an open technique and a 10-mm trocar under the direct vision. Intra-abdominal pressure was maintained at about 12 mmHg with carbon dioxide. Five trocars were usually used (Fig. 1a); one 10-mm umbilicus trocar for the laparoscope, one 12-mm trocar on the left midclavicular line for the left hand of the operator, and three 5-mm trocars (one on the mid-epigastrium for the right hand of the first assistant, one at the subxiphoid for stomach traction, and the other at the left flank for the right hand of the operator). Operative procedures and range of dissection were similar to or the same as those of the open method described by Strasberg et al. [9]. We inspected the intraperitoneal cavity carefully after entry. The lesser sac was entered after dividing the gastro-colic and gastro-splenic ligaments close to the stomach to remove the gastrosplenic nodes. We generally hung the stomach using direct sutures to the abdominal wall to create a working space under the stomach (Fig. 1b). The lymph nodes along the common hepatic artery (CHA) and gastroduodenal artery were removed after sufficient mobilization of the pancreas through dissecting the tissue around the upper border of the pancreas (Fig. 2a). The right gastric artery was divided routinely for proper dissection of the lymph node along the CHA and gastroduodenal artery during open RAMPS, but we did not need to divide the right gastric artery routinely during the laparoscopic approach because the laparoscope could be passed in the space created beneath the stomach. The

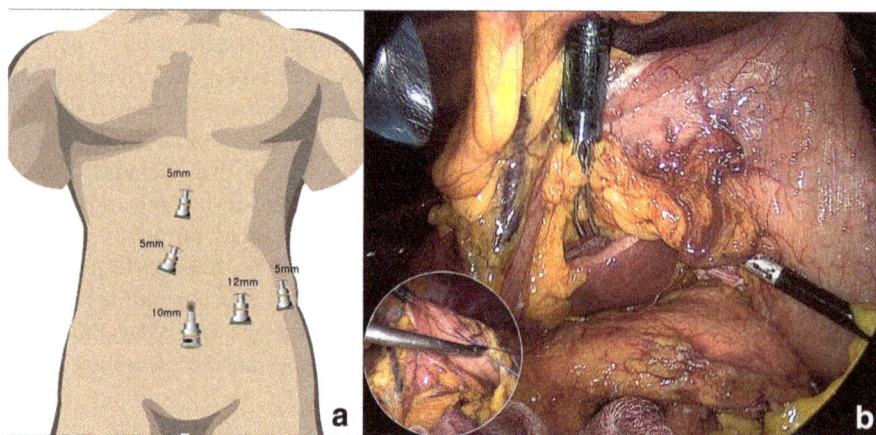

Fig. 1 Trocar positions (a) and intraoperative view of the working space for laparoscopic radical antegrade modular pancreatosplenectomy (RAMPS) (b)

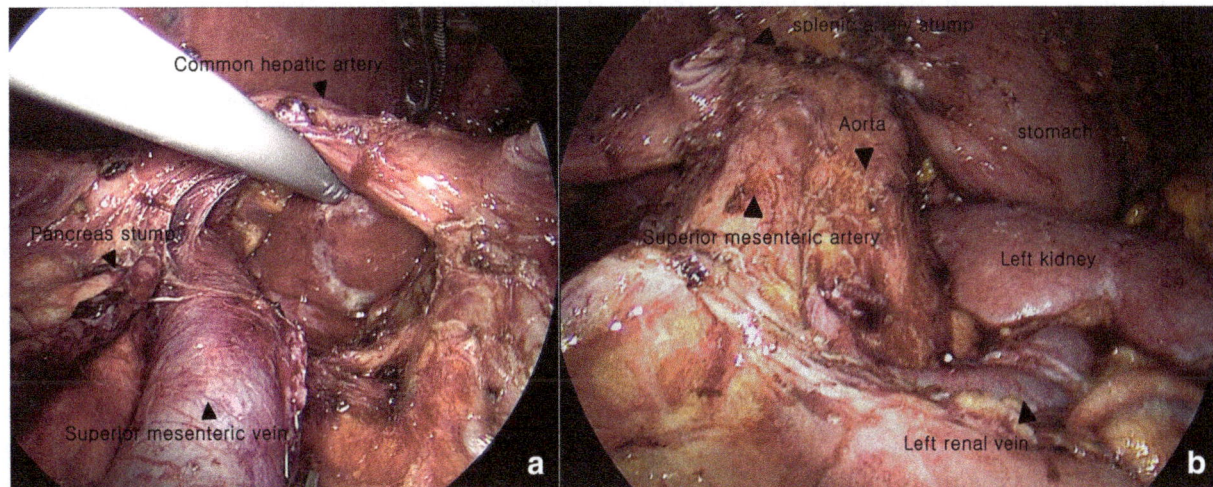

Fig. 2 Completion of lymph node dissection. Lymph nodes along the common hepatic artery (CHA) and gastroduodenal artery (GDA) were removed after sufficient mobilization of the pancreas by dissecting the tissue around the upper border of the pancreas (**a**). The lymph nodes dissected around the celiac axis, the superior mesenteric artery, the left adrenal gland, and Gerota's fascia were completely resected in a case of posterior radical antegrade modular pancreatosplenectomy (RAMPS) (**b**)

pancreatic neck was elevated off the superior mesenteric vein (SMV) and portal vein (PV) and a window was created between the posterior surface of the pancreas and the confluence of the SMV, PV and splenic vein. The pancreatic neck was transected with straight endoscopic linear staples (Echelon Endopath™ Stapler, Ethicon Endo-Surgery, Inc., Cincinnati, OH, USA) after sufficient peri-firing compression. Staple size depended on the hardness or thickness of the pancreas. Lymph nodes around the celiac axis were dissected to expose the origin of the splenic artery (Fig. 2b). The splenic artery was ligated and divided using a laparoscopic ligation system (Hem-o-lok® Ligation System, Teleflex Medical, Boston, MA, USA) and the splenic vein was also resected using the endo-GIA (white cartilage). The lymph nodes were dissected medial-to-lateral and the resection range was up to the diaphragmatic crus, down to the left renal vein, and to the left lateral portion of the aorta on the posterior side. The dissection continued more laterally to the left of Gerota's fascia, and the inferior mesenteric vein was divided after detaching the distal pancreas with the underlying fascial layer from the retroperitoneum. The operator used either the anterior or posterior RAMPS procedure to maximize the chance of achieving a negative tangential margin. The decision was based on the principles emphasized by Strasberg et al. [9]; therefore, the left adrenal gland and Gerota's fascia were completely resected concomitantly during posterior RAMPS (Fig. 2b). After completely resecting the distal pancreas with *en bloc* lymph node dissection, the specimen was bagged and retrieved through the umbilical port site with minimal extension. Two closed suction drains were used; one for the pancreatic

stump through the 5-mm port mid-epigastric incision and the other for the splenectomy site through the left flank port site.

Postoperative management and outcome assessment

The medical records and follow-up data of all patients were reviewed retrospectively for patient demographics, operative results (operative time, estimated blood loss, and type of RAMPS), tumor characteristics (tumor differentiation, tumor size, number of retrieved lymph nodes, TNM stage, and margin status), postoperative outcomes (pain score, length of postoperative hospital stay, start of soft diet, postoperative complications, and mortality), and follow-up data. Tumor size and differentiation and the number of retrieved lymph nodes were recorded from the pathology report. Margin status included negative (R0) and positive margin resection (R1 or R2), and these margins included the superior and inferior borders and the posterior surface of the specimen. The transected surface at the neck of pancreas and all tangential margins of the specimen that were not covered with peritoneum were marked with ink on the back table after retrieving the specimen to assess margin status. TNM cancer stage was evaluated based on the AJCC Caner Staging Manual, 7th edition. We checked postoperative pain using a visual analog scale (VAS) from 0 (no pain) to 10 (worst pain imaginable) on postoperative days 1, 3, 5, and 7, and length of stay was estimated from the day of the operation to the day of discharge. Postoperative complications were reviewed and analyzed according to the Clavien–Dindo classification [12]. A postoperative pancreatic fistula was graded as A, B, or C based on the International Study Group of Pancreatic Fistula definition [13]. We also assessed the incidence of digestive complications, such as prolonged diarrhea defined as loose stools for at least 4 weeks after surgery. Wound infection was established as any complication of a trocar site with tenderness or erythema requiring opening, drainage, or antibiotics although a seroma or hematoma was not considered a wound infection. Postoperative mortality was defined as mortality within 30 days of surgery or within the same hospital stay as the surgery. Patients with acceptable postoperative physical status were treated with adjuvant chemotherapy by the oncologist under our institutional policy.

Results

Patient demographics and perioperative outcomes

The demographics and perioperative outcomes of laparoscopic RAMPS are summarized in Table 1. Six men (40%) and nine women (60%) were included, with mean age of 68.1 ± 9.2 years (range, 50–79) and mean body mass index of 21.9 ± 3.8 kg/m^2 (range, 16.4–28.1 kg/m^2). Mean operative time was 219.3 ± 53.8 min (range, 119–305 min) and mean estimated blood loss was 250 ± 70 mL (range, 150–400 mL). Three patients (20%) received intraoperative transfusions, no case was converted to open surgery, and no postoperative mortality occurred. Posterior RAMPS was performed in eight cases (53.3%) because preoperative CT scans showed that the tumor had penetrated the posterior capsule of the pancreas. The VAS pain score decreased gradually over time from 4.1 ± 1.8 on postoperative day 1 to 2.5 ± 1.1, 1.5 ± 1.1, and 0.7 ± 0.6 on postoperative days 3, 5, and 7, respectively. It took a mean of 2.6 ± 0.6 postoperative days (range, 2–4 days) for patients to return to an oral diet, and the mean number of postoperative hospital days was 6.1 ± 1.2 (range, 5–9 days). Postoperative urinary retention complications developed in two patients (13.3%) who were treated conservatively. No case of digestive complications, such as prolonged diarrhea or ileus, or pulmonary complications, such as atelectasis or pleural effusion, occurred that required additional management.

Oncological outcomes

All 15 patients were diagnosed with ductal adenocarcinoma on the pathology report. Mean tumor size was 3.8 ± 1.8 cm (range, 1.8–4.5 cm), and mean length of the resected pancreas was 10.1 ± 1.8 cm (range, 6.7–13.2 cm). Tumor differentiation stages were three well differentiated (20%), eleven moderately differentiated (73.3%), and one poorly differentiated (6.7%). The median number of lymph nodes retrieved was 18.1 ± 6.2 (range, 10–30), and six patients (40%) had malignant-positive lymph nodes.

Thirteen patients (86.7%) had T3 tumors that had invaded the peripancreatic tissue from outside the pancreatic capsule. All of these cases achieved a negative tangential margin and R0 resection on the permanent pathological report.

Survival and follow-up outcomes

Mean and median follow-up times were 46.6 and 46.0 months, respectively. Four patients (26.7%) developed disease recurrence; two patients (13.3%) had a local recurrence in the pancreatic bed, one patient (6.7%) had a recurrence around the celiac axis and the other patient (6.7%) had a recurrence around the SMA. One patient with a pancreatic bed recurrence presented with carcinomatosis peritonei 25 months after surgery. The 1-year disease free survival rate (DFS) was 100%, and the 3-year DFS was 56.3%. Median survival was 40.0 months, and 1-year and 3-year overall survival (OS) rates were 100% and 74.1%, respectively (Table 2). Five patients (33.3%) died 16–41 months after surgery. The Kaplan–Meier survival curve of laparoscopic RAMPS is presented in Fig. 3.

Discussion

Laparoscopic surgery has been widely accepted due to its minimally invasive approach and advantages, such as less bleeding, smaller transfusion requirement, and shorter incisions with less pain. Consequently, laparoscopic surgery has been expanded to various fields of surgery and these advantages also applied to laparoscopic RAMPS. Conventional open RAMPS usually requires a long midline abdominal incision or left subcostal incision that could cause severe pain and easily develop infection. Prolonged wound pain can be associated with difficulties coughing or expectoration and disturb ambulation and can cause postoperative morbidities, such as atelectasis and ileus, which prevent early recovery of normal activities. In our study, postoperative pain improved rapidly over time, and no postoperative morbidities, such as wound infection, atelectasis, or ileus, were observed. We also showed favorable outcomes in terms of starting an oral diet and length of hospital stay [1, 7, 14–17]. We expect that the early return to an oral diet improved nutritional status, which would shorten recovery and advance the commencement of adjuvant treatment.

Although the safety and oncological feasibility of laparoscopic surgery for pancreatic cancer remains controversial, several studies have reported favorable outcomes of laparoscopic approaches to the pancreatic cancer as experience has accumulated [3, 18, 19]. We have applied laparoscopic RAMPS to selected cases of left-sided pancreatic cancer since 2011 and our early experience showed acceptable oncological outcomes with adequate

Table 1 Results of all patients who underwent laparoscopic radial antegrade modular pancreaticosplenectomy for left-sided pancreatic cancer

Characteristics	Total (n = 15)
(a) Patient demographics and perioperative outcomes	
Age (range, yr)	68.1 ± 9.2 (50–79)
Sex (M/F)	7/8
BMI (range, kg/m²)	21.9 ± 3.8 (16.4–28.1)
ASA class (%)	
Class I	5 (33.3)
Class II	7 (46.7)
Class III	3 (20)
Operative procedure (%)	
Anterior RAMPS	7 (46.7)
Posterior RAMPS	8 (53.3)
Conversion to laparotomy (%)	0
Operative time (range, min)	219.3 ± 53.8 (119–305)
Estimated blood loss (range, ml)	250 ± 70 (150–400)
Intraoperative transfusion (%)	3 (20)
Postoperative pain[a]	
POD 1	4.1 ± 1.8
POD 3	2.5 ± 1.1
POD 5	1.5 ± 1.1
POD 7	0.7 ± 0.6
Postoperative hospital stay (range, day)	6.1 ± 1.2 (5–9)
Return to oral diet (range, day)	2.6 ± 0.6 (2–4)
Overall complications (%)	2 (13.3)
urinary retention	2 (13.3)
Hospital mortality (%)	0
(b) Oncologic outcomes	
Tumor differentiation (%)	
well differentiated	3 (20)
moderately differentiated	11 (73.3)
poorly differentiated	1 (6.7)
T stage (%)	
T2	2 (13.3)
T3	13 (86.7)
N stage (%)	
N0	9 (60)
N1	6 (40)
TNM staging (%)	
stage IB	1 (6.7)
stage IIA	8 (53.3)
stage IIB	6 (40)
Tumor size (range, cm)	3.8 ± 1.8 (1.8–4.5)
Count of retrieving lymph node (range)	18.1 ± 6.2 (10–30)

Table 1 Results of all patients who underwent laparoscopic radial antegrade modular pancreaticosplenectomy for left-sided pancreatic cancer (Continued)

R0 resection (%)	15 (100)
Negative tangential margin (%)	15 (100)
Recurrence (%)	4 (26.7)
Metastasis (%)	3 (20)

[a] estimated by visual analog scale (VAS) score

lymph node harvest and negative margin status. Our results are mainly attributed to the properties of RAMPS and feasibility for a laparoscopic approach. First, RAMPS does not require complex reconstruction of an anastomosis unlike pancreaticoduodenectomy, so the entire procedure is relatively simple, which is favorable for a laparoscopic approach. Second, the dissection proceeds from right to left, which is familiar to operators with conventional laparoscopic distal pancreatectomy experience for benign or borderline malignancies. An operator accustomed to laparoscopic distal pancreatectomy can easily adapt to a RAMPS laparoscopic approach. The familiar manipulations during the surgery are helpful for reducing burden on the operator, which and produces fewer tissue injuries. Third, RAMPS uses a more objective dissection plane, and some difficulties determining the overall anatomic structure at a glance can occur during laparoscopic surgery because the magnified view is provided for a limited area, unlike open surgery. This disadvantage could be complemented during RAMPS because the objective dissection plane allows for an easier operative process without the need to capture the whole anatomy. We believe these RAMPS characteristics contributed to the safe and feasible outcomes in laparoscopic approach.

The right-to-left dissection with a magnified view during laparoscopic RAMPS provides a posterior dissection plane that can assist acquiring a sufficient margin. Actually, our results revealed successful tumor margin status and survival outcomes over the long-term. We obtained a negative tangential margin and R0 resection in all cases. We also achieved favorable 1- and 3-year DFS (100% and 56.3%, respectively) and 1- and 3-year OS rates (100% and 74.1%, respectively). Additionally, trocar site metastasis and wound recurrence which are

Table 2 Survival outcomes of laparoscopic radical antegrade modular pancreatosplenectomy (RAMPS) in well-selected cases of left pancreatic cancer (n = 15)

	n	Disease free survival (%)			Overall survival (%)		
		1-year	2-year	3-year	1-year	2-year	3-year
Lap. RAMPS	15	100	75.0	56.3	100	88.9	74.1

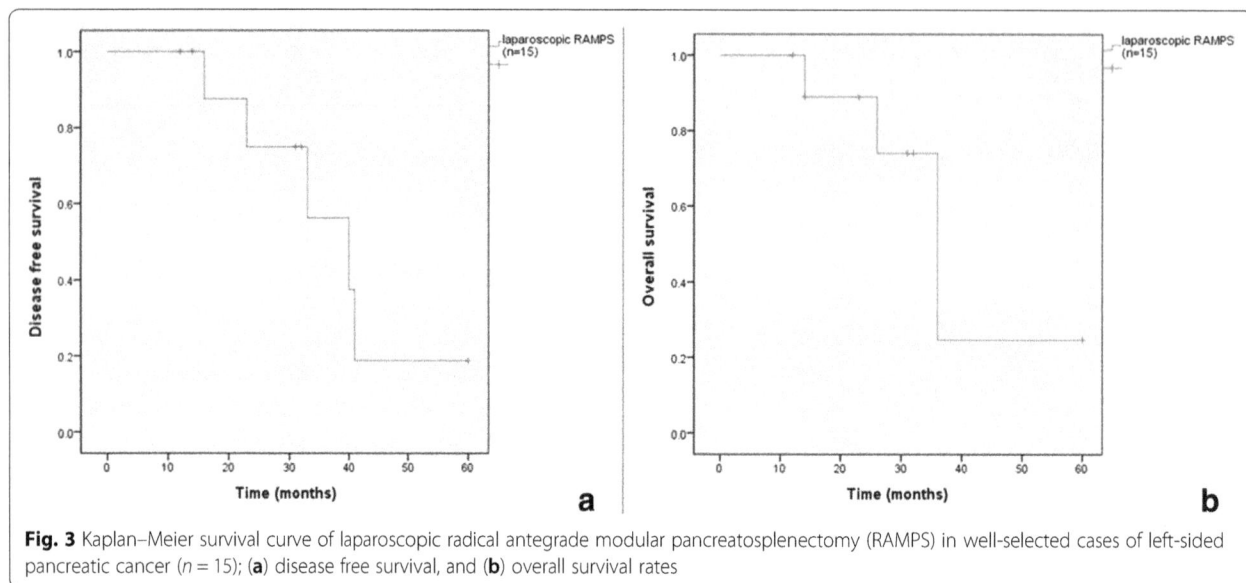

Fig. 3 Kaplan–Meier survival curve of laparoscopic radical antegrade modular pancreatosplenectomy (RAMPS) in well-selected cases of left-sided pancreatic cancer (*n* = 15); (**a**) disease free survival, and (**b**) overall survival rates

concerns for malignancy during laparoscopic surgery, were not observed in our study. The oncological outcomes of our study and those of previous reports using RAMPS are summarized in Table 3 [10, 19–24].

The mean number of retrieved lymph nodes in this study was 18.1 ± 6.2, which is comparable with previous RAMPS reports (Table 3). The magnified angular laparoscopic view facilitated the delicate manipulation around lymph nodes (Fig. 2). Moreover, we suspended the posterior wall of the stomach using direct sutures to the abdominal wall, and we also used a 30°-sloped laparoscope. These allowed sufficient working space beneath the stomach. As a result, we were able to approach the lymph nodes around the gastroduodenal artery and common hepatic artery more easily without routinely resecting the right gastric artery, unlike during open RAMPS.

Our surgical outcomes should be interpreted with caution because of limitations. We are only presenting our early experience of laparoscopic RAMPS and did not compare the results with those of conventional open RAMPS. However, the surgical outcomes for left-sided pancreatic cancer are shown in oncologic safety and survival outcomes results, accompanied by reduced pain and a shorter hospital stay. A comparative study composed of more samples and with conventional open RAMPS should be performed to confirm the feasibility of laparoscopic RAMPS for left-sided pancreatic cancer.

Conclusions

We achieved feasible survival outcomes accompanied by successful negative resection margins and radical lymph node dissection during laparoscopic RAMPS. Our data

Table 3 Previously reported laparoscopic radical antegrade modular pancreatosplenectomy (RAMPS) or open RAMPS trials or series

Publication	No. of patients	Year of publication	Mean tumor size (cm)	Operative time (min)	EBL (ml)	Length of hospital stay (day)	Count of retrieved lymph nodes	Margin status, RO (tangential) (%)	Median survival (month)
Open RAMPS									
Strasberg et al. [10]	23	2007	5.1	378	630	11	15	87 (91)	21
Mitchem et al. [19]	47	2011	4.4	244	744	11.3	18	81 (89)	26
Chang et al. [20]	24	2012	4.1	305	_a	_a	21	92 (92)	18.2
Park et al. [21]	38	2014	3.1	210	325	11.5	14	89.4 (-)a	24.6
Kitagawa et al. [22]	24	2014	3.5	387	371	11.5	28	88 (92)	_b
Laparoscopic RAMPS									
Choi et al. [23]	4	2012	_a	390	475	7	9	100 (100)	24
Lee et al. [24]	12	2014	2.8	324	446	12	11	100 (100)	60
Kim et al. c	10	2015	4.1	290	284	9	20	100 (100)	40

a Data not described in this report
b Five-year overall survival rate was 53%
c Current study

show reduced postoperative pain, which hastened recovery. We suggest that laparoscopic RAMPS is a safe and oncologically feasible procedure in well-selected cases of left-sided pancreatic cancer. However, a further prospective comparative trial with open RAMPS should be conducted.

Abbreviations
CHA: Common hepatic artery; CT: Computed tomography; DFS: Disease free survival; OS: Overall survival; PV: Portal vein; RAMPS: Radical antegrade modular pancreatosplenectomy; SMA: Superior mesenteric artery; SMV: Superior mesenteric vein.

Acknowledgements
No additional investigators were involved in this research project.

Funding
This investigation and manuscript preparation received no external funding.

Authors' contributions
EYK collected the data and wrote the paper and THH designed the research and revised the paper. Both authors read and approved the final manuscript.

Competing interests
The authors declare that they have no competing interests.

References
1. Sui CJ, Li B, Yang JM, Wang SJ, Zhou YM. Laparoscopic versus open distal pancreatectomy: a meta-analysis. Asian J Surg. 2012;35(1):1–8.
2. Song KB, Kim SC, Park JB, Kim YH, Jung YS, Kim MH, et al. Single-center experience of laparoscopic left pancreatic resection in 359 consecutive patients: changing the surgical paradigm of left pancreatic resection. Surg Endosc. 2011;25(10):3364–72.
3. Kang CM, Kim DH, Lee WJ. Ten years of experience with resection of left-sided pancreatic ductal adenocarcinoma: evolution and initial experience to a laparoscopic approach. Surg Endosc. 2010;24(7):1533–41.
4. Kooby DA, Chu CK. Laparoscopic management of pancreatic malignancies. Surg Clin North Am. 2010;90(2):427–46.
5. Kooby DA, Hawkins WG, Schmidt CM, Weber SM, Bentrem DJ, Gillespie TW, et al. A multicenter analysis of distal pancreatectomy for adenocarcinoma: is laparoscopic resection appropriate? J Am Coll Surg. 2010;210(5):779–85. 86-7.
6. Christein JD, Kendrick ML, Iqbal CW, Nagorney DM, Farnell MB. Distal pancreatectomy for resectable adenocarcinoma of the body and tail of the pancreas. J Gastrointest Surg. 2005;9(7):922–7.
7. Abu Hilal M, Takhar AS. Laparoscopic left pancreatectomy: current concepts. Pancreatology. 2013;13(4):443–8.
8. Choi SH, Kang CM, Lee WJ, Chi HS. Multimedia article. Laparoscopic modified anterior RAMPS in well-selected left-sided pancreatic cancer: technical feasibility and interim results. Surg Endosc. 2011;25(7):2360–1.
9. Strasberg SM, Fields R. Left-sided pancreatic cancer: distal pancreatectomy and its variants: radical antegrade modular pancreatosplenectomy and distal pancreatectomy with celiac axis resection. Cancer J. 2012;18(6):562–70.
10. Strasberg SM, Linehan DC, Hawkins WG. Radical antegrade modular pancreatosplenectomy procedure for adenocarcinoma of the body and tail of the pancreas: ability to obtain negative tangential margins. J Am Coll Surg. 2007;204(2):244–9.
11. Strasberg SM, Drebin JA, Linehan D. Radical antegrade modular pancreatosplenectomy. Surgery. 2003;133(5):521–7.
12. Dindo D, Demartines N, Clavien PA. Classification of surgical complications: a new proposal with evaluation in a cohort of 6336 patients and results of a survey. Ann Surg. 2004;240(2):205–13.
13. Bassi C, Dervenis C, Butturini G, Fingerhut A, Yeo C, Izbicki J, et al. Postoperative pancreatic fistula: an international study group (ISGPF) definition. Surgery. 2005;138(1):8–13.
14. Abraham NS, Young JM, Solomon MJ. Meta-analysis of short-term outcomes after laparoscopic resection for colorectal cancer. Br J Surg. 2004;91(9):1111–24.
15. Viñuela EF, Gonen M, Brennan MF, Coit DG, Strong VE. Laparoscopic versus open distal gastrectomy for gastric cancer: a meta-analysis of randomized controlled trials and high-quality nonrandomized studies. Ann Surg. 2012;255(3):446–56.
16. Briggs CD, Mann CD, Irving GR, Neal CP, Peterson M, Cameron IC, et al. Systematic review of minimally invasive pancreatic resection. J Gastrointest Surg. 2009;13(6):1129–37.
17. Kooby DA, Gillespie T, Bentrem D, Nakeeb A, Schmidt MC, Merchant NB, et al. Left-sided pancreatectomy: a multicenter comparison of laparoscopic and open approaches. Ann Surg. 2008;248(3):438–46.
18. Fernandez-Cruz L, Cosa R, Blanco L, Levi S, López-Boado MA, Navarro S. Curative laparoscopic resection for pancreatic neoplasms: a critical analysis from a single institution. J Gastrointest Surg. 2007;11(12):1607–21. discussion 21-22.
19. Mitchem JB, Hamilton N, Gao F, Hawkins WG, Linehan DC, Strasberg SM. Long-term results of resection of adenocarcinoma of the body and tail of the pancreas using radical antegrade modular pancreatosplenectomy procedure. J Am Coll Surg. 2012;214(1):46–52.
20. Chang YR, Han SS, Park SJ, Lee SD, Yoo TS, Kim YK, et al. Surgical outcome of pancreatic cancer using radical antegrade modular pancreatosplenectomy procedure. World J Gastroenterol. 2012;18(39):5595–600.
21. Park HJ, You DD, Choi DW, Heo JS, Choi SH. Role of radical antegrade modular pancreatosplenectomy for adenocarcinoma of the body and tail of the pancreas. World J Surg. 2014;38(1):186–93.
22. Kitagawa H, Tajima H, Nakagawara H, Makino I, Miyashita T, Terakawa H, et al. A modification of radical antegrade modular pancreatosplenectomy for adenocarcinoma of the left pancreas: significance of en bloc resection including the anterior renal fascia. World J Surg. 2014;38(9):2448–54.
23. Choi SH, Kang CM, Hwang HK, Lee WJ, Chi HS. Robotic anterior RAMPS in well-selected left-sided pancreatic cancer. J Gastrointest Surg. 2012;16(4):868–9.
24. Lee SH, Kang CM, Hwang HK, Choi SH, Lee WJ, Chi HS. Minimally invasive RAMPS in well-selected left-sided pancreatic cancer within Yonsei criteria: long-term (>median 3 years) oncologic outcomes. Surg Endosc. 2014;28(10):2848–55.

33

A case of complete splenic infarction after laparoscopic spleen-preserving distal pancreatectomy

Kenjiro Kimura*, Go Ohira, Ryosuke Amano, Sadaaki Yamazoe, Ryota Tanaka, Jun Tauchi and Masaichi Ohira

Abstract

Background: Laparoscopic spleen-preserving distal pancreatectomy (LSPDP), a newly developed operative procedure, is indicated for benign and low-grade malignant disease of the pancreas. However, few studies have reported on postoperative splenic infarction after LSPDP.

Case presentation: We report a case of complete splenic infarction and obliteration of the splenic artery and vein after LSPDP. The patient was a 69-year-old woman with a 35-mm cystic tumor of the pancreatic body who underwent LSPDP. Although the operation was completed with preservation of the splenic artery and vein, postoperative splenic infarction was revealed with left back pain and fluid collection around the stump of the pancreas on postoperative day 9. Fortunately, clinical symptoms disappeared within days and additional splenectomy was not needed. Splenic infarction was attributed to scattered micro-embolizations within the spleen after drawing strongly on the tape encircling the splenic vessels.

Conclusion: Preserving splenic vessels in LSPDP is a demanding procedure. To prevent splenic infarction in LSPDP, we should carefully isolate the pancreatic parenchyma from the splenic vessels, and must avoid drawing tightly on the vessel loop encircling splenic vessels.

Keywords: Laparoscopic spleen-preserving distal pancreatectomy, Splenic infarction, Kimura's method

Background

Laparoscopic spleen-preserving distal pancreatectomy (LSPDP), a newly developed operative procedure, is indicated for benign and low-grade malignant disease of the pancreas. Preservation of the spleen is preferred over routine combined splenectomy not only to avoid the risk of postoperative infectious complications after splenectomy, but also to provide longer survival with malignancy [1, 2].

LSPDP can be carried out with either preservation of the splenic vessels, as Kimura's method [3], or with division of these vessels, as Warshaw's method [4]. Kimura et al. provided the first report of splenic vessel-conserving spleen-preserving distal pancreatectomy for benign tumor [3]. Very few studies have evaluated outcomes for conserved splenic vessels and spleen [5–7]. Hwang et al. recently reported that 17.2% of SPDP patients showed

obliteration of the splenic vein and 13.8% eventually developed collateral venous circulation around the gastric fundus and spleen [8]. Partial splenic infarction was reported in their previous reports. However, no cases of complete spleen infarction have been described.

In our institute, LSPDP using Kimura's method was performed for 10 cases of benign pancreatic tumor. We encountered one case of complete splenic infarction and obliteration of both the splenic artery and vein. This report offers the first description of complete splenic infarction after LSPDP using Kimura's method.

Case presentation

A pancreatic cystic lesion was incidentally detected in a 69-year-old woman during a clinical survey. She had no symptoms and her past history was unremarkable. Computed tomography (CT) and magnetic resonance imaging (MRI) revealed a cystic lesion with solid component in the pancreatic body (Fig. 1). Cyst diameter was 35 mm. Endoscopic ultrasonography showed this cystic

---

* Correspondence: kenjiro@med.osaka-cu.ac.jp
Department of Surgical Oncology, Osaka City University School of Medicine, 1-4-3 Asahi-machi, Abeno-ku, Osaka 545-8585, Japan

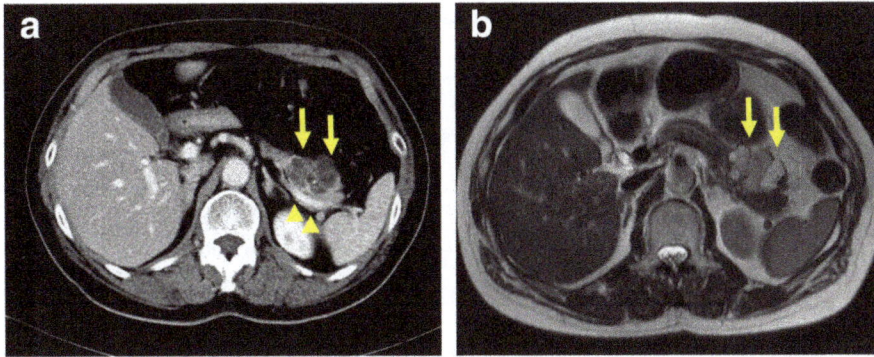

Fig. 1 Findings from preoperative CT and MRI. CT and MRI show a cystic neoplasm (*arrow*) in the pancreatic body. Cyst diameter is 35 mm. **a** CT. **b** T2-weighted MRI. Splenic vein was normal status (*arrowhead*)

lesion as a polycystic lesion with a 5-mm mural nodule. Serous cystadenoma was considered the most likely preoperative diagnosis, with a small possibility of MCN or serous cystadenocarcinoma. Because the size was beyond 3-cm and it included solid component, we decided it to be operative indication. However the risk of malignant disease was considered low, we planned to perform LSPDP using Kimura's method.

Surgery was performed supine, 30° reverse Trendelenburg position with left-side-up adjustment. After creation of carbon dioxide pneumoperitoneum via a 12-mm umbilical port, 4 additional trocars were inserted.

After trocar placement, the greater omentum was divided using ultrasonic shears (Harmonic scalpel®; Ethicon, Cincinnati, OH) from the middle to the spleen. With the stomach elevated, the pancreatic tumor was visible from the pancreatic body to the tail. The retroperitoneum was opened along the inferior pancreatic border and further dissection was performed on the avascular plane posterior to the pancreas until the splenic vein and artery were identified. The splenic vein and artery were encircled and taped at the right side of the cystic tumor of the pancreas. When the pancreatic parenchyma was isolated from the splenic vessels, small branches from the splenic vessels were divided using

ultrasonic shears and polymer ligation clips (Hem-o-lok®, Teleflex, Research Triangle Park, NC). VIO soft-coagulation system (VIO 300D; ERBE Elektromedizin, Tübingen, Germany) was used for hemostasis against oozing. Pancreatic transection was achieved using the Endo GIA™ Reinforced Reload with Tri-Staple™ Technology (Medtronic, Minneapolis, MN) with sufficient surgical margins. As the cystic tumor was tightly adherent to splenic vessels, the encircled tape was pulled to separate the tumor from the splenic vessels.

The splenic artery and vein were preserved without dissection of the short gastric artery and vein, including left gastroepiploic vessels. The spleen was successfully conserved. The surgical specimen was retrieved in a vinyl bag and extracted through a small incision created by extending the umbilical port site. Operation time was 304 min and total blood loss was 80 g. Although the operation time was relatively long, no particular difficulties were encountered during the operation (Fig. 2).

For several days after the operation, the patient showed a slight fever, but abdominal pain appeared to be within the acceptable range. Concentration of amylase in the drain discharge fluid was 2225 IU/L on postoperative day 1 and 170 IU/L on postoperative day 3. The drainage tube was removed on postoperative day 5.

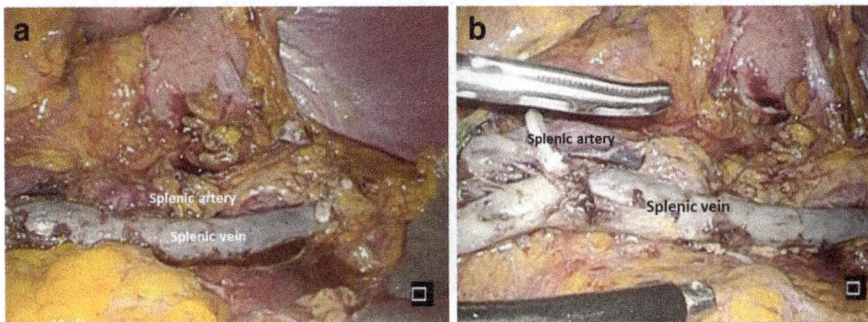

Fig. 2 Postoperative imaging. Imaging after removal of the specimen. The splenic artery and vein are preserved along with the spleen, and they are indicated by panel labels in the Fig. 2a and b

On postoperative day 9, the patient reported left back pain and abdominal CT revealed fluid collection around the stump of the pancreas (Fig. 3a). Because postoperative pancreatic fistula was considered the most likely cause, antibiotics and octreotide were administered and eating was stopped. Clinical symptoms disappeared within a few days after this specific treatment. Contrast-enhanced CT on postoperative day 15 demonstrated obliteration of the splenic artery and vein and complete splenic infarction (Fig. 3b and c). Clinical course subsequently progressed satisfactorily. Eating was restarted on postoperative day 15, and the patient was discharged from hospital on postoperative day 25. White blood cell count was 10,100, 16,500, and 8600 /mm^3, respectively on postoperative day 1, 3, and 6. After postoperative day 6, white blood cell count was within normal range. Infectious symptom was not obvious in the clinical course. Because we recognize the incidence of the splenic infarction at postoperative 15 days, we considered to be late to do add pharmacotherapy. So we did not added any treatment for splenic infarction. Contrast-enhanced CT at 3 months postoperatively showed organization of the infarcted spleen (Fig. 3d). As of 1 year postoperatively, the patient has shown no particular complications.

Discussion and conclusions

LSPDP is increasingly being applied for benign and low-malignant pancreatic tumors, thanks to significant progress in laparoscopic procedures. Although the patency of conserved splenic vessels and the rate of splenic infarction are important issues for LSPDP, few studies have reported on this problem.

Kimura et al. provided the first report of splenic vessel-conversing spleen-preserving distal pancreatectomy for a benign tumor [3]. To preserve the splenic artery and vein, careful ligation of the pancreatic tributaries was demanded, and the procedure is technically difficult and time-consuming. On the other hand, Warshaw's method for the LSPDP procedure involves removal of the splenic artery and vein with the left pancreas, but meticulous preservation of the collateral blood supply from the short gastric and left gastroepiploic vessels.

Xinzhe et al. reported a meta-analysis of Warshaw's methods found a significantly shorter operation time, but no difference between Warshaw's method and Kimura's method in the overall rate of complications, including the rate of pancreatic fistula. However, the frequencies of gastric varices and splenic infarction were significantly higher with Warshaw's method [9]. Although no definitive consensus has been reached on which is the superior procedure, we prefer Kimura's method due to the lower risk of splenic complications. Several reports have described splenic infarction after spleen-preserving distal pancreatectomy. Beane et al. reported 1 case of splenic infarction among a total of 45

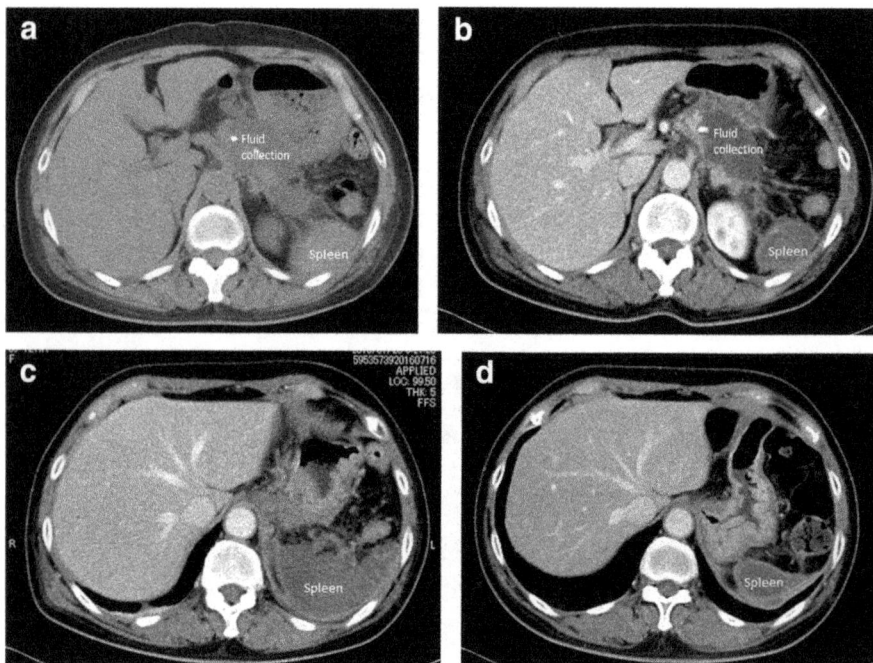

Fig. 3 CT findings after surgery. **a** Fluid collection is evident around stump of the pancreas on postoperative day9. **b**, **c** Contrast-enhanced CT on postoperative day 15 revealed that the splenic artery and vein have been obliterated and complete splenic infarction is apparent. **d** Contrast-enhanced CT on 3 months post-operatively showed that the spleen has become atrophic and organized

Table 1 Recent studies about incident of splenic infarction after laparoscopic distal pancreatectomy

Author	Year	Country	Reference No.	Study type	Technique	No. of patients	Splenic infarction (%)
Zhou ZQ	2014	China	6	R	Kimura	206	33 (16.0%)
					Warshaw	40	21 (52.5%)
Beane JD	2011	USA	10	R	Kimura	45	1 (2.2%)
					Warshaw	41	16 (39%)
Worhunsky	2014	USA	7	R	Kimura	13	2 (15.4%)
					Warshaw	15	7 (46.7%)
Butturini	2012	Italy	11	R	Kimura	36	1 (2.8%)
					Warshaw	7	1 (14.3%)
Hwang HK	2012	Korea	8	R	Kimura	29	0 (0%)
Yoon YS	2009	Korea	5	R	Kimura	22	4 (18.2%)
Lee LS	2016	Simgapore	13	R	Kimura	63	2 (3.2%)
					Warshaw	26	9 (34.6%)

R Retrospective, *Kimura* LSPDP with conserving splenic vessels, *Warshaw* LSPDP with division of splenic vessels

cases, for a rate of 4.5% [10]. Worhunsky et al. reported 2 cases among a total of 13 cases (15.4%) [7], and Zhou et al. reported 33 cases among a total of 206 cases (16%) [6]. However, all of those involved partial infarction. We found a report stating that postoperative splenectomy was needed for splenic infarction after LSPDP using Kimura's method [11]. That group reported three cases of re-operation and 1 case of postoperative splenectomy among 36 cases of LSPDP using Kimura's procedure. We summarized recent studies about incident of splenic infarction after LSPDP in Table 1 [5–8, 10–12].

In the current case, we preserved the splenic artery and vein and the collateral blood supply from the short gastric and left gastroepiploic vessels. Even if obliteration of the splenic vessels had occurred, the splenic blood supply was expected to be maintained via the short gastric and left gastroepiploic vessels. However, splenic infarction still occurred. In our series of 10 LSPDPs, although another two cases showed obliteration of the splenic vessels, splenic infarction was not seen in either of those two cases. Two possible mechanisms were considered for the splenic infarction in the current case. The first was scattered micro-embolization to the spleen resulting from intraoperative procedures. Because the tumor was widely attached to the splenic vessels, we needed to draw on the tape encircling the splenic vessels to separate the tumor from the splenic vessels. Drawing on the tape strongly and for an extended period may have resulted in micro-emboli within the splenic artery flowing into the spleen, subsequently causing complete splenic infarction. The second mechanism might have involved the postoperative pancreatic fistula. Locally intense inflammation around the spleen might have contributed to splenic infarction, leading to obliteration of not only the splenic artery, but also the short gastric and left epigastric artery [13]. Overall, the first mechanism was considered more likely.

Conservation of splenic vessels in LSPDP is a demanding procedure. To prevent splenic infarction in LSPDP using Kimura's method, the possibility of splenic infarction should be kept in mind and drawing tightly on the vessel loop encircling the splenic vessels should be avoided. If splenic infarction might have occurred intraoperatively, splenic arterial flow should be checked by intraoperative ultrasonography and splenectomy added if needed. Fortunately, the current splenic infarction did not require additive splenectomy after LSPDP.

To the best of our knowledge, this represents the first report of complete splenic infarction after LSPDP using Kimura's method. Preventing splenic infarction in LSPDP requires careful isolation of the pancreatic parenchyma from the splenic vessels, and avoidance of drawing tightly on the vessel loop encircling the splenic vessels.

Abbreviations
CT: Computed tomography; LSPDP: Laparoscopic spleen-preserving distal pancreatectomy; MRI: Magnetic resonance imaging

Acknowledgements
We wish to thank the patient and her family, who agreed to allow publication of the clinical data.

Funding
No funding was obtained for this study.

Authors' contributions
KK, GO, and RA were involved in data collection, case analysis, and the writing of the manuscript. SY, RT, JT, and MO assisted in drafting the manuscript and reviewed the article. All authors read and approved the final manuscript.

Competing interests
The authors declare that they have no competing interests.

References

1. Mellemkjoer L, Olsen JH, Linet MS, Gridley G, McLaughlin JK. Cancer risk after splenectomy. Cancer. 1995;75(2):577–83.
2. Di Sabatino A, Carsetti R, Corazza GR. Post-splenectomy and hyposplenic states. Lancet. 2011;378(9785):86–97.
3. Kimura W, Inoue T, Futakawa N, Shinkai H, Han I, Muto T. Spleen-preserving distal pancreatectomy with conservation of the splenic artery and vein. Surgery. 1996;120(5):885–90.
4. Warshaw AL. Conservation of the spleen with distal pancreatectomy. Arch Surg. 1988;123(5):550–3.
5. Yoon YS, Lee KH, Han HS, Cho JY, Ahn KS. Patency of splenic vessels after laparoscopic spleen and splenic vessel-preserving distal pancreatectomy. Br J Surg. 2009;96(6):633–40.
6. Zhou ZQ, Kim SC, Song KB, Park KM, Lee JH, Lee YJ. Laparoscopic spleen-preserving distal pancreatectomy: comparative study of spleen preservation with splenic vessel resection and splenic vessel preservation. World J Surg. 2014;38(11):2973–9.
7. Worhunsky DJ, Zak Y, Dua MM, Poultsides GA, Norton JA, Visser BC. Laparoscopic spleen-preserving distal pancreatectomy: the technique must suit the lesion. J Gastrointest Surg. 2014;18(8):1445–51.
8. Hwang HK, Chung YE, Kim KA, Kang CM, Lee WJ. Revisiting vascular patency after spleen-preserving laparoscopic distal pancreatectomy with conservation of splenic vessels. Surg Endosc. 2012;26(6):1765–71.
9. Yu X, Li H, Jin C, Fu D, Di Y, Hao S, Li J. Splenic vessel preservation versus Warshaw's technique during spleen-preserving distal pancreatectomy: a meta-analysis and systematic review. Langenbeck's Arch Surg. 2015;400(2):183–91.
10. Beane JD, Pitt HA, Nakeeb A, Schmidt CM, House MG, Zyromski NJ, Howard TJ, Lillemoe KD. Splenic preserving distal pancreatectomy: does vessel preservation matter? J Am Coll Surg. 2011;212(4):651–7. discussion 657-658
11. Butturini G, Inama M, Malleo G, Manfredi R, Melotti GL, Piccoli M, Perandini S, Pederzoli P, Bassi C. Perioperative and long-term results of laparoscopic spleen-preserving distal pancreatectomy with or without splenic vessels conservation: a retrospective analysis. J Surg Oncol. 2012;105(4):387–92.
12. Lee LS, Hwang HK, Kang CM, Lee WJ. Minimally invasive approach for spleen-preserving distal pancreatectomy: a comparative analysis of postoperative complication between splenic vessel conserving and Warshaw's technique. J Gastrointest Surg. 2016;20(8):1464–70.
13. Kang CM, Chung YE, Jung MJ, Hwang HK, Choi SH, Lee WJ. Splenic vein thrombosis and pancreatic fistula after minimally invasive distal pancreatectomy. Br J Surg. 2014;101(2):114–9.

34

Comparison of pancreatojejunostomy techniques in patients with a soft pancreas: Kakita anastomosis and Blumgart anastomosis

Shoji Kawakatsu, Yosuke Inoue, Yoshihiro Mise, Takeaki Ishizawa, Hiromichi Ito, Yu Takahashi and Akio Saiura[*]

Abstract

Background: Postoperative pancreatic fistula (PF) is the main cause of operative mortality in patients who undergo pancreatoduodenectomy. Various pancreatoenteric anastomosis techniques have been reported to minimize the postoperative PF rate. However, the optimal method remains unknown. This study was performed to clarify the impact of pancreatojejunostomy on clinically relevant PF (CR-PF) between Blumgart anastomosis and Kakita anastomosis in patients with a soft pancreas.

Methods: In total, 620 consecutive patients underwent pancreatoduodenectomy at our institute from January 2010 to December 2016, and 282 patients with a soft pancreas were analyzed (Blumgart anastomosis, $n = 110$; Kakita anastomosis, $n = 176$). Short-term outcomes were assessed, and univariate and multivariate analyses of several clinicopathological variables were performed to analyze factors affecting the incidence of CR-PF.

Results: The CR-PF rate was 42.7% (122/286). The CR-PF rate was not significantly different between the Blumgart and Kakita groups (42.7% and 42.6%, respectively; $p = 0.985$). The morbidity rate (Clavien–Dindo grade ≥ IIIa) was 24.5% (70/286), and the operation-related mortality rate was 0.7% (2/286). In the multivariate analysis, male sex ($p = 0.0245$) and a body mass index of ≥22 kg/m^2 ($p < 0.0001$) were statistically significant risk factors for CR-PF.

Conclusions: The CR-PF rate was not significantly different between patients treated with Kakita versus Blumgart anastomosis.

Keywords: Pancreatoduodenectomy, Pancreatojejunostomy, Pancreatic fistula

Background

Recent advances in surgical techniques and perioperative management have made it possible to reduce the postoperative mortality rate after pancreatoduodenectomy. A nationwide survey from Japan reported that the mortality rate after pancreatoduodenectomy was 2.9% [1]. The recently reported mortality rate after pancreatoduodenectomy in the US was 1.4% [2]. However, pancreatoduodenectomy remains a complex and technically demanding procedure, and postoperative pancreatic fistula (PF) is an unsolved

problem. Most cases of mortality after pancreatoduodenectomy result from the development of postoperative PF, such as septic complications or intra-abdominal hemorrhage [3] from ruptured aneurysms. Although numerous pancreatoduodenectomy techniques have been proposed, there is no standardized procedure for preventing postoperative PF, especially in patients with a soft pancreas.

To minimize the incidence of postoperative PF, which is closely associated with subsequent mortality, we have contrived various pancreatoenteric anastomosis techniques, and several methods of pancreatojejunostomy (PJ) have been proposed in the literature. Among them, Kakita anastomosis, originally described by Kakita et al.

[*] Correspondence: akio.saiura@jfcr.or.jp
Department of Gastroenterological Surgery, Cancer Institute Hospital, Japanese Foundation for Cancer Research, 3-10-6 Ariake, Koto-ku, Tokyo 135-8550, Japan

[4] in 1996, is one of the most widely accepted procedures for PJ in Japan. In recent decades, a new standardized U-suture technique, which was originally described by Blumgart et al. [5, 6] in 2000, has been improved and rapidly accepted. Several studies have demonstrated the superiority of Blumgart anastomosis over Kakita anastomosis [7, 8].

Based on these reports, we hypothesized that the purse-string–like suture used in Blumgart anastomosis would be superior to Kakita anastomosis in achieving a surer water-tight anastomosis and lower incidence of PF, although such a suture might cause ischemic change of the pancreatic stump and a higher rate of latent PF. Beginning in July 2014, we changed the PJ method from modified Kakita anastomosis to modified Blumgart anastomosis in a phased manner. A soft pancreas texture was recently reported to be the most influential factor for postoperative PF [9–12]. From January 2010 to June 2014, the clinically relevant PF (CR-PF) rate after pancreatoduodenectomy reconstructed with Kakita anastomosis at our institute was 44.7% (76/170) among patients with a soft pancreas and 7.2% (11/152) among those with a hard pancreas. In the present large-scale retrospective cohort study, we analyzed the incidence of CR-PF between Kakita and Blumgart anastomosis for patients with a soft pancreas.

Methods
Patient selection
From January 2010 to December 2016, 620 consecutive patients underwent pancreatoduodenectomy at the Department of Gastroenterological Surgery, Cancer Institute Hospital, Japanese Foundation for Cancer Research, Tokyo, Japan. The institutional review board approved this study protocol. Among the 620 patients, 319 with a soft pancreas texture were enrolled in this study. Five patients who underwent pancreatogastrostomy and six who underwent a combination of Kakita and Blumgart PJ were excluded. Twenty-two patients who underwent concomitant resection of the adjacent colon were also excluded. In total, 286 patients were analyzed. Patient allocation in this study is summarized in Fig. 1.

Surgical procedure
Resection
We basically performed subtotal stomach-preserving pancreatoduodenectomy. Systematic mesopancreas dissection using a supracolic anterior artery-first approach was performed as previously reported [13]. Before pancreas transection, the proximal side of the pancreas was ligated with 2–0 polyglactin, and the distal side was gently clamped by an intestinal forceps to control bleeding from the pancreatic stump. The method of pancreas transection was left to the surgeon's discretion, and various methods were

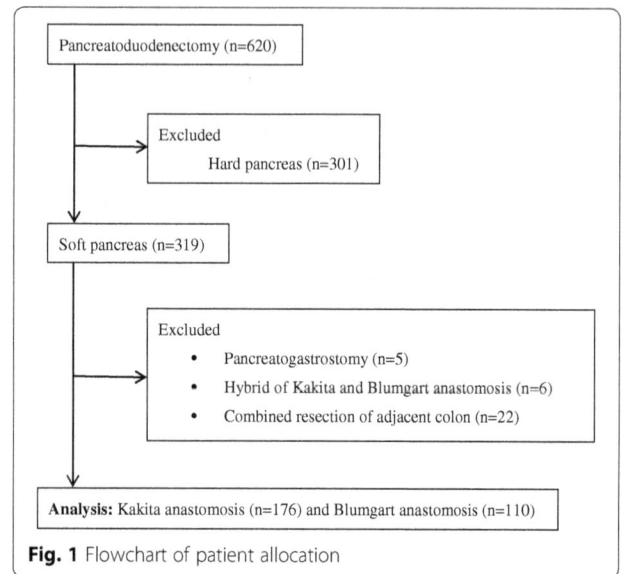

Fig. 1 Flowchart of patient allocation

employed, such as the clamp-crushing method [14] or transection by a scalpel, ultrasonically activated device, or stapler.

Reconstruction
Reconstruction was performed according to the modified Child's technique. After the jejunal limb was brought up through the retrocolic root, PJ (8 interrupted sutures with single-armed 6–0 polydioxanone for anastomosis of the main pancreatic duct to the jejunal mucosal layer and several interrupted sutures with double-armed 3–0 polydioxanone for anastomosis of the pancreatic parenchyma to the jejunal seromuscular layer [modified Kakita anastomosis (Fig. 2a) or modified Blumgart anastomosis (Fig. 2b)]) was performed about 15 cm away from the end of the jejunal limb. An external drainage tube was inserted into the main pancreatic duct and brought out through the jejunal limb and abdominal wall. Choledochojejunostomy was then performed with 5–0 polyglyconate suture (interrupted sutures on the posterior wall and a running suture on the anterior wall) about 10 cm distal to the PJ. An external drainage tube was also inserted into the intrahepatic duct and brought out through the jejunal limb and abdominal wall. Gastrojejunostomy was then performed with a stapling device, and the insertion hole was closed with a hand-sewn Albert–Lembert suture (a running Albert suture with 4–0 polydioxanone and interrupted Lembert sutures with 4–0 polyglactin 910) about 40 cm distal to the choledochojejunostomy. Braun anastomosis was added with a 4–0 polydioxanone running suture. A feeding tube was routinely inserted into the jejunum. The round ligament was mobilized and wound around the stump of the gastroduodenal artery. Silicone drains with a diameter of 8 mm were routinely placed at the foramen of Winslow and the superior sides of the PJ in patients with a soft pancreas.

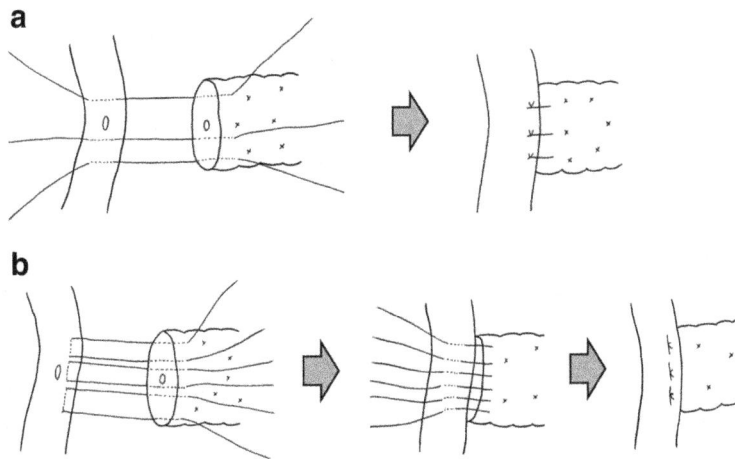

Fig. 2 Pancreatojejunostomy method. Eight interrupted sutures with single-armed 6–0 polydioxanone for anastomosis of the main pancreatic duct to the jejunal mucosal layer (omitted from this schema) and several interrupted sutures with double-armed 3–0 polydioxanone for anastomosis of the pancreatic parenchyma to the jejunal seromuscular layer [(**a**) modified Kakita anastomosis or (**b**) modified Blumgart anastomosis]

Modified Kakita anastomosis (Fig. 2a)

The parenchyma of the remnant pancreas was fixed to the jejunal seromuscular layer with two or three double-armed 3–0 polydioxanone penetrating sutures using gentle force to prevent laceration of the pancreatic parenchyma. The knots were placed on the jejunal serosa.

Modified Blumgart anastomosis (Fig. 2b)

The parenchyma of the remnant pancreas was fixed to the jejunal seromuscular layer with two or three double-armed 3–0 polydioxanone horizontal mattress sutures. One of the sutures strode across the main pancreatic duct to bind it.

Definition of PF

Postoperative PF was diagnosed and graded in accordance with the International Study Group on Pancreatic Fistula classification [15]. PF was diagnosed when the amylase concentration in the drainage fluid on postoperative day 3 was more than three times the upper limit of the normal serum level. PF with an elevated inflammatory response on the blood examination and intravenous administration of antibiotics was defined as Grade B PF caused by infection. PF that required drain placement for > 22 days without an elevated inflammatory response or administration of antibiotics was defined as Grade B PF caused by long drain placement. Latent PF [16] was defined as PF that initially lacked amylase-rich effluent but ultimately progressed to CR-PF.

Management of drainage tube

The amylase concentration of the drainage fluid was measured every day. When PF was evident, the drainage tube was exchanged on postoperative day 7, maintained with regular exchange until the drainage tube tract matured, and removed after the drainage fluid had nearly disappeared. In patients without postoperative PF, the drainage tube placed through the foramen of Winslow was removed on postoperative day 4, and the tube on the superior side of the PJ was removed on postoperative day 5.

Analysis

All clinical data in the medical records were retrospectively reviewed. In this study, two major issues were analyzed using these data. First, short-term outcomes were compared among the patients who underwent Kakita anastomosis (Kakita group) and those who underwent Blumgart anastomosis (Blumgart group). Subgroup analyses of risk-stratified patients were also performed for CR-PF. Second, univariate and multivariate analyses of several clinicopathological variables were performed to analyze factors affecting the incidence of CR-PF. The texture of the pancreatic parenchyma was assessed by the operator's palpation. The size of the main pancreatic duct was measured at the presumed surgical transection line on preoperative contrast-enhanced computed tomography.

Statistical analysis

All statistical analyses were performed using JMP software version 10.0.2 (SAS Institute, Cary, NC). Categorical variables were analyzed using Pearson's chi-square test or Fisher's exact test as appropriate. Continuous variables were compared using the Mann–Whitney U test. Continuous data are presented as a range of median values. To identify prognostic factors in the study population, the clinicopathological variables were analyzed in a univariate proportional hazard model, and all variables associated with survival with a p value of < 0.1 were subsequently entered into a Cox multivariate regression model. Values of $p < 0.05$ were considered statistically significant.

Results

Baseline characteristics and short-term outcomes

Table 1 summarizes the baseline characteristics of the 286 patients and their short-term outcomes. The CR-PF rate was 42.7% (122/286). A drain placement duration of ≥22 days was the most common cause of Grade B PF, accounting for 48.4% (59/122) of cases. Twelve patients (4.2%) developed Grade C PF; reoperation was required for 6 patients, and arterial embolization for intra-abdominal bleeding was required for 6 patients. The median length of drain placement was 18.5 (4–127) days. The median postoperative hospital stay was 30 (8–127) days. The morbidity rate (Clavien–Dindo grade ≥ IIIa) was 24.5% (70/286), and the operation-related mortality rate was 0.7% (2/286). The readmission rate within 30 days after discharge and 90 days after the operation was 4.9% (14/286) and 7.0% (20/286), respectively. The most common reason for readmission was cholangitis (12/20 readmissions). Only one patient required readmission because of PF; this patient develop a pseudoaneurysm after conservative treatment for PF. Among the patients with operation-related mortality, one died of liver failure caused by postoperative bleeding arising from the PF and another died of aspiration pneumonia without development of PF.

Comparison between Kakita and Blumgart groups

Table 1 also compares the baseline characteristics and surgical outcomes between the Kakita and Blumgart groups. There was no significant difference in short-term outcomes, such as the incidence of CR-PF and latent PF, between the Kakita group ($n = 176$) and the Blumgart group ($n = 110$). The diameter of the main pancreatic duct was significantly larger in the Blumgart group.

Univariate and multivariate analysis of clinicopathological variables

The results of the univariate and multivariate analyses of clinicopathological variables are shown in Table 2. The multivariate analysis showed that male sex ($p = 0.0245$)

Table 1 Patients characteristics and short-term outcomes

Variables	Total (n = 286)	Kakita (n = 176)	Blumgart (n = 110)	p
Patients characteristics				
Age (years)	67 (21–87)	66 (32–87)	69 (21–86)	0.143
Male	166 (58.0)	100 (56.8)	66 (60.0)	0.594
BMI	22.3 (15.9–32.0)	22.3 (15.9–32.0)	22.2 (16.1–31.6)	0.560
History of DM	47 (16.4)	27 (15.3)	20 (18.2)	0.530
Diameter of MPD (mm)	3 (1–16)	2 (1–8)	3 (1–16)	0.0001*
Thickness of the pancreas (mm)	10 (5–18)	10 (5–18)	10 (6–18)	0.203
Shor-term outcomes				
Operative time (min)	481 (254–920)	487 (295–834)	477 (254–920)	0.782
Blood loss (mL)	450 (20–3530)	400 (20–3530)	490 (60–1875)	0.551
Pancreatic fistula (≥ Grade B)	122 (42.7)	75 (42.6)	47 (42.7)	0.985
Grade B	110 (38.5)	69	41	0.744
Length of drain placement ≥ 22	59 (20.6)	39	20	0.416
Infection	51 (17.8)	30	21	0.661
Grade C	12 (4.2)	6 (3.4)	6 (5.5)	0.407
Re-operation	6 (2.1)	4	2	0.792
Intraabdominal bleeding (IAB)	4 (1.4)	2	2	0.637
Leakage of pancreatojejunostomy	2 (0.7)	2	0	0.163
Arterial embolization for IAB	6 (2.1)	2	4	0.158
Latent pancreatic fistula (≥ Grade B)	17 (5.9)	14 (8.0)	3 (2.7)	0.055
Morbidity (≥ Clavien-Dindo Grade IIIa)	70 (24.5)	45 (25.6)	25 (22.7)	0.586
Postoperative hospital stay	30 (16–127)	30 (16–108)	31 (16–127)	0.290
Length of drain placement	18.5 (4–127)	18 (4–85)	19 (4–127)	0.204
Mortality	2 (0.7)	1 (0.5)	1 (0.9)	0.740

All the data are shown as median (range) or the number (percentage)
*Indicates statistically significant

Table 2 Univariate and multivariate analysis for risk factors of CR-PF

Variable	Univariate analysis			Multivariate analysis		
	OR	95% CI	P	OR	95% CI	P
Age ≥ 70	1.40	0.87–2.25	0.1693			
Male	2.35	1.45–3.88	0.0005*	1.90	1.12-3.23	0.0170*
BMI ≥ 22	3.75	2.28–6.26	< 0.0001*	2.85	1.69–4.88	< 0.0001*
Disease (pancreatic cancer)	1.19	0.69–2.03	0.5295			
History of DM	1.66	0.89–3.14	0.1121			
Pancreatojejunostomy (Blumgart)	1.00	0.62–1.63	0.9849	1.05	0.62–1.80	0.8465
Portal vein resection	1.14	0.59–2.18	0.6840			
SMD level (III)	1.41	0.71–2.80	0.3279			
Diameter of MPD > 3 mm	0.52	0.30–0.88	0.0144*	0.57	0.32-1.01	0.0543
Thickness of the pancreas > 10 mm	1.32	0.82–2.12	0.2522			
Operative time ≥ 500 min	1.88	1.17–3.04	0.0096*	1.15	0.66-1.98	0.6184
Blood loss ≥ 500 mL	2.48	1.54–4.04	0.0002*	1.58	0.91-2.76	0.1043

OR Odds ratio, CI Confidence interval, SMD Systemic mesopancres dissection
*Indicates statistically significant

and a body mass index (BMI) of ≥22 kg/m^2 ($p < 0.0001$) were statistically significant risk factors for CR-PF. There was no significant difference in the incidence of CR-PF between the Kakita and Blumgart groups.

Risk-stratified subgroup analysis of CR-PF between the Kakita and Blumgart groups

A subgroup analysis of high-risk subsets for CR-PF (age of ≥70 years, male, BMI of ≥22 kg/m^2, main pancreatic duct diameter of ≤3 mm, and pancreatic thickness of ≥10 mm) as estimated by univariate and multivariate analyses was performed between the groups (Table 3). There were no significant differences in the rate of CR-PF between the two groups.

Discussion

Several attempts to reduce the incidence of postoperative PF have been made in recent years, but no standard methods with which to minimize the incidence of postoperative PF have yet been established. According to a recent study, a soft pancreas texture is probably the most influential factor for postoperative PF [9–12]. In the current study, we compared the rate of CR-PF between the Kakita and Blumgart anastomosis groups of patients with a soft pancreas texture.

As shown in previous reports, male sex and a BMI of > 22 kg/m^2 were risk factors for CR-PF [17] in our study. Unlike in previous reports [7, 8, 18], there was no significant difference in the incidence of CR-PF between the Kakita and Blumgart anastomosis groups. Our hypothesis that Blumgart anastomosis is associated with a lower incidence of whole PF and higher incidence of latent PF was denied in this study. In Blumgart anastomosis, the use of transpancreatic, full-thickness, mattress U-sutures instead of tangential sutures reportedly eliminates tangential tension and shear force at the stitch points of the pancreatic parenchyma because the pancreatic stump and stitch points are theoretically coved by jejunal serosa [18]. In Kakita anastomosis, the tangential suture through the pancreatic capsule may result in the development of shear forces at the stitch points of the pancreatic parenchyma, and more careful ligation is required. However, it is possible to completely cover the pancreatic cut end with jejunal serosa and protect the knots from cutting through the pancreatic parenchyma by consciously placing the knot on the jejunal side. Moreover, when the pancreas is too thick for the diameter of the jejunum, it is very difficult to perform Blumgart anastomosis. Therefore, Kakita anastomosis may have

Table 3 Risk-stratified subgroup analysis of clinically relevant pancreatic fistula between Kakita and Blumgart groups

Subgroup	Kakita	Blumgart	p
Age of ≥70 years	51.5% (34/66)	42.3% (22/52)	0.3195
Male sex	53.0% (53/100)	48.5% (32/66)	0.5690
Body mass index of ≥22 kg/m^2	53.1% (51/96)	62.7% (37/59)	0.2406
Main pancreatic duct diameter of ≤3 mm	44.7% (59/132)	52.2% (36/69)	0.3135
Pancreatic thickness of > 10 mm	53.9% (35/65)	40.8% (20/49)	0.1673

broader utility. In spite of these minor differences between mattress U-sutures and tangential sutures, the sutures are placed through the full thickness of the pancreas in the same fashion. We believe that both Kakita and Blumgart anastomosis are basically the same method. In addition, blood flow at the pancreatic anastomosis is important to optimize healing of the pancreatic reconstruction [19], and our results indicate that even in Blumgart anastomosis with mattress U-sutures, the rate of latent PF due to ischemia was not higher than that in Kakita anastomosis, as was reported previously [20].

Various strategies to reduce the occurrence and morbidity of postoperative PF are required for optimal outcomes in high-risk patients. The rate of postoperative PF cannot be reduced to zero, especially in patients with a soft pancreas. Previous reports have indicated that it would be possible to abandon routine prophylactic drainage tube placement after pancreatic resection [21–23]. Another prospective randomized controlled multicenter trial strongly demonstrated that routine placement of an intraperitoneal drainage tube in patients undergoing pancreatoduodenectomy reduces the mortality rate [24]. Intraperitoneal drains are routinely placed in our institute. When postoperative PF was evident, the drainage tube was exchanged and maintained with regular exchange until the drainage fluid was nearly absent. Although our method of drainage tube management increased the rate of Grade B PF due to prolonged drain placement, extension of the drain placement duration to avoid intra-abdominal fluid collection did not induce clinically relevant problems, as demonstrated by our low mortality and readmission rates compared with previous reports [1, 2, 25–27]. Our CR-PF rate in patients with a soft pancreas (42.7%) was relatively higher than that in previous reports restricted to high-risk cohorts [17, 27]. However, nearly half of CR-PF cases resulted from extension of the drain placement duration, and no patients developed fever or abdominal pain. Our strategy seems too heterodox and more wasteful than the Western style of early drain removal followed by early discharge. However, we have demonstrated lower mortality and readmission rates than those reported in Western countries, even in an exclusive cohort of patients with a soft pancreas. Although further investigation and validation would be needed to optimize the indication for our drainage tube management in patients with a soft pancreas cohort, our strategy is a promising choice for significantly high-risk patients.

This study does have limitations. First, although the sample size was considerably large, this was a single-institution retrospective study with several operators. However, this study was the largest-scale analysis to date restricted to patients with a soft pancreas who had a high risk of CR-PF. In such a situation, which is similar to the practical setting of each hospital, we have achieved a low mortality rate in high-risk cohorts for postoperative PF. Second, texture of the pancreas was subjective parameter, and potential selection bias could not be eliminated. Third, Kakita anastomosis was our original method, and we were therefore familiar with it. Conversely, Blumgart anastomosis was a new procedure for us. Therefore, our results should be carefully interpreted, considering the difference in the learning curve between the two methods. A large-scale prospective randomized trial is warranted to determine the superiority of the two techniques.

Conclusions

In conclusion, there was no significance difference in the CR-PF rate between patients who underwent Kakita versus Blumgart anastomosis. Regardless of the anastomosis technique, an accurate and meticulous procedure is essential to achieve a low rate of postoperative PF.

Abbreviations
CR-PF: Clinically relevant pancreatic fistula; PF: Pancreatic fistula; PJ: Pancreatojejunostomy

Acknowledgments
We thank Angela Morben, DVM, ELS, from Edanz Group (www.edanzediting.com/ac), for editing a draft of this manuscript.

Authors' contributions
SK and YI designed the study. SK was involved with writing the manuscript. YI, YM, TI, HI, and YT contributed to the conception and critically revised the manuscript. AS was responsible for the study conception, design, data analysis and drafting of the manuscript. All authors read and approved the final manuscript.

Competing interests
The authors declare that they have no competing interests.

References
1. Kimura W, Miyata H, Gotoh M, Hirai I, Kenjo A, Kitagawa Y, et al. A pancreaticoduodenectomy risk model derived from 8575 cases from a national single-race population (Japanese) using a web-based data entry system: the 30-day and in-hospital mortality rates for pancreaticoduodenectomy. Ann Surg. 2014;259(4):773–80.
2. Cameron JL, He J. Two thousand consecutive pancreaticoduodenectomies. J Am Coll Surg. 2015;220(4):530–6.

3. Yekebas EF, Wolfram L, Cataldegirmen G, Habermann CR, Bogoevski D, Koenig AM, et al. Postpancreatectomy hemorrhage: diagnosis and treatment: an analysis in 1669 consecutive pancreatic resections. Ann Surg. 2007;246(2):269–80.

4. Kakita A, Takahashi T, Yoshida M, Furuta K. A simpler and more reliable technique of pancreatojejunal anastomosis. Surg Today. 1996;26(7):532–5.

5. Brennan M. Pancreatojejunostomy. In Blumgart LH, Fong Y, eds. Surgery of the liver and biliary tract, 3rd ed. Philadelphia: Saunders, 2000;pp1073–89.

6. Grobmyer SR, Kooby D, Blumgart LH, Hochwald SN. Novel pancreaticojejunostomy with a low rate of anastomotic failure-related complications. J Am Coll Surg. 2010;210(1):54–9.

7. Fujii T, Sugimoto H, Yamada S, Kanda M, Suenaga M, Takami H, et al. Modified Blumgart anastomosis for pancreaticojejunostomy: technical improvement in matched historical control study. J Gastrointest Surg. 2014;18(6):1108–15.

8. Oda T, Hashimoto S, Miyamoto R, Shimomura O, Fukunaga K, Kohno K, et al. The tight adaptation at pancreatic anastomosis without parenchymal laceration: an institutional experience in introducing and modifying the new procedure. World J Surg. 2015;39(8):2014–22.

9. Kawai M, Kondo S, Yamaue H, Wada K, Sano K, Motoi F, et al. Predictive risk factors for clinically relevant pancreatic fistula analyzed in 1,239 patients with pancreaticoduodenectomy: multicenter data collection as a project study of pancreatic surgery by the Japanese Society of Hepato-Biliary-Pancreatic Surgery. J Hepatobiliary Pancreat Sci. 2011;18(4):601–8.

10. Ansorge C, Strommer L, Andren-Sandberg A, Lundell L, Herrington MK, Segersvard R. Structured intraoperative assessment of pancreatic gland characteristics in predicting complications after pancreaticoduodenectomy. Br J Surg. 2012;99(8):1076–82.

11. El Nakeeb A, Salah T, Sultan A, El Hemaly M, Askr W, Ezzat H, et al. Pancreatic anastomotic leakage after pancreaticoduodenectomy. Risk factors, clinical predictors, and management (single center experience). World J Surg. 2013;37(6):1405–18.

12. Callery MP, Pratt WB, Kent TS, Chaikof EL, Vollmer CM Jr. A prospectively validated clinical risk score accurately predicts pancreatic fistula after pancreatoduodenectomy. J Am Coll Surg. 2013;216(1):1–14.

13. Inoue Y, Saiura A, Yoshioka R, Ono Y, Takahashi M, Arita J, et al. Pancreatoduodenectomy with systematic Mesopancreas dissection using a Supracolic anterior artery-first approach. Ann Surg. 2015;262(6):1092–101.

14. Koga R, Yamamoto J, Saiura A, Natori T, Katori M, Kokudo N, et al. Clamp-crushing pancreas transection in pancreatoduodenectomy. Hepato-Gastroenterology. 2009;56(89):89–93.

15. Bassi C, Dervenis C, Butturini G, Fingerhut A, Yeo C, Izbicki J, et al. Postoperative pancreatic fistula: an international study group (ISGPF) definition. Surgery. 2005;138(1):8–13.

16. Pratt WB, Callery MP, Vollmer CM Jr. The latent presentation of pancreatic fistulas. Br J Surg. 2009;96(6):641–9.

17. Sugimoto M, Takahashi S, Kojima M, Kobayashi T, Gotohda N, Konishi M. In patients with a soft pancreas, a thick parenchyma, a small duct, and fatty infiltration are significant risks for pancreatic fistula after Pancreaticoduodenectomy. J Gastrointest Surg. 2017;21(5):846–54.

18. Kleespies A, Rentsch M, Seeliger H, Albertsmeier M, Jauch KW, Bruns CJ. Blumgart anastomosis for pancreaticojejunostomy minimizes severe complications after pancreatic head resection. Br J Surg. 2009;96(7):741–50.

19. Strasberg SM, Drebin JA, Mokadam NA, Green DW, Jones KL, Ehlers JP, et al. Prospective trial of a blood supply-based technique of pancreaticojejunostomy: effect on anastomotic failure in the Whipple procedure. J Am Coll Surg. 2002;194(6):746–58 discussion 59-60.

20. Wang SE, Chen SC, Shyr BU, Shyr YM. Comparison of modified Blumgart pancreaticojejunostomy and pancreaticogastrostomy after pancreaticoduodenectomy. HPB. 2016;18(3):229–35.

21. McMillan MT, Malleo G, Bassi C, Allegrini V, Casetti L, Drebin JA, et al. Multicenter, prospective trial of selective drain Management for Pancreatoduodenectomy Using Risk Stratification. Ann Surg. 2017;256(6):1209–18.

22. Mehta VV, Fisher SB, Maithel SK, Sarmiento JM, Staley CA, Kooby DA. Is it time to abandon routine operative drain use? A single institution assessment of 709 consecutive pancreaticoduodenectomies. J Am Coll Surg. 2013;216(4):635–42 discussion 42-4.

23. Correa-Gallego C, Brennan MF, D'Angelica M, Fong Y, Dematteo RP, Kingham TP, et al. Operative drainage following pancreatic resection: analysis of 1122 patients resected over 5 years at a single institution. Ann Surg. 2013;258(6):1051–8.

24. Van Buren G 2nd, Bloomston M, Hughes SJ, Winter J, Behrman SW, Zyromski NJ, et al. A randomized prospective multicenter trial of pancreaticoduodenectomy with and without routine intraperitoneal drainage. Ann Surg. 2014;259(4):605–12.

25. Sutton JM, Wilson GC, Wima K, Hoehn RS, Cutler Quillin R 3rd, Hanseman DJ, et al. Readmission after Pancreaticoduodenectomy: the influence of the volume effect beyond mortality. Ann Surg Oncol. 2015;22(12):3785–92.

26. Ahmad SA, Edwards MJ, Sutton JM, Grewal SS, Hanseman DJ, Maithel SK, et al. Factors influencing readmission after pancreaticoduodenectomy: a multi-institutional study of 1302 patients. Ann Surg. 2012;256(3):529–37.

27. Ecker BL, McMillan MT, Asbun HJ, Ball CG, Bassi C, Beane JD, et al. Characterization and optimal Management of High-Risk Pancreatic Anastomoses during Pancreatoduodenectomy. Ann Surg. 2018;267(4):608–16.

Embryological etiology of pancreaticobiliary system predicted from pancreaticobiliary maljunction with incomplete pancreatic divisum

Yukihiro Sanada[1,2*], Yasunaru Sakuma[1] and Naohiro Sata[1]

Abstract

Background: The genesis of the "complex type" classification of pancreaticobiliary maljunction (PBM) is unclear, and the pancreaticobiliary anatomy is also varied according to each case. We encountered a patient with PBM and incomplete pancreatic divisum (PD). We herein discussed about the embryological etiology of pancreaticobiliary system predicted from PBM with incomplete PD.

Case presentation: A 67-year-old man was found to have a dilatation of the common bile duct (CBD) during a medical examination at 62 years of age. The dilatation of the CBD subsequently progressed, and he was admitted to our hospital for surgical treatment. Magnetic resonance cholangiopancreatography revealed a dilatation from the common hepatic duct to the middle bile duct with PBM. Endoscopic retrograde cholangiopancreatography from the papilla of Vater revealed the pancreatic main duct via the pancreatic branch duct, and PBM with dilatation of the CBD and incomplete PD were revealed. We performed an extrahepatic bile duct resection and hepaticojejunostomy because of high risk of malignant transformation. Taping and transection of the bile duct without dilatation on the pancreatic side were performed, and thereafter, two orifices of the common channel and ventral pancreatic duct were ligated. The level of amylase in the bile was 7217 IU/L, and a histological examination of the CBD showed an inflammatory change of CBD, not a malignant transformation.

Conclusion: It is somewhat easy to identify the pancreatobiliary anatomy when the cause of embryology of both PBM and PD is thought to be an abnormal embryology of the ventral pancreas.

Keywords: Pancreaticobiliary maljunction, Incomplete pancreatic divisum, Embryology, Ventral pancreas, Endoscopic retrograde cholangiopancreatography

Background

The "complex type" classification of pancreaticobiliary maljunction (PBM) is rare, [1] and in particular, PBM with pancreatic divisum (PD) is classified a "complex type" of PBM. The genesis of the "complex type" classification of PBM is unclear, and the pancreaticobiliary anatomy is also varied according to each case. Therefore, it is occasionally difficult to understand the anatomy and pathophysiology of patients with PBM and PD. In addition, the misunderstanding of pancreaticobiliary anatomy affects a decision of the transection line during biliary diversion procedure.

We encountered a patient with PBM and incomplete PD. We herein discussed about the embryological etiology of pancreaticobiliary system predicted from PBM with incomplete PD in order to understand the pancreaticobiliary anatomy.

Case presentation

A 67-year-old man was found to have a dilatation of the common bile duct (CBD) (19 mm) during a medical examination at 62 years of age. The dilatation of the

* Correspondence: yuki371@jichi.ac.jp
[1]Department of Surgery, Jichi Medical University, 3311-1 Yakushiji, Shimotsuke City, Tochigi 329-0498, Japan
[2]Department of Transplant Surgery, Jichi Medical University, Shimotsuke, Japan

CBD subsequently progressed (26 mm), and he was admitted to our hospital for surgical treatment. Abdominal computed tomography revealed a dilatation of the CBD with no tumor or stone. Magnetic resonance cholangiopancreatography revealed a dilatation from the common hepatic duct (CHD) to the middle bile duct (Fig. 1a and b) with PBM (Fig. 1c). Endoscopic retrograde cholangiopancreatography (ERCP) from the papilla of Vater revealed the pancreatic main duct via the pancreatic branch duct (Fig. 2a and b). PBM with dilatation of the CBD (26 mm) and incomplete PD were revealed (Fig. 2c). Figure 3 shows a schema of this case with dilatation of the CBD and PBM, and incomplete PD in which the ventral pancreatic duct joined the dorsal pancreatic branch duct was observed.

We planned an extrahepatic bile duct resection and hepaticojejunostomy because of high risk of malignant transformation. Laparotomy was performed by a right hypochondrium incision. Taping and transection of the bile duct without dilatation on the pancreatic side were performed, and thereafter, two orifices of the common channel and ventral pancreatic duct were ligated (Fig. 3). The transection line of the CHD without dilatation was identified using cholangiography (Fig. 3), and then, the CBD was resected. The level of amylase in the bile was 7217 IU/L, and a histological examination of the CBD showed an inflammatory change of CBD, not a malignant transformation.

The postoperative course was good and uneventful, and the patient was discharged from the hospital on postoperative day 9. The patient is doing well at 1.5 years after surgery.

Discussion

The "complex type" classification of PBM is rare, [1] and in particular, PBM with PD is considered a "complex type" classification of PBM. The embryological mechanism of PBM is unclear; however, there are strong arguments for an abnormal embryology of the ventral pancreas until embryonic week four [2, 3]. In contrast, it is conceivable that the embryological mechanism of PD occurs by an abnormal fusion of the ventral and dorsal pancreatic ducts because the ventral pancreas fuses with the dorsal pancreas at embryonic weeks 6–7 [4]. That is, PBM and PD are congenital anomalies that develop in the embryo at an early stage, and they may be the result of bile and pancreatic duct misarrangement. However, the genesis of the "complex type" classification of PBM is unclear, and the anatomy is also varied according to each case. In addition, few patients have been reported with PBM and PD [5]. Therefore, it is occasionally difficult for physicians and surgeons to understand the anatomy and pathophysiology of patients with PBM and PD. We herein encountered a patient with PBM and incomplete PD, and we considered that PBM and incomplete PD occurred in this case due to abnormal embryology of the ventral pancreas. If the embryological etiology of PBM and PD is an abnormal embryology of the ventral pancreas, the genesis and anatomy of the "complex type" classification of PBM is easy to understand. This case supports the idea that the embryology of PBM and PD is based on abnormal embryology of the ventral pancreas.

Although the recommended treatment for a biliary dilatation with the "complex type" classification of PBM is an extrahepatic bile duct resection and hepaticojejunostomy (biliary diversion procedure), [3] selecting the transection lines of the CBD is occasionally difficult. It is important to leave as little as possible of the bile duct unresected, and in this case, the bile duct on the pancreatic side was transected at the bifurcation of the common channel and ventral pancreatic duct so as not to leave the bile duct because drainage from the ventral pancreatic duct to the dorsal pancreatic duct can be identified by ERCP. The patient is doing well without

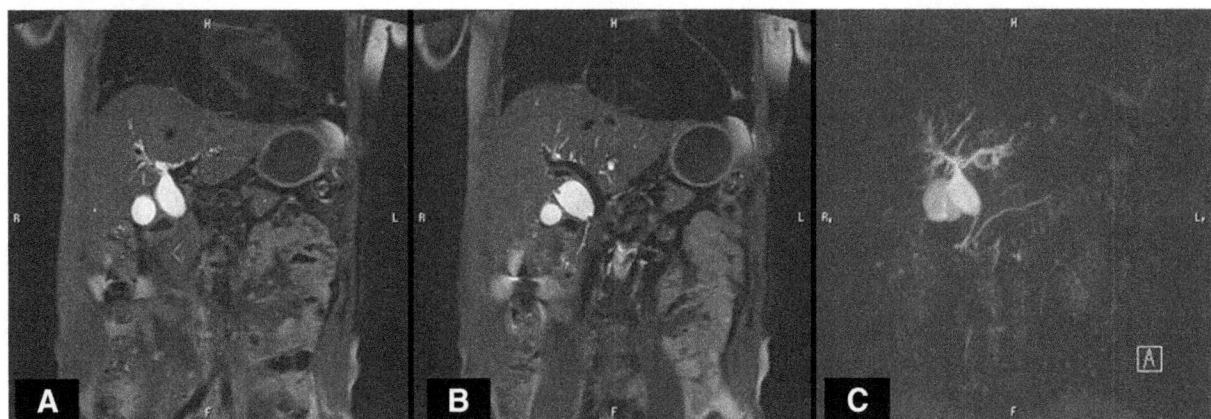

Fig. 1 Magnetic resonance cholangiopancreatography (MRCP). MRCP revealed a dilatation from the common hepatic duct to the middle bile duct (**a** and **b**) with pancreaticobiliary maljunction (**c**)

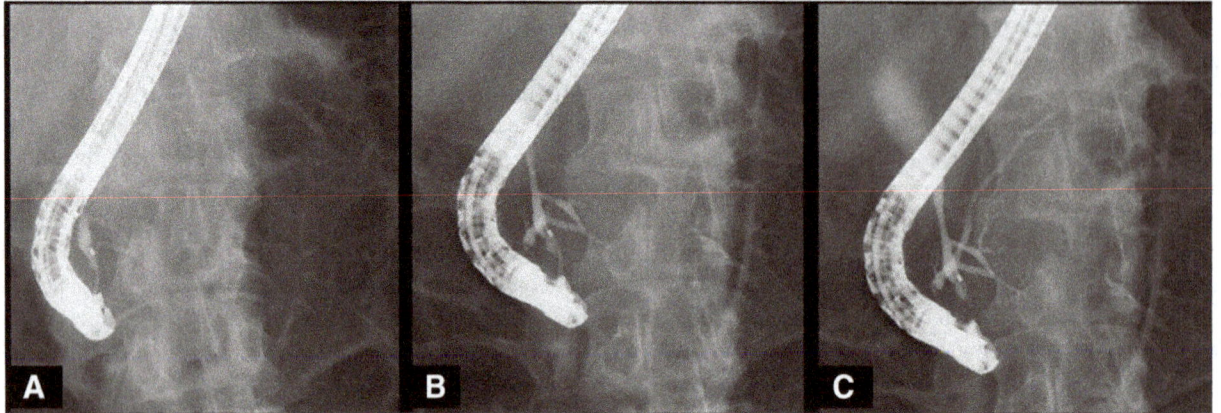

Fig. 2 Endoscopic retrograde cholangiopancreatography (ERCP). ERCP from the papilla of Vater revealed the pancreatic main duct via the pancreatic branch duct (**a** and **b**). Pancreaticobiliary maljunction with dilatation of the common bile duct (26 mm) and incomplete pancreas divisum were revealed (**c**)

having an acute pancreatitis due to insufficient drainage of the ventral pancreatic duct. Therefore, it is important for patients with the "complex type" classification of PBM to clear the dynamics of the ventral pancreatic juice by preoperative ERCP, and it is possible to undergo a complete resection of the bile duct on the pancreatic side.

Conclusion

It is difficult to identify the "complex type" pancreatobiliary anatomy of PBM; however, it is somewhat easy to identify when the cause of embryology of both PBM and PD is thought to be an abnormal embryology of the ventral pancreas.

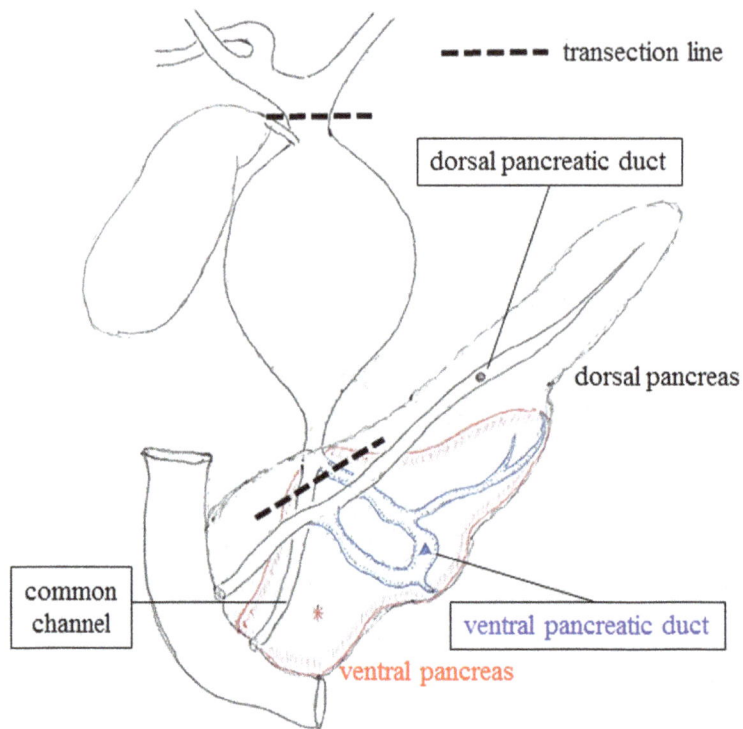

Fig. 3 Anatomical schema of the pancreaticobiliary system in this patient. This patient was diagnosed with the "complex type" classification of pancreaticobiliary maljunction with incomplete pancreas divisum. Extrahepatic bile duct resection and hepaticojejunostomy were performed based on the transection line of this schema

Abbreviations
CBD: Common bile duct; CHD: Common hepatic duct; ERCP: Endoscopic retrograde cholangiopancreatography; PBM: Pancreaticobiliary maljunction; PD: Pancreas divisum

Acknowledgements
We thank Kazue Morishima, Naoya Kasahara, Yuji Kaneda, Atsushi Miki, Kazuhiro Endo, Masaru Koizumi, Hideki Sasanuma, and Yoshikazu Yasuda (Department of Surgery, Jichi Medical University) for helpful advices regarding medical examination and treatment. No financial support has been received.

Authors' contributions
SanaY: study design, acquisition of data, analysis and interpretation of data, and drafting of the manuscript. Saku Y: acquisition of data, analysis and interpretation of data, critical revision of the manuscript for important intellectual content. SN: analysis and interpretation of data, and critical revision of the manuscript for important intellectual content. All authors read and approved the final manuscript.

Competing interests
The authors declare that they have no competing interests.

References
1. The Japanese Study Group on Pancreaticobiliary Maljunction (JSPBM) and The Committee of JSPBM for Diagnostic Criteria. Diagnostic criteria of pancreaticobiliary maljunction. J Hepato-Biliary-Pancreat Surg. 1994;1:219–21.
2. Odgers PNB. Some observations on the development of the ventral pancreas in man. J Anat. 1930;65:1–7.
3. Kamisawa T, Ando H, Suyama M, Shimada M, Morine Y, Shimada H, Working Committee of Clinical Practice Guidelines for Pancreaticobiliary Maljunction, Japanese study group on Pancreaticobiliary Maljunction. Japanese clinical practice guidelines for pancreaticobiliary maljunction. J Gastroenterol. 2012; 47(7):731–59.
4. Kamisawa T, Takuma K, Egawa N, Tsuruta K, Sasaki T. A new embryological theory of the pancreatic duct system. Dig Surg. 2010;27(2):132–6.
5. Kamisawa T, Tu Y, Egawa N, Tsuruta K, Okamoto A, Matsukawa M. Pancreas divisum in pancreaticobiliary maljunction. Hepato-Gastroenterology. 2008; 55(81):249–53.

Continuous or interrupted suture technique for hepaticojejunostomy? A national survey

Maximilian Brunner*[iD], Jessica Stockheim, Christian Krautz, Dimitrios Raptis, Stephan Kersting, Georg F. Weber and Robert Grützmann

Abstract

Background: Hepaticojejunostomy is commonly used in hepato-bilio-pancreatic surgery and a crucial step in many surgical procedures, including pancreaticoduodenectomy. The most frequently used techniques are the interrupted suture and the continuous suture technique. Currently, there is no data available in regard to the utilization of these techniques.

Methods: In total, 102 hospitals in Germany were invited between September and November 2017 to participate in this survey. Using a paper-based questionnaire, data were collected on surgical technique and complication rates of hepaticojejunostomies.

Results: A total of 77 of the 102 addressed hospitals (76%) participated in the survey. On average, each hospital performed 71 hepaticojejunostomies per year - most often in the context of pancreaticoduodenectomy (71%). 24 (31%) hospitals exclusively use an interrupted suture technique, 7 (9%) hospitals solely a continuous suture technique, 3 (4%) hospitals perform a combination of continuous and interrupted suture technique and 43 (56%) hospitals decide on one of both techniques depending on intraoperative findings. According to the participants in this survey, the continuous suture technique is significantly faster than the interrupted suture technique in hepaticojejunostomy ($p = 0,015$). There were no significant differences in the overall complication rate ($p = 0,902$) and insufficiency rate ($p = 1,000$).

Conclusions: In Germany, there is a heterogeneity in the technique used to create a hepaticojejunostomy. As our survey suggests that the use of continuous suture technique may offer an advantage in time without jeopardizing patient outcomes, the different techniques should be compared in a randomized controlled study.

Keywords: Hepaticojejunostomy, Pancreatic surgery, Hepatic surgery, Surgical technique, Survey

Background

The surgical technique of the hepaticojejunostomy represents the "surgical school" in a unique way and while some of us use either continuous or interrupted sutures depending on the situation and the operative situs, others adhere very much to their surgical education be it interrupted or continuous suturing for all cases.

Hepaticojejunostomies represent an important step in pancreatic resections, liver resections, liver transplantations and bile duct resections, are used as a palliative procedure for non-resectable tumors of the pancreatic head and distal bile duct and are performed in bile duct injuries. Failure of this anastomosis leads to considerable morbidity and even mortality [1, 2].

After various methods of anastomosing the biliary system with the gastrointestinal tract (cholecystocolostomy, cholecystojejunostomy, hepaticoduodenostomy) had been published at the end of the nineteenth century, Dahl was the first to report a hepaticojejunostomy in 1909 [3–6]. Over the years, various modifications have been described [7]. Since then, hepaticojejunostomy has been established as an important component of many surgical procedures and all other techniques have been more or less abandoned.

Basic principles for the successful implementation of a hepaticojejunostomy are [8]:

* Correspondence: Maximilian.Brunner@uk-erlangen.de
Department of General Surgery, University Hospital of Friedrich-Alexander-University, Krankenhausstraße 12, 91054 Erlangen, Germany

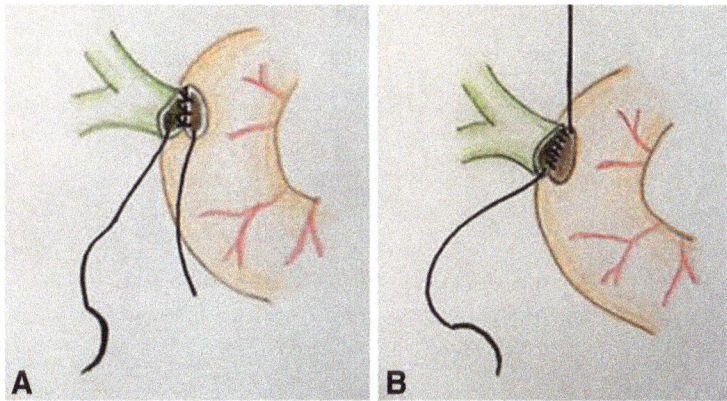

Fig. 1 Hepaticojejunostomy with interrupted suture technique (**a**) and continuous suture technique (**b**); own figures

- A tension-free reconstruction
- Anastomosis in the area of intact, well-perfused bile duct and small bowel mucosa
- Precise mucosal adaptation between the bile duct and jejunum
- Creation of hepaticojejunostomy near to the hepatic duct bifurcation

The most important complications following a hepaticojejunostomy are bile duct leakage and anastomotic stenosis. In the literature leakage rates after hepaticojejunostomies vary between 2.3 and 5.6% [9, 10]. Although this is a relatively rare postoperative complication, bile duct leakage can have far-reaching consequences with a high risk of prolonged hospitalization and need for interventional drainage or re-laparotomy, which is associated with high morbidity and mortality, even in high volume centers [1, 2]. For the development of anastomotic stenosis, studies report rates between 3.7 and 8.0% [11, 12].

There are various surgical techniques available for the creation of a hepaticojejunostomy. Figures 1, 2 and 3 show the most commonly used techniques: interrupted suture technique and continuous suture technique. A combination of both techniques is also possible (posterior and anterior wall in different techniques). The advantage of the interrupted suture technique is the universal use even for small bile ducts, whereas the costs and the operating time for this technique should be higher in comparison to the continuous suture technique (Table 1). Especially for larger bile ducts, the continuous technique might offer a better sealing of the anastomosis. Conversely, advocates of the interrupted technique allege that the continuous suture might lead in long term to a higher rate of stenosis at the anastomosis.

Despite the frequent necessity of hepaticojejunostomies in surgery and the relevant consequences for the patient with leakage or stenosis, there are no randomized studies to compare the different surgical techniques.

In preparation of a randomized trial, the aim of the current questionnaire-based survey was to determine the status quo of the surgical techniques used for hepaticojejunostomies in Germany.

Methods

In September 2017, a total of 102 surgical hospitals in Germany were addressed to take part in this survey.

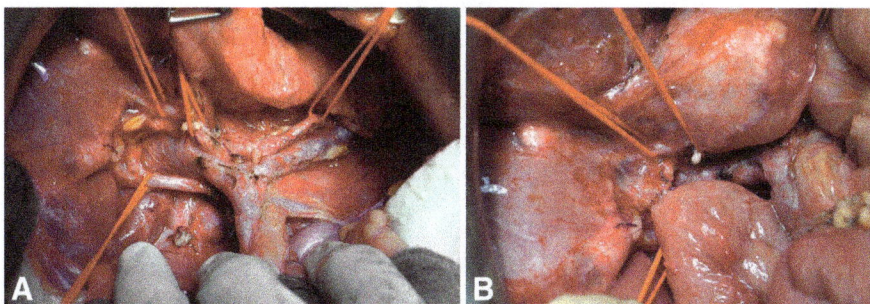

Fig. 2 Hepaticojejunostomy with interrupted suture technique; intraoperative pictures: situs after pancreaticoduodenectomy and before hepaticojejunostomy (**a**) and situs after hepaticojejunostomy in interrupted suture technique (**b**); pictures are examples for the interrupted suture technique from our institute, other versions of the technique are possible

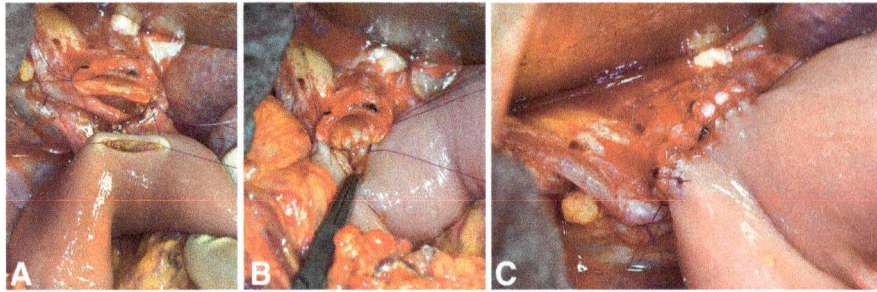

Fig. 3 Hepaticojejunostomy with continuous suture technique; intraoperative pictures: situs before hepaticojejunostomy (**a**), situs after reconstruction of the posterior wall in continuous suture technique (**b**) and situs after complete hepaticojejunostomy in continuous suture technique (**c**); pictures are examples for the continuous suture technique from our institute, other versions of the technique are possible

Since most hepaticojejunostomies are constructed as part of pancreatic surgery and these are more likely to be performed in larger institutions, all hospitals in Germany that treat least 30,000 cases per year were selected for inclusion in this survey. In November 2017, a reminder letter was sent to all hospitals that had not responded by then. The collection of data was paper-based to make the answer to the questionnaire as simple as possible.

In the questionnaire the following aspects were queried:

- Number of hepaticojejunostomies per year
- Surgical technique used for hepaticojejunostomy
- Criteria for the choice of technique (if several techniques were used)
- Sutures used for hepaticojejunostomy
- Estimated duration of hepaticojejunostomy
- Estimated overall complication rate after hepaticojejunostomy
- Estimated leakage rate after hepaticojejunostomy

Statistical analysis

The statistical analysis of the collected data was done using the SPSS statistical program package (SPSS inc., Chicago, USA). To compare categorical data, the chi-square test was used. For comparison of quantitative data the Mann-Whitney U-test or the t-test were used. A p-value of less than 0.05 was considered significant.

Table 1 Advantages and disadvantages of interrupted suture technique and continuous suture technique during hepaticojejunostomy

	Interrupted suture technique	Continuous suture technique
Advantages	Always possible	Lower costs
		Shorter operating time
Disadvantages	Higher costs	Difficult for very small bile ducts
	Longer operating time	

Results

Of the 102 German surgical hospitals addressed, 77 hospitals (25 university hospitals (33%), 52 other hospitals (68%)) responded. The average number of hepaticojejunostomies performed per year was 71 [range 17–300]. Open surgical approach was used for all hepaticojejunostomies. Hepaticojejunostomies were performed with a significantly higher frequency in university hospitals than in other hospitals (115 vs. 51 on average, $p < 0.001$). Mostly hepaticojejunostomies were done during pancreatic resections (71%), followed by bile duct resections (15%) and liver resections (14%) (Table 2).

Depending on the individual situation, most hospitals (56%) use both, either the interrupted suture technique or the continuous suture technique, to create a hepaticojejunostomy. 31% of the hospitals always apply an interrupted suture technique, whereas 9% always utilize a continuous suture technique. Only 4% use a combination of both techniques in the same anastomosis (Table 3). The surgical technique used for hepaticojejunostomy did not differ between university hospitals and other hospitals ($p = 0.620$) and between hospitals above and below the median of 54 hepaticojejunostomies per year ($p = 0.833$). Hospitals using both suturing techniques indicated in 95% of the cases the bile duct

Table 2 Characteristics of the participating hospitals

Response rate		77 / 102 (76%)
Hospitals	University hospitals	25 / 76 (33%)
	Other hospitals	52 / 76 (68%)
Mean number of hepaticojejunostomies per year [range]	All	71 [17–300]
		median 54
	- University hospitals	115 [40–300]
	- Other hospitals	51 [17–190]
Hepaticojejunostomies during … (in %) [range]	Pancreatic resection	71 [40–100]
	Bile duct resection	15 [0–40]
	Liver resection	14 [0–49]
	Other surgical procedures	1 [0–33]

Table 3 Techniques of hepaticojejunostomy; HJ = hepaticojejunostomies

		All (n = 76)	University hospitals (n = 24)	Other hospitals (n = 52)	p-value	Hospitals with < 54 HJ/year (n = 38)	Hospitals with ≥54 HJ/Jahr (n = 39)	p-value
Technique used	Interrupted suture technique	24 (31%)	10 (40%)	14 (27%)	0,620	11 (29%)	13 (33%)	0,833
	Continuous suture technique	7 (9%)	1 (4%)	6 (12%)		3 (8%)	4 (10%)	
	Interrupted + continuous suture technique	43 (56%)	13 (52%)	30 (58%)		23 (61%)	20 (51%)	
	Combination of interrupted and continuous suture technique	3 (4%)	1 (4%)	2 (4%)		1 (3%)	2 (5%)	
Technique used in cases of S + C (%) [range]	Interrupted suture technique	48 [5–95]	49 [10–90]	48 [5–95]	1,000	47 [5–95]	49 [5–90]	1,000
	Continuous suture technique	52 [5–95]	51 [10–90]	52 [5–95]		53 [5–95]	51 [10–95]	
Decision criteria for the choice of technique (in cases of I + C)*	Bile duct diameter	41 (95%)	12 (92%)	29 (97%)		22 (96%)	19 (95%)	
	Bile duct wall thickness	16 (37%)	6 (46%)	10 (33%)		8 (35%)	8 (40%)	
	Other reason	11 (26%)	6 (46%)	5 (17%)		3 (17%)	7 (35%)	
Suture material used*	Monofilament suture	76 (100%)	24 (100%)	52 (100%)	< **0,001**	38 (100%)	39 (100%)	0,052
	Absorbable suture	76 (100%)	24 (100%)	52 (100%)		38 (100%)	39 (100%)	
	Strength 3.0	1 (1%)	0 (0%)	1 (2%)		1 (3%)	0 (0%)	
	Strength 4.0	26 (34%)	4 (16%)	22 (42%)		15 (39%)	11 (28%)	
	Strength 5.0	60 (78%)	23 (92%)	37 (71%)		25 (66%)	35 (90%)	
	Strength 6.0	17 (22%)	13 (52%)	4 (8%)		4 (8%)	14 (36%)	

*Multiple answers possible

diameter, in 37% the bile duct wall thickness and in 26% other reasons to be criteria for the choice of technique. Other decision criteria were: surgeon's preference, the presence of infection, the quality of exposure of the site, the extent of surgery, the location of the anastomosis (central vs. peripheral), the underlying diagnosis, the age of the patient (pediatric vs. adult) and whether it is a redo procedure.

Interestingly, all of the hospitals surveyed uniformly use monofilament absorbable sutures for the hepaticojejunostomy. University hospitals used significantly thinner sutures than other hospitals ($p < 0.001$) (Table 3).

The duration of the continuous suture technique was estimated to be significantly shorter than the time estimated for the interrupted suture technique ($p = 0.002$). Regarding the estimated overall complication rate and leakage rate, there were no significant differences between the techniques ($p = 0.695$ and $p = 0.258$) (Table 4).

Discussion

Hepaticojejunostomies are a common surgical procedure with a low complication rate, but relevant consequences in the event of complications. Various surgical techniques exist for the creation of a hepaticojejunostomy. So far, there is no randomized controlled comparison of techniques in the literature. Comparative data on the different techniques of

hepaticojejunostomy are currently only available in the context of liver transplants (Table 5) [13, 14]. The results of these liver transplant studies suggest that an interruptedly sutured hepaticojejunostomy is associated with a higher leakage rate and the continuous sutured hepaticojejunostomy with a higher rate of stenosis [8]. Due to the small number of cases and the distinct indication, these results are likely to include relevant uncertainty and are therefore not transferable to common hepaticojejunostomies.

This survey provides an overview of the surgical technique used for the creation of a hepaticojejunostomy in Germany. The results of the survey show a strong heterogeneity in the techniques used. The majority of respondents used both the interrupted suture as well as the continuous suture technique. This shows that even within most hospitals there is no standardization, but intraoperative reasons play the decisive role. The most common decision criterion among hospitals using both techniques is the bile duct diameter. This reflects the experience that in very small hepatic ducts the continuous suture technique can be very demanding. Moreover, the own particular surgical school will certainly play a crucial role.

The current survey suggests that the continuous suture technique is considered to be significantly faster, and both suture techniques are considered equivalent in terms of morbidity and, in particular, leakage rate. This

Table 4 Estimated duration and morbidity of hepaticojejunostomy

		Interrupted suture technique	Continuous suture technique	Interrupted + continuous suture technique		p-value
				Interrupted technique	Continuous technique	
Duration	Number	24	7	43	43	**0,002**
	- < 10 min	1 (4%)	5 (71%)	6 (14%)	11 (26%)	
	- 10-20 min	19 (79%)	2 (29%)	20 (47%)	25 (58%)	
	- 20-30 min	4 (17%)	0 (0%)	13 (30%)	6 (14%)	
	- > 30 min	0 (0%)	0 (0%)	4 (9%)	1 (2%)	
Morbidity	Number	23*	7	41*	41*	0,695
	- < 3%	7 (30%)	4 (57%)	9 (22%)	10 (24%)	
	- 3-5%	11 (48%)	1 (14%)	17 (41%)	16 (39%)	
	- 5-10%	5 (22%)	2 (29%)	9 (22%)	11 (27%)	
	- 10-15%	0 (0%)	0 (0%)	3 (7%)	2 (5%)	
	- 15-20%	0 (0%)	0 (0%)	3 (7%)	2 (5%)	
	- > 20%	0 (0%)	0 (0%)	0 (0%)	0 (0%)	
Leakage rate	Number	23*	7	42*	42*	0,258
	- < 3%	13 (57%)	5 (71%)	14 (33%)	15 (36%)	
	- 3-5%	10 (44%)	2 (29%)	19 (45%)	20 (48%)	
	- 5-10%	0 (0%)	0 (0%)	7 (17%)	6 (14%)	
	- 10-15%	0 (0%)	0 (0%)	2 (5%)	1 (2%)	

*Partially missing data due to incomplete answers

Table 5 Existing literature comparing hepaticojejunostomies in various techniques (Combi = combination of interrupted and continuous suture technique)

Author	Indication	Number	Follow-up	Technique	Number	Bile leak	Stenosis
Kasahara (2006) [13]	Liver transplantation	121	Median 60 months [7–80]	Interrupted	68	14,7%	7,4%
				Continuous	48	8,3%	10,4%
				Combi	5	20,0%	0,0%
Soejima (2006) [14]	Liver transplantation	76	3-year rate	Interrupted	53		31,8%
				Continuous	5		0,0%
				Combi	18		22,0%

raises the question why not all hepaticojejunostomies with adequate bile duct diameter are performed with the continuous suture technique. An adequate bile duct diameter should be present in most cases, since the bile duct is dammed up in the majority of cases due to the tumor. A randomized controlled comparison of the suturing techniques of interrupted suture technique and continuous suture technique is absolute necessary to answer this question.

An interesting aspect of the survey is the fact that university hospitals use significantly thinner sutures. In a review by Heidenhain in 2011, thin sutures are considered to be one of the decisive factors in the performance of a hepaticojejunostomy without complications [8]. However, the estimated complication rates of university hospitals and other hospitals do not differ in our survey. In addition, there are no comparative studies concerning the suture material.

This study has crucial limitations that need to be appropriately taken into consideration. Since data on the duration and complication rate of hepaticojejunostomies in this survey were given as estimates to facilitate participation in the survey, the validity of these data is limited. However, a very high response rate of 76% was achieved by a low threshold for participation in the survey. In addition, the estimated overall complication rate and the estimated insufficiency rate in the current survey are 3–5%. This value is comparable to the data published in the previous literature. This can underline a realistic assessment of the own complication rates and thus the value of the collected data. However, this could also be a sign that many respondents have answered the survey with known values from the literature and not their own realistic complication rate.

Conclusion

In summary, heterogeneous techniques for hepaticojejunostomy are used in Germany. The most important decision criterion for the choice of technique is the bile duct diameter. The different techniques should be compared in a randomized controlled study.

Authors' contributions

MB created the survey, analyzed the data, conducted the literature search, wrote the paper and approved the final manuscript. GFW and RG created the survey, wrote the paper and approved the final manuscript. JS made substantial contributions to conception and design of the study, was involved in revising the manuscript critically for important intellectual content and approved the final manuscript, CK, DR and SK made substantial contributions to analysis and interpretation of data, were involved in revising the manuscript critically for important intellectual content and approved the final manuscript. All authors agreed to be accountable for all aspects of the work in ensuring that questions related to the accuracy or integrity of any part of the work are appropriately investigated and resolved. All authors read and approved the final manuscript.

Competing interests

The authors declare that they have no competing interests.

References

1. Akamatsu N, Sugawara Y, Hashimoto D. Biliary reconstruction, its complications and management of biliary complications after adult liver transplantation: a systematic review of the incidence, risk factors and outcome. Transpl Int. 2011;24:379–92.
2. Chok KS, Ng KK, Poon RT, et al. Impact of postoperative complications on long-term outcome of curative resection for hepatocellular carcinoma. Br J Surg. 2009;96:81–7.
3. Von Winiwarter A, Bidder A. Ein Fall von Galleretention bedingt durch Impermeabilität des Ductus choledochus: Anlegung einer Gallenblasen-Darmfistel: Heilung. Zentralbl Chir. 1882;9:581–2.
4. Monastyrski ND, Tilling G. Zur Frage von der chirurgischen Behandlung der vollständigen Undurchgängigkeit des Ductus choledochus. Zentralbl Chir. 1888;15:778–9.
5. Sprengel O. Über einen Fall von Exstirpation der Gallenblase mit Anlegung einer Kommunikation zwischen Duodenum und Ductus choledochus. Zentralbl Chir. 1891;18:121–2.
6. Dahl R. Eine neue Operation an den Gallenwegen. Zentralbl Chir. 1909; 36:266–7.
7. Cole WH, Ireneus C, Reynolds JT. Strictures of the common duct. Ann Surg. 1951;133:684–96.
8. Heidenhain C, Rosch R, Neumann UP. Hepatobiliary anastomosis techniques. Chirurg. 2011;82(1):7–10 12-3.
9. Antolovic D, Koch M, Galindo L, Wolff S, Music E, Kienle P, Schemmer P, Friess H, Schmidt J, Büchler MW, Weitz J. Hepaticojejunostomy—analysis of risk factors for postoperative bile leaks and surgical complications. J Gastrointest Surg. 2007;11(5):555–61.
10. de Castro SM, Kuhlmann KF, Busch OR, van Delden OM, Laméris JS, van Gulik TM, Obertop H, Gouma DJ. Incidence and management of biliary leakage after hepaticojejunostomy. J Gastrointest Surg. 2005;9(8):1163–71 discussion 1171-3.
11. Asano T, Natsume S, Senda Y, Sano T, Matsuo K, Kodera Y, Hara K, Ito S, Yamao K, Shimizu Y. Incidence and risk factors for anastomotic stenosis of continuous hepaticojejunostomy after pancreaticoduodenectomy. J Hepatobiliary Pancreat Sci. 2016;23(10):628–35.
12. Kadaba RS, Bowers KA, Khorsandi S, Hutchins RR, Abraham AT, Sarker SJ, Bhattacharya S, Kocher HM. Complications of biliary-enteric anastomoses. Ann R Coll Surg Engl. 2017;99(3):210–5.

Permissions

The contributors of this book come from diverse backgrounds, making this book a truly international effort. This book will bring forth new frontiers with its revolutionizing research information and detailed analysis of the nascent developments around the world.

We would like to thank all the contributing authors for lending their expertise to make the book truly unique. They have played a crucial role in the development of this book. Without their invaluable contributions this book wouldn't have been possible. They have made vital efforts to compile up to date information on the varied aspects of this subject to make this book a valuable addition to the collection of many professionals and students.

This book was conceptualized with the vision of imparting up-to-date information and advanced data in this field. To ensure the same, a matchless editorial board was set up. Every individual on the board went through rigorous rounds of assessment to prove their worth. After which they invested a large part of their time researching and compiling the most relevant data for our readers.

The editorial board has been involved in producing this book since its inception. They have spent rigorous hours researching and exploring the diverse topics which have resulted in the successful publishing of this book. They have passed on their knowledge of decades through this book. To expedite this challenging task, the publisher supported the team at every step. A small team of assistant editors was also appointed to further simplify the editing procedure and attain best results for the readers.

Apart from the editorial board, the designing team has also invested a significant amount of their time in understanding the subject and creating the most relevant covers. They scrutinized every image to scout for the most suitable representation of the subject and create an appropriate cover for the book.

The publishing team has been an ardent support to the editorial, designing and production team. Their endless efforts to recruit the best for this project, has resulted in the accomplishment of this book. They are a veteran in the field of academics and their pool of knowledge is as vast as their experience in printing. Their expertise and guidance has proved useful at every step. Their uncompromising quality standards have made this book an exceptional effort. Their encouragement from time to time has been an inspiration for everyone.

The publisher and the editorial board hope that this book will prove to be a valuable piece of knowledge for researchers, students, practitioners and scholars across the globe.

List of Contributors

Marius Distler, Maximilian Hunger, Stephan Kersting, Christian Pilarsky, Hans-Detlev Saeger and Robert Grützmann
Department of General, Thoracic and Vascular Surgery, University Hospital Carl Gustav Carus, Technical University Dresden, Fetscherstrasse 74, Dresden 01307, Germany

Felix Rückert
Surgical Department, University Hospital Mannheim, Heidelberg University, Mannheim, Germany

Jon Arne Søreide
Department of Gastrointestinal Surgery, Stavanger University Hospital, N-4068 Stavanger, Norway
Department of Clinical Medicine, University of Bergen, Bergen, Norway

Ole Jakob Greve
Department of Radiology, Stavanger University Hospital, Stavanger, Norway

Einar Gudlaugsson
Department of Pathology, Stavanger University Hospital, Stavanger, Norway

Ulrich Nitsche, Tara C Müller, Christoph Späth, Dirk Wilhelm, Helmut Friess and Jörg Kleeff
Department of Surgery, Klinikum rechts der Isar, Technische Universität München, Ismaninger Strasse 22, 81675 Munich, Germany

Lynne Cresswell
Institute of Medical Statistics and Epidemiology, Klinikum rechts der Isar, Technische Universität München, Munich, Germany

Christoph W Michalski
Division of Surgical Oncology, Department of Surgery, Oregon Health and Science University, Portland, OR, USA

Stefan M Brunner, Jens M Werner, Ayman Agha, Stefan A Farkas, Hans J Schlitt and Matthias Hornung
Department of Surgery, University Medical Center Regensburg, Franz-Josef-Strauss-Allee 11, 93053 Regensburg, Germany

Florian Weber
Institute of Pathology, University Medical Center Regensburg, Regensburg, Germany

Johannes Baur and U. Steger
Department of General, Visceral, Vascular and Pediatric Surgery, University Hospital Wuerzburg, Wuerzburg, Germany

Ulla Schedelbeck
Institute of Radiology, University Hospital Wuerzburg, Wuerzburg, Germany

Christina Bluemel
Department of Nuclear Medicine, University Hospital Wuerzburg, Wuerzburg, Germany

Alina Pulzer
Department of Internal Medicine I, Endocrinology, University Hospital Wuerzburg, Wuerzburg, Germany

Martin Fassnacht
Department of Internal Medicine I, Endocrinology, University Hospital Wuerzburg, Wuerzburg, Germany
Comprehensive Cancer Center Mainfranken, University of Wuerzburg, Wuerzburg, Germany

Vanessa Wild
Comprehensive Cancer Center Mainfranken, University of Wuerzburg, Wuerzburg, Germany
Institute of Pathology, University Wuerzburg, Wuerzburg, Germany

Bruno Cacopardo, Marilia Rita Pinzone and Giuseppe Nunnari
Department of Clinical and Molecular Biomedicine, Division of Infectious Diseases, University of Catania, 95125 Catania, Italy

Salvatore Berretta, Rossella Fisichella, Maria Di Vita, Guido Zanghì, Alessandro Cappellani and Antonio Zanghì
Department of Surgery, General Surgery Unit, University of Catania, 95100 Catania, Italy

Masaaki Murakawa, Toru Aoyama, Masahiro Asari, Yusuke Katayama, Koichiro Yamaoku, Amane Kanazawa, Akio Higuchi, Manabu Shiozawa, Takaki Yoshikawa and Soichiro Morinaga
Department of Gastrointestinal Surgery, Kanagawa Cancer Center, 2-3-2 Nakao, Asahi-Ku, Yokohama 241-8515, Japan

Satoshi Kobayashi, Makoto Ueno and Manabu Morimoto
Department of Gastrointestinal medicine, Kanagawa Cancer Center, Yokohama, Japan

Naoto Yamamoto, Yasushi Rino and Munetaka Masuda
Department of Surgery, Yokohama City University, Yokohama, Japan

Masamichi Matsuda, Shusuke Haruta, Hisashi Shinohara, Kazunari Sasaki and Goro Watanabe
Department of Surgery, Toranomon Hospital, 2-2-2 Toranomon Minato-ku, Tokyo 105-8470, Japan

Dietrich A. Ruess, Frank Makowiec, Sophia Chikhladze, Olivia Sick, Ulrich T. Hopt and Uwe A. Wittel
Department of Surgery, University of Freiburg, Freiburg, Germany

Hartwig Riediger
Department of Surgery, Vivantes-Humboldt-Clinic, Berlin, Germany

Dianbo Yao, Shuodong Wu, Yongnan Li, Yongsheng Chen, Xiaopeng Yu and Jinyan Han
Department of General Surgery, Shengjing Hospital, China Medical University, Shenyang 110004, China

Roberto L Meniconi, Roberto Caronna, Dario Borreca, Monica Schiratti and Piero Chirletti
Department of Surgical Sciences, Sapienza University of Rome, Viale del Policlinico 155, Rome 00161, Italy

Georg Wiltberger, Hans-Michael Hau and Michael Bartels
Department of Visceral, Transplantation, Thoracic, and Vascular Surgery, University Hospital Leipzig, 04103 Leipzig, Germany

Julian Nikolaus Bucher
Department of Surgery, University Hospital Großhadern (LMU), Munich, Germany

Felix Krenzien, Christian Benzing, Georgi Atanasov and Moritz Schmelzle
Department of General, Visceral, and Transplant Surgery, Charité - Universitätsmedizin Berlin, Campus Virchow Klinikum, Augustenburger Platz 1, 13353 Berlin, Germany

Julie Ahn
Division of Surgery, University of Western Sydney, Sydney, Australia

Manju D Chandrasegaram, Benjamin L Woodham and Neil D Merrett
Division of Surgery, University of Western Sydney, Sydney, Australia
Upper Gastrointestinal Unit, Bankstown Hospital, Sydney, Australia

Khaled Alsaleh, Adrian Teo, Amithaba Das and Christos Apostolou
Upper Gastrointestinal Unit, Bankstown Hospital, Sydney, Australia

Marius Distler, Stephan Kersting, Peggy Kross, Hans-Detlev Saeger, Jürgen Weitz and Robert Grützmann
Department of General, Thoracic and Vascular Surgery, University Hospital Carl Gustav Carus, TU, Dresden, Germany

Felix Rückert
Department of Surgery, University Hospital Mannheim, Mannheim, Germany

Bo Kong, Carsten Jäger, Silke Kloe, Barbara Beier, Helmut Friess and Jorg Kleeff
Department of Surgery, Technische Universität München, Ismaningerstrasse 22, 81675 Munich, Germany

Christoph W. Michalski
Department of Surgery, Technische Universität München, Ismaningerstrasse 22, 81675 Munich, Germany
Current address: Department of Surgery, University of Heidelberg, Heidelberg, Germany

Mert Erkan
Department of Surgery, Technische Universität München, Ismaningerstrasse 22, 81675 Munich, Germany
Current address: Department of Surgery, Koc University School of Medicine, Istanbul, Turkey

Rickmer Braren
Institute of Radiology, Technische Universität München, Munich, Germany

Irene Esposito
Institute of Pathology, Technische Universität München, Munich, Germany
Current address: Institute of Pathology, Heinrich Heine University Düsseldorf, Düsseldorf, Germany

Ying-Jui Chao, Edgar D Sy and Hui-Ping Hsu
Division of General Surgery, Department of Surgery, National Cheng Kung University Hospital, Tainan, Taiwan

Yan-Shen Shan
Division of General Surgery, Department of Surgery, National Cheng Kung University Hospital, Tainan, Taiwan
Institute of Clinical Medicine, College of Medicine, National Cheng Kung University, Tainan, Taiwan

Łukasz Dobosz, Tomasz Stefaniak, Małgorzata Dobrzycka, Jagoda Wieczorek, Paula Franczak, Dominika Ptaszyńska, Katarzyna Zasada and Peter Kanyion
Department of General, Endocrine and Transplant Surgery, Medical University
of Gdansk, ul. Smoluchowskiego 17, 80-214 Gdansk, Poland

Knut Jørgen Labori and Kristoffer Lassen
Department of Hepato-Pancreato-Biliary Surgery, Oslo University Hospital, Oslo, Norway

Dag Hoem
Department of Acute and Digestive Surgery, Haukeland University Hospital, Bergen, Norway

Jon Erik Grønbech
Department of Gastrointestinal Surgery, St. Olavs Hospital, Trondheim University Hospital, Trondheim, Norway
Department of Clinical and Molecular Medicine, Norwegian University of Science and Technology, Trondheim, Norway

Jon Arne Søreide
Department of Gastrointestinal Surgery, Stavanger University Hospital, Stavanger, Norway
Department of Clinical Medicine, University of Bergen, Bergen, Norway

Kim Mortensen
Department of Gastrointestinal and Hepatobiliary Surgery, University Hospital of Northern Norway, Tromsø, Norway

Rune Smaaland
Department of Haematology and Oncology, Stavanger University Hospital, Stavanger, Norway

Halfdan Sorbye
Department of Oncology, Haukeland University Hospital, Bergen, Norway
Department of Clinical Science, Haukeland University Hospital, University of Bergen, Bergen, Norway

Caroline Verbeke
Department of Pathology, Oslo University Hospital, Oslo, Norway
Institute of Clinical Medicine, University of Oslo, Oslo, Norway

Svein Dueland
Department of Oncology, Oslo University Hospital, Oslo, Norway

Benoît Bédat, Cosimo Riccardo Scarpa, Samira Mercedes Sadowski, Frédéric Triponez and Wolfram Karenovics
Thoracic and Endocrine Surgery, University Hospitals of Geneva, 1211 Geneva, Switzerland

Ophélie Aumont, Adeline Abjean, Julie Veziant and Bertrand Le Roy
Department of Digestive and Hepatobiliary Surgery, Estaing University Hospital, 1, place Lucie et Raymond Aubrac, 63000 Clermont-Ferrand, France

Denis Pezet, Emmanuel Buc and Johan Gagnière
Department of Digestive and Hepatobiliary Surgery, Estaing University Hospital, 1, place Lucie et Raymond Aubrac, 63000 Clermont-Ferrand, France
UMR 1071 INSERM/ Clermont Auvergne University, Clermont-Ferrand, France

Aurélien Dupré
Department of Surgical Oncology, Léon Bérard Cancer Center, Lyon, France

Bruno Pereira
Biostatistics, Délégation à la Recherche Clinique et à l'Innovation, University Hospital of Clermont-Ferrand, Clermont-Ferrand, France

Kosei Takagi, Ryuichi Yoshida, Takahito Yagi, Yuzo Umeda, Daisuke Nobuoka, Takashi Kuise and Toshiyoshi Fujiwara
Department of Gastroenterological Surgery, Okayama University Graduate School of Medicine, Dentistry, and Pharmaceutical Sciences, 2-5-1 Shikata-cho, Kita-ku, Okayama 700-8558, Japan

Eirik Kjus Aahlin and Kristoffer Lassen
Department of GI and HPB surgery, University Hospital of Northern Norway,
9038 Breivika, Tromsø, Norway
Department of Clinical Medicine, University of Tromsø - The Arctic University of Norway, Tromsø, Norway

Frank Olsen and Bård Uleberg
Centre of Clinical Documentation and Evaluation, Northern Norway Regional Health Authority, Tromsø, Norway

Bjarne K. Jacobsen
Centre of Clinical Documentation and Evaluation, Northern Norway Regional Health Authority, Tromsø, Norway
Department of Community Medicine, University of Tromsø - The Arctic University of Norway, Tromsø, Norway

Andrea Lauretta, Claudio Belluco, Matteo Olivieri, Marco Forlin, Stefania Basso, Bruno Breda and Giulio Bertola
Department of Surgical Oncology. Surgical oncology Unit, National Cancer institute-Centro di Riferimento Oncologico IRCCS, Aviano (PN), Italy

Gian Piero Guerrini
Department of Surgical Oncology. Surgical oncology Unit, National Cancer institute-Centro di Riferimento Oncologico IRCCS, Aviano (PN), Italy
Hepato-Pancreato-Biliary Surgery and Liver Transplantation Unit, University of Modena and Reggio Emilia, Modena, Italy

Fabrizio Di Benedetto
Hepato-Pancreato-Biliary Surgery and Liver Transplantation Unit, University of Modena and Reggio Emilia, Modena, Italy

Feng Cao, Jia Li, Ang Li and Fei Li
Department of General Surgery, Xuanwu Hospital, Capital Medical University,
Beijing 100053, People's Republic of China

Giovanni Ramacciato, Giuseppe Nigri and Niccolo' Petrucciani
Department of Medical and Surgical Sciences and Translational Medicine, Faculty of Medicine and Psychology, St Andrea Hospital, Sapienza University, General Surgery Unit, Via di Grottarossa 1037, 00189 Rome, Italy

Antonio Daniele Pinna and Matteo Ravaioli
Department of Medical and Surgical Sciences-DIMEC, S. Orsola-Malpighi Hospital, Alma Mater Studiorum, University of Bologna, General Surgery and Transplantation Unit, Bologna, Italy

Elio Jovine
General Surgery Unit, 'Maggiore' Hospital, Bologna, Italy

Francesco Minni
Department of Medical and Surgical Sciences (DIMEC), Alma Mater Studiorum, S. Orsola-Malpighi Hospital, University of Bologna, General Surgery Unit, Bologna, Italy

Gian Luca Grazi
Regina Elena National Cancer Institute IFO, Hepato-pancreato-biliary Surgery Unit, Rome, Italy

Piero Chirletti
Department of Surgical Sciences, Sapienza University of Rome, Policlinico Umberto I Hospital, General Surgery Unit, Rome, Italy

Giuseppe Tisone
Department of Experimental Medicine and Surgery, Liver Unit, Tor Vergata University of Rome, Rome, Italy

Fabio Ferla
Division of General Surgery and Transplantation Surgery, Niguarda Hospital, Milan, Italy

Niccolo' Napoli and Ugo Boggi
Division of General Surgery and Transplantation Surgery, Pisa University Hospital, Pisa, Italy

Tim R. Glowka, Hanno Matthaei, Nico Schäfer, Jörg C. Kalff and Steffen Manekeller
Department of Surgery, University of Bonn, Sigmund-Freud-Str. 25, 53105 Bonn, Germany

Markus Webler
Department of Orthopedic and Trauma Surgery, University of Bonn, Sigmund-Freud-Str. 25, 53105 Bonn, Germany

Volker Schmitz
Department of Gastroenterology, St. Marienwörth Hospital, Mühlenstr. 39, 55543 Bad Kreuznach, Germany

Jens Standop
Department of Surgery, Maria Stern Hospital, Am Anger 1, 53424 Remagen, Germany

Masahide Fukaya, Tetsuya Abe and Masato Nagino
Division of Surgical Oncology, Department of Surgery, Nagoya University Graduate School of Medicine, 65 Tsurumai-cho Showa-ku, Nagoya 466-8550, Japan

Evangelos Tagkalos, Hauke Lang and Stefan Heinrich
Department of General, Visceral and Transplantation Surgery, Johannes Gutenberg University Hospital, Langenbeckstrasse 1, 55131 Mainz, Germany

Florian Jungmann
Department of Diagnostic and Interventional Radiology, Johannes Gutenberg University Hospital, Mainz, Germany

Alexander Betzler, Soeren T. Mees, Josefine Pump, Sebastian Schölch, Carolin Zimmermann, Jürgen Weitz, Thilo Welsch and Marius Distler
Department of General, Thoracic and Vascular Surgery, University Hospital Carl Gustav Carus, TU Dresden, Fetscher Str. 74, 01037 Dresden, Germany

Daniela E. Aust
Institute for Pathology, University Hospital Carl Gustav Carus, TU Dresden, Fetscher Str. 74, 01307 Dresden, Germany

Zhihui Tong, Lu Ke, Baiqiang Li, Gang Li, Jing Zhou and Xiao Shen
SICU, Department of General Surgery, Jinling Hospital, Nanjing University School of Medicine, Nanjing 210002, People's Republic of China

Weiqin Li
SICU, Department of General Surgery, Jinling Hospital, Nanjing University School of Medicine, Nanjing 210002, People's Republic of China

Department of SICU, Research Institute of General Surgery, Jinling Hospital, 305 East Zhongshan Road, Nanjing 210002, Jiangsu Province, China

Ning Li and Jieshou Li
Department of General Surgery, Jinling Hospital, Nanjing University School of Medicine, Nanjing 210002, People's Republic of China

Kosei Takagi, Takahito Yagi, Yuzo Umeda, Ryuichi Yoshida, Daisuke Nobuoka, Takashi Kuise and Toshiyoshi Fujiwara
Department of Gastroenterological Surgery, Okayama University Graduate School of Medicine, Dentistry and Pharmaceutical Sciences, 2-5-1 Shikata-cho, Kita-ku, Okayama 700-8558, Japan

Takehiro Tanaka
Department of Diagnostic Pathology, Okayama University Hospital, 2-5-1 Shikata-cho, Kita-ku, Okayama 700-8558, Japan

Eun Young Kim and Tae Ho Hong
Department of Hepato-biliary and Pancreas Surgery, Seoul St. Mary's Hospital, College of Medicine, The Catholic University of Korea, 222, Banpo-daero, Seocho-gu, Seoul 06591, Republic of Korea

Kenjiro Kimura, Go Ohira, Ryosuke Amano, Sadaaki Yamazoe, Ryota Tanaka, Jun Tauchi and Masaichi Ohira
Department of Surgical Oncology, Osaka City University School of Medicine, 1-4-3 Asahi-machi, Abeno-ku, Osaka 545-8585, Japan

Shoji Kawakatsu, Yosuke Inoue, Yoshihiro Mise, Takeaki Ishizawa, Hiromichi Ito, Yu Takahashi and Akio Saiura
Department of Gastroenterological Surgery, Cancer Institute Hospital, Japanese Foundation for Cancer Research, 3-10-6 Ariake, Koto-ku, Tokyo 135-8550, Japan

Yasunaru Sakuma and Naohiro Sata
Department of Surgery, Jichi Medical University, 3311-1 Yakushiji, Shimotsuke City, Tochigi 329-0498, Japan

Yukihiro Sanada
Department of Surgery, Jichi Medical University, 3311-1 Yakushiji, Shimotsuke City, Tochigi 329-0498, Japan
Department of Transplant Surgery, Jichi Medical University, Shimotsuke, Japan

Maximilian Brunner, Jessica Stockheim, Christian Krautz, Dimitrios Raptis, Stephan Kersting, Georg F. Weber and Robert Grützmann
Department of General Surgery, University Hospital of Friedrich-Alexander-University, Krankenhausstraße 12, 91054 Erlangen, Germany

Index

www.ingramcontent.com/pod-product-compliance
Lightning Source LLC
Chambersburg PA
CBHW061305190326
41458CB00011B/3769

9 781632 416018